QV 137
H 297
2010

Tobacco or Health?

Knut-Olaf Haustein† · David Groneberg

Tobacco or Health?

Second Edition

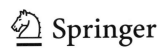
Springer

Prof. Dr. Knut-Olaf Haustein†
Fritz-Lickint-Institut für
Nikotinforschung und
Raucherentwöhnung
Johannes Str. 85–87
99084 Erfurt
Germany

Prof. Dr. Dr. h.c. mult. David Groneberg
Charité - Universitätsmedizin Berlin
Institut für Arbeitsmedizin
Thielallee 73
14195 Berlin
Germany
david.groneberg@charite.de

ISBN: 978-3-540-87576-5   e-ISBN: 978-3-540-87577-2

DOI: 10.1007/978-3-540-87577-2

Springer Heidelberg Dordrecht London New York

Library of Congress Control Number: 2009931695

© Springer-Verlag Berlin Heidelberg 2010

Cover design: eStudioCalamar, Figueres/Berlin

Printed on acid-free paper

Springer is part of Springer Science+Business Media (www.springer.com)

Dedication

This book is dedicated to all the unborn who suffer from the negative effects of tobacco. They cannot protect themselves, and often, they suffer a lifetime.

Preface

This book comprehensively summarizes the adverse effects of tobacco smoking on human health. The current second edition has integrated a large set of new data that have been published in numerous scientific studies and meta-analyses over the past few years.

Unfortunately, the harmful sequelae of tobacco smoking are played down by the industry and politicians in many industrialized countries. However, about 800,000 people/year in the EU die from the immediate consequences of smoking. The particularly insidious feature of tobacco consumption is that smoking-attributable harmful effects on health do not generally become apparent until three or four decades after smoking initiation.

Although some positive changes in the legislative handling of tobacco have appeared in the past five years, we still need to form a pact, sealed by politicians, the medical professionals, teachers and the media, to target the problem across nations. In this respect, a minority of countries, including the US and the UK, have given positive examples.

There are four areas that need to be improved in future: (1) strict bans on tobacco advertisement on a global level, (2) better measures to protect against side-stream (passive) smoke exposure, (3) establishment of prevention programs, especially for children and (4) treatment of tobacco addiction.

While preparing the second edition of the German version of this book, the founding author Knut-Olaf Haustein deceased. After the fall of the Berlin wall, he was one of the first Germans to take an active part in the battle against tobacco in the united Germany and it is the author's hope that the present edition continues the thoughts of Knut-Olaf Haustein on how to approach the numerous problems. As a comprehensive work, the book is intended to meet the needs of a large readership, including all medical professionals and scientists, as well as teachers, sociologists, the media and politicians.

First and foremost, I am grateful to all the scientists who provided the data. I also gladly acknowledge the help of Springer, Heidelberg, and the assistance of Dr. Carolin Kreiter, Dr. Julia-Anik Börger, Dr. David Quarcoo, Dr. Alexander Gerber, Bianca Kusma, Stefania Mache, Karin Vitzthum and Silvana Kölzow. Without the help of my family and the family of Knut-Olaf Haustein, this book could not have been realized.

I trust that this book will meet with a good reception both within and outside the field of medicine.

Berlin, Germany
Prof. Dr. David Groneberg

Contents

History of Tobacco

We like to look in the future, because the undetermined in it, which may be affected this or that way, we feel as if we could guide by our silent wishes in our own favour.

(J. W. Goethe, Novels and tales. 1854)

1.1
Tobacco Plants and Their Origin

Nicotiana tabacum, the tobacco plant used since ancient times in the Central and South America, does not occur naturally but is a product of human cultivation [1], being a hybrid of *Nicotiana sylvestris* and *Nicotiana tomentosifosa* [2]. *Nicotiana rustica* (developed later in Russia as machorka) was the variety cultivated in North America, and has a higher nicotine content than the other tobacco plants. Illustrations of tobacco plant appeared under the name of *Nicotiana major* in the seventeenth-century herbals (Fig. 1.1) because tobacco was believed to possess healing properties [3]. The nicotine content of the tobacco leaves is increased if the leading stem of the plant and its lateral shoots are removed (a process known as "topping and suckering"), and drying improves the flavour of the leaves [1]. The juice of lime is used to enhance the flavour of some tobacco varieties [4], and in the process the nicotine release as a free base is improved [5].

1.2
Use of Tobacco for Religious Purposes

Ten thousand years ago, the tobacco plant was used for ceremonial religious purposes among the indigenous peoples of North and Central America. The Mayan priests lit sacred fires [6], blew repeatedly on the embers to kindle them into life, inhaled the smoke, and thus experienced the effects of the ingredients of the plant. Tobacco became a sacred plant [4]. Later, the tobacco plant attained a ceremonial religious status in the context of bringing a sacrificial offering to the gods. The indigenous peoples of North America smoked tobacco

K.-O. Haustein, D. Groneberg, *Tobacco or Health?*
DOI: 10.1007/978-3-540-87577-2_1, © Springer Verlag Berlin Heidelberg 2010

Fig. 1.1   Illustration of a tobacco plant from the
herbal of Tabernaemontanus (1664)

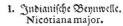

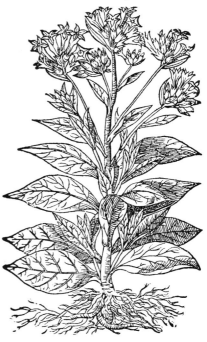

in a "peace-pipe" to set the seal on treaties and friendships, while those of Central and
South America used tobacco in a rolled form, rather similar to present-day cigars and cigarettes. These people also attributed the healing properties to the tobacco plant (for example,
the shaman or medicine man would apply tobacco leaves to wounds). In South America,
tobacco was used preferentially for medicinal purposes, but it was also taken as snuff,
chewed, and used as a liquid brew. The appetite-suppressing quality of tobacco was recognised even at that time. Beyond the American continent, tobacco plants were found only in
Australia, and in some parts of the Sunda Islands of Indonesia.

1.3
The Appropriation of Tobacco by Europeans

For obvious reasons, until Columbus landed on San Salvador in 1492, the tobacco plant
did not attract the interest of Europeans, although it may be noted that the Amerindians
used the word *tabago* to describe the pipe used for tobacco smoking rather than the plant
itself. On his second voyage to the New World, Columbus was presented with a bunch of
tobacco leaves, but had no inkling of their intended use. In 1527, the first bishop of the new

colony, Fray Bartolomé de Las Casas, wrote a description of the properties of the tobacco plant [7]. Although the Amerindians presented the Spaniards with tobacco leaves as a gesture of friendship and devotion, the plant lost all its ceremonial religious significance over the ensuing centuries in the hands of the Spaniards and other Europeans, and tobacco became a luxury commodity that was exploited solely for commercial purposes.

After his return from sea voyages, Spaniard Rodrigo de Jerez – credited with being the first European tobacco smoker – used to walk the streets of his home port of Ayamonte, with smoke billowing from his mouth and nose. Believing he was consorting with the Devil, the local clergy handed Rodrigo over to the Inquisition, and he was imprisoned for 10 years! This was in stark contrast to the extremely liberal attitude of the Spanish colonial rulers outside Spain as far as tobacco smoking was concerned. After his second voyage to the New World, Columbus brought a number of tobacco plants back to Spain where they were used initially as ornamental plants in the gardens of the aristocracy. Jean Nicot (1530–1600), French ambassador to the Portuguese court, conducted a number of "experiments" which identified the healing effects of tobacco. In 1559, on the strength of this conviction, he sent some plants to Paris for Catherine de Medici who had them processed as snuff powder, and successfully administered them to her son, Charles IX, as a remedy for his headaches [8]. The Spaniard Nicolas Monardes, a physician at the University of Seville, wrote a treatise in 1571 on the medicinal use of tobacco, and his compendium was very rapidly translated into other languages [9]. By 1590, the plant was already known as *Nicotiana*, and since 1828 Nicot has given his name to the principal alkaloid, nicotine.

Tobacco arrived at the English court of Queen Elizabeth I in 1573, and by 1614 there were already more than 7,000 tobacco retail outlets in London [10]. Benefiting from the extensive trading relationships with the Spaniards and the Portuguese, the tobacco plant was carried to the Philippines, to the Southeast and East Asia, as well as to Africa and, by the beginning of the seventeenth century, even further afield to Japan, Korea and China, from where it also entered Tibet, Mongolia, and Siberia [11]. Tobacco became an immensely valuable commercial commodity, comparable with cocaine and other illegal drugs at the present time.

1.4
Worldwide Spread of Tobacco

In the beginning of the eighteenth century, tobacco was found in all corners of the world. This spread of tobacco, and its use as a luxury commodity also led to the secularisation of society [12]. The use of tobacco was prohibited in numerous countries (Turkey, Russia, Vatican City, and Germany). In contrast, the English King James I became an ardent champion of the tobacco trade because it brought him considerable financial revenue through import duties. Nevertheless, in 1603, King James I published his treatise "A counterblaste to tobacco" in which he argued against the cultivation of tobacco [13]. The Spanish monopoly on tobacco was broken when the English obtained tobacco seeds from Virginia, and James I placed a ban on imports from Spain to encourage his country's own production. After 1630 the prohibition policy for tobacco products became a taxation policy [14], one of the first attempts at indirect prohibition.

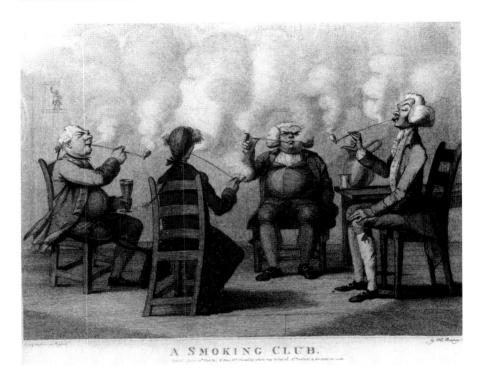

Fig. 1.2 A Smoking Club. Etching from an original by Bunbury Esq. (1750–1811), in S.W. Fores No. 3, Piccadilly, where all of Mr. Bunbury & Rowlandsons' works are stored [15]

Smoking clubs became increasingly commonplace. Henry Bunbury's etching *A Smoking Club* (Fig. 1.2) depicts four gentlemen of differing build enjoying the ritual pleasures of the pipe. They adopted an almost statuesque pose, and their exaggerated look of rapture had something ridiculous about it. Frowned upon for a long period, the activity of smoking was condemned, and was restricted to the lower social strata (soldiers), becoming socially acceptable only toward the end of the eighteenth century. Normally, smoking was permitted only in specifically designated rooms; the ban on smoking in public persisted in many places until the nineteenth century.

In addition to tobacco smoking, the practice of snuff taking (witnessed by the Spaniards during their seafaring voyages of discovery) was also taken from the Amerindians. In France, snuffing was widespread before the French Revolution, with some 90% of tobacco being consumed in this way. The *tabatière* or snuffbox was the status symbol of the aristocracy. As a result, olfactory disturbances or total loss of the sense of smell were widespread in the eighteenth century, particularly in France. By contrast, the chewing of fermented tobacco leaves was less common, even though it was claimed to alleviate the pangs of hunger. In Europe, the custom of tobacco chewing survived longest among seafarers and mineworkers. In 1742, King Frederick the Great of Prussia issued an edict "against tobacco smoking as a risk of fire" which was not completely repealed until 1848.

1.4.1
Development of the Cigar

Cigars were the commonest form of processed tobacco in the eighteenth century, with the earliest *tabacerias* for the production of cigars having emerged in Spain in the seventeenth century. In the USA in the nineteenth century, two varieties of tobacco were developed which dominated the tobacco market of the future – hot-air, flue-cured Bright (or Virginia) tobacco, and air-cured, yellowish-red Burley tobacco from other plants [11, 16]. This tobacco was then used for chewing because, owing to its coarse plant structure, it could absorb more sugars and other flavouring agents without appearing moist.

The first tobacco manufactory was established in Seville, and in 1788 the first cigar factory based on the Spanish model was built in Hamburg by Schlottmann [7]. The cigars produced by Schlottmann sold poorly, prompting him to transport them to Cuxhaven so that they could then be fetched back as "imports" with great commercial success. Napoleon brought the cigar to France from where it crossed into Germany. The cigar became the status symbol of the socially ambitious middle classes, and later became the hallmark of the capitalist (George Grosz: "The Face of the Ruling Class", 1921). The *tabacerias* which originated in Cuba were also involved in the manufacture of cigars, with 100–300 workers being employed in a single factory.

In some European countries, cigar was perceived as the symbol of foreign influence and of opposition tendencies, for example, in the nineteenth century Prussia. The *Neue Preussische Kreuzzeitung* wrote in 1848: *"The cigar is the visible symbol of recklessness. With a cigar in his mouth, a young man says and dares quite different things than he would say and dare without a cigar"*. During the revolutionary confrontations in March 1848, the middle classes in Berlin demanded "Freedom to smoke in the Zoological Gardens". The cigar was the dominant tobacco product for virtually 100 years.

1.4.2
Development of the Cigarette

The development of the cigarette coincided with the beginning of the transformation of tobacco into a product of mass consumption. *Cigaritos*, pencil-thin paper wrappers filled with Virginia tobacco, were common in Spain, Portugal, and their colonies. They were also rolled in Seville by *cigarreras*, the women who worked in the tobacco factories. In the middle of the nineteenth century in North Carolina, a high-temperature drying method came into use for tobacco leaves [16]. Since the tobacco leaves have a relatively high sugar content, the dried material became relatively acidic. Nicotine was, thus, present in the form of its salts and was distributed in droplets in the smoke aerosol. This smoke can be inhaled more easily [17]. In 1913, Reynolds used Burley tobacco for the production of his Camel cigarettes [18]. This tobacco blend became the prototype for the American cigarette, whereas British cigarettes were also produced with Virginia tobacco.

Compared with the acrid and strong-tasting smoke of cigars, cigarette smoke is more pleasant, and this can be attributed to the pH of the smoke [17]. Where pH is in the alkaline range, nicotine in the smoke is present predominantly in its free form but is not found in the gaseous phase. This smoke is difficult to inhale because of the acrid taste of nicotine. The fact that nicotine is nevertheless absorbed when a cigar is smoked is due to its slower passage across the buccal mucosa, the membrane lining the mouth [5].

Cigarette smoking first became widespread during the Crimean War (1853–1856): soldiers became accustomed to smoking strong Russian cigarettes, and took the habit back with them to their own countries when hostilities ended. One St. Petersburg cigarette factory (the Yenidse Company) opened its first subsidiary in Dresden in 1862. The first cigarette-making machine, with an hourly output of 3,600 cigarettes, was displayed by the Susini Company from Havana at the Paris World Exhibition in 1867. By the 1880s, US companies followed suit with their own cigarette-making machines. As a result, production costs fell dramatically, new markets opened up, and young people around the age of 18 became a major consumer market for the first time [19]. Thus, smoking took on a new face: smoking as a leisurely pastime was replaced by smoking at short intervals, mainly as a means of coping with stress. Unlike the cigar or a pipe, a cigarette can be smoked in 3–5 min: the smoking break can be equated with "the time it takes to smoke a cigarette". The cigarette came to symbolise modern twentieth century living (see Table 1.1).

Because smoking was always subject to certain restrictions, it both represented something "special" and, in the nineteenth century, was invariably associated with political freedom movements. Following the outbreak of Asian influenza in the summer of 1831, cigar smoking in public places was permitted as a protection against infection [7], and the right to smoke in public was on the list of demands at the Hambach Festival in 1832. During the student protests of 1968, it was even demanded that the ban on smoking in lecture theatres be lifted and that smokers' corners be set up in schools or universities. In wartime too, the soldiers of all armies have always been liberally supplied with cigarettes to boost their fighting morale and readiness for battle [8].

Within about 100 years, the cigarette industry rose to become one of the foremost branches of industry [20] (see Table 1.1).

Table 1.1 Cigarette consumption in various countries during the first third of the twentieth century

Country	Before 1914	1927	1928
Germany	195	302	499
England	201	811	–
France	96	248	326
Holland	–	341	–
Italy	104	372	–
Sweden	115	233	–
USA	143	798[a]	840[a]

Per-capita statistics (from [7])
[a]In the USA 97,000 million cigarettes were smoked in 1927 and 106,000 million in 1928

1.5
Objections to Smoking on Health Grounds

In the nineteenth century, smoking was not viewed from the standpoint of enjoyment. After the prohibition on smoking was abolished, the respectable middle-classes started to voice their criticism on smoking which, even then, were intended primarily to protect young people. In one of his paintings from 1885/1886 (*Skull with burning cigarette*, see Fig. 1.3), the Dutch artist Vincent van Gogh (himself a pipe smoker) foreshadowed the role the cigarette was to play in the century to come. Even then, with smoking perceived as a specific social problem prevalent among 10–12-year-old boys [8], there were complaints about "wayward" young smokers. Parents, teachers and educators were told that they had: ... "*a serious duty to make young people aware of the great dangers of premature use of the narcotic tobacco, an activity that destroys their physical and mental well-being*" [8].

In the second half of the nineteenth century, both in the USA and in Europe (including Germany and Austria), anti-tobacco associations were formed because newer insights into the chemical processes of nature and of human life itself had raised concerns about the health-related consequences of smoking [21]. Education was required concerning the

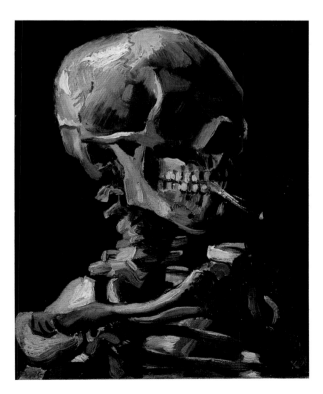

Fig. 1.3 Vincent van Gogh: Skull with burning cigarette (1885/1886)

dangers of tobacco use and misuse [22]. As a result, smoking perceptions have undergone a complete transformation – the "sophisticated" habit of the 1930s is a lethal addiction in the new millennium. What was considered an appropriate social behaviour, frequently endorsed by the medical profession (cf. Fig. 1.4), has now been established as an antisocial behaviour. Nevertheless, the tobacco industry unrestrainedly advertised its products in the medical journals (cf. Fig. 1.4) and among young people who were very soon familiar with all the major cigarette brands (Fig. 1.5).

In 1821, the physician Posselt and the chemist Reimann described a milky distillate obtained from fresh and dried tobacco leaves [24] and in 1828, they isolated nicotine as the principal alkaloid of tobacco [8, 25]. Trommsdorff also studied extracts from tobacco plants [26], but his research was not as fruitful as that of Posselt and Reimann. At that time, this (poisonous) alkaloid fuelled numerous debates about the harmfulness of smoking, based on evidence from various experiments on animals with nicotine dating back to the seventeenth century [8]: Conrad Gesner had observed that dogs vomited when they were administered a small quantity of powdered, dried tobacco leaves. The first Bocarme poisoning trial before a Belgian court in 1850 attracted great interest, particularly when the chemist Stas detected the alkaloid nicotine in the corpse [8]. This case prompted numerous animal experiments with nicotine to permit further elucidation of its effects. The animal experiments described by Tiedemann, working in conjunction with the anatomist Bischoff in Gießen, were conducted in frogs, rabbits, and dogs after he had received nicotine base from Dr. Merck of Darmstadt [8]. These experiments described the high toxicity and rapid onset of poisoning followed by the death of animals. In a letter to Theodor Zwinger, Conrad Gesner described the pattern of poisoning following excessive tobacco consumption in the following terms: "*folii particula fumum haurientem subito inebriat, ut ipse non semel expertus sum*" [8].

Concepts such as acute and chronic nicotine poisoning were introduced. Symptoms described in humans included agitation, stupor, cough, accelerated breathing, nausea, and vomiting etc. [8]. Long-term damage (chronic glossitis, pharyngitis, tonsillitis, and cancer of the tongue) was already being reported as early as 150 years ago [8, 27].

By 1927, more than 50% of the tobacco users in the USA were already smoking cigarettes (97,000 million, rising to 106,000 million in the following year, Table 1.1); even then such consumption was associated with illness on a fairly large scale. Statistics on the incidence of lung cancer were collected in Great Britain as early as 1920. At that time it was still unclear whether a third (genetic) factor was involved alongside smoking and lung cancer. Despite evidence to the contrary, the tobacco industry continued to dispute this fact into the 1950s [28]. The tobacco industry did not shy away from advertising its products even when diseases caused by cigarettes were reported (Fig. 1.6).

1.6
Women Won Over by the Cigarette

In the nineteenth century, smoking was the exclusive privilege of men. Even today, cigar and pipe smoking are still considered to be a predominantly male attribute. Before the 1920s, cigarette was not considered to be the dominant tobacco product. The image it projected was not

THE PENNSYLVANIA MEDICAL JOURNAL   FEBRUARY, 1939

VERIFY THE FACTS
FOR YOURSELF

Just as important as *how many* cigarettes — is *what brand* of cigarettes your patient smokes.

Researches on the subject of irritation of the nose and throat due to smoking have proved conclusively that . . .

> *When smokers changed to* PHILIP
> *MORRIS every case of irritation cleared*
> *completely or definitely improved.*

Smoke Philip Morris. Enjoy the advantages of a better cigarette. Verify for yourself the superiority of Philip Morris.

Reprints of studies, as published in leading medical journals will gladly be sent you on request.*

Tune in to "JOHNNY PRESENTS" on the air Coast-to-Coast Tuesday evenings, NBC Network . . . Saturday evenings, CBS Network . . . Johnny presents "What's My Name" Friday evenings — Mutual Network

PHILIP MORRIS & CO.

- -

☐ Proc. Soc. Exp. Biol. and Med., 1934, 32, 241-245

☐ Laryngoscope, 1935, XLV, 149-154

☐ N. Y. State Jour. Med., 1935, 35-No. 11, 590

☐ Laryngoscope, 1937, XLVII, 58-60

Philip Morris & Co. Ltd., Inc.
119 Fifth Avenue, New York

* Please send me copies of the reprints checked.

NAME_____

ADDRESS_____

CITY_____STATE___ _____

Fig. 1.4 Cigarette advertisement seeming to indicate physician's approval [23]. Philip Morris & Co. advertises with four articles for their products

Fig. 1.5 Example of the tobacco industry's covert yet obvious advertising targeted at young people

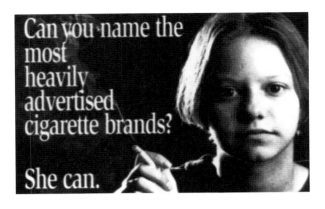

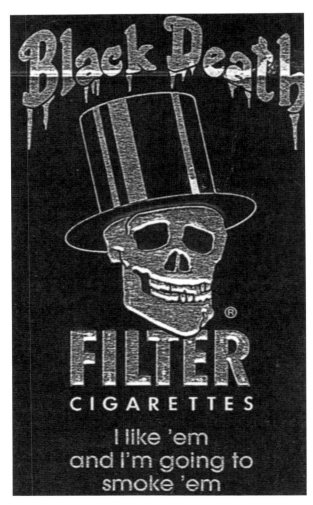

Fig. 1.6 The tobacco industry did not even shy away from using macabre methods to advertise its products, as illustrated by this cigarette pack. Insert for the above cigarette brand

as prestigious as that of chewing tobacco or the cigar. Cigars were thought of as male domain. In 1904, a New York woman was arrested for smoking and simultaneously driving her car [29]. After the First World War, cigarettes also became increasingly popular with women. The dancer Lola Montez and the writer George Sand may be cited as prominent examples of women who smoked. In the USA, the habit was observed mainly among well-to-do women, especially in New York. The cigarette brands of the day, such as *Herbe de la Reine*, were aimed mainly at a female clientele. The London tobacco house Philip Morris developed a cork tip for the cigarette, and advertised this modified cigarette for women. However, since these cigarettes were rolled by hand, they were too expensive to capture broad segments of the market. This situation changed again when it became customary for women also to take employment and, as they became increasingly emancipated, to smoke in public. The US firm American Tobacco produced *Lucky Strike*, which became the best selling cigarette brand. Using testimonials from female celebrities, such as the aviatrix Amelia Earhart, slogans like "*To keep a slender figure – reach for a Lucky instead of a sweet*", or endorsements from film stars Constance Talmadge and Jean Harlow, who appeared from 1929 onwards smoking *Lucky Strike* cigarettes in public, advertisements for cigarette smoking were systematically targeted at women. Even in those days, advertising used slogans extolling the virtues of mild smoking: "*Easier on your throat*", "*I prefer Luckies, and so does my daughter*", "*For your digestion – smoke Camel*" or "*Camels never jangle your nerves*" [2, 30]. In its advertising, the Chesterfield company directed the following slogan at older women: "*To help the country, I think I'll try one*".

With these advertising practices, the US cigarette industry succeeded in the 1930s and 1940s in stylising the cigarette as an integral part of life. During the First World War, the US General Pershing had stated: "*Tobacco is as indispensable* (to the soldiers) *as the daily ration* (of food)" [31] and President Roosevelt later declared the cigarette to be just as essential as food. Smoking was a conspicuously common feature in countless Hollywood movies (e.g. Humphrey Bogart and his female co-stars). Marlene Dietrich and Greta Garbo were further prime examples for this advertising campaign which influenced countless women to become smokers [32].

The Second World War brought a further boost for the cigarette industry as uniformed women in the Allied Forces joined male soldiers in smoking either *Camel* or *Chesterfield*. Cigarette consumption during this period quadrupled worldwide. The women, like their male counterparts, were permitted to smoke in public. In addition, this period saw the arrival of king-size and mentholated cigarettes created especially for women. When the first studies on the lung cancer-producing properties of cigarettes were published, the cellulose mouthpiece was introduced in the 1950s with the advertising slogans "*Pure white, wonderful*" or "*Just what the doctor ordered*", alongside arguments from the cigarette industry refuting the link between smoking and lung cancer. In 1961 in England filter cigarettes were already being bought by some 33% of female smokers but by only 17% of male smokers. In the 1970s, the purchase of filter cigarettes by both sexes had risen to 90% in the hope that this would sidestep the risk of cancer. The development of "*light*" cigarettes with a reduced tar yield, and therefore considered "more healthy", may be regarded as a miscalculation on the part of the cigarette industry for the smoker [33]. What the cigarette industry did achieve by this development was to ensure that, by 1990, 47% of women aged between 29 and 41 in the USA had become smokers.

1.7
The Medical Use of Tobacco in the Nineteenth Century

In the nineteenth century, tobacco was cultivated for medicinal purposes in the Alsace and the Palatinate, and was sold in the form of extracts, powders, ointments and aqueous solutions [10]. Bartholin from Copenhagen used tobacco as an enema and into the nineteenth century tobacco preparations were occasionally prescribed as remedies for strychnine poisoning and tetanus (lockjaw). In the monograph by Müller [34], tobacco and its formulations (decoctions, ointments, tinctures, wine, vinegar, pills) were recommended for dropsy in the lower abdomen. Fowler [34] claimed to have cured 18 out of 31 patients this way. However, the dose was selected in such a way that, as far as possible, neither salivation nor dizziness occurred. Other physicians in the seventeenth and eighteenth centuries also used tobacco preparations for the treatment of oedema. Nicotine preparations were further prescribed for "spastic dysuria" (a category which included gonorrhoea). Other authors from this period described its useful administration as a remedy for neuroses and tetanus, for strangulated hernias (primarily in the form of enemas) as well as for disorders of the lower abdomen associated with constipation, spastic colitis and spastic ileus (in this case using the so-called smoke enemas), and many other conditions [34].

As late as 1837, an infusion of tobacco leaves was recommended as an antidote to arsenic poisoning, and this was tested in dogs. The effect of tobacco preparation was achieved by inducing vomiting several hours after arsenic poisoning [34]. In the mid-nineteenth century, Tiedemann [8] was credited with publishing a comprehensive monograph on tobacco and its history from the earliest beginnings.

1.8
Tobacco Research in the Twentieth Century

In the twentieth century, the interest stimulated in tobacco research paralleled the spread of cigarette consumption coupled with the means for increased production, and the identification of the first harmful effects (Table 1.1). Dr. John Hill, a London physician and botanist, first suggested a relationship between the development of cancer and the long-term use of snuff. He made these comments in 1761 and reported six cases of "polypusses" related to excessive indulgence in tobacco snuff. One such "polypus" was described as a swelling in one nostril that was hard, black and adherent on a broad base. It later developed the symptoms of an open cancer [35]. The huge increase in the number of male smokers was precipitated by the First World War and its consequences [7]. Most men who took up smoking then continued with the habit as they were already addicted. Schoolboys then smoked to a far lesser extent than 50 years later (Fig. 1.7). Even at that time the anti-tobacco lobby was in the minority because it was inevitable that it would lose the struggle against a superpower. Before the outbreak of the Second World War, the Dresden internist Lickint deserved recognition for summarising what was then known about tobacco and its harmful

Fig. 1.7 Age distribution
for cigarette consumption
among 1,058 students
attending higher educational
establishments (data from a
1933 survey) [22]

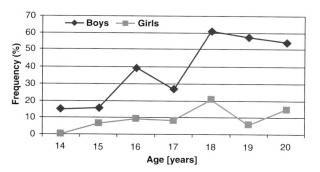

Table 1.2 Lickint's demands in 1939 for the regulation of tobacco consumption [21]

Ban on tobacco consumption for young people below the age of 18
Strong warnings against tobacco consumption by women
Cultivation of nicotine-free or low-nicotine tobacco for "less toxic smoking"
Protection of non-smokers
Creation of counselling centres for tobacco addicts in major cities
Government-sponsored information campaign
Government support for the "German League to Combat the Dangers of Tobacco" funded by
revenue raised from tobacco duty

properties in a comprehensive monograph that is still available [22]. He was also one of the first clinicians to publicise the connection between smoking and the development of bronchial carcinoma in his numerous lectures, a state that he described in detail in his book. His demands at the end of the book for stemming the consumption of tobacco are understandable even today, with one exception (cultivation of low-nicotine tobacco varieties) (Table 1.2). Because of the Second World War, German research into the causal relationship between smoking and the development of bronchial carcinoma [36–40] could not be shared with the international scientific community, and was also ignored after the end of the war. The text of the article by Schairer and Schöninger was not published in English translation until 2001 when it appeared in the *International Journal of Epidemiology* [41], together with several commentaries [42, 43].

All countries, irrespective of the prevailing form of government, "encouraged and promoted in every conceivable way their people's passion for smoking simply for the sake of the national purse" [7]. Following the failure of the bans on smoking in the USA in the 1920s, with Kansas the last state to lift such prohibition in 1927, the European countries never seriously considered similar regulations; in the view of those in power, such action might have an adverse if not disastrous effect on the economic and political situation. After the Second World War this attitude continued, with cigarettes being rationed on "stamps" for the many smokers in Germany (see Chap. 14). In the immediate post-war period, the Americans offered aid in the form of the Marshall Plan, but at the same time they gave the Germans 97,000 tons of tobacco [44] – a gift with immense potential for harm.

Fig. 1.8 An example for
advertising encouraging
women to smoke and
incorporating a historical
reference to emancipation
"You've come a long way
baby"

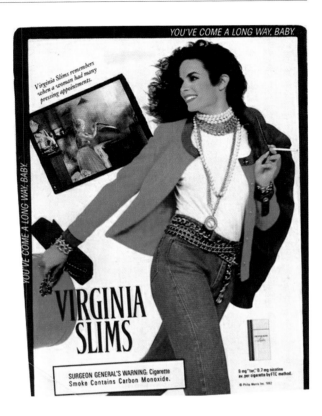

1.9
Concluding Remarks

- As with other luxury commodities (opium, alcohol), tobacco has developed over the
  course of 500 years from being a drug with religious and ceremonial connotations to a
  product of mass consumption (in the case of opium, only the Law on Anaesthetics
  blocks its illegal spread).
- If the tobacco plant had not contained nicotine, it would never have attained its worldwide significance. However, since it does, the tobacco companies in a small number of
  countries earn an estimated hundreds of billions at the expense of the health of billions
  of smokers throughout the world.
- Even 200–300 years ago, attitude of Europeans towards tobacco were clearly ambivalent, as reflected in the actions of monarchs (e.g. James of England) and statesmen. On
  the one hand, economic controls were used to ban tobacco, while on the other regulatory mechanisms were successfully exploited to make capital from the sale of tobacco.
  In the Europe of past centuries, a variety of methods were selected to achieve these
  ends: import and export taxes, monopolies on the manufacture of tobacco products,
  leasing of factories by the state or transfer of rights to these, taxation of land set aside
  for tobacco cultivation, etc.

- The German government and its politicians have adopted this ambivalent attitude from the past and have denied protection from the dangers of smoking to the majority of its electorate, the non-smokers. They have also failed to protect the majority of smokers from the increasingly apparent dangers of smoking.
- In most countries in the world, cigarette smoking is the number 1 killer. Worldwide, more people die from the consequences of cigarette smoking than from any other disease. Despite these problems, the tobacco industry has been able to increase its annual turnover by wooing new smokers of both sexes (Fig. 1.8). Under these circumstances, it is expected that in the year 2025 more than 2 million people in the European Union alone will die from the consequences of cigarette smoking if this trend is not halted soon.

References

1. Akuhurst BC (1981) Tobacco. Longman, London
2. Japan Tobacco Plant Breeding & Genetic Research Laboratory (1994) The genus *Nicotiana* illustrated
3. Tabernaemontanus DIT (1664) New vollkommen Kräuter-Buch. Johann Königs, Basel
4. Wilbert J (1987) Tobacco and Shamanism in South America. Yale University Press, New Haven
5. Travell J (1940) The influence of the hydrogen ion concentration on the absorption of alkaloids from the stomach. J Pharmacol Exp Ther 69:23–33
6. Robicsek F (1978) The smoking gods. Tobacco in Maya art, history and religion. The University of Oklahoma Press, Norman
7. Corti ECC (1930) Die trockene Trunkenheit: *Ursprung, Kampf und Triumph des Rauchens.* Insel, Leipzig
8. Tiedemann F (1854) Geschichte des Tabaks und anderer ähnlicher Genussmittel. H. L. Brömmer, Frankfurt
9. Monardes N (1970) Joyful Newes Out to the Newe Founde Worlde. London. 1577 (reprint). Da Capo Press, Amsterdam
10. Laufer B (1924) Introduction of tobacco into Europe. Field Museum of Natural History, Chicago
11. Brooks JE (1952) The mighty leaf. In: Little B (ed) Tobacco through the centuries. Little Brown, Boston
12. Sandgruber R (1994) Genussmittel. Ihre reale und symbolische Bedeutung im neuzeitlichen Europa. In: Jahrbuch für Wirtschaftsgeschichte. Akademie, Berlin, pp 73–88
13. Jacob. (1603) MBR. Misocapnus seu de abusu tabaci lusus regius. London
14. Precht K, Baumgartner HJ (1993) Tabak. Gewohnheiten, Konsequenzen. Edition diá, St. Gallen
15. Bunbury H (1794) A Smoking Club. S.W. Fores No. 3, Piccadilly
16. Tilley NM (1948) The bright-tobacco industry, 1860–1929. University of North Carolina Press, Chapel Hill
17. Slade J (1993) Nicotine delivery devices. In: Orleans CT, Slade J (eds) Nicotine addiction: principles and management. Oxford University Press, New York, pp 3–23
18. Tilley NM (1985) The R.J. Reynolds Tobacco Company. University of North Carolina Press, Chapel Hill
19. Kluger R (1996) Ashes to ashes. America's Hundred-Year Cigarette War, the Public Health, and the Unabashed Triumph of Philip Morris. Alfred A. Knopf, New York
20. Lorillard P Jr (1895) American tobacco factories. In: Depew CM (ed) One hundred years of American commerce. Haynes, New York

21. Goodman J (1993) Tobacco in history. The cultures of dependence. Routledge, London
22. Lickint F (1939) Tabak und Orgnaismus. In: Handbuch der gesamten Tabakkunde. Hippokrates, Stuttgart, pp 1232
23. (1938–1939) Pennsylvania Med J 42:471
24. Posselt WH, Reimann KL (1821) Bemerkungen Nicotinanin und seine Eigenschaften. Schweigger u Meinicke Neues Journal für Chemie und Physik, pp 1–442
25. Posselt WH, Reimann KL (1828) Chemische Untersuchung des Tabaks und Darstellung des eigenthümlichen wirksamen Prinzips dieser Pflanze. Geigers Magazin f Pharmacie 6(23): 138–161
26. Trommsdorff JB (1829) Beiträge zur chemischen Kenntnis des Tabaks. Neues Journal der Pharmacie (Leipzig) 19:129–155
27. Hartwich C (1911) Die menschlichen Genußmittel. Ihre Herkunft, Verbreitung, Geschichte, Bestandteile, Anwendung und Wirkung. Tauchnitz, Leipzig
28. Bentley HR (1997) Report on visit to USA and Canada, 17 April–12 May 1958. Tob Prod Litigation Rep 12:383–389
29. Goodman J (1993) Tobacco in history.Routledge, London
30. Kellogg JH (1946) Tobaccoism. Battle Creek/Mich. The Good Health Publishing, Michigan
31. Hamilton AE (1927) The smoking world. Century, New York
32. Blum D (1997) Auf leichten Flügeln ins Land der Phantasie. Tabak und Kultur – Columbus bis Davidoff. Transit, Berlin
33. Hurt RD, Robertson CR (1998) Prying open the door to the tobacco industry's secrets about nicotine: the Minnesota Tobacco Trial. JAMA 280:1173–1181
34. Müller J (1842) Der Tabak in geschichtlicher, botanischer, chemischer, medicinischer und diätetischer Hinsicht. von Gebrüder Daams, Emmerich
35. Redmond DE Jr (1970) Tobacco and cancer: the first clinical report, 1761. N Engl J Med 282: 18–23
36. Glinski von (1939) Untersuchungen über die Zunahme des primären Lungenkrebses unter Berücksichtigung der Pathogenese. Dtsch Arch klin Med 185:75–88
37. Müller FH (1939) Tabakmissbrauch und Lungencarcinom. Zschr Krebsforsch 49(1):57–85
38. Haustein KO (2004) Fritz Lickint (1898–1960) – Ein Leben als Aufklärer über die Gefahren des Tabaks. Suchtmed 6(3):249–255
39. Schöninger E (1944) Lungenkrebs und Tabakrauch. Inaugural-Dissertation, Universität Jena, pp 1–25
40. Schairer E, Schöninger E (1943) Lungenkrebs und Tabakverbrauch. Zschr Krebsforsch 54: 261–269
41. Schairer E, Schoniger E (2001) Lung cancer and tobacco consumption. Int J Epidemiol 30(1): 24–27
42. Ernst E (2001) Commentary: The Third Reich – German physicians between resistance and participation. Int J Epidemiol 30:37–42
43. Proctor RN (2001) Commentary: Schairer and Schoniger's forgotten tobacco epidemiology and the Nazi quest for racial purity. Int J Epidemiol 30(1):31–34
44. Wachter T (2001) Befleckte Kampagne gegen das Rauchen. Der Bund (Zürich) 2:16

Epidemiology of Tobacco Dependence

2

The twentieth century has witnessed the birth and development of a new epidemic - tobacco dependence [1–3]. In the last 40 years, due to the rise in tobacco consumption (Fig. 2.1; Table 2.1), tobacco use has become a particular health hazard, as documented in numerous reports [2, 3, 7–13]. It has become clear that the nicotine dependence (nicotine being produced through the tobacco plant), a fact now confirmed by the World Health Organization (WHO), is responsible for the adverse effects on health [14]. Nicotine itself is known to be a powerful poison – similar to prussic acid [15]. Nevertheless, most health-related consequences are attributable to the 2,500 toxins in the tobacco plant and to some 4,000 substances present in tobacco smoke [16–18]. In the USA and many European Union (EU) countries, tobacco causes more deaths than any other dependence-producing substance (Table 2.2) [4, 19]. The developing countries will be suffering this if they continue to increase their tobacco consumption [20].

In Europe, more than 30% of the population smoke cigarettes; cigar and pipe smoking and the use of chewing or snuff tobacco are of secondary importance. In Germany, where more than 17 million people currently smoke, 309 people die each day from the direct consequences of smoking, whereas road traffic accidents claim a "mere" 21 deaths/day. If an airliner with 309 passengers on board crashes every day in Germany, there would be a

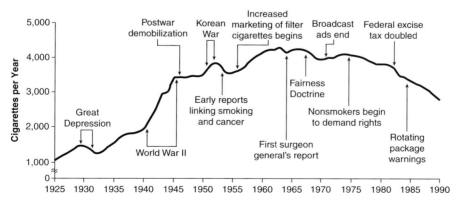

Fig. 2.1 Annual per capita cigarette consumption in the USA during the period from 1925 to 1990 (from [4])

K.-O. Haustein, D. Groneberg, *Tobacco or Health?*
DOI: 10.1007/978-3-540-87577-2_2, © Springer Verlag Berlin Heidelberg 2010

Table 2.1 Methods of tobacco consumption in the USA from 1900 to 1991 [5, 6]

Tobacco type	1900	1952	1991
Tobacco in general (kg/person)	3.4	5.9	2.3
Cigarettes (%)	2	81	87
Snuff, chewing tobacco (%)	4	3	5
Cigars (%)	27	10	4
Pipe or hand-rolled (%)	19	1	1

Table 2.2 Avoidable deaths in the USA in 1990 [4]

Death due to	Deaths	Percentage
Tobacco	400,000	19
Poor diet, sedentary lifestyle	300,000	14
Alcohol	100,000	5
Bacterial infections	90,000	4
Poisoning	60,000	3
Firearms	35,000	2
Sexual deviancy	30,000	1
Road traffic accidents	25,000	1
Illicit drugs	20,000	<1

national outcry and the government would be compelled to take action. During the period from 1925 to the 1960s, tobacco consumption in the USA showed a 4.2-fold increase, before falling again to 2.5 times the 1925 level by the start of the 1990s (Fig. 2.1).

In the USA, cigarette smoking is responsible for one in every five deaths (400,000 deaths per annum, see Table 2.2), chiefly as a result of coronary heart disease, lung cancer and other respiratory tract diseases which would be avoidable in principle by smoking cessation [21]. As an exotic commodity, therefore, the cigarette has advanced to become the commonest cause of death. The problem has reached similar dimensions in Europe [4].

2.1
Tobacco Consumption in the Twentieth Century

The first two decades of the twentieth century laid the foundation for huge growth in the cigarette industry, with cigarettes in the 1920s not so much producing dependence, but rather being highly toxic for the respiratory tract. In the 1920s and 1930s, cigarette consumption was boosted particularly when women were included as targets of the increasingly successful advertising efforts of the tobacco industry, with Camel cigarettes gaining widespread popularity [5, 22]. Following the recognition even during these years of the adverse effects of cigarettes on health [7, 9, 13, 23], the cigarette industry developed the filter cigarette as a kind of safety "guarantee" in the 1950s and the "low-tar" cigarette in the 1960s [2, 5]. The percentage share of filter cigarettes increased from 0.3% in 1949 to 97% in 1992 [24].

In men born between 1911 and 1930, the prevalence of cigarette smoking in the USA reached peak levels of 67% in the 1940s and 1950s [25], with a maximum prevalence of

Fig. 2.2 Smoking prevalence among men and women as a function of age. Data from the Microcensus Study 1999 [27], by kind permission of the German Federal Statistics Office

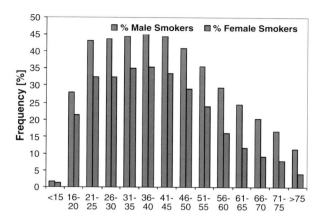

44% recorded for women in the 1960s. The number of smokers fell only in response to the massive anti-smoking campaigns of the 1970s, with a greater decline among men than among women [26]. Smoking prevalence in Germany was confirmed in the latest Microcensus Study (Fig. 2.2). The national Youth Risk Behavior Survey (YRBS) 2003 of the United States indicates that the prevalence of current cigarette use has declined substantially since the late 1990s and is at the lowest level since YRBS was initiated in 1991 [28].

2.2
Cigarette Smoking in the USA Since 1965

Over the period from 1965 to 1993, smokers in the USA and their tobacco-use behaviour were monitored in a survey of all smokers above the age of 18 years with a minimum annual consumption of 100 cigarettes [6]. With effect from 1991 and 1992, the survey included all those who smoked daily [29, 30]. Defined in these terms, the annual prevalence of cigarette smoking in the USA was 42% in 1965 and 25% in 1993 [6, 30]. Smoking cessation was achieved by 24% in 1965 compared with 50% in 1993 [30]. In the 30–39-year-old category, 89% first tried smoking before the age of 18 and 71% became regular smokers [21]. The average age at which smoking was first tried was 14.6 years and the age at which survey respondents became regular smokers was 17.7 years [21]. In contrast, after 1980, the survey revealed that the transition to regular smoking did not occur until after the age of 20 [31].

Smoking was initially a male preserve; however, from 1965 to 1993, smoking prevalence among men declined from 52 to 28%. Smoking prevalence among women was 34% in 1965, falling to 22% in 1993. Overall, the prevalence of cessation among ex-smokers in 1993 was 52% for men and 47% for women [30]. Nevertheless, the prevalence of male pipe and cigar smoking, chewing tobacco and using snuff rose continuously [3, 32]. Among adolescent smokers, there was gender equality. From 1967 onwards in particular, there was an increase in the number of female smokers following the introduction of "female cigarettes" [31], whereas smoking prevalence among young women with a college education declined over the period from 1983 to 1991 [6].

Differences in educational level are also apparent among smokers: 37% of individuals in education for 9–11 years were smokers compared with only 14% of those who were in education for 16 years [30]. Higher educational levels were correlated with a willingness to quit smoking [6, 33]. Willingness to quit smoking also increased with age, with educational level also being a decisive factor in this context [21, 34, 35].

Smoking prevalence was highest among people living below the poverty line [30], blue-collar workers [2, 36], single or divorced people [13] and military personnel [37, 38]. Tobacco use declined most rapidly among the medical professionals; at the beginning of the 1990s, only 3% of doctors in the USA were smokers [35], compared with some 20% of doctors in Germany [27]. However, there seems to be a rethinking of smoking habits in the United States. The prevalence of cigarette smoking among US adults has declined by almost half since 1965, with positive trends observed among people in almost all sociodemographic groups and efforts to reduce disparities recognized as an important goal in public health [39].

2.3
Smoking Habits in Germany

In Germany, in people between the age of 21 and 50 years, smoking prevalence is about 33% in women and 44% in men (Fig. 2.2). Simultaneously, as direct consequences of cigarette smoking, approximately 80,000–90,000 new cases of cardiovascular disease and 30,000 new cases of bronchial carcinoma are recorded every year. Above the age of 35, tobacco-attributable mortality rates in the federal German states range from 5.6 to 13.2% for women and from 24.3 to 29.2% for men. The highest mortality statistics are recorded for women in Hamburg, Berlin and Bremen [27]. With an overall mortality rate in Germany of 17%, smoking represents the commonest avoidable and exclusively behaviour-related cause of death [40].

According to the Microcensus Study, a representative survey conducted in 1995 among the population in Germany, interesting conclusions can be drawn concerning smoking behaviour as a function of gross income and educational level (see Fig. 2.3). Similar results are also evident from the latest Microcensus Study [27] with regard to the postulated connection between school and university education and smoking behaviour (Fig. 2.3). The influence of the educational level on smoking pattern in different social classes might be explained by the efficiency of anti-smoking campaigns and the awareness about health effects of smoking among persons with different educational levels [41].

Thus, according to self-reported information in April 1995, 30.9% of men and 18.2% of women were regular cigarette smokers. In both sexes, smoking prevalence fell with increasing age: among men and women over the age of 64, smoking prevalence was only 12.9 and 4.9%, respectively [42]. The data summarised in Figs. 2.4 and 2.5 indicate that the relationship between monthly income and smoking behaviour applies more for men than for women. Smoking prevalence is higher (42.6%) among men in the lowest income category (< 700 EUR) than among those with a high monthly income (>6,500 DM), though the rate is still 23.1%. For women, the most pronounced income-specific differences are found in the youngest age group (18–29-year olds). Here too there is a considerable difference in smoking prevalence (41.4 vs. 18.5%) for the lowest and highest income groups [42].

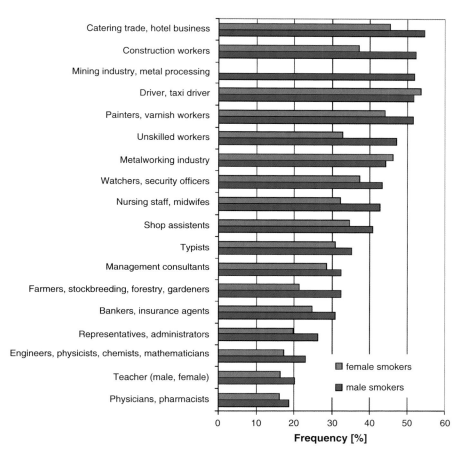

Fig. 2.3 Smoking prevalence in different occupational groups [27]. By kind permission of the German Federal Statistics Office

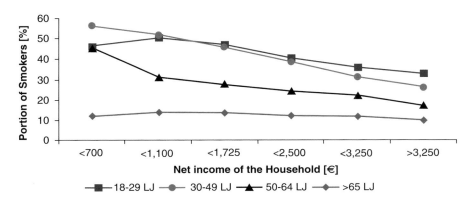

Fig. 2.4 Correlations between smoking behaviour and average gross monthly income for men. Results of the Microcensus Study [42]

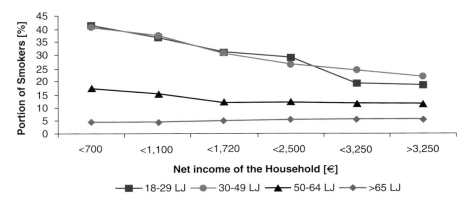

Fig. 2.5 Correlations between smoking behaviour and average gross monthly income for women. Results of the Microcensus Study [42]

Overall, it may be concluded that a very highly pronounced social gradient exists in terms of smoking behaviour [39]. Smokers tend to be particularly from households with a very low income and/or from people whose primary income is based on social welfare or unemployment benefit. In addition, the Microcensus Study reveals that ex-smokers are mainly from households with a higher net monthly income [42].

2.4
Cigarette-Related Mortality in Different Countries

While prospective studies potentially providing evidence of the number of deaths related to cigarette smoking would be unambiguous, they are too time-consuming and costly in practice and are, therefore, problematic to conduct. Nevertheless, this difficulty can be overcome by using survival statistics, e.g., by comparing data from different countries on lung cancer mortality among smokers and non-smokers. The correlation between smoking and lung cancer mortality is clearer in developing countries than in industrialised countries because environmental factors are more influential in the latter (Tables 2.3 and 2.4).

A survey of trends for mortality from smoking over the past 50 years among men and women in the age category from 35 to 69 years reveals a pattern that gives pause for thought: when extrapolated to the coming decades, smoking-related mortality for men and women is expected to be identical (Figs. 2.6 and 2.7) [43]. In addition, when calculated with reference to age, mortality attributable to smoking rises disproportionately more rapidly than mortality without such harmful exposure [43]. The data summarised in Tables 2.3 and 2.4 show that smoking-related mortality in the former socialist economies of Eastern Europe is lower than that in the industrialised countries, though it should be remembered that the data for the former Eastern Bloc countries may be incomplete. It is clear that all state initiatives to stem the smoking tide have not resulted in a reduction in smoking-related mortality in middle age. Even though the age of 70 is regarded as a significant

Table 2.3 Numbers and percentages of smoking-related deaths in OECD countries in 1990

Country	Men			Women		
	35–69 years	>70 years	All ages	35–69 years	>70 years	All ages
Australia	6.7 (28)	7.3 (21)	14.0 (22)	1.9 (15)	3.1 (8)	5.0 (9)
Austria	4.0 (28)	3.6 (16)	7.5 (20)	0.6 (7)	1.5 (4)	2.0 (5)
Belgium	7.9 (41)	8.6 (28)	16.5 (31)	0.7 (6)	0.6 (1)	1.2 (2)
Canada	13.5 (35)	14.1 (24)	27.6 (27)	5.0 (23)	7.0 (11)	12.1 (14)
Denmark	3.3 (32)	4.3 (22)	7.6 (25)	1.8 (27)	2.6 (11)	4.4 (15)
Finland	2.6 (25)	2.7 (21)	5.3 (21)	0.2 (5)	0.5 (3)	0.8 (3)
France	32.6 (32)	24.5 (16)	57.1 (21)	1.0 (2)	1.2 (1)	2.2 (1)
Germany	52.0 (32)	43.3 (18)	95.3 (22)	6.2 (7)	10.4 (3)	16.5 (3)
Greece	5.2 (33)	5.2 (17)	10.4 (21)	0.4 (5)	0.9 (3)	1.3 (3)
Ireland	1.7 (31)	2.5 (24)	4.2 (25)	0.7 (20)	1.6 (15)	2.3 (16)
Italy	37.8 (37)	34.9 (21)	72.7 (26)	2.7 (5)	7.4 (4)	10.1 (4)
Japan	26.8 (16)	41.5 (16)	68.3 (15)	3.6 (4)	15.4 (6)	19.0 (5)
Luxemburg	0.2 (34)	0.3 (25)	0.5 (27)	<0.1 (9)	<0.1 (1)	0.1 (3)
Netherlands	8.6 (38)	13.0 (32)	21.6 (32)	1.4 (11)	1.3 (3)	2.7 (4)
New Zealand	1.4 (28)	1.7 (22)	3.1 (22)	0.7 (21)	0.8 (9)	1.4 (11)
Norway	1.4 (21)	1.9 (12)	3.4 (14)	0.4 (12)	0.6 (3)	1.0 (5)
Portugal	4.0 (21)	2.8 (9)	6.5 (13)	0.0 (0)	0.0 (0)	0.0 (0)
Spain	20.5 (33)	19.4 (19)	40.0 (23)	0.0 (0)	0.0 (0)	0.0 (0)
Sweden	2.1 (16)	3.2 (9)	5.3 (11)	0.7 (10)	1.3 (3)	2.0 (4)
Switzerland	3.1 (31)	3.7 (18)	6.8 (21)	0.3 (6)	0.9 (3)	1.2 (4)
United Kingdom	37.2 (35)	52.1 (27)	89.4 (28)	16.4 (24)	32.1 (13)	48.5 (15)
USA	150.0 (36)	136.2 (23)	286.3 (26)	72.7 (28)	102.1 (14)	174.9 (17)
Total	423.5 (32)	427.8 (20)	851.3 (23)	117.7 (16)	191.6 (7)	309.3 (9)

Numbers of deaths in 1,000s; percentages in parentheses [43]

"milestone" in various countries, only one in five smokers survives this milestone. The opposite picture is found in the OECD countries: without the use of tobacco one-fifth of people die before reaching the age of 70, and deaths among non-smokers before the age of 70 are declining all the time [43].

The statistics calculated for 1990 are impressive: for all countries together, mortality from smoking was 24% and in the 35–69-year-old age group, mortality was 35% for men and 12% for women [43]. The loss of life for a smoker is calculated at 5–7 years. In several countries (France, the Netherlands, Sweden), there has been an increase in cigarette consumption in young women in particular, with the result that increased mortality must be anticipated in the decades ahead [40] (Figs. 2.6 and 2.7). The summarised data indicate that no smoking-related deaths occurred in people below the age of 35 [43]. Approximately half of all smokers from the developing countries suffered from their smoking behaviour. Teenagers or young adults who become regular smokers must expect to forfeit 8 years of life [43], as also shown by a study among British doctors conducted over a 40-year period [23].

Table 2.4 Numbers and percentages of smoking-related deaths in the former socialist countries in 1990

Country	Men			Women		
	35–69 years	>70 years	All ages	35–69 years	>70 years	All ages
Armenia	2.2 (38)	0.5 (13)	2.8 (23)	0.2 (6)	<0.1 (1)	0.3 (3)
Azerbaijan	2.7 (24)	0.5 (8)	3.1 (14)	0.0 (0)	0.0 (0)	0.0 (0)
Belarus	1.0 (39)	3.1 (16)	14.1 (26)	0.3 (2)	0.1 (<1)	0.4 (1)
Bulgaria	8.2 (30)	2.2 (7)	10.4 (17)	0.5 (3)	0.4 (1)	0.9 (2)
Czech Republic	13.3 (42)	6.1 (19)	19.4 (29)	1.4 (9)	1.5 (3)	2.9 (5)
Estonia	1.9 (38)	0.5 (15)	2.4 (26)	0.2 (6)	0.1 (2)	0.3 (3)
Georgia	2.8 (24)	0.7 (9)	3.5 (15)	0.1 (2)	<0.1 (<1)	0.1 (1)
Hungary	16.0 (41)	6.5 (19)	22.5 (29)	3.1 (14)	3.1 (7)	6.0 (9)
Kazakhstan	15.2 (43)	3.7 (22)	18.9 (28)	2.3 (12)	1.9 (6)	4.2 (7)
Kirghizstan	2.0 (28)	0.7 (17)	2.7 (17)	0.2 (4)	0.3 (5)	0.5 (4)
Latvia	3.3 (38)	1.0 (15)	4.3 (25)	0.3 (6)	0.3 (2)	0.6 (3)
Lithuania	3.8 (38)	1.4 (17)	5.2 (25)	0.2 (3)	0.4 (3)	0.6 (3)
Moldavia	3.5 (31)	0.7 (10)	4.3 (20)	0.3 (3)	0.3 (3)	0.6 (3)
Poland	44.6 (42)	15.3 (18)	59.9 (29)	5.1 (10)	4.4 (4)	9.5 (5)
Romania	19.6 (32)	4.2 (8)	23.8 (18)	2.2 (6)	0.8 (1)	2.9 (3)
Russia	191.9 (42)	48.6 (20)	240.5 (30)	16.4 (7)	19.3 (3)	35.7 (4)
Slovakia	5.8 (38)	1.9 (15)	7.7 (26)	0.3 (4)	0.4 (2)	0.7 (3)
Tadzhikistan	0.7 (14)	0.2 (6)	1.0 (5)	0.0 (0)	0.0 (0)	0.0 (0)
Turkmenistan	1.1 (22)	0.2 (6)	1.3 (9)	0.0 (0)	0.0 (0)	0.0 (0)
Ukraine	64.4 (40)	19.5 (17)	83.9 (28)	5.9 (6)	8.5 (4)	14.5 (4)
Uzbekistan	4.7 (20)	0.9 (5)	5.6 (8)	0.7 (5)	0.5 (2)	1.3 (2)
Yugoslavia	19.4 (36)	6.3 (13)	25.7 (23)	2.0 (6)	1.6 (2)	3.6 (4)
Total	441.2 (39)	126.3 (17)	567.5 (26)	42.1 (7)	44.4 (3)	86.5 (4)

Numbers of deaths in 1,000s; percentages in parentheses [43]

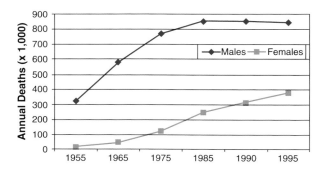

Fig. 2.6 Annual death rates from lung cancer in men and women in OECD countries [43]

It is estimated that in the year 2000, smoking caused 4.83 million premature deaths in the world, 2.41 million in developing countries and 2.43 million in industrialised countries. There were 3.84 million male deaths and 1.00 million female deaths associated with smoking. The leading causes of death from smoking were cardiovascular diseases, COPD and lung cancer [44].

Fig. 2.7 Annual death rates from lung cancer in men and women in the former socialist countries [43]

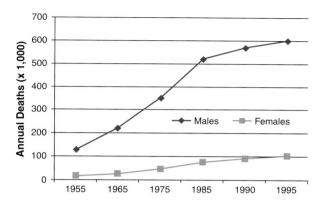

Smoking-related deaths in the industrialised countries will also continue to increase in the coming years, a fact that is of course attributable to the huge increase in cigarette consumption. In the light of these developments, the WHO convened a conference back in 1989 [1]. According to the data listed in Tables 2.3 and 2.4, the number of smoking-related deaths in 1990 was 1.8 million, and on this basis, a total of some 20 million deaths may be assumed for the 1990s. Males predominated numerically, but this pattern is set to change in the coming years.

The calculation of smoking-related mortality is difficult for the majority of developing countries: a spectacular increase has been recorded in China in recent years, particularly since smoking prevalence among men in that country has exceeded the 50% limit. The incidence of illness in Asia and Latin America is very high [40]. Taking all countries together (the industrialised plus the developing countries), 3 (2–4) million people die annually from the consequences of cigarette smoking.

Currently, there are 2,300 million children and teenagers in the world, of whom 30–40% (i.e. 800 million young people) smoke. If smoking doubles in all age groups, this could result in the death of 50% of all smokers [43].

During the period 1978–1992, cigarette production in China increased from 500,000 million to 1.7 billion, and the cigarettes had very high tar values. Research in China into the health-related consequences of this development (lung cancer, COPD and oesophageal cancer) has already been conducted, but the results remain unpublished [43].

According to extrapolations for the period 2020–2030, it is estimated worldwide that 3–10 million deaths a year would be attributable to smoking [43]!

2.5
Other Forms of Tobacco Use

Cigar smoking has increased again in recent years in the belief that it represents a smaller risk than cigarette smoking (Fig. 2.8) [45, 46]. Cigar consumption increased by 66% between 1964 and 1993 and by 46.4% between 1993 and 1997 [46]. Consumption of

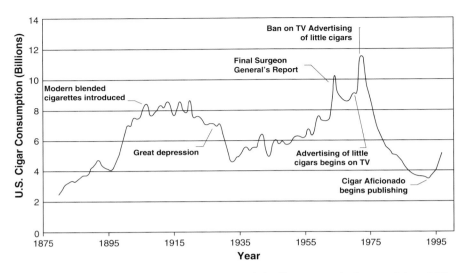

Fig. 2.8 Total U.S. cigar consumption 1880–1997 and significant events in the use of cigars [45]

large cigars and cigarillos increased by 69% between 1993 and 1997 [47]. According to research conducted in California, between 1990 and 1996, more young adult male than female high-school graduates preferred to smoke cigars [48] and this activity has since overtaken smokeless tobacco use in the USA [49]. Some young people also replace the inner tobacco of the cigar with marijuana or other illegal drugs (a practice known as blunting) [50].

According to several studies, cigar smoking is perceived to be less dangerous than cigarette smoking in terms of carcinogenicity [51–53]. Aside from notions of reduced carcinogenicity, however, differing smoking behaviours, duration of smoking, extent of inhalation and age at smoking initiation must also be taken into account [51, 54, 55]. Overall, no studies have been conducted among larger numbers of smokers using tobacco products other than cigarettes. According to a meta-analysis of seven studies involving 7,200 controls and 5,600 male smokers (pipe and cigar), there was a dose-dependent increase in lung cancer risk, with cigarillo smokers having the same increased risk as cigarette smokers (odds ratio (OR): 12.7 vs. 14.7; cigarillo vs. cigarette) [56], obviously a consequence of the inhalation of tobacco smoke. In a cohort study in 17,774 men between the age of 30 and 85 years, cigar smokers were also found to have an increased risk of developing coronary heart disease (OR 1.27), COPD (OR 1.45) and cancers of the upper respiratory and gastrointestinal tract (OR 2.02). Cigar smokers clearly underestimate their cancer risk, with only 7.8% believing that cigar smoking will damage their health. They also underplay the damage to the health of those around them as a result of passive smoking [57–59].

The use of other forms of tobacco is more common among men than women [6, 21]. Snuff tobacco has been consumed increasingly during the last 25 years. A recently published study from Sweden indicates that taking snuff contributes to increased smoking.

Therefore, one should not encourage the use of the less harmful snuff in smoking cessation programmes [60].

Water pipe smoking is familiar to approximately 1 billion people around the world. It is widely encountered in Turkey and Arabic and Middle East countries.

A study in the year 2003 shows that one single smoking session increased oxidation injury (8-epi-PGF2alpha: $p = 0.03$; MDA: $p = 0.001$) and 11-DH-TXB2 ($p = 0.00003$) significantly. Repeated daily smoking induced a persistent long-lasting oxidation injury reflected by elevated pre-values. These results indicate a significant increase of in vivo oxidative stress by regular water pipe smoking [61].

In the USA, there are regional differences for chewing tobacco, with the black population in the Southern states using it more than whites in the North [62]. The consumption of smokeless tobacco has clearly increased among white male adults during the period 1970–1985 [6], though here too a higher educational level is associated with lower consumption [28]. In 1992, this tobacco form was used by 11.9% of 12–17-year olds. In contrast, pipe or cigar smoking has declined continuously since 1970, for example, from 16 to 4% within 20 years [6].

2.6
Smokers and Other Risk Factors

University graduates smoked more commonly if they did not engage in any sporting or other physical activity or if they had increased numbers of sexual relationships [21]. Furthermore, smoking was more prevalent among those individuals who slept for less than 7 h at night, did not take breakfast in the morning and did not eat their meals until later in the day [63–65]. It is also shown that the parental smoking habits are a consistent risk factor for adolescent smoking. The relative risk of adolescent daily smoking (adjusted for age and sex) was significantly higher for maternal only smoking compared with paternal only smoking in each ethnic group [66].

A Swedish prospective population-based cohort study pointed out the cumulative influence of multiple socio-economic and psychosocial chains of risks experienced during childhood. One major finding was the fact that being from a divorced family and having poor contact with their parents influenced the smoking directly.

Adolescents with adverse socio-economic status were also likely to be unpopular in school and consequently, their smoking behaviour was affected directly [67].

In an international study conducted in six countries from 1985 to 1995, the level of dependence in smokers (Fagerström test) was compared with smoking prevalence in the countries concerned [68]. It was found that smokers showed a higher average level of dependence in countries with a low smoking prevalence (USA, Finland) compared with countries where smoking was more prevalent (Poland, Austria, France). One possible explanation is that, in countries with a low smoking prevalence, the "occasional smokers" or those with a low dependence level had already stopped smoking in response to external influences (educational campaigns etc.), whereas the remaining smokers were more highly dependent.

2.7
Smoking Behaviour and Educational Level in the EU

As a part of a study conducted in 12 European countries, smoking behaviour in men and women (aged 20–44 years and 45–74 years) was compared with educational level by country – something that had only rarely been done before [69–71]. In this study, smokers in several countries were classified in terms of the highest level of education completed by the individual [72]. This classification comprised five levels where "5" was tertiary education, including university: levels 1–3 formed the "lower educated" group, while levels 4 and 5 were the "higher educated" group. The data (education vs. smoking behaviour) were processed using regression analyses and ORs were calculated to indicate an association. If the OR was clearly greater than 1.0, an association was to be accepted between low educational level and smoking behaviour. As is apparent from the data summarised in Fig. 2.9, considerable differences existed between the 12 countries studied. Among the younger men (20–44-years old), the proportion of current smokers ranged from 32 to 64%, while among the older men (45–74-years old), it ranged from 28 to 55%. The ORs for current smoking were greater than 1.00, indicating an association between (lower) educational level and smoking prevalence (Fig. 2.10). The ORs among the younger men were usually higher than among the older men [64], with values >2.00 being calculated. The highest ORs among younger men were observed in Norway, Sweden, France and Great Britain. Among the older men, the highest ORs (>2.00) were observed in Great Britain and Norway, indicating that smoking was more prevalent in the lower educated group in those countries. By contrast, in Portugal more than in Spain, smoking was more prevalent in higher educated men (OR <1.00); at the same time, the prevalence of smoking among women was <5%. In the more Southerly countries of the EU (France, Italy, Spain, Portugal), smoking was more prevalent among higher educated older women (OR <1.00) (Fig. 2.9, Table 2.5).

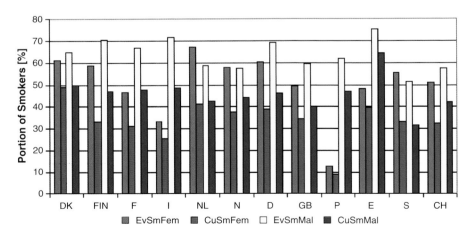

Fig. 2.9   Smoking prevalence among men (Mal) and women (Fem) in 12 European Union (EU) and Switerzland countries. Data shown for ever smoking (EvSm) and current smoking (CuSm) [72]

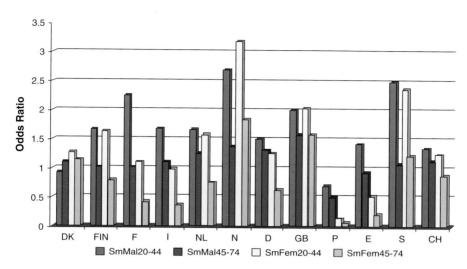

Fig. 2.10 Odds ratios (ORs) in 12 EU countries for male (SmMal) and female (SmFem) smokers, each in two age groups (20–44 years and 45–74 years) [72]. ORs greater than 1.0 are indicative of an association between smoking and low educational level

Table 2.5 Stages of smoking behaviour in 12 European Union countries [72]

Stage 1	Smoking is an exceptional behaviour and is mainly a habit of higher socio-economic groups
Stage 2	Smoking becomes ever more common. Rates among men peak at 50–80%, irrespective of socio-economic group. In women, these patterns usually lag 10–20 years behind those of men, but smoking is first adopted by women from higher socio-economic groups (Portugal)
Stage 3	Smoking prevalence rates among men decrease to about 40% since many men stop smoking. Women reach their peak rate (35–40%), but at the end of this stage, their rates start to decline too (starting to happen in Spain, Italy, France)
Stage 4	Prevalence rates decline gradually for both men and women, and smoking becomes progressively more a habit of lower socio-economic groups (northern European countries: Norway, Sweden, Great Britain)

According to data from the 1995 Microcensus Study published in 1998, a definite social differentiation for smokers of both sexes can also be identified in Germany. Smoking was 2–3 times more prevalent among men and women with a low educational level than among those with a higher educational level or in the graduate professions (Fig. 2.3) [73]. The highest smoking prevalences were found among men with simple manual jobs (building site labourers, road construction workers, etc.). The highest rates among women were found for workers in the hotel and restaurant trade, care assistants for the elderly and cleaners, etc. (Fig. 2.3). These results are consistent with findings from international surveys.

Overall, it is concluded that cigarette smoking is taken up in stage 1 by people with a higher educational level and who are financially better off (as in the USA in the early years of the twentieth century; see Table 2.5). In stage 2, smoking is taken up by all strata of the population. In stage 3, educational initiatives cause a decline in prevalence rates, firstly among men and some time later, among women (emancipation, "equality problems"). In stage 4, smoking remains the preserve of people with a low level of education (and reduced social status). These data are also confirmed by research conducted as part of the Microcensus Study [42, 73].

2.8
Concluding Remarks

- Worldwide, there has been an increase in smoking and hence, in tobacco-associated diseases and deaths.
- In all the industrialised countries, as well as in the developing countries, cigarette consumption is the dominant form of smoking.
- In many countries, smoking prevalence is determined by educational level and monthly income, with smoking being more common among the socially disadvantaged.
- The growing frequency of smoking among children and women is most alarming, entailing increases in rates of morbidity and mortality.
- Regardless of how they are used (e.g. inhalation), cigars and cigarillos also carry a greater risk than was thought previously.

References

1. Peto R, Lopez AD (1990) The future worldwide health effects of current smoking patterns. 1990 report on the seventh World Conference on Tobacco or Health, on the behalf of the WHO consultative group on statistical aspects of tobacco-related mortality. In: Durston B, Jamrozik K (eds) The global war. Proceedings of the seventh World Conference on Tobacco or Health. Health Department of Western Australia, Perth
2. US Department of Health and Human Services. Public Health Service (1989) Reducing the health consequences of Smoking: 25 years of progress: a report of the Surgeon General. 1989 executive summary. Centers for Disease Control. Center for Chronic Disease Prevention and Health Promotion, Office an Smoking and Health, Rockville, MD. DHHS publication no. (CDC) 89–8411
3. US Department of Health and Human Services, Public Health Service, Centers for Disease Control, Center for Chronic Diseuse Prevention und Health Promotion, Office an Smoking and Health (1990) The health benefits of smoking cessation: a report of the Surgeon General. US Department of Health and Human Services, Public Health Service, Centers for Disease Control, Center for Chronic Diseuse Prevention und Health Promotion, Office an Smoking and Health, Rockville, MD. DHHS publication no. (CDC) 90–8416
4. Bartecci CT, MacKenzie TD, Schrier RW (1995) The global tobacco epidemic. Sci Am 272:26–33
5. Oleans CT, Slade J (eds) (1993) Nicotine addiction: principles and management. Oxford University Press, New York
6. Giovino GA, Schooley MW, Zhu BP, Chrismon JH, Tomar SL, Peddicord JP, et al (1994) Surveillance for selected tobacco-use behaviors – United States, 1900–1994. Mor Mortal Wkly Rep CDC Surveill Summ 43(3):1–43

7. Doll R, Hill AB (1999) Smoking and carcinoma of the lung. Preliminary report. 1950. Bull World Health Organ 77(1):84–93
8. Doll R, Peto R, Hall E, Wheatley K, Gray R (1994) Mortality in relation to consumption of alcohol: 13 years' observations on male British doctors. BMJ 309(6959):911–918
9. Hammond CE, Horn D (1954) The relationship between human smoking habits and death rates: a follow-up study of 187.766 men. J Am Med Assoc 155:1316–1338
10. Ochsner A (1973) Corner of history. My first recognition of the relationship of smoking and lung cancer. Prev Med 2(4):611–614
11. Ochsner A (1971) The health menace of tobacco. Am Sci 59(2):246–252
12. Stolley PD (1991) When genius errs: R.A. Fisher and the lung cancer controversy. Am J Epidemiol 133(5):416–425
13. Wynder EL, Graham EA (1985) Landmark article May 27, 1950: tobacco smoking as a possible etiologic factor in bronchiogenic carcinoma. A study of six hundred and eighty-four proved cases. By Ernest L. Wynder and Evarts A. Graham. JAMA 253(20):2986–2994
14. World Health Organization (1993) International statistical classification of diseases und related health Problems, Tenth revision, vol 1. World Health Organization, Geneva, Switzerland
15. Beemann IA, Hunter WC (1937) Fatal nicotine poisoning: a report of twenty four cases. Arch Pathol 24:481–485
16. Dube MF, Green CR (1982) Methods of collection of smoke for analytical purpose. Recent Adv Tobacco Sci 8:42–102
17. Hecht SS, Hoffmann D (1988) Tobacco-specific nitrosamines, an important group of carcinogens in tobacco and tobacco smoke. Carcinogenesis 9(6):875–884
18. Hoffmann D, Hecht SS (1990) Advances in tobacco carcinogenesis. In: Cooper CS GPLe (ed) Chemical carcinogenesis und mutagenesis.Springer, Berlin, pp 63–102
19. McGinnis JM, Foege WH (1993) Actual causes of death in the United States. JAMA 270(18): 2207–2212
20. Lopez AD, Collishaw NE, Piha T (1994) A descripitive model of the cigarette epidemic in developed countries. Tobacco Control 3:242–247
21. US Department of Health und Human Services, Public Health Service, Centers for Disease Control und Prevention, National Center for Chronic Disease Prevention und Health Promotion, Office on Smoking und Health. (1994) Preventing tobacco use among young people: a report of the Surgeon General. US Department of Health und Human Services, Public Health Service, Centers for Disease Control und Prevention, National Center for Chronic Disease Prevention und Health Promotion, Office on Smoking und Health, Atlanta, GA
22. Slade J (1989) The tobacco epidemic: lessons from history. J Psychoactive Drugs 21(3):281–291
23. Doll R, Peto R, Wheatley K, Gray R, Sutherland I (1994) Mortality in relation to smoking: 40's years observations on male British doctors. Br Med J 309:901–911
24. US Federal Trade Commission (1994) Federal trade commission report to Congress for 1992: pursuant to the federal Ciagarette labeling and advertising Act. US Federal Trade Commission, Washington, DC
25. Tolley HD, Crane L, Shipley N (1991) Smoking prevalence and lung cancer death rates. In: Strategies to control tobacco use in the United States: a blueprint for public health action in the 1990's. US Department of Health and Human Services, Public Health Service, National Institutes of Health, National Cancer Institute, Bethesda, MD, pp 75–144. NIH publication no. 92-3316
26. Warner KE (1989) Effects of the antismoking campaign: an update. Am J Public Health 79(2):144–151
27. Anon (1999) Statistisches Bundesamt, Mikrozensus-Studie (bisher unveröffentlicht)
28. Centers for Disease Control and Prevention (CDC) (2004) Cigarette use among high school students – United States 1991–2003. MMWR Mob Mortal Wkly Rep 53:499–502
29. Centers for Disease Control and Prevention (CDC) (1994) Cigarette smoking among adults – United States, 1992, and changes in the definition of current cigarette Smoking. MMWR Morb Mortal Wkly Rep 43:342–346

30. Centers for Disease Control and Prevention (CDC) (1993) Cigarette smoking among adults – United States. MMWR Mob Mortal Wkly Rep 43:925–930
31. Gilpin EA, Lee L, Evans N, Pierce JP (1994) Smoking initiation rates in adults and minors: United States, 1944–1988. Am J Epidemiol 140(6):535–543
32. Jarvis M (1984) Gender and smoking: do women really find it harder to give up? Br J Addict 79(4):383–387
33. Pierce JP, Fiore MC, Novotny TE, Hatziandreu EJ, Davis RM (1989) Trends in cigarette smoking in the United States. Projections to the year 2000. JAMA 261(1):61–65
34. Johnson LD, O'Malley PM, Bachmann JG (1994) National survey results on drugs use from the monitoring the Future study, 1975–1993, vol I, Secondary school students. US Department of Health and Human Services, Puplic Health Service, National Institut of Health, National Institut on Drug Abuse, Rockville, MD. NIH puplication no 94–3809
35. Nelson DE, Giovino GA, Emont SL, Brackbill R, Cameron LL, Peddicord J et al (1994) Trends in cigarette smoking among US physicians and nurses. JAMA 271(16):1273–1275
36. Nelson DE, Emont SL, Brackbill RM, Cameron LL, Peddicord J, Fiore MC (1994) Cigarette smoking prevalence by occupation in the United States. A comparison between 1978 to 1980 and 1987 to 1990. J Occup Med 36(5):516–525
37. Ballweg JA, Li L (1989) Comparison of health habits of military personnel with civilian populations. Public Health Rep 104(5):498–509
38. Bray RM, Marsden ME, Peterson MR (1991) Standardized comparisons of the use of alcohol, drugs, and cigarettes among military personnel and civilians. Am J Public Health 81(7):865–869
39. Giovino, GA (2002) Epidemiology of tobacco use in the United States. Oncogene 21: 7326–7340
40. John U, Hanke M (2001) [Tobacco smoking attributable mortality in Germany]. Tabakrauch-attributable Mortalitat in den deutschen Bundeslandern. Gesundheitswesen 63(6):363–369
41. Rohrmann S, Becker N, Kroke A, Boeing H (2003) Trends in cigarette smoking in the German centers of the European Prospective Investigation into Cancer and Nutrition (EPIC): the influence of the educational level. Prev Med 36:448–454
42. Helmert U (1999) [Income and smoking behavior in Germany – a secondary analysis of data from the 1995 microcensus]. Gesundheitswesen 61(1):31–37
43. Peto R, Lopez AD, Boreham J, Thun M, Heath C, Doll R (1996) Mortality from smoking worldwide. Br Med Bull 52(1):12–21
44. Ezzati M, Lopez AD (2004) Regional, disease specific patterns of smoking-attributable mortality in 2000. Tob Control 13(4):388–395
45. Baker F, Ainsworth SR, Dye JT, Crammer C, Thun MJ, Hoffmann D, et al (2000) Health risks associated with cigar smoking. JAMA 284(6):735–740
46. National Cancer Institute (1998) Cigars: health effects and trends. US Dept of Helath and Human Services, Bethesda, MD, pp 98–4302. Smoking and tobacco control monographs no. 9, NHI publication
47. US Dept of Agriculture Tobacco (1998) Situation and outlook report. US Dept of Agriculture, Commodity Economics Division, Economic Research Service, Washington, DC. Publication TBS-241
48. Pierce JP, Gilpin EA, Farkas AJ, et al (1998) Tobacco Control in California: Who's winning the war? An evaluation of tobacco control program, 1989.1996. University of California, San Diego, La Jolla
49. Centers for Disease Control and Prevention (CDC) (1998) Tobacco use among high school students – United States, 1997. MMWR Morb Mortal Wkly Rep 47:229–233
50. US Dept of Health and Human Services, OoIG (1999) Youth use of cigars: patterns of use and perceptions of risk. US Department of Health and Human Services OoIG, Washington, DC
51. Burns DM, Shanks TG (1998) Disease consequence of sigar smoking. In Cigars: health effects and trends (Smoking and Tobacco Control Monograph 9). US Department of Health and Human Services, Washington, DC, pp 105–158. DHHS Publication no. (NIH) 98-4302

52. US Department of Health and Human Services. (1979) Smoking and health. Other forms of tobacco use. Report of the Surgeon General. United States. Public Health Service. Office on Smoking and Health, Rockville, MD. DHHS Publication no (PHS) 79-50066
53. Zaridze D, Peto R (eds) (1986) Tobacco: a major international health hazard (IARC Scientific Publication 74). International Agency for Research on Cancer, Lyon, France
54. Peto R (1986) Influence of dose and duration of smoking on lung cancer rates. IARC Sci Publ (74):23–33
55. Wald NJ, Watt HC (1997) Prospective study of effect of switching from cigarettes to pipes or cigars on mortality from three smoking related diseases. BMJ 314(7098):1860–1863
56. Boffetta P, Pershagen G, Jockel KH, Forastiere F, Gaborieau V, Heinrich J et al (1999) Cigar and pipe smoking and lung cancer risk: a multicenter study from Europe. J Natl Cancer Inst 91(8):697–701
57. Strecher VJ, Kreuter MW, Kobrin SC (1995) Do cigarette smokers have unrealistic perceptions of their heart attack, cancer, and stroke risks? J Behav Med 18:45–54
58. Weinstein ND (1987) Unrealistic optimism about susceptibility to health problems: conclusions from a community-wide sample. J Behav Med 10:481–500
59. Baker F, Dye JT, Ainsworth SR, Denniston M (1998) Risk perception and cigar smoking behaviour. In: American Cancer Society's Cigar Smoking Health Risks, State-of-the-Science Conference, Washington DC, 15 June 1998
60. Bask M, Melkersson M (2003) Should one use smokeless tobacco in smoking cessation programs? A rational addiction approach. Eur J Health Econ 4:263–270
61. Wolfram RM., Chehne F, Oguogho A, Sinzinger H (2003) Narghile (water pipe) smoking influences platelet function and (iso-)eicosanoids. Life Sci 74:47–53
62. Centers for Disease Control and Prevention (CDC) (1993) Use of smokeless tobacco among adults – United States, 1991. MMWR Morb Mortal Wkly Rep 42:263–266
63. La Vecchia C, Negri E, Franceschi S, Parazzini F, Decarli A (1992) Differences in dietary intake with smoking, alcohol, and education. Nutr Cancer 17(3):297–304
64. Benson V, Schoenborn CA (1988) Relationship between smoking and other unhealthy habits: United States, 1985: advance data. US Department of Health and Human Services. Public Health Service, Centers for Disease Control National Center for Health Statistics, Hyattsville, MD. Publication no.154
65. Shah M, French SA, Jeffery RW, McGovern PG, Forster JL, Lando HA (1993) Correlates of high fat/calorie food intake in a worksite population: the Healthy Worker Project. Addict Behav 18(5):583–594
66. Scragg R, Glover M (2007) Parental and adolescent smoking: does the association vary with gender and ethnicity? N Z Med J 120(1267):U2862
67. Novak M, Ahlgren C, Hammarstrom A (2007) Inequalities in smoking: influence of social chain of risks from adolescence to young adulthood: a prospective population-based cohort study. Int J Behav Med 14(3):181–187
68. Fagerstrom KO, Kunze M, Schoberberger R, Breslau N, Hughes JR, Hurt RD, et al (1996) Nicotine dependence versus smoking prevalence: comparisons among countries and categories of smokers. Tob Control 5(1):52–56
69. Helmert U, Mielck A, Classen E (1992) Social inequities in cardiovascular disease risk factors in East and West Germany. Soc Sci Med 35(10):1283–1292
70. Pierce JP (1989) International comparisons of trends in cigarette smoking prevalence. Am J Public Health 79(2):152–157
71. Pierce JP (1991) Progress and problems in international public health efforts to reduce tobacco usage. Annu Rev Public Health 12:383–400
72. Cavelaars AE, Kunst AE, Geurts JJ, Crialesi R, Grotvedt L, Helmert U, et al (2000) Educational differences in smoking: international comparison. BMJ 320(7242):1102–1107
73. Helmert U, Borgers D (1998) Rauchen und Beruf: eine Analyse von 100000 Befragten des Mikrozensus 1995. Bundesgesundheitsblatt 3:102–107

Tobacco Constituents and Additives

3

Tobacco users opinion: *Chewing tobacco is tobacco's body, smoke is the ghost, snuff is tobacco's soul.*

B.C. Stevens, *The collector's book of snuff bottles* 1976

Until 1995, it was not possible for the medical world to gain access to information held by cigarette manufacturers concerning the mode of action of nicotine, its addictive properties and its harmful effects on health [1–6]. In 1994, the State of Minnesota instituted legal proceedings against the tobacco companies and confiscated millions of internal documents from the tobacco industry. The anti-social attitude – in some respects – of this industry sector was revealed in these legally certified documents whose content was related to addiction issues, cigarettes with reduced tar content, and information on cigarette design and nicotine manipulation. The documents originated from various tobacco companies, though they were confiscated from Brown & Williamson (B&W), and also included material relating to cigarette advertising targeted at children [7–10] and described attempts to influence tobacco research [11–14]. Additionally, the confiscated material revealed the activities of lawyers in contributing to the manipulation of information.

3.1
Non-Disclosure of Findings by the Tobacco Industry

The first confidential meeting within the tobacco industry was held in 1953 when the problem of a relationship between cigarette smoking and lung cancer emerged [15–18]. For decades thereafter, the tobacco industry persisted in casting doubts on these findings, as also reflected in a written statement to cigarette smokers [19, 20]. Shortly before the statement was published, however, the following sentence was deleted: "*We will never produce and market a product shown to be the cause of any serious human ailment*" [17]. It was replaced by the wording: "*We accept an interest in people's health as a basic responsibility, paramount to every other consideration in our business*" [19], an undertaking which the tobacco industry has failed to keep. Even at that time, the tobacco industry was aware of the carcinogenic effects of cigarettes and also knew that smokers cannot quit (… "*a habit they can't break*") [17]. The cigarette industry also believed then that, if such an association were to prove true [17], it was capable of producing a "cancer-free" cigarette.

K.-O. Haustein, D. Groneberg, *Tobacco or Health?*
DOI: 10.1007/978-3-540-87577-2_3, © Springer Verlag Berlin Heidelberg 2010

3.2
Constituents of Tobacco

Cigarettes are smoked because of nicotine, the substance which is responsible for the desired psychological reactions and for the dependence that develops within a few years. Apart from nicotine, tobacco leaves also contain some 2,500 constituents such as polynuclear aromatic hydrocarbons (benzanthracene, benzo*[a]*pyrene), aza-arenes (dibenzacridine, dibenzcarbazole), *N*-nitrosamines, aromatic amines (2-toluidine, 4-aminobiphenyl, 2-naphthylamine), acrylonitrile, crotonaldehyde, vinyl chloride, formaldehyde, benzene as well as inorganic compounds (CO, CN, CS_2, As, Ni, Cd, Cr, Pb, ^{210}Po etc.) (see Tables 3.1 and 3.2).

However, the smoker inhales a mixture of more than 4,000 [21] varyingly toxic substances, some of which are listed in Table 3.1. These include carcinogens, various organic compounds, solvents, heavy metals as well as gaseous substances also possessing health-damaging properties, with carbon monoxide (CO) at the top of the list. In addition, there are the 600 or so substances added by the tobacco companies during the cigarette manufacturing process [21, 22]. Table 3.3 lists the major toxic agents in mainstream smoke.

The combustion products that are formed during smoking differ in composition, depending on whether they are formed by pyrolysis in mainstream or side-stream smoke. Temperatures of 860–900°C are attained in the burning zone for mainstream smoke compared with only 500–650°C for side-stream smoke (cf. Fig. 3.1). Side-stream smoke should

Table 3.1 Constituents (a select list from some 4,000 compounds) of fresh, undiluted mainstream tobacco smoke, produced using a smoking machine (1 puff/min, puff duration 2 s, 35 ml smoke volume, i.e. 10 puffs/cigarette) [106]

Compounds in the gas phase	Amount in mainstream smoke (µg/cigarette)	Compounds in the gas phase	Amount in mainstream smoke (µg/cigarette)
Carbon monoxide	10,000–23,000	*Nicotine*	1,000–2,500
Carbonyl sulphide	18–42	*Phenol*	60–140
Benzene	12–48	Hydroquinone	110–300
Toluene	160	*Aniline*	0.36
Formaldehyde	70–100	2-Toluidine	0.16
Acrolein	60–100	Benz[o]anthracene	0.02–0.07
Acetone	100–250	Benz[o]pyrene	0.02–0.04
Pyridine	16–40	γ-Butyrolactone	10–22
Ammonium	50–130	Harmane	1.7–3.1
3-Methylpyridine	12–36	*N'*-Nitrosonornicotine	0.2–3
3-Vinylpyridine	11–30	NNK	0.1–1
Prussic acid	400–500	*Cadmium*	0.1
Nitric oxides	100–600	Nickel	0.02–0.08
N-Nitrosodimethylamine	0.01–0.04	Zinc	0.06
N-Nitrosopyrrolidine	0.006–0.03	^{210}*Polonium*	0.04–0.1 pCi

The table does not take into account the toxic substances in side-stream smoke, which also constitute a danger for the smoker and passive smoker. Particularly toxic substances are shown in *italic* typeface
NNK 4-(*N*-methyl-*N*-nitrosamino)-1-(3 pyridyl)-1-butanone

Table 3.2   Selected carcinogens in tobacco smoke of non-filter cigarettes (NFC)

Agent	Concentration/ NFC	IARC evaluation, evidence of carcinogenity in		
		Lab animals	Humans	Group
PAH				
Benz(a)anthracene	20–70 ng	S		2°
Benzo(a)pyrene	20–40 ng	S	P	2A
Indeno(1,2,3-cd)pyrene	4–20 ng	S		2B
Heterocyclic compounds				
Dibenz(a,j)acridine	3–10 ng	S		2B
Furan	18–37 ng	S		2B
N-Nitrosoamines				
N-Nitrosodimethylamine	2–180 ng	S		2A
N-Nitrosodiethylamine	ND-2.8 ng	S		2A
N-Nitrosopyrrolidine	3–110 ng	S		2B
4-(Methylnitrosoamino)-1-(pyridyl)-1-butanone	80–770 ng	S		2B
Aromatic amines				
2-naphthylamine	1–334 ng	S	S	1
4-Aminobiphenyl	2–5.6 ng	S	S	1
N-heterocyclic amines				
AaC	25–260 ng	S		2B
PhIP	11–23 ng	S	P	2A
Aldehyde				
Formaldehyde	70–100 µg	S	L	2A
Acetaldehyde	500–1,400 µg	S	I	2B
Volatile hydrocarbons				
1,3-Butadiene	20–75 µg	S	I	2B
Benzene	20–70 µg	S	S	1
Miscellaneous organic compounds				
Acrylonitrile	3–15 µg	S	L	2A
Vinyl chloride	11–15 ng	S	S	1
DDT	800–1,200 µg	S	P	2B
DDE	200–370 µg	S		2B
Catechol	100–360 µg	S		2B
Ethylene oxide	7 µg	S	S	1
Propylene oxide	12–100 µg	S		2B
Inorganic compounds				
Hydrazine	24–43 ng	S	I	2B
Arsenic	40–120 µg	I	S	1
Nickel	ND-600 ng	S	S	1
Chromium (only hexavalent)	4–70 ng	S	S	1
Cadmium	7–350 ng	S	S	1
Cobalt	0.13–0.2 ng	S	I	2B
Lead	34–85 ng	S	I	2B
Polonium-210	0.03–1.0 pCi	S	S	1

S sufficient; *I* inadequate; *P* probable, possible; *L* limited; *ND* not detected; *PAH* polynuclear aromatic hydrocarbons; *AaC* 2-Amino-9H-pyrido[2, 3-b]indole; *PhIP* 2-Amino-1-methyl-6-phenylimidazo [4, 5-b]pyridine; IARC Monographs on the Evaluation of Carcinogenic Risks: 1: Human carcinogen; 2A: probably carcinogenic in humans; 2B: possibly carcinogenic to humans [23]

Table 3.3 Major toxic agents in cigarette smoke (incomplete list) [23]

Agent	Concentration/NFC	Toxicity
Carbon monoxide	10–23 mg	Binds to haemoglobin, inhibits respiration, induces atherosclerosis
Ammonia	10–130 µg	Irritation of respiratory tract
Nitrogen oxide (NO_x)	100–600 µg	Inflammation of the lung
Hydrogen cyanide	400–500 µg	Highly ciliatoxic, inhibits lung clearance
Hydrogen sulfide	10–90 µg	Irritation of respiratory tract
Acrolein	60–140 µg	Ciliatoxic, inhibits lung clearance
Methanol	100–250 µg	Toxic upon inhalation and ingestion
Pyridine	16–40 µg	Irritates respiratory tract
Nicotine	1–3 mg	Induces dependence, affects some endocrine functions
Phenol	80–160 µg	Tumour promoter in laboratory animals
Catechol	200–400 µg	Co-carcinogen in laboratory animals
Aniline	360–655 µg	Forms methaemoglobin, and this affects respiration
Maleic hydrazine	1.16 µg	Mutagenic agent

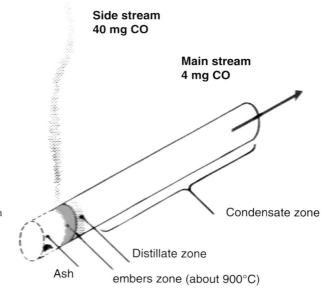

**Side stream
40 mg CO**

**Main stream
4 mg CO**

Fig. 3.1 Schematic illustration of burning cigarette. Mainstream and side-stream smoke differ in terms of the temperatures at which they are formed and the composition of their toxic constituents (cf. CO content of a cigarette)

Condensate zone

Distillate zone

Ash

embers zone (about 900°C)

be regarded as more toxic than mainstream smoke because the amounts of various sub-stances in side-stream smoke (benzo[*a*]pyrene, CO, benzene, formaldehyde, hydrazine, cadmium etc.) are higher by several multiples. In contrast, however, mainstream smoke contains approximately 1,000 times more particles than side-stream smoke (5×10^9 vs. 1×10^5–1×10^6). Mean particle size in mainstream smoke is 0.2 µm (0.1–1.0 µm) and is clearly smaller than that in side-stream smoke at 0.5 μm (0.1–1.5 μm), resulting in a higher proportion of particles in mainstream smoke having a toxic effect on tissues. Furthermore, mainstream smoke contains 2–3 × 10^10 radicals per ml. The majority of naphthalines and polynuclear hydrocarbons are formed in mainstream and side-stream smoke as a result of the combustion process (Table 3.2).

The tar content of cigarettes has been an important issue for more than 50 years. The tobacco industry has recognised that tar constituents, such as are also formed by the burning of tobacco in the mainstream and side-stream smoke of a cigarette, are extremely hazardous to health. Ever since 1950s, the tobacco industry has striven to reduce the tar yield of cigarettes (cf. Fig. 3.2). Aside from lowering tar yields, however, the tobacco industry is also concerned with nicotine release during the smoking process, particularly since lowering the tar yield also reduces the nicotine content (Fig. 3.3). As a result of

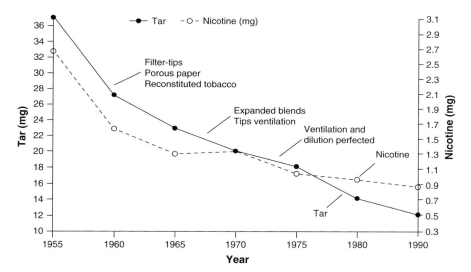

Fig. 3.2   Tar and nicotine yields of US cigarettes over the past 35 years and measures to reduce the tar content. Cigarette industry data [23, 24]

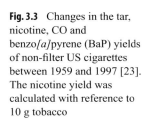

Fig. 3.3   Changes in the tar, nicotine, CO and benzo[a]pyrene (BaP) yields of non-filter US cigarettes between 1959 and 1997 [23]. The nicotine yield was calculated with reference to 10 g tobacco

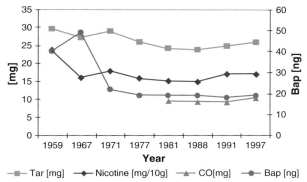

efforts by the tobacco industry laboratories, tar yields in US cigarettes have been lowered from 38 mg to <12 mg [23, 24]. US cigarettes currently have a nicotine yield of 0.95 mg. Tar yields have been similarly reduced in Great Britain, but the quantities of nicotine in the cigarette have been kept at a higher level [25].

Various modifications to the cigarette have been made to achieve these changes as follows:

- Cigarette length has been altered
- Modern filters have been incorporated into cigarettes [26]
- Aromatic agents (terpenoids, pyrroles, pyrazines) have been introduced into tobacco
- Porous (citrate-treated) paper has been used increasingly
- New tobacco mixtures employ a reduced tobacco volume
- Manufacturing technology has been optimised (e.g. glycerol and propylene glycol are more suitable than diethylene glycol and sorbitol etc. for moistening the tobacco [27])

Filter dimensions were important for the partial removal of toxic substances from mainstream cigarette smoke: charcoal filters reduced the content of ciliatoxic substances (cyanide, formaldehyde, acrolein, acetaldehyde) by up to 66% [28–30] and were superior to cellulose acetate filters. By combining the two, even better results were achieved in terms of the absorption of toxic substances (e.g. volatile phenols and nitrosamines) from mainstream smoke [31–33].

The porosity of the paper reduces the inhalation of various gases (hydrogen, NO, CO, CO_2, methane, ethane, ethylene) by outward diffusion, whereas the diffusion of N_2 and O_2 into the tobacco is increased [23]. The reduction of nitrogen oxides in the inhaled smoke lowers the formation of tobacco-specific N-nitrosamines [34].

One previously neglected aspect has been the question of the occurrence of bacterial endotoxin as an active component of cigarette smoke [35]. The *Limulus* amebocyte lysate (LAL) assay was used to measure the lipopolysaccharide (LPS) content of the tobacco portion and filter tip components of unsmoked "light" cigarettes, as well as in mainstream and side-stream smoke. In addition, blood LPS activity and plasma cytokine concentrations (TNFα, IL-6) were measured in smokers and non-smokers. Bioactive LPS was detected in the "light" cigarettes, in their filter tips, and in both mainstream and side-stream smoke; no differences in blood LPS levels were detected between smokers and non-smokers. In terms of adverse effects on health, however, it is estimated that the LPS dose delivered from smoking one pack of cigarettes/day is comparable to the level of LPS exposure of cotton textile workers (dust from textile manufacture) and that, in addition, LPS release may be one factor responsible for the development of chronic lung diseases (chronic bronchitis) [35].

3.3
Nicotine and Dependence

The addictive effects of nicotine were known within the industry as early as 1963 [2], but were denied publicly until 1980 because the simultaneous admission of carcinogenic and addictive effects would not have been defensible [36]. Studies in rats showed that only some of the animals became dependent as a result of the tobacco smoke. The dependence-inducing effect was linked to the rate of nicotine delivery to the CNS [37, 38]. The delivery of nicotine and the associated "kick" were enhanced by the addition of K_2CO_3 [39].

Even in the early 1970s, in the face of growing concern over the harmful effects of cigarettes, the tobacco industry was considering a strategy on three major fronts: "Litigation – Politics – Public Opinion" [40]. The decisive steps were to create doubt about the health charge without actually denying it, seek allies in Congress to manipulate public opinion and argue in the media that cigarette smoking may not be the decisive risk to health, and that environmental factors, for example, might be responsible [40]. This resulted in the development of "low-tar and low-nicotine cigarettes" (Fig. 3.2), purportedly to provide increasing safety for smokers [41]. The intention was to open up a new market with improved and "healthier" cigarettes [41].

3.3.1
The Cigarette as a Vehicle for Nicotine Release

Because smokers can regulate the release of nicotine by modifying the frequency and volume of their puffs, cigarette becomes an interesting model for the release of an active substance. Representatives of tobacco companies have also expressed themselves along these lines in describing the cigarette as an ideal vehicle for the release of nicotine [42]. Thus, the tobacco industry embarked upon research to identify a minimally effective nicotine dose per cigarette and discover how the effect of nicotine might be improved by additives, pH changes, etc. [42]. Their intention was also to intensify the dependence-inducing effect. Nicotine and the cigarette were viewed as a drug or as a drug formulation [12]. The FDA itself was interested in classifying tobacco more as a food and luxury commodity, rather than as a drug [43]. The cigarette industry came to view the manufacture and marketing of its goods as nicotine-release products [44, 45]. The smoke was regarded as the optimal vehicle for nicotine and the cigarette as the optimal dispenser for smoke [46].

3.3.2
Modifications of Nicotine Release

The overriding objectives of the tobacco industry in the 1980s were to increase the release of nicotine and enhance the effectiveness of its action [47]. At that time, therefore, efforts were made to control the nicotine content of smoke [47] and the addition of nicotine to cigarette tobacco was even considered [48]. The tobacco industry invested a great deal of research into optimising nicotine release by improving the availability of nicotine from the cigarette through modifications to tobacco blends, cigarette size, filters, ventilation, paper porosity, additives and the ratio of cut tobacco to tobacco weight per cigarette. Smoke development was "improved" temporarily by the addition of freon, from which phosgene is formed on combustion [47]. In addition, attempts were made to use genetic engineering (project code: Y1) to increase the nicotine yield of tobacco plants while leaving tar yield unchanged [49].

3.3.3
Maintaining Nicotine Dependence

The cigarette industry produced "low-tar" and "low-nicotine" cigarettes, imagining them to be a product that would be less harmful to health. It recognised very early that there is a major difference in smoke constituents measured on a Federal Trade Commission (FTC) smoking machine and in a human smoker (Tables 3.4–3.6). The FTC machines "inhale" constant smoke volumes at regular set intervals, whereas smokers individually regulate their depth and frequency of smoking. The smoker smokes a low-tar or low-nicotine cigarette quite differently from a regular cigarette [50], a fact that is also apparent from the earliest medical studies [51]. When smokers are offered different types of cigarettes, they are able to obtain approximately the same nicotine dose, irrespective of the nicotine yield of the cigarette, by varying the frequency of puffs and the depth of inhalation [50]. The "light" cigarette was also one reason why the dependence-inducing effect of nicotine was repeatedly and vociferously disputed by the cigarette industry [52].

Table 3.4 Declared tar and nicotine yields of two cigarette brands and the effect of increasing blocking of the lateral filter vents during smoking (measured with a Filtrona SM 400 cigarette testing machine) [107]

Filter blocking	Silk cut ultra		Marlboro light	
	Tar (mg)	Nicotine (mg)	Tar (mg)	Nicotine (mg)
Declaration on the pack	1.0	0.1	6.0	0.5
Smoking without blocking	1.4	0.16	6.3	0.54
Smoking with 50% blocking	4.5	0.56	7.6	0.62
Smoking with complete blocking	12.3	1.21	10.5	0.77

Table 3.5 Declared tar yields of several cigarette brands (mg/cigarette), together with yields measured using the ISO method (smoking machine) compared with realistic yields following inhalation of cigarette smoke [108]

Cigarette brands	Tar yield declared on the pack	Standard ISO test	Realistic "smoking test"
DuMaurier king size	15	15.2	36.9
DuMaurier light king size	12	14.4	38.25
Player's regular	16	16.5	37.2
Player's light king size	13	13.7	33.3
Player's extra light regular	11	11.8	31.4
Matinee extra mild king size	4	4.7	26.0
Rothmans king size	15	15.8	34.2
Export A regular	16	15.0	34.0
Export A light regular	13	13.0	28.0

Table 3.6   A comparison of smoke data for two low-yield US filter cigarettes smoked according to the FTC method and by smokers [109]

Parameters	FTC machine smoking	Cigarette smokers	
		FTC 0.6–0.8 nicotine	FTC 0.9–1.2 nicotine
Puff			
Volume (ml)	35.0	48.6 (45.2–52.3)[a]	44.1 (40.8–46.8)[b]
Interval (s)	58.0	21.3 (19.0–23.8)[a]	18.5 (16.5–20.6)[b]
Duration (s)	2.0	1.5 (1.4–1.7)[a]	1.5 (1.4–1.6)[b]
Nicotine	0.7 (0.6–0.8)	1.74 (1.54–1.98)[c]	2.39 (2.20–2.60)[d]
(mg/cigarette)	0.1 (1.09–1.13)		
Tar (mg/cigarette)	8.5 (7.7–9.5)	22.3 (18.8–26.5)[e]	29.0 (25.8–32.5)[f]
	15.4 (14.2–14.9)		
CO (mg/cigarette)	9.7 (9.0–10.4)	17.3 (15.0–20.1)[g]	22.5 (20.3–25.0)[h]
	14.6 (14.2–14.9)		
BaP (ng/cigarette)	10 (8.2–12.3)	17.9 (15.3–20.9)[i]	21.4 (19.2–23.7)[j]
	14 (10.1–19.4)		
NNK (ng/cigarette)	112.9 (96.6–113.0)	186.5 (158.3–219.7)[i]	250.9 (222.7–282.7)[j]
	146.2 (132.5–165.5)		

Test groups: [a]56, [b]71, [c]30, [d]42, [e]18, [f]19, [g]15, [h]16, [i]6 and [j]3 smokers

3.3.4
Marketing of Cigarettes with a "Reduced" Health Risk

By even discussing technical aspects of cigarette production, the tobacco industry used every endeavour to make the purchaser believe that the modern cigarette represented less of a health risk than cigarettes in the past. Thus, it pointed to the installation of the cigarette filter [53] and has repeatedly cited the minimal health risk associated with this product. For the consumer, however, the tobacco industry has never communicated clearly where the health risk actually lies. At most it is stated that the newer "low-nicotine and low-tar" cigarettes (light and ultralight cigarettes) are "healthier" than regular cigarettes (e.g. *Viceroy, Marlboro, Winston*) [54] (Tables 3.4–3.6). With the cigarette industry making such claims, light and ultralight cigarettes are smoked more frequently than "orthodox" brands [41]. The actual concentrations of toxic substances (CO, benzo*[a]*pyrene) have since been published (Tables 3.5 and 3.6).

3.3.5
Compensatory Behaviour by Smokers

The tobacco industry realised relatively soon that light cigarettes are smoked differently from regular cigarettes, a fact that was also evident from a comparison of human smoking behaviour patterns with those of a smoking machine [55]. The dependent smoker immediately detects the modified release pattern of nicotine from the new cigarettes. Cigarettes with a reduced nicotine yield are inhaled more deeply to obtain the same nicotine dose. In many cases, especially in situations of stress or altered psychological mood, either stronger cigarettes are used or two or more cigarettes are smoked in rapid succession [56]. Observations of this kind were made with the Marlboro Light brand [57]. In fact, observations and findings obtained with light cigarettes have often been the subject of publications [25, 54, 58, 59]. The health-related consequences of long-term use of these cigarettes cannot yet be foreseen, especially because they are smoked with greater intensity, deeper inhalation and larger inhaled and exhaled volumes [60]. Many smokers were previously unaware that light cigarettes have (or had) vents in the filter to improve ventilation (e.g. the Winston "*Reds*" brand) [61–64]. The tobacco industry argued unofficially that as the cigarette increasingly burns down, the holes become blocked and hence, the release of nicotine is increased [65].

Cigarettes with selective reductions in nicotine delivery have been considered as potential tools to prevent or treat nicotine dependence or reduce harm by virtue of reduced nicotine and nitrosamine delivery. An important question is whether individuals smoke these products more intensively, as has been shown to occur with ventilated-filter cigarettes. To investigate this issue, we compared conventional highly ventilated filter cigarettes, having very low tar and nicotine yields when smoked by Federal Trade Commission method (1 mg tar, 2 mg carbon monoxide [CO], 2 mg nicotine), with low nicotine content cigarettes, manufactured from a genetically modified strain of tobacco, which had higher tar but lower nicotine yield (14 mg tar, 13 mg CO, 02 mg nicotine). A total of 16 cigarette smokers participated in two 8-h sessions (order counterbalanced) during which they smoked each type of cigarette ad libitum. Expired-air CO, plasma nicotine and smoking topography measures were collected. Subjects showed significant increases in smoking when using the highly ventilated filter cigarettes and puff volume was significantly greater than with the low nicotine content cigarettes. Subjects achieved an expired-air CO level of as high as 74% with the low nicotine content cigarettes; the latter produced CO levels similar to those measured at baseline when subjects smoked their habitual brands of cigarettes. Plasma nicotine levels obtained when subjects smoked the highly ventilated filter cigarettes also were significantly higher than when they smoked the low nicotine content cigarettes. These results indicate that the delivery of substantial amount of smoke, with selective reductions in nicotine yield, appears to prevent compensatory smoking behaviour. Further studies should determine whether similar results are obtained in naturalistic environments [66].

3.3.6
Optimising Nicotine Release

According to the tobacco industry, one of its crucial research objectives was to increase the availability of nicotine released from tobacco to smokers as the free base: the pH of tobacco has an important function in this context. Depending on pH, nicotine is present in the form of a diprotonated or monoprotonated salt and as the free base [67]. The former is the bound form ($pK_1 = 3.02$) and the latter is the freely available form ($pK_1 = 8.02$). The free form penetrates biological membranes very rapidly and extensively, whereas the penetration of the bound form is very much slower and less quantitative. Because the nicotine base reaches the brain far more rapidly, the tobacco industry became aware of this property of free nicotine at a very early stage [68]. The higher the pH, the greater the amount of extractable nicotine [69]. The pH of cigarette smoke is between 6.5 and 7.0, a range in which nicotine is absorbed primarily in the lungs, whereas the nicotine from alkaline cigar smoke is absorbed primarily in the mouth, not least because of the larger doses of nicotine involved [70].

3.3.7
Importance of Absorption Rate

Since physiological effects are to be anticipated very much more rapidly from non-bound (free) nicotine (as the ammonium ion) than from bound nicotine (as ammonium chloride), smoke with a high pH is richer in nicotine. Consequently, the nicotine yield of cigarette smoke may be considered as a measure of the strength of the cigarette [71] because more rapid absorption is then to be expected [72]. Nevertheless, nicotine is absorbed in the following three forms:

- As salt from the particulate phase (1)
- As free base in the particulate phase (2)
- As free base in the gas phase (3)

The ratio (2)/(3) has long been considered to be important for the nicotine effect [73]. Altering the pH of cigarette tobacco was intended to provide an extra "kick" [74, 75]. Moreover, this objective was to be achieved by (a) increasing the Burley content in the tobacco blend, (b) reducing the sugar casing used for the tobacco, (c) using alkalis – especially ammonium compounds – for the tobacco blend, (d) adding nicotine to the tobacco blend, (e) removing acid constituents from the tobacco, (f) using special filter systems which permit removal of acids and addition of alkalis to mainstream smoke and (g) using filter systems that dilute the inhaled air to a major extent. Some of these considerations have already been tested at Philip Morris [76].

3.3.8
Ammonium and pH Manipulation

During cigarette smoking, the free nicotine base is absorbed in the pulmonary alveoli. In many cases, nicotine is found only in trace amounts in the particles of exhaled mainstream smoke. The intensity of nicotine delivery was further increased by the addition of ammonium salts (cf. the practices of Philip Morris) [9]. At the same time, the measurements of tar and nicotine in the FTC smoking machines were no longer representative (Tables 3.5 and 3.6) because the ratio of free to bound nicotine could not be determined; also the tar yields measured were lower than in reality (Tables 3.5 and 3.6) [77]. The use of ammonium technology permitted the downward manipulation of nicotine yields measured in the smoking machines, but the smoker still got the expected "kick" [78]. This was the decisive finding: the greater the alkalinity of mainstream smoke, the faster the build-up of nicotine in the blood (and hence the "kick"). The tobacco industry declared the added ammonium salts as "flavour correction agents" and not as additives to enhance the nicotine effect. Seen in these terms, no objection to these pH manipulations can be serious enough.

3.4
Tobacco Additives

In the EU, more than 600 additives are used in the manufacture of tobacco products (Table 3.7). Although these additives are subjected to toxicological testing, it is unclear what effects they have on smoking behaviour: if such products when added to tobacco lead to accelerated dependence, hasten the craving to smoke or initiate an increased craving, then this is a major problem [79]. With more than 1 million people dying annually from smoking-related causes, a mere 1% increase due to the addition of a chemical to tobacco may result in the premature death of hundreds or thousands of smokers. For this reason, additives in tobacco products are a major public health issue in their own right.

Some 600 additives have been approved as admixtures to tobacco products. However, only the tobacco companies can disclose which additives appear in which cigarette brands. Not even the European Commission, which is responsible for the regulation of tobacco products, can provide this information or has the power to demand it.

Additives are put into tobacco (see Table 3.7; [80]) for the following reasons:

- To increase the free nicotine portion because this boosts the "kick". Ammonium compounds have been found to fulfil this role because they increase the alkalinity of the smoke.
- To improve the flavour of tobacco and to make the product more desirable.
- Sweeteners and chocolate are used as additives to make the flavour of tobacco more appealing to children and first-time users. Eugenol and menthol are added to "mask" the harmful effects on the respiratory tract.
- Cocoa is added as a bronchodilator with the goal of achieving deeper inhalation so that more nicotine (and tar) reaches the alveoli in the lower pulmonary segments.
- Additives are used to make the smell and visibility of side-stream smoke less annoying and mask its dangerous nature and thus, to make it more difficult for passive smokers to protect themselves from smoking.

Various additives are already toxic alone or in combination with other additives and pharmacologically active or toxic products are also formed during the combustion process.

Substances intended to keep the tobacco moist (see above) may account for up to 5% of the tobacco weight in a cigarette: one such example is glycerol (which undergoes transformation to the ciliatoxic substances acrolein and propylene glycol) [81]. Propylene oxide has been detected in the tobacco smoke of cigarettes treated with propylene glycol [82]. Ethylene glycol has also been used to moisten cigarette tobacco; however, this practice has been banned because of the formation of carcinogenic ethylene oxide following combustion [83]. In addition, traces of N-hydroxyethylvaline haemoglobin (217–690 pmol/g haemoglobin) have been detected in the blood of smokers [84], whereas non-smokers have only about 15% of such levels.

Tobacco aroma is intensified by tobacco-specific terpenoids, pyrroles and pyrazines [85, 86], but this effect is attenuated in turn by filter tips. Tobacco aroma has been modified by the addition of mint, wood, spices, fruits and flower essences (coumarins), but also of

Table 3.7 Select list of tobacco constituents used in cigarette production and their effects on the smoker [80]

Principles	Substance	Effects
Additives with a pharma-cologi-cal effect	Free nicotine base	Ammonium technology increases release in smoke [110]
	Ammonium	Dissociation of increasing nicotine effect and tar yield (reduction) [14]
Additives that enhance the effect of nicotine	Acetaldehyde (produced by the burning of sugars)	Increases the addictive effects of nicotine [110, 111], optimised sugar content of the cigarette provides the basis for optimal formation of acetaldehyde and thus for an optimal nicotine/acetaldehyde ratio [110]
	Laevulinic acid (degradation product of starch, cane sugar and cellulose)	Nicotine laevulinate removes the harshness from the tobacco flavour while preserving the aroma, the salt also intensifies binding to the high-affinity nicotine receptors by about 30% [112]
	Cocoa and theobromine	Cocoa contains alkaloids which modify the effects of nicotine: one such alkaloid is theobromine (1%), which has bronchodila-tor activity and thus improves absorption on inhalation [113]
	Glycyrrhizin (an ingredient of liquorice)	Possesses bronchodilator activity, to date this effect is suspected during smoking
	Pyridine (from tobacco)	Acts like nicotine but is less reliable. Has a central calming action. Like nicotine, pyridine is formed on pyrolysis. Both substances have CNS-antagonist activity [114]
Flavour modifiers (required to improve the taste of nicotine)	Sugar	Improves flavour, particularly due to the sugar-ammonium reaction [115] by giving smoke a mild and natural flavour
	Liquorice	Added to sugar to improve the flavour of the smoke (more mellow, woody) [116]
	Chocolate	Harsh tobacco flavour is rounded off by traces of chocolate
	Cocoa butter	Makes tobacco smoke less harsh [117]
Additional toxins	Coumarins	Powerful aromatic agents, but hepatotoxic, use now mostly abandoned
	Acetaldehyde	Mutagenic, embryotoxic, causes tumours in the respiratory tract
Additional toxins	Furfural (acetate)	Mutagenic, has a synergistic carcinogenic effect in conjunction with benzo[a]pyrene
	Maltol	Mutagenic only in vitro
	Eugenol	As a phenol, its carcinogenic activity is uncertain [118]; tests required
Substances that alter side-stream smoke	Sodium acetate	Used in cigarette paper instead of tripotassium citrate, hence less visible side-stream smoke through the paper [119]
	Calcium hydroxide	Less irritating for non-smokers after impregnation of cigarette paper [120], milder aroma

synthetic substances [87, 88]. Cigarette additives have also been found to reduce the perception of environmental tobacco smoke (ETS; [87]).

Legislators and consumers falsely assume that additives make it easier for the consumer to accept cigarettes with a low tar yield and that the health risks are, thus, also reduced. These cigarettes have perforated filters in order to dilute the inhaled air. However, smokers very quickly learn to cover these perforations with their hands in order either to regulate nicotine delivery or to achieve deeper inhalation.

The modern US cigarette contains 10% additives (calculated with reference to weight), mostly in the form of sugar, aromatic agents and moistening agents. They contain further additives that modify the effects of nicotine and make the (inhaled) mainstream and (evaporating) side-stream smoke appear more pleasant and less annoying. In this context, it is important to remember that side-stream smoke sometimes contains higher levels of toxic substances than mainstream smoke; CO levels in side-stream smoke, for example, are 4–14 times higher than those in mainstream smoke (see Fig. 3.2).

3.5
Cigarettes with Reduced Tar Yield

If cigarettes are labelled "Light" and "Ultralight", smokers imagine that there are a number of advantages: reduced tar and nicotine yields, lesser risk to health and milder flavour. A considerable proportion of smokers believe that lower-tar cigarettes are less dangerous than regular cigarettes. According to the representative judgement of smokers of ultralight (45.7%), light (32.2%) and regular cigarettes (22%), ultralight cigarettes reduce the risk of cancer [88]. In a survey of 12,371 Canadians, the label "Light" was associated with "less tar" (20.1%), "less nicotine" (36.2%), "greater safety" or "induces less dependence" (3.2%), "milder taste" (6.7%) and "nothing" or "marketing trick" (14.1%). The term did not convey anything at all to a large proportion of survey respondents [89]. For the most part, smokers are unaware of the tar and nicotine yields of the cigarettes they smoke and believe that they are reducing the risk to their health by smoking light (40%) and ultralight cigarettes (60%) [87, 89]. In the context of other surveys, lower scores were reported for these questions (see also [88]). According to the Canadian survey, in fact, more smokers complained of health problems (emphysema, asthma, lung cancer, stroke) after switching from regular to light cigarettes compared with smokers who stayed with regular cigarettes (2.13 vs. 1.94%) [89].

Smokers frequently ignore the existence of cigarettes with a reduced tar yield, despite the declaration on the packs. Consumers interpret these figures as a reflection of varying levels of damage to health. Table 3.5 presents details of the tar and nicotine yields of different cigarette brands. Various studies indicate that there are no reliable data to show that switching from regular to light cigarettes reduces cigarette consumption or the desire to smoke [89]. Also, switching from regular to light cigarettes as a deliberate interim strategy does not ultimately improve success rates for smoking cessation.

From the lawsuits against the tobacco industry in the USA, it has emerged that the tobacco companies knew for decades about the discrepant and distorted results obtained with smoking machines based on criteria defined by the ISO (International Organization for Standardization, founded in 1946 to promote worldwide trade and collaboration). Agencies in the USA (including the Federal Trade Commission, the FDA and the National Cancer Institute) are now working towards a useful solution to the problem. The European Commission is also preparing proposals for the correct measurement of tar and nicotine yields in cigarettes.

A few smokers may actually benefit minimally from low-tar cigarettes, but the health consequences in a positive sense have not yet been demonstrated. However, it has been shown that deeper inhalation is associated with an increase in adenocarcinomas, a type of cancer rarely seen in the past and affecting the deep sections of lung tissue. One study published in 1997 presented summary data on smokers who had smoked light and ultra-light cigarettes over the period from 1959 to 1991 and who were found to have an increased incidence of adenocarcinomas; these tumours were found to occur 17 times more commonly in women and 10 times more commonly in men [90, 91].

In 2003, Kabat published a review on 50 years' experience of reduced-tar cigarettes and posed the question about the known health effects [92]. It was stated that since 1950s, cigarettes sold in the United States have undergone a progressive modification, including the addition of filters and a reduction in the average machine-measured tar and nicotine yield per cigarette by over 60%. These and other temporal changes in manufactured cigarettes, coupled with the complexity of smoking behaviour, make it difficult to assess the impact of the newer cigarettes on health. Some researchers have suggested that the newer products, marketed as being less harmful, may in fact provide no benefit compared to the older, higher tar cigarettes. Kabat critically evaluated the available epidemiologic evidence on the health effects of low-tar cigarettes. After identifying important methodological problems confronting research in this area, studies of lung cancer, coronary heart disease, chronic obstructive pulmonary disease and total mortality were examined in terms of their strengths and weaknesses and their results. Thirty-five studies of lung cancer were found to be suggestive that smokers of low tar cigarettes have a lower risk (by 20–30%) compared to smokers of higher tar cigarettes. Only a minority of studies of heart disease provided evidence of a reduction in risk, on the order of 10%. Studies concerning chronic obstructive pulmonary disease (COPD) were inconsistent, but the majority suggest decreased risk in smokers of lower tar cigarettes. Finally, studies that included total mortality indicated with a high degree of consistency that the total death rate is reduced in smokers of lower tar cigarettes, on the order of 10–20% [92].

However, there are also studies that indicate that there are no major changes and additional analyses of existing data sets could further clarify the impact of low-tar cigarettes. In this respect, a further analysis by Thun and Burns also examined the epidemiological evidence relevant to the health consequences of "reduced yield" cigarettes [93]. They conclude that some epidemiological studies have found attenuated risk of lung cancer, but not other diseases, among people who smoke "reduced yield" cigarettes compared to smokers of unfiltered, high yield products. These studies probably overestimated the magnitude of any association with lung cancer by overadjusting for the number of cigarettes smoked per day (one aspect of compensatory smoking) and by not fully considering other differences between smokers of "high yield" and "low yield" cigarettes. Selected cohort studies in the USA and UK were found that showed that lung cancer risk continued to increase among older smokers from the 1950s to the 1980s, despite the widespread adoption of lower yield cigarettes. The change to filter tip products was found not to prevent a progressive increase in lung cancer risk among male smokers who began smoking during and after the second world war compared to the first world war era smokers [93].

National trends in vital statistics data showed declining lung cancer death rates in young adults, especially males, in many countries, but the extent to which this is attributable to "reduced yield" cigarettes remained unclear. No studies have adequately assessed whether health claims used to market "reduced yield" cigarettes delay cessation among smokers who might otherwise quit, or increase initiation among non-smokers. Thun and Burns stated that there is no convincing evidence that past changes in cigarette design have resulted in an important health benefit to either smokers or the whole population [93].

3.6
Snuff Tobacco

Snuff tobacco has been used in England since the seventeenth century and had already gained worldwide popularity by the eighteenth century. In eighteenth-century France, snuff taking was so intensive that olfactory disturbances through to total loss of the sense of smell were widespread [94]. For the most part, dark, strong tobacco varieties (Kentucky or Virginia) are used for the preparation of snuff tobacco: in earlier times, after crushing, drying and multiple fermentation, these were stored for 4–7 years as "*carottes*" (pressed and shaped tobacco). Only then was the tobacco ground down to a fine powder and perfumed with a variety of aromatic substances (oil of roses, lavender, garlic and jasmine, menthol, etc.). Larger quantities of nicotine are absorbed slowly from snuff tobacco across the nasal mucosa (Table 4.5).

As with cigarette smoking, the desired effect of snuff-taking is for nicotine to reach the central nervous system (Chap. 4.3). Snuff users very often report a calming or stimulating effect, as well as an increased ability to concentrate and a sense of wish-fulfilment as part of a reward system (see Chap. 7.1.2).The content of various nitrosamines (Box 3.1–3.3) in the snuff of different origin shows great differences (Table 3.8).

In Germany, snuff tobacco use is encountered only in a few individuals, most commonly still in Bavaria. By contrast, snuff use is widespread in India and the Sudan, and considerable adverse effects on health are encountered in the population also because of the type of snuff tobacco used (known as "toombak" in the Sudan) [95]. In India, 2.8 million kg of snuff tobacco are consumed annually, corresponding to an annual consumption of 1.1–1.2 kg per adult [96].

The tobacco used in India is produced from *Nicotiana rustica* mixed with a solution of bicarbonate and has a pH of 8–11. The moisture content is between 6 and 60% and the nicotine content ranges from 8 to 102 mg/g dried weight. Snuff tobacco brands differ in terms of the tobacco variety used, fermentation method, ageing process, tobacco-specific nitrosamines present and expression of the p53 suppressor gene (important for cancer development).

Due to its nicotine content, snuff tobacco initially causes increased secretion followed by a long-lasting reduction in mucus production. In addition, the vessels in the venous networks in the middle and deeper layers of the nasal mucosa undergo constriction,

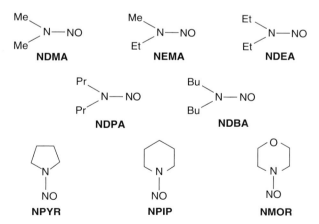

Box 3.1 Tobacco-specific nitrosamines (TSNA). *NNN* nitrosonornicotine; *NAT* N-nitrosoanatabine; *NAB* N-nitrosoanabatine; *iso-NNAL* 4-(N-nitrosomethylamino)-4-(3-pyridyl)-1-butanol; *NNK* 4-(N-nitrosomethylamino)-4-(3-pyridyl)-butanone; *NNAL* 4-(N-nitrosomethylamino)-1-(3-pyridyl)-1-butanol

Box 3.2 Volatile nitrosamines in tobacco: *NDMA* dimethylamine; *NEMA* ethylmethylamine; *NDEA* diethylamine; *NDPA* dipropylamine; *NDBA* dibutylamine; *NPYR* pyrrolidine; *NPIP* piperidine; *NMOR* morpholine

Box 3.3   Non-volatile nitrosamines in tobacco: *NSAR* N-nitrosarcosine; *NMPA* 3-(N-nitroso-N-methylamino)-propionic acid; *NMBA* 3-(N-nitroso-N-methylamino)-butyric acid; *NPYRAC* N-nitroso-pyrrolidine-2-acetic acid; *NPIPAC* N-nitroopiperidine-2-acetic acid; *NazCA* N-nitrosoa-zetadine-2-carboxylic acid; *NPRO* N-nitrosoproline; *NPIC* N-nitrosopipecolic acid; *NHPRO* N-nitrosohydroxypyroline; *NTCA* N-nitrosothiazolidine-4-carboxylic acid

Table 3.8   N-Nitroso compounds in oral tobaccos and their carcinogenic potency

Nitros-amine	English moist snuff (mg/a*)	Swedish moist snuff (mg/a)	Indian zarda (mg/a)	Target organ (cancero-genity), (results from experiments in the rat)
NDMA	0.07	0.16	0.04	Liver, kidney (lung)
NDELA	0.40	0.16	0.04	Liver, nasal cavity
NSAR	0.50	0.10	0.20	Esophagus
NMBA	3.5	0.4	0.6	Urinary bladder
NAB/NAT	45.4	15.3	59.0	Esophagus
NNN	37.2	19.5	49.0	Esophagus, nasal cavity
NNK**	8.1	4.6	14.7	Liver, lung, nasal cavity

The Indian zarda is a partially fermented tobacco produced by boiling small pieces of tobacco leaves in water with various spices and lime until evaporation. Exposures basel on the following daily use: English moist snuff: 4.5 g/day; Swedish moist snuff: 14.3 g/day; Indian zarda tobacco: 10 g/day [100]
*mg/a: annual uptake; **tested only by subcutaneous injection

causing an ischaemic reaction in the nose. This reaction may become less pronounced in the sense of tachyphylaxis. Studies conducted in Indian snuff tobacco users indicate that mucociliary clearance (a cleansing function) is depressed [28]. Using a saccharin test, it has been demonstrated that following intranasal application of a small saccharin crystal, the time to reporting a sweet taste in the mouth may be 3 times as long in users of Indian snuff tobacco compared with control subjects [97]. Tissue damage was detected macroscopically and histologically in the affected mucosal areas of the nose. The risk of cancer development is increased many times if this type of tobacco ("toombak") is placed in the oral cavity (relative risk increased 7.3–73.0-fold). The snuff tobacco sold in Germany is less dangerous than "toombak".

The nitroso compounds in Indian tobacco include:

- N-nitroso-nicotine (NNN; 136 mg/g snuff tobacco)
- N-nitroso-ana-tabanine (NAT; 113 μg/g)
- 4-(N-methyl-N-nitrosamino)-1-(3-pyridyl)-1-butanone (NNK; 110–680 mg/g)
- N-nitroso-pyrrolidine (NPYR)
- N-nitrosodimethylamine (NDMA) [98]

In animal studies, the purified components display carcinogenic activity [99, 100] (cf. Table 3.8), initially producing a reduction in nasal ciliary cells in the mucosa and irreversible damage to the remaining cells. Moreover, changes (metaplasias) occur in the various epithelial cells. Due to the dependence-inducing effect of nicotine, the consumed doses of snuff tobacco are continuously increased, in turn damaging mucociliary clearance because of the increased tobacco dose and the prolonged contact with the mucosa [101]. These reactions may develop into malignant changes. In rats, too, exposure to the tobacco-specific nitrosamines NNK and NDMA has led to DNA damage to cells of the nasal mucosa and to lymphocyte changes, with the overall result that these animal studies indicate genotoxic effects of tobacco constituents not only in the nose, but also in the liver [102].

A recent meta-analysis addressed the relation between European and American smokeless tobacco and oral cancer [103]. Following a literature review, a meta-analysis was conducted of 32 epidemiological studies published between 1920 and 2005, including tests for homogeneity and publication bias by Weitkunat et al. Based on 38 heterogeneous study-specific estimates of the odds ratio or relative risk for smokeless tobacco use, the random-effects estimate was 1.87 (95% confidence interval 1.40–2.48). The authors showed that the increase was mainly evident in studies conducted before 1980. No increase was found in studies in Scandinavia. Restricting attention to the seven estimates adjusted for smoking and alcohol eliminated both heterogeneity and excess risk (1.02; 0.82–1.28). Estimates also varied by sex (higher in females) and study design (higher in case-control studies with hospital controls), but more clearly in studies where estimates were unadjusted, even for age. From the pattern of estimates, the authors suggested some publication bias. Based on limited data specific to non-smokers, the random-effects estimate was 1.94 (0.88–4.28), and based on few exposed cases, the eight individual estimates were heterogeneous. It was concluded that smokeless tobacco, as used in America or Europe, carries at most a minor increased risk of oral cancer. However, the authors stated that elevated risks in specific populations or from specific products cannot definitely be excluded [103].

Overall, in Germany, there are too few consumers of snuff tobacco to demonstrate the adverse effects of snuff tobacco on health in larger epidemiological studies. Harmful effects on the nasal mucosa have mainly been proven for foreign varieties of snuff tobacco; it remains open to conjecture to what extent the lungs are also affected by the inhalation of

Table 3.9 Tobacco-specific nitrosamine levels in the saliva of habitual tobacco chewers

Tobacco habit	NAT/(NAB)[a]	NNN	NNK
Snuff-dipping women (USA)	187 (12.5–470)	154 (26–420)	32.6 (<10–96)
Students (USA)	204 (48–555)	99 (37.4–222)	3.4 (ND-60.6)
Inuit snuff dippers (Canada)	1318 (123–4560)	980 (115–2601)	56 (ND-201)
Snuff dippers (Sweden)	18.5 (5–37)	36.5 (6–65)	2.6 (ND-9)
Betel quid + tobacco (India)	4.8 (1.0–10.9)	7.5 (1.6–14.7)	0.3 (ND-2.3)
Tobacco chewers (India)	29.8 (13.5–51.7)	33.4 (16.5–59.7)	ND
Masheri, women (India)	ND	28.3 (14.3–43.5)	ND
Tobacco + lime (India)	30.4 (ND-133)	113 (10–430)	3.8 (ND-28.5)

NAT/NAB N-nitrosoanatabine/N-nitrosoanabatine; *NNN;* N-nitrosonornicotine; *NNK* 4-(N-nitrosomethylamino)-1-(3-pyridyl)-1-butanone. Results from users of tobacco products even when placed in the mouth between the gum and check without chewing [100]. *ND* not detected
[a]Refers primarily to NAT, NAB may be present in some cases

snuff tobacco. Larger-scale epidemiological studies should help to clarify this question, but "without the support of the tobacco industry." Analysis of saliva obtained from tobacco chewers shows that tobacco-specific nitrosamines (TSNA) are rapidly extracted from oral tobacco products, even when placed between the gum and cheek without chewing. In Inuit Indians, large differences have been observed for the extraction of TSNA in snuff (Table 3.9). Following 15 min snuff dipping of 0.5–1.5 g tobacco, 22-fold differences in the amount of NNN and 37-fold differences in the amounts of NAB/NAT in saliva were detected. Under extreme conditions, the total exposure to TSNA approaches 440 µg/day [94]. Furthermore, the carcinogenic risk due to oral intake of TSNA increases as a function of gastric pH [100]. Nitrosation of tobacco alkaloids produces a greater increase in the formation of carcinogen NNN than of NAB and NAT under stimulated gastric conditions (pH from 2.0 to 3.5; Fig. 3.4) [108]. In addition, slight decomposition of 4-(N-nitrosomethylamino)-1-(3-pyridyl)-1-butanone due to transnitrosation has been reported [104].

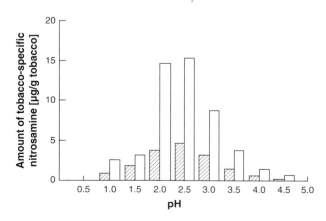

Fig. 3.4 The effect of pH on the nitrosation of tobacco alkaloids under simulated gastric conditions. Nitrosation resulted in the formation of NAB and NAT (*striped columns*) and NNN (*open columns*) [104]

A study published in 2007 by scientists of the Swedish Karolinska Institute addressed the long-term use of Swedish moist snuff and the risk of myocardial infarction amongst men [105]. The scientists aimed at studying whether long-term use of snuff affects the risk of myocardial infarction. A cohort was created with information on tobacco use and other risk factors, collected through questionnaires from construction workers. Between 1978 and 1993, all construction workers in Sweden were offered repeated health check-ups by the Swedish Construction Industry's Organization for Working Environment Safety and Health. In total, 118,395 non-smoking men without a history of myocardial infarction were followed through 2004 by the researchers. Information on myocardial infarction morbidity and mortality was obtained from national registers and relative risk estimates were derived from Cox proportional hazards regression model, with adjustment for age, body mass index and region of residence. It was found that almost 30% of the men had used snuff. In total, 118,395 non-smoking men without a history of myocardial infarction were followed through 2004. The multivariable-adjusted relative risks for ever-snuff users were 0.91 (95% confidence interval, 0.81–1.02) for non-fatal cases and 1.28 (95% confidence interval, 1.06–1.55) for fatal cases. Heavy users ($>$or $= 50$ g day(1)) had a relative risk of fatal myocardial infarction of 1.96 (95% confidence interval, 1.08–3.58). Snuff use increased the probability of mortality from cardiovascular disease among non-fatal myocardial infarction patients. The authors concluded that their results indicate that snuff use is associated with an increased risk of fatal myocardial infarction [105].

3.7
Concluding Remarks

- Between 1950 and 1975, important changes to the cigarette were already being made and attempts were also made (e.g. by the installation of cigarette filters) to reduce the toxic and carcinogenic potential of the cigarette that had been demonstrated in experimental animal work.
- Changes in the cultivation and production of cigarette tobacco led to an increase in tobacco-specific nitrosamines in tobacco smoke, which are also responsible for the increased incidence of adenocarcinomas.
- Efforts to lower the nicotine content of cigarettes to about one-third were ostensibly successful on the basis of measurements of tobacco smoke in FTC machines. As a result of changes in smoking behaviour (depth and frequency of inhalation), 2–3-fold yields of tar, nicotine and CO were achieved.
- Smokers of various filter and light cigarettes intensify their smoking behaviour in order to obtain the amounts of nicotine they require from cigarette smoke. Likewise, compared with regular cigarettes, light and ultralight cigarettes do not assist smoking cessation.
- The use of smokeless tobacco (snuff dipping, chewing tobacco) facilitates the oral uptake of TSNA, which are transformed in the stomach to potent carcinogens by an acidic pH. The same scenario is likely when smokers consume cigars and cigarillos preferentially containing dark tobacco types.

References

1. Barnes DE, Hanauer P, Slade J, Bero LA, Glantz SA (1995) Environmental tobacco smoke. The Brown and Williamson document. J Am Med assoc 274:248–253
2. Slade J, Bero LA, Hanauer P, Barnes DE, Glantz SA (1995) Nicotine and addiction. The Brown and Williamson documents. J Am Med assoc 274:225–233
3. Todd JS, Rennie D, McAfee RE, Bristow LR, Painter JT, Reardon TR, Johnson DH Jr, Corlin RF, Coble YD Jr, Dickey NW, et al (1995) The Brown and Willamson documents: Where we go from here? J Am Med assoc 274:256–258
4. Bero L, Barnes DE, Hanauer P, Slade J, Glantz SA (1995) Lawyer control of the tobacco industry's external research program. The Brown and Williamson documents. JAMA 274:241–247
5. Hanauer P, Slade J, Barnes DE, Bero L, Glantz SA (1995) Lawyer control of internal scientific research to protect against products liability lawsuits. The Brown and Williamson documents. JAMA 274:234–240
6. Glantz SA, Barnes DE, Bero L, Hanauer P, Slade J (1995) Looking through a keyhole at the tobacco industry. The Brown and Williamson documents. JAMA 274:219–224
7. Dukes CA (1975) Marketing plans presentation to RJRI board of directors. Trial exhibit 12493. 30-9-1974. RJR
8. Hind JF (1975, Jan 23) Memo to CA Tucker. Trial exhibit 12865
9. Johnson RL (1973, Feb 21) Memo to RA Pittman, B & W. Trial exhibit 13820
10. Long GH (1980, Jun 22) MDD report on teenage smokers (14–17). Memo to EA Horrigan Jr. Trial exhibit 13101
11. Colby FG (1973, Dec 04) Cigarette concept to assure RJR a larger segment of the youth market. Memo to R A Blevins Jr. Trial exhibit 12464
12. Dann WL (1980, Mar 21) The nicotine receptor program. Memo to RB Seligman, Philip Morris. Trial exhibit 26227
13. Senkus M (1969) Invalidation of some reprints in the research department. Memo to Max Crohn (Legal department). Trial exhibit 26216. RJR
14. Stanford LE (1993, Dec 02) Memo to Phillip Morris, Document collection file regarding Phillip Morris USA product research performed at INBOFO laboratory in COLOGNE; Germany. Carbon copied to Alfred T. McDonell (A&P) among others. Trial exhibit 26277. Philip Morris
15. Doll R, Hill AB (1950) Smoking and carcinoma of the lung, a preliminary report. Br Med J 2: 739–748
16. Wynder EL, Graham EA (1950) Landmark article, May, 27: tobacco smoking as a possible etiologic factor in bronchiogenic carcinoma. A study of six hundred and eighty-four proved cases. By Ernest L. Wynder and Evarts A. Graham. J Am Med Assoc 113:329–336
17. Hanners D (1998, Feb 15) Tobacco's promise exemplifed early PR: PR firm hired to go on offensive when health concerns surfaced. [1A, 12A]. St Paul Pionieer
18. Wynder EL, Graham EA, Croninger AB (1953) Experimental production carcinoma with cigarette tar. Cancer Res 13:856–864
19. Tobacco Industrie Research Committee (1954, Jan 04) A frank statement to cigarette smokers. Trial exhibit 14115
20. Tobacco Industrie Research Committee meeting (1954, Jan 18) Trial exhibit 14127
21. Green DR, Rodgman A (1996) The Tobacco Chemists' Research Conference. A half-century of advances in analytical methodology of tobacco and its products. Recent Adv Tob Sci 22: 131–304
22. Doull J, Frawley JP, George W (1994) List of ingredients added to tobacco in the manufacture of cigarettes by six major American cigarette companies. Tob J Int 196:32–39

23. Hoffmann D, Hoffmann I (1997) The changing cigarette, 1950–1995. J Toxicol Environ Health 50(4):307–364
24. Hoffmann D, Djordjevic M, Brunnemann K (1995) Changes in cigarette design and composition over time and how they influence the yields of smoke constituents. J Smoking Rel Disord 6:9–23
25. Henningfield JE (1997, Jan 30) Verbal Testimony
26. Haag HB, Larson PS, Finnegan JK (1959) Effect of filtration on the chemical and irritation properties of cigarette smoke. AMA Arch Otolaryngol 69:261–265
27. Voges E (1984) Tobacco Encyclopedia. Tobacco Journal International, Mainz, Germany
28. Kensler CJ, Battista SP (1963) Components of cigarette Smoke with ciliary depressant activity. N Engl J Med 269:1161–1166
29. Battista SP (1975) Ciliatoxic components in cigarette smoke. In: Wynder EL, Hoffmann D, Gori GB (eds) Smoking and health. I. Modifying the risk for the smoker. DHEW Publ. No. (NIH) 76-1221. U.S. Department of Health Education, and Welfare, New York, pp. 517-534. Proceedings of the Third World Conference on Smoking and Health
30. Tiggelbeck D (1976) Vapor phase modification. An underutilized technology, Modifying the Risk for the Smoker. 1, 507–514. DHEW publication NO. (NIH) 76–1221
31. Shepherd RJK (1994) New charcoal filters. Tob Report 121(2):10–14
32. Wynder E, Mann JA (1957) Study of tobacco carcinogenesis III. Filtered cigarettes. Cancer 10:1201–1205
33. Wynder E, Hoffmann DA (1961) Study of tobacco carcinogenesis. VIII. The role of acidic fractions as promoters. Cancer 14:1306–1315
34. Brunnemann KD, Hoffmann D, Gairola CG, Lee BC (1994) Low ignition propensity cigarettes: smoke analysis for carcinogens and testing for mutagenic activity of the smoke particulate matter. Food Chem Toxicol 32:917–922
35. Hasday JD, Bascom R, Costa JJ, Fitzgerald T, Dubin W (1999) Bacterial endotoxin is an active component of cigarette smoke. Chest 115:829–835
36. Knopick PC (1980, Sep 09) Memo to W Kluepfer, Tobacco Institute. Trial exhibit 14303
37. Ellis C (1962, Feb 13) The effects of smoking: proposal for further research contracts with Battelle. Trial exhibit 11938
38. Henningfield JE, Keenan RM (1992) Nicotine delivery kinetics and abuse liability. J Consult Clin Paychol 61:743–750
39. Anderson HD (1964, Aug 07) Potassium Carbonate. Memo to R F Dobson. [10356]. Trial exhibit
40. Panzer F (1972, May 01) The Roper proposal. Memo to H Kornegay. Trial exhibit 20987
41. Nowland Org. SHF Cigarette Marketplace Opportunities Search and Situation (1976) Analysis, II. Trial exhibit 17994. 1976. Lorillard. Management Report
42. Teague CE Jr (1972, Apr 14) The nature of tobacco business and the crucial role of nicotine therein. Research planning memorandum. Trial exhibit 12408. RJR
43. MacCormick AD (1974, May 03) Smoking and health. Trial exhibit 10602. BAT
44. Osdene TS (1980, Aug 12) Evaluation of major R&D programs. Letter to RB Seligman, Philip Morris. Trial exhibit 10255
45. Roberts DL (1983, Oct 13) Memo to flavour and biobehavioral divisions regarding brainstorming Session. RJR. Trial exhibit 12743. RJR
46. Dunn W Jr (1972) Motives and incentives in cigarette smoking. Philip Morris. Trial exhibit 18089
47. R&D views on potential marketing opportunities (1984, Dec 09) Trial exhibit. 11275
48. Slawen RW (1982, Feb 25) A progress report on nicotine migration and manipulation. Trial exhibit 10019. Lorillard
49. Anonym. Y1 product. Trial exhibit 13671. 1000. B&W

50. Robinson JH (1983) Criticque of smokers of low yield cigarettes do not consume less nicotine. To A Rodgman, RJR. Trial exhibit 12648
51. Benowitz NL, Hall SM, Herning RI, Jacob P III, Jones RT, Osman AL (1983) Smokers of low-yield cigarettes do not consume less nicotine. N Engl J Med 309:139–142
52. Robinson JH, Pritchard WS (1992) The meaning of addiction: reply to West. Psychopharmacology 108:411–416
53. Smoking and Health (1964, Feb 18) Significance of the Report of the Surgeon Generals Committee to Phillip Morris Incorporated. Memo to Dr. H Wakeham, Mr Hugh Cullman. Trial exhibit 10322. Philip Morris
54. Short PL (1977, Apr 14) Smoking and health item, 7: The effect on marketing. Memo to Fred Haslam. Trial exhibits 10584 and 10585. BAT
55. Creighton DE (1978, Jun 27) Compensation for changed delivery. Trial exhibit 11089. BAT
56. Greig CC (1970) Structured creativity group, thoughts by CC Greig – R&D Southampton marketing scenario, 1: low CO product; 2: high expanded tobacco cigarette. Trial exhibit 10683. BAT
57. Goodmann B (1975, Sep 17) Marlboro-Marlboro Lights study delivery data. Report to L I Meyer, Philip Morris. Trial exhibit 11564
58. Smith RE (1950, Feb 13) Memo to JR Ave, JG Flinn and AW Spaers. Trial exhibit 10170. Lorillard
59. Wood DJ (1977, Jan 19) Smoking products research. Trial exhibit 11203. BAT
60. Oldman M (1981, May 19) Products/consumer interaction: The role of human smoking studies in subjective testing, with particular reference to machine vs. human smoking. Trial exhibit 11357
61. Centers for Disease Control and Prevention (1997) Filter ventilation levels in selected U.S. cigarettes, 1997. Morb Mortal Wkly Rep 46:1043–1047
62. Townsend D (1991) Deposition of Davis Townsend, in the Circuit Cort, 4th Judicial Circuid, Duval County, Florida, case No. 9501820-CA, Division CV-C. Jean Connor, plaintiff, vs RJ Reynolds Tobacco Company, etc, et al, defendants. October 3th 1994: 1–102. Cited by: Kozlowski IT, Goldberg ME, Yost BA, Ahern FM, Aronson KR, Sweeney CT: Smokers are unaware of the filter events now on most cigarettes: result of a national survey. Tob Control 5: 265–270
63. US Department of Health an Human Services (1996) The FTC Cigarette Test Method for determining tar, nicotine carbon monoxide Yields of US Cigarette report of the NCI Expert Committee. Public Health Service, Washington DC, 96–4028
64. Kozlowski LT, Goldberg ME, Yost BA, Ahern FM, Aronson KR, Sweeney CT (1996) Smokers are unaware of the filter vents now on most cigarettes: results of a national survey. Tob Control 5:265–270
65. Hirji T (1987, Jul 23) Effect of ventilation on tar delivery. To AL Heard. Trial exhibit 12110. BAT
66. Rose J, Behm F (2004) Effects of low nicotine content cigarettes on smoke intake. Nicotine Tob Res 6(2):309–319
67. Creighton DE (1988) The significance of pH in tobacco and tobacco smoke. Report issued by T Hirji. Trial exhibit 12228. BAT
68. Blackhurst JD (1966, Sep 30) Further work on "extractable" nicotine. Report issued by IW. Hughes. Trial exhibit 17825
69. Williams R (1971, Dec 16) Development of a cigarette with increased smoke pH. Trial exhibit 11903. Liggett
70. Ihrig AM (1973, Feb 08) pH of particulate-phase. Memo to CI Tucker Jr, Lorillard. Trial exhibit 10095
71. Woods RJ, Hartlee GC (1973, May 10) Historical review of smoke pH data and sales trends for competitive Brand filter cigarettes. Trial exhibit 12337. RJR
72. BAT Cigarette design. Trial exhibit 11973. 1000
73. Riehl T, McMurtrie D, Heemann V (1984, Nov 05) Project SHIP: review of progress November 5–6th 1984. Trial exhibit 13430

74. Colby FG (1981, Dec 09) Weekly highlights. Memo to J Giles. Trial exhibit 26229
75. McKenzie JL (1976, Sep 21) Product characterization definitions an implications. Memo to AP Ritchy. Trial Exhibit 12270
76. Teague CE (1973) Implications and activities arising from correlation of smoke pH with nicotine impact, other smoke qualities, and cigarette sales. Trial exhibit 13155. RJR
77. Schori TR (1979, Oct 22) Free nicotine: its implication on smoke impact. Trial exhibit 2590. B&W
78. Blackman I, Heath A (1984, Jul 30) Proceedings of the smoking behavior-marketing conference. Trial exhibit 13430
79. Haustein KO (2000) Tabakzusätze in Zigaretten. Dt Ärztebl 97:A-1520
80. Bates C, Jarvies M, Conolly G (1999) Tobacco additives, cigarette engineering and nicotine addition
81. Cundiff RH, Greene GH, Laurene AH (1964) Column elution of humecatants from tobacco and determination by vapor chromatography. Tob Sci 8:163–170
82. Kagan MR, Cunningham JA, Hoffmann D (1999) Propylene glycol. A precursor of propylene oxide in cigarette smoke. 53rd Tobacco Science Research Conference
83. International Agency for Research on Cancer (1994) Ethylene oxide. IARC Monographs on the Evaluation of Carcinogenic. [60]. Some Industrial Chemicals, Lyon, France, pp 73–159
84. Tornqvist M, Osterman-Golkar S, Kautiainen A, Jensen S, Farmer PB, Ehrenberg L (1986) Tissue doses of ethylene oxide in cigarette smokers determined from adduct levels in hemoglobin. Carcinogenesis 7:1519–1521
85. Leffingwell JC (1987) Chemical and sensory aspects of tobacco flavor. Recent Adv Tab Sci 14:1–218
86. Roberts D, Rowland RL (1962) Macrocyclic diterpenes a- and b- 4, 8, 13-duvatriene-1,3-diol from tobacco. J Org Chem 27:3989–3995
87. Connolly GN, Wayne GD, Lymperis D, Doherty MC (2000) How cigarette additives are used to mask environmental tobacco smoke. Tob Control 9(3):283–291
88. Giovino GA, Tomar SL, Reddy MN, Peddicord JP, Zhu B, Escobedo LG, et al (1996) Attitudes, knowledge and beliefs about low-yield cigarettes among adolescents and adults. NIH Publication No. 96–4028. The FTC Cigarette Test Method for Determining Tar, Nicotine and Carbon Monoxide Yields of U.S. Cigarettes; Smoking and Tobacco Control Monograph No. 7
89. Health Canada (1995) Survey on smoking in Canada. Cycle 4. Health Canada, Ottawa
90. Kozlowski LT, Goldberg ME, Yost BA, White EL, Sweeney CT, Pillitteri JL (1998) Smokers' misperceptions of light and ultra-light cigarettes may keep them smoking. Am J Prev Med 15:9–16
91. Gazdar AF, Minna JD (1997) Cigarettes, sex, and lung adenocarcinoma. J Natl Cancer Inst 89:1563–1565
92. Kabat GC (2003 Sep 15) Fifty years' experience of reduced-tar cigarettes: what do we know about their health effects? Inhal Toxicol 15(11):1059–102
93. Thun MJ, Burns DM (2001) Health impact of "reduced yield" cigarettes: a critical assessment of the epidemiological evidence. Tob Control 10(Suppl 1):i4–i11
94. Haustein KO (2000) Geschichte des Tabaks und die Folgen des Tabakrauchens für die Menschheit. Arzneimittel-Therapiekritik 32:321–330
95. Idris AM, Ibrahim SO, Vasstrand EN, Johannessen AC, Lillehaug JR, Magnusson B, et al (1998) The Swedish snus and the Sudanese toombak: are they different? Oral Oncol 34:558–566
96. Sanghvi LD (1989) Tobacco related cancers. In: Sanghvi LD, Notani P (eds) Tobacco and health: the Indian scene. Tata Memorial Centre, Bombay, pp 9–15
97. Chetan S (1993) Nasal muco-ciliary clearance in snuff users. J Laryngol Otol 107:24–26
98. Bhide SV, Padma PR, Amonkar AJ, Maru GB, Nair J, Kulkarni JR (1989) Studies on tobacco specific nitroamines and other carcinogetic agents in smokers tobacco products. In: Sanghvi LD MP (ed) In tobacco and health: the Indian scene. UICC Workshop, Tata Memorial Centre, Bombay, pp 121–131

99. Hoffmann D, Djordjevic MV (1997) Chemical composition and carcinogenicity of smoke-less tobacco. Adv Dent Res 11:322–329

100. Tricker AR, Preussmann R (1989) Preformed nitrosamines in smokeless tobacco. In: Maskens AP (ed) Tobacco and cancer. Perspectives in preventive research. Elsevier Science Publishers B. V, Amsterdam, pp 35–47

101. Jaffe JH (1990) Drug addiction and drug abuse. In: Gilman AG, Rall TW, Nies AS(eds) Goodmann and Gilman: the pharmacological basics therapeutics. Pergamon, NewYork, pp 522–753

102. Pool-Zobel BL, Klein RG, Liegibel UM, Kuchenmeister F, Weber S, Schmezer P (1992) Systemic genotoxic effects of tobacco-related nitrosamines following oral and inhalational administration to Sprague-Dawley rats. Clin Investig 70:299–306

103. Weitkunat R, Sanders E, Lee PN (2007 Nov 15) Meta-analysis of the relation between European and American smokeless tobacco and oral cancer. BMC Public Health 7(1):334

104. Tricker AR, Haubner R, Spiegelhalder B, Preussmann R (1988) The occurrence of tobacco-specific nitrosamines in oral tobacco products and their potential formation under simulated gastric conditions. Food Chem Toxicol 26:861–865

105. Hergens MP, Alfredsson L, Bolinder G, Lambe M, Pershagen G, Ye W (2007) Long-term use of Swedish moist snuff and the risk of myocardial infarction amongst men. Intern Med 262(3):351–359

106. Air Quality and Safety (1986) The airliner cabin environment. Washington DC, pp 135–136

107. Darall KG, Figgins JA (1998) The blocking of cigarette filter ventilation holes. EH40M007/98. Laboratory of the Government Chemist Report

108. Jarvis M, Bates C (1999) Why low tar cigarettes don't work and how the tobacco industry has fooled the smoking public. Action on Smoking and Health UK online bulletin: www.ash.org.uk/html/regulation/html/big-one.html

109. Djordjevic MV, Stellman SD, Zang E (2000) Doses of nicotine and lung carcinogens delivered to cigarette smokers. J Natl Cancer Inst 92:106–111

110. Phillip M (1982) Evaluation of the DeNoble nicotine acetaldehyde data. BN 2056144727-4728. Tobacco Resolution

111. Phillip M Termination of chronic acetaldehyde administration does not result in a physical dependence syndrome. BN 1000060695-60704. 1000. Tobacco Resolution

112. Lippiello PM, Fernandes K (1989, Sep 25) "Enhancement of nicotine bindung to nicotinic receptors by nicotine levulinate an levulinic acid". BN 508295794. RJR

113. Phillip Morris. BN 2060535081-85. 1000

114. BAT The absorbtion and mechanism of action of pyridine and its interaction with nicotine. BN 402419398-9486, FN AW 2730. 1000

115. BAT (1985) The Unique Differences of Phillip Morris Cigarette Brands. BN 109359953, FN K762

116. BAT Tobacco flavouring for smoking products. [FN 1500]. 1000. BN 104805407

117. BAT (1967) Cocoa butter as a tobacco additive. BN 105534584, FN B263

118. BAT (1962, Dec 12) Letter regarding Eugenol. FN M456. BN 110090779-110090785

119. BAT (1987, Jun 15) Studies into alternative burn additives that reduce visible sidestream. FN AW 1428, BN 402385586-402385589

120. BAT (1983, Sep 09) The addition of sugar solution of CA(OH)2 in sugar to cigarette paper. BN 100480228-0229 FN J562

Pharmacology and Pharmacokinetics of Nicotine

4

Nicotine is the principal alkaloid of the tobacco plant. Alkaloids from other plants, e.g. coniine (from hemlock), cytisine (from laburnum) and lobeline (from *Lobelia inflata* or Indian tobacco), possess actions partly resembling those of nicotine (Box 4.1). Nicotine was first isolated from the leaves of tobacco, *Nicotiana tabacum*, by Posselt and Reimann in 1828, and Orfila performed the earliest pharmacological analysis of its effects in 1843.

Nicotine is one of the few alkaloids with a liquid-oily consistency at room temperature (pK_a = 7.9). It takes on a brownish discolouration and acquires the odour of tobacco on exposure to air. As a therapeutic agent in medicine, nicotine is used exclusively to achieve smoking cessation. Approximately 25% of the alkaloid is present in the blood in non-ionised, free-base form. The two optical isomers differ in potency, with the L-form being more potent than the D-form.

4.1
The Nicotine Receptor

The nicotinic acetylcholine receptor (nAChR) is the receptor with the longest tradition as an object of experimental research. It is the prototype ligand-gated ion channel (LGIC). The earliest investigations into the specific binding of nicotinic agonists date back to

(-)-Cytisine

(±)-Anatoxin A

Box 4.1 Compounds with nAChR-agonistic efficacy: cytisine, epibatidine, anatoxin A, lobeline

(±)-Epibatidine

Lobeline

K.-O. Haustein, D. Groneberg, *Tobacco or Health?*
DOI: 10.1007/978-3-540-87577-2_4, © Springer Verlag Berlin Heidelberg 2010

Langley and Anderson [1] and Dale [2]. Detailed analyses of the receptor and its subunits were made possible in the wake of studies of the electric organ of the *Torpedo* and the identification of α-neurotoxins.

nAChRs consist of pentameric LGICs, are found in the central nervous system (CNS) and in peripheral nerve structures, and comprise an α- and a β-subunit with a large number of variants (α2–α9, β2–β4, γ, δ, ε) (Fig. 4.1) [3, 4]. In contrast to their central role in autonomic neurotransmission and the triggering of muscle contraction, nAChRs in the CNS display several modulatory reactions [3]. The importance of nAChRs in the pathophysiology of various disorders, such as Alzheimer's disease, Parkinson's disease, schizophrenia, Tourette syndrome, etc., is now established [5]. Furthermore, they also play a key role in smoking cessation, analgesia, anxiolysis and neuroprotection [5]. Important subtypes of nAChR are found in the central and peripheral nervous system and another subtype is found in both systems (Fig. 4.1).

The nAChR of mammalian brain consists predominantly (about 90%) of $2\alpha_4$ and $3\beta_2$ subunits [6] and binds [H]-cytisine and nicotine with high affinity [7, 8] (Table 4.1)[10]. Another form of nAChR occurring both in the CNS and the peripheral nervous system is made up exclusively of α_7 subunits [11] (Fig. 4.1). The α subunits contain a cysteine pair in positions 192–193 of the C loop (Figs. 4.2 and 4.3). These loops accommodate the binding site for agonists and also contain aromatic side-chains (tryptophan, tyrosine), which trigger cationic π-interactions with the agonists [13]. The polypeptide chain of the nAChR subunits contains four hydrophobic transmembrane domains (M1–M4), which span the plasma membrane (Fig. 4.2). M2 is an α-helix that includes the cation channel.

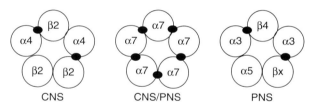

Fig. 4.1 Schematic illustration of the structure of nAChRs in the central and peripheral nervous system

Table 4.1 Binding affinities (K_i) and functional potencies (EC_{50}) reported at brain thalamic synaptosomes $\alpha_4\beta_2$-nAChRs or heterogenously expressed nAChRs for nicotinic agonists at native or recombinant $\alpha_4\beta_2$- and α_7-nAChRs and recombinant $\alpha_3\beta_4$-nAChRs [9]

	Binding affinity K_i (nM)			Functional potency EC_{50} (µM)		
	α4β2	α7	α3β4	α4β2	α7	α3β4
(–)-Nicotine	1–11	400–8,900	300–475	0.3–15	18–91	5–410
(–)-Cytisine	0.14–2.7	1,400–3,883	56–195	0.019–71.4	n.d.	72–134
(–)-Epibatidine	0.01–0.06	3.1–350	n.d.	0.004–0.02	1.1–2.2	0.009
Acetylcholine	6.8–57	4,000–10,830	560–881	0.48–3	79–316	53–210
Choline	112,000	2,380,000	n.d.	n.d.	1,600	n.d.
Lobeline	4–50	11,000–13,100	480	n.d.	no activ.	n.d.
Carbachol	207–582	18,000–580,000	3,839	2.5–29	296	n.d.
DMPP	9.4–400	160–2,300	1,300	0.07–18	19–75	10–92

DMPP dimethylphenylpiperazine; *n.d.* not determined; *no activ.* no activation

Fig. 4.2 Structure of a nAChR subunit (segments M1 to M4) [12]

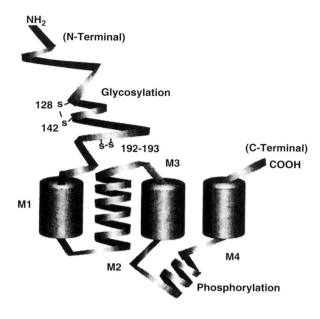

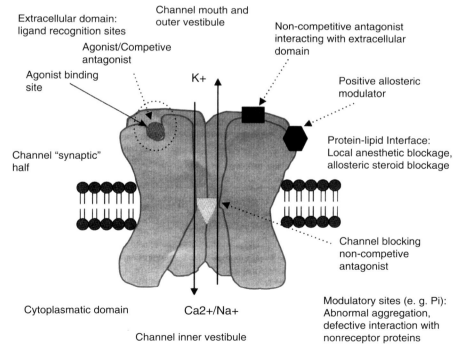

Fig. 4.3 Structural overview of a nAChR with one subunit removed revealing channel lumen. Demonstrated are binding sites for agonists, competitive and non-competitive antagonists and positive allosteric modulators (e.g. ACh esterase inhibitors) [5]

A study published in 2004 in *Science* analysed the identity of nicotinic receptor subtypes sufficient to elicit both the acute and chronic effects of nicotine dependence is unknown. The researchers engineered mutant mice with a4 nicotinic subunits containing a single point mutation, Leu9'→Ala9', in the pore-forming M2 domain, rendering a4* receptors hypersensitive to nicotine. Selective activation of a4* nicotinic acetylcholine receptors with low doses of agonist recapitulates nicotine effects thought to be important in dependence, including reinforcement in response to acute nicotine administration, as well as tolerance and sensitisation elicited by chronic nicotine administration. The data indicated that activation of a4* receptors is sufficient for nicotine-induced reward, tolerance and sensitisation [14].

M3 and M4 are separated from each other by a long intracellular loop that contains centres for the phosphorylation of serine/threonine kinases [15]. During binding of the agonist (e.g. nicotine), the nAChRs undergo allosteric modulation [16] in which there is a transition from the resting conformation to an open state in which the cations Na^+, K^+ and Ca^{2+} are transported. When nAChRs are in the open state, agonists are bound with low affinity (Figs. 4.2 and 4.3). The permanent presence of an agonist results in channel closure and desensitisation of the receptor, which becomes refractory for activation (Fig. 4.4) [17]. The various nAChR subtypes differ considerably in terms of extent of desensitisation and recovery: the α_7 nAChR becomes desensitised very rapidly [18] and the permanent presence of an agonist results in inactivation followed by only slow recovery. The neuronal $\alpha_4\beta_2$ nAChR is very susceptible to inactivation in response to chronic nicotine exposure [19]. The transitions from the resting, open and inactive states are reversible, and various ligands are able to stabilise the conformational receptor state. Agonists initially stabilise the activated (open) state, whereas competitive antagonists preferentially stabilise the closed (resting or inactive) state (Fig. 4.4).

Tables 4.1 and 4.2 present details of the activity of a small number of agonists and antagonists on various nAChR subtypes.

As well as the muscle nicotine receptor, the neuronal nicotine receptor has also been largely characterised. The nAChRs in the various brain regions display differences in their

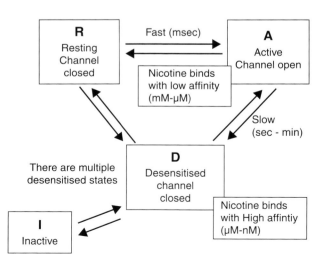

Fig. 4.4 Relationship between major states occupied by a nAChR

Table 4.2   Binding affinities (K_i) for nicotinic antagonists in competition binding assays at native or recombinant $\alpha4\beta2$ and $\alpha7$-nAChRs and recombinant $\alpha3\beta4$-nAChRs

nAChR-subtype/ antagonist	K_i (nM)		
	$\alpha4\beta2$	$\alpha7$	$\alpha3\beta4$
d-Tubocurarine	1,000–25,000	3,400–7,700	22,929
Dihydro-β-erythroidine	13.9–1,900	25,000–57,900	218,622
Methyllycoconitine (MLA)	3,700–6,100	0.69–10.3	3,700
Decamethonium	460–120,000	124,000–200,000	n.d.
Mecamylamine	822,000–>1,000,000	>1,000,000	>1,000,000

Binding affinities reported for competition binding assays of [H]-agonist binding to brain membranes ($\alpha4\beta2$-nAChRs) and [?H]-agonist binding to heterologously expressed $\alpha4\beta2$-nAChRs [9]. *n.d.* not determined

binding kinetics to nicotine and in their reactivity to electrophysiological stimuli [3, 4, 20]. Permanent desensitisation of the receptor may explain the occurrence of tachyphylaxis (Fig. 4.4). In addition, up-regulation of nicotine receptors occurs in response to prolonged nicotine exposure [21, 22].

4.2
Agonists and Antagonists of the nAChR and its Subtypes

Nicotine agonists react with the different nAChR subtypes by attaching themselves to the various binding sites and causing allosteric modulation of the pentameric complex with opening of the ion channel. The changes measured for some agonists are summarised in Table 4.1. Apart from nicotine, naturally occurring agonists include cytisine, anatoxin A, epibatidine and anabasine (Box 4.1). The binding affinity of these substances to the $\alpha4\beta2$ nAChR subtypes is 100–1,000 times higher than to the $\alpha7$ subtypes (Table 4.1). Their binding affinities (K_i) are 100–1,000 times higher than their functional potencies (EC_{50}) for the activation of the nAChR subtypes (Table 4.1). Nicotine is the prototype nAChR agonist: it binds with high affinity to the $\alpha4\beta2$ nAChR (Table 4.1), while the $\alpha7$ nAChR reacts 1,000 times less sensitively [23]. The binding activities of the nicotine metabolite, cotinine, are scarcely measurable [24].

Competitive antagonists act reversibly with the nAChR by stabilising the conformation of the binding site and thereby blocking the action of agonists. However, this effect can be abolished by high doses of the agonist. D-tubocurarine (d-TC; Box 4.2) and dihydro-β-erythroidine are classic examples of such substances (see Table 4.2). This group includes various snake venoms such as bungarotoxin and a range of α-conotoxins. d-TC does not discriminate between the various nAChR subtypes, and is active at concentrations of 10 µM [25].

Non-competitive antagonists produce their effect away from the binding centre and therefore, do not interact with agonists. Their effect is achieved as a result of binding in the vicinity of the ion channel, and consequently, these substances can also be used to predict possible concentrations at the receptor. In this category, the classic example is

Mecamylamine   **d-Tubocurarine**

Box 4.2 Compounds with nAChR-antagonistic efficacy: mecamylamine, d-tubocurarine

mecamylamine (Box 4.2; Table 4.2), which has IC_{50} values in the lower μM range [25]; in this case, the α7 nAChR subtypes react somewhat less sensitively than the α–β heteromers. In addition, N-methyl-D-aspartate (NMDA) receptors are blocked at concentrations in the higher μM range [26]. Similar effects are also produced by other ganglionic blocking agents, such as hexamethonium, decamethonium and chlorisondamine (Table 4.2). At concentrations in the low μM range, the antidepressant bupropion also inhibits various nAChR subtypes (α3β2, α4β2, α7) in the rat as well as nAChR-mediated rubidium efflux of a human cell line (SH-SY5Y) [27, 28]. The effect of bupropion on human cells was voltage-independent, with the result that an effect via the channel lumen may be excluded. Further substances with non-competitive effects include the neuroleptic drug chlorpromazine and the anaesthetics phencyclidine and ketamine [29]. Various steroid hormones, such as corticosterone, aldosterone, oestradiol and cortisol, are able to inhibit neuronal nAChR subtypes from a human cell line (SH-SY5Y) at concentrations in the upper nM to lower μM range [30]. Progesterone inhibits the α4β2 nAChR subtype at concentrations of only 9 μM (IC_{50}) [31, 32]. A β-amyloid polypeptide$_{1-42}$ also inhibits the α7 nAChR subtype in the pM range [33], prompting speculation concerning an association with the pathogenesis of Alzheimer's disease and the role of nAChRs in its development. Section 7.1 in Chap. 7 includes a discussion of the association between smoking and slowing of the progression of Alzheimer's disease.

4.3
Pharmacology

Like acetylcholine, nicotine stimulates receptors of the parasympathetic nervous system, and a distinction is drawn between nicotinic and muscarinic receptors (N and M receptors) and effects.

4.3.1
Effects of Nicotine on Receptors in Different Organs

Nicotine predominantly stimulates presynaptic nACh receptors, thereby producing an excitatory action [4, 20]. If these receptors are located on dopaminergic neurons, they promote the metabolism of this transmitter in mesolimbic and nigrostriatal structures [6, 34]. The density of nicotine receptors is higher in the cerebral structures of smokers than of non-smokers and in contrast to the situation following nicotine infusions, the smoking of single cigarettes leads to the formation of additional nACh receptors, preferentially in the hippocampus, gyrus rectus and cerebellar cortex [35].

In the persistent presence of nicotine (as in heavy smoking), *up-regulation of the nicotine receptors* occurs in numerous regions of the brain (hippocampus, neocortex, gyrus rectus, cerebellar cortex, median raphe) [21, 36–38], probably due to reduced internalisation and/or degradation (Fig. 4.4) [39]. The density of the receptors is altered (doubled), but not their affinity for the ligand. The excess nicotine is probably bound to desensitised or inactivated receptors [6].

nAChR density is particularly high in the nucleus accumbens [40], the structure which is also the centre for the reward system and plays an important role with regard to caloric intake, among other things [41]. In animal experiments, dopamine is released by nicotine administration. Clearly, the nucleus accumbens is crucial for the development of dependence [34, 42]. The combination of nicotine administration with stimulation of the dopaminergic system, especially in the mesoaccumbens, seems to be exceptionally important in that there is a regionally selective down-regulation of the control of dopaminergic neurons localised in the mesoaccumbens and these are additionally inhibited by NMDA-glutamate receptors [43]. It is suggested that sensitisation is related to enhanced burst firing of mesoaccumbens neurons, which results in enhancement of dopamine release into the extracellular space and hence, potentiates the effect on extrasynaptic dopamine receptors [43]. According to Wise and Bozarth [44], the dependence-producing effect of nicotine and other substances is also determined by whether they influence dopaminergic synapses in the mesolimbic system. However, this hypothesis is not without its opponents [45].

4.3.2
Organ Effects and Toxicity

Nicotine stimulates sympathetic cardiac ganglia via the N-receptors, leading to an increase in *heart rate* (see Table 4.3). This effect may also be achieved by paralysis of parasympathetic

Table 4.3   Pharmacological effects of nicotine [46]

Release of adrenaline from the adrenals, of noradrenaline (NA) in the hypothalamus (central increase in sympathetic tone) and of dopamine in the mesolimbic system
Increased catecholamine levels in the bloodstream affecting blood pressure, heart rate and blood coagulation factors
Varying increase in gastric acid secretion, ulcerogenic effect (peptic ulcer) as a result of reduced mucosal perfusion
Stimulant effect on the CNS (low doses): tremor, blunting of emotions, increased ability to concentrate
Stimulant effect on respiration via the carotid and aortic bodies
Stimulation of the vomiting centre
Intoxication: circulatory collapse, depolarisation block of neuromuscular transmission, respiratory paralysis (central)

cardiac ganglia or by the discharge of adrenaline from the adrenal medulla. Conversely, nicotine may slow the heart rate by paralysis of sympathetic or stimulation of parasympathetic cardiac ganglia or by a combination of the two mechanisms. These opposite effects – in some respects – are dependent on dose, route of administration, and time after dosing. Small nicotine doses or moderate smoking produce a slight increase in heart rate and *blood pressure*.

The effect of nicotine on the *gastrointestinal tract* is intensified by acetylcholine, catecholamines and peptide hormones. Gastric acid secretion is not regularly stimulated, and yet, tobacco smoking may be assumed to possess an ulcerogenic effect. Intestinal peristalsis is clearly stimulated and this may lead to multiple bowel movements [46], often a reason why smokers do not want to do without their morning cigarette.

Respiration is stimulated and the *vomiting centre* is activated by stimulation of nAChRs in the carotid and aortic bodies.

Nicotine is classed as a powerful poison that is effective in almost the same doses as prussic acid (HCN). For an individual who is not accustomed to nicotine, it is estimated that a single dose of 60 mg will have a lethal effect [47]. Relatively high doses of nicotine elicit convulsions. Ingestion of toxic doses leads to central stimulation, respiratory paralysis and circulatory collapse. Furthermore, nicotine causes depolarisation with blockade of neuromuscular transmission; if the nicotine dose is sufficiently high, death may ensue within a few minutes due to respiratory paralysis (see Table 4.3).

4.3.3
Metabolic and Hormonal Effects of Nicotine

Smokers are known to have a lower body weight than non-smokers, and this difference is (over)compensated for following smoking cessation. Weight reduction associated with smoking is caused by the reduced intake of calories, especially sweets, as well as by an increased metabolic rate and the increased secretion of catecholamines from the adrenal medulla and steroid hormones from the adrenal cortex [48]. Besides apparently playing a crucial role in these reactions [49, 50], nicotine also stimulates the secretion of anti-diuretic hormone and β-endorphin.

A similar reaction is observed in terms of the secretion of anterior pituitary lobe hormones (e.g. ACTH) [51], though nicotine has much smaller effects than smoking per se in this context. Moreover, in female smokers, differences in oestrogen secretion and premature onset of menopause are thought to be related to smoking [52].

4.3.4
Central Nervous System Effects of Nicotine

Nicotine in low doses stimulates the CNS, an effect that is frequently accompanied by a fine tremor. Emotions are blunted and the ability to concentrate is reported to be enhanced.

The dependence-producing effects of nicotine have been beyond doubt now for a number of years. The degree of nicotine dependence of smokers can be deduced on the basis of their daily cigarette consumption, the time when the first cigarette is smoked in the morning and possibly their need to smoke during the night.

Although the relationship between nicotine and changes in heart rate and blood pressure has been demonstrated, the relationship between nicotine and subjective effects such as decreased craving, relaxation, sickness and decreased nervousness is less well-delineated. Therefore, Guthrie et al. performed a study in which arterial nicotine levels were observed in 21 smokers who smoked two average nicotine (AN) cigarettes and one low nicotine (LN) cigarette [53]. Craving for a cigarette, relaxation, sickness and decreased nervousness were rated on a visual analogue scale (VAS) before and after smoking each cigarette. None of these subjective measures except craving for a cigarette was changed significantly by smoking. The change in craving was significantly correlated with the area under the plasma nicotine concentration vs. time curve ($r = -0.57$, $p = 0.01$) calculated from the arterial nicotine samples drawn up to 20 min after the initiation of smoking the first AN cigarette. Although well-documented behavioural manipulations such as smoking denicotinised cigarettes reduce craving, increases in plasma arterial nicotine concentrations after smoking the first cigarette of the day also reduce craving. The authors concluded that both the psychology and pharmacology of nicotine/tobacco smoking are involved in craving reduction [53].

The characteristics of nicotine are also very clearly different from those of other "addictive" substances. Dependence in the context of smoking is produced by the ultra-rapid delivery of the alkaloid to the brain and can be abolished by the administration of nicotine preparations over the course of several weeks in a gradually diminishing dosage regimen (see Chap. 11). The effects of nicotine can be blocked with the antihypertensive ganglion blocking drug mecamylamine, but not with substances with antimuscarinic, anticholinergic or anti-adrenergic activity [54]. Experimental animal work may indicate that nicotine promotes memory performance and lowers aggressive behaviour [54]. Smokers also confirm that the first cigarette smoked in the day produce general relaxation, especially in stressful situations [49].

4.4
Pharmacokinetics of Nicotine

Nicotine is absorbed at varying rates from different tobacco preparations. As a result of tobacco chewing or snuffing, large quantities of the alkaloid are absorbed more slowly than from a cigarette (see Fig. 4.5). During cigar or pipe smoking, varying amounts of nicotine are absorbed through the mucosa, depending on the length of time for which the smoke is held in the oral cavity. In contrast, nicotine from inhaled cigarette smoke is absorbed extremely rapidly across the epithelium of the pulmonary alveoli and bypasses the liver to reach the brain (Fig. 4.6). There is a corresponding rise in CO-haemoglobin levels in the blood (Fig. 4.7) [58].

Nicotine is metabolised in the liver by oxidative processes (see Fig. 4.8) and is eliminated with a half-life of 1.5 h. Only about 10% of absorbed nicotine leaves the body in unchanged form. The breakdown product cotinine, which is pharmacologically inactive,

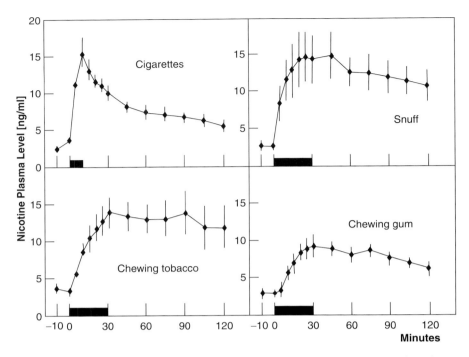

Fig. 4.5 Changes in plasma nicotine levels in response to cigarettes, snuff tobacco, chewing tobacco and nicotine chewing gum (single dose) [52, 55]. Consumption of one cigarette (12 puffs over 9 min), 2.5 g tobacco (kept in the mouth for 30 min), 8 g chewing tobacco (chewed for 30 min) and 4 mg chewing gum (chewed for 30 min)

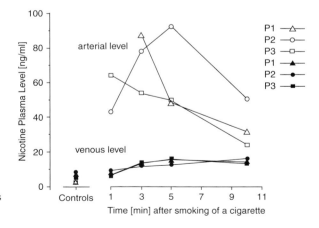

Fig. 4.6 Arterial and venous plasma levels of nicotine following inhalation of one cigarette. Data for three smokers; *open symbols*: arterial, *solid symbols*: venous plasma levels of nicotine [56]

Fig. 4.7 Mean nicotine plasma levels and CO-haemoglobin levels in cigarette smokers. The subjects smoked one cigarette of low (*dotted lines*) and high nicotine content (*solid line*) every 30 min from 08:30 to 23:00 (a total of 30 cigarettes/day). The cigarettes in question were produced for research purposes [57]

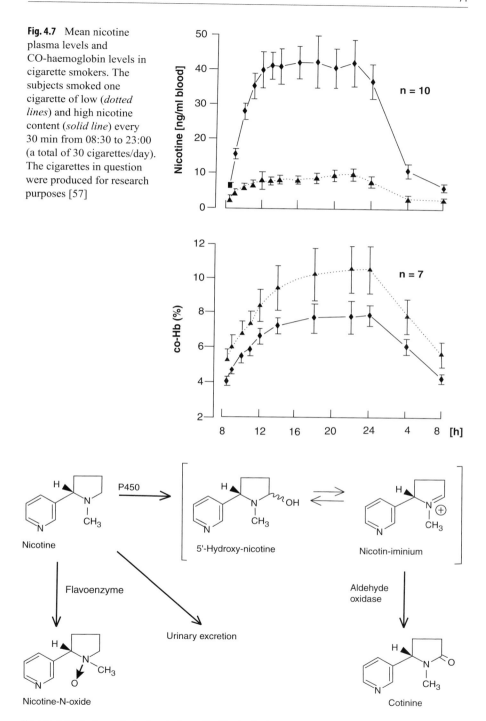

Fig. 4.8 Metabolism of nicotine (schematic illustration)

accumulates and is eliminated much more slowly (half-life 20–30 h), with the result that it can be used for assay purposes in smokers and passive smokers [59]. Quantitative methods (e.g. gas chromatography/mass spectrometry or GC/MS) for measuring urine cotinine, which has a longer half-life, are valid and reliable, though costly and time-consuming. Recently developed semi-quantitative urine cotinine measurement techniques (i.e. urine immunoassay test strips or ITS) address these disadvantages, though the value of ITS as a means of identifying abstaining smokers has not been evaluated. Therefore, Acosta et al. examined ITS as a measure of smoking status in temporarily abstaining smokers [60]. A total of 236 breath and urine samples were collected from smokers who participated in two separate studies involving three independent, 96-h (i.e. Monday–Friday), Latin-square-ordered, abstinence or smoking conditions; a minimum 72-h washout separated each condition. Each urine sample was analysed with GC/MS and ITS. Under these study conditions, CO demonstrated moderate sensitivity (83.1%) and strong specificity (100%), whereas ITS assessment showed strong sensitivity (98.5%) and weak specificity (58.5%). In this study of short-term abstinence, ITS classified as non-abstinent nearly half of the samples collected from abstaining smokers. However, it classified nearly all non-abstinent smokers as currently smoking. The researches concluded that the validation of ITS using GC/MS results from smokers undergoing more than 96 h of abstinence may be valuable [60].

Nicotine N-oxide is not of pharmacological interest [58]. The extensive hepatic metabolism of nicotine may mean that elimination is delayed where liver function is clearly impaired; the administration of nicotine should, therefore, be assessed with caution in individuals with very marked impairment of hepatic and renal function.

The specialist literature contains accurate descriptions of the pharmacokinetic properties of nicotine from cigarettes, one particular feature being that its extremely rapid delivery to the CNS is not achieved by any product used for nicotine replacement therapy (Figs. 4.5, 4.9 and Figs. 11.1–11.3 in Chap. 11) [62, 63]. The amount of nicotine absorbed daily as a result of cigarette smoking depends on the number of cigarettes smoked, their nicotine yield, the number of puffs taken and the depth to which the smoke is inhaled. Within a few hours, a "dependent smoker" can attain plasma nicotine levels that are perceived as sufficient for a whole day. The body absorbs nicotine more slowly from nicotine preparations (inhalers > nasal spray > chewing gum > patch) than from cigarette smoking (Fig. 4.9). These products never achieve the peak nicotine levels attained by smoking, although considerable inter-individual differences exist.

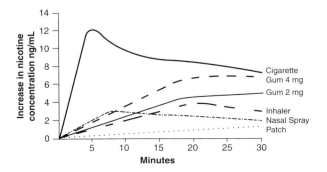

Fig. 4.9 Comparison of plasma nicotine levels following inhalation of one cigarette with levels following nasal spray (1 mg), inhaler (1 mg) and chewing gum (2 mg) [61]

For the most part, pharmacokinetic studies with nicotine preparations take account of plasma nicotine levels over time, whereas in clinical studies, plasma cotinine or thiocyanate levels also yield important information.

4.5
Nicotine Dependence

The German word for dependence ("Sucht") comes from the verb "siechen" (cognate with our English word "sick") and thus, implies an illness requiring medical assistance. The tobacco industry has known for about 50 years that nicotine is an addictive substance. None of the other constituents of tobacco smoke are responsible for the development of dependence [64].

4.5.1
Types of Dependence

Nicotine stimulates the release of mediator substances, such as noradrenaline (NA), acetylcholine, dopamine, 5-hydroxytryptamine (5-HT), γ-aminobutyric acid (GABA) and endorphins. As a reward system, the dopaminergic system is primarily influenced by nicotine [65].

Unlike alcohol or heroin, nicotine possesses hardly any psychotoxic activity; among other things, this also means that even the heavily dependent smoker is only minimally conspicuous socially. The psychological effects of nicotine are summarised in Table 4.4. A magnetic resonance imaging (MRI) study showed that intravenous administration of nicotine (in doses from 0.75 to 2.25 mg/70 kg of weight) to 16 active smokers induced a dose-dependent increase in behavioural parameters, including feelings of "rush," "high" and "drug liking." Likewise, there was an accumulation of nicotine in various brain regions, including the nucleus accumbens, amygdala, cingulate and frontal lobes. The activation of these structures

Table 4.4   Effects of nicotine associated with dependence

Effects	Consequences
Binds to nicotine receptors in the CNS	Facilitates release of transmitter substances (dopamine, NA, acetylcholine, 5-hydroxytryptamine, γ-aminobutyric acid, β-endorphin)
Mood	Increases sensation of pleasure, has a stimulant and anxiolytic effect
Performance	Increases attention, improves performance for repetitive tasks
Body weight	Suppresses appetite, accelerates metabolic processes, weight reduction
Neuroadaptation of nicotine receptors (repeated doses)	Development of tolerance, withdrawal symptoms (irritability, restlessness, drowsiness, difficulty concentrating, diminished performance, anxiety, hunger, weight gain, sleep disturbances, craving for cigarettes)

is consistent with nicotine's behaviour-arousing and behaviour-reinforcing properties, especially since the identified brain regions participate in the reinforcing, mood-elevating and cognitive properties [66].

Van Den Eijnden et al. addressed in 2003 that besides nicotine, other chemicals in tobacco smoke such as norharman may contribute to the addictive properties of cigarettes [67]. More specifically, elevated blood plasma levels of norharman may reduce feelings of craving among tobacco-dependent individuals. To test this hypothesis, plasma concentrations of norharman were measured in 38 male smokers (at least 15 cigarettes/day) at three time-points on 3 different days spread over a 4-month period. The first measurement (T0) was conducted in the morning at 8.30 a.m., after 12 h of smoking abstinence. The T1 and T2 measurements were conducted at 13.00 p.m. and 16.30 p.m., respectively, during a period of ad libitum smoking (after the T0 measurement, participants were not restricted in their smoking behaviour) [67]. At each of the nine time-points, craving was assessed by means of a shortened version of the Questionnaire of Smoking Urges. The Fagerström Test of Nicotine Dependence was used to obtain an indication of nicotine dependence. The study showed that, after a period of smoking abstinence, craving was stronger in those with a high tobacco dependence than in those with a low tobacco dependence. After resumption of smoking, craving declined to a similar low level in both low and high dependent smokers. The authors conclude that measurements during periods of ad libitum smoking indicate that plasma levels of norharman are related negatively to craving among LN-dependent smokers, but not among high dependent smokers [67].

Approximately 17% of smokers are heavily dependent [68], with the result that smoking cessation in this group of people is also only achievable with great difficulty and generally, not without medical help.

Different dependence types can be identified among cigarette smokers:

1. Those who smoke one cigarette at regular intervals throughout the day,
2. Those who smoke by preference during the hours of the morning or evening,
3. Those who even get up during the night in order to smoke
4. Those who smoke in phases, e.g. at weekends, while on holiday or at other social events.

The Fagerström Test for Nicotine Dependence (FTDN) permits assessment of the degree of dependence on the basis of six questions (Table 4.5) [68]. This can be estimated from the scores achieved (maximum 10), with scores > 7 being associated with very high dependence [68]. According to the Diagnostic and Statistical Manual (DSM-IV; [69]) of the American Psychiatric Association, nicotine dependence is assumed to be present if three or more of the following six assessment criteria are satisfied:

- Tolerance
- Withdrawal symptoms
- Compulsive desire to consume tobacco
- Reduced ability to control the start, end and quantity of tobacco consumption
- Progressive neglect of other interests or recreational activities due to tobacco consumption
- Smoking larger amounts than actually intended, smoking despite detailed knowledge of the harmful effects on health.

Table 4.5   Fagerström test for nicotine dependence (FTDN) [68]

Questions		Responses	Scores
1	How soon after you wake up do you smoke your first cigarette?	Within 5 min	3
		6–30 min	2
		31–60 min	1
		After 60 min	0
2	Do you find it difficult to refrain from smoking in places where it is forbidden? (e.g. in the cinema, at meetings etc.)	Yes	1
		No	0
3	Which cigarette would you hate most to give up?	The first in the morning	1
		Any other	0
4	How many cigarettes/day do you smoke?	10 or less	0
		11–20	1
		21–30	2
		31 or more	3
5	Do you smoke more frequently during the first hours after awakening than during the rest of the day?	Yes	1
		No	0
6	Do you smoke if you are so ill that you are in bed most of the day?	Yes	1
		No	0
		Total :	[__]

Each smoker "titrates" his/her own plasma nicotine level in terms of the number of cigarettes smoked, the number of puffs and the depth of inhalation. Smokers, thus, largely avoid the signs of intoxication (tachycardia, perspiration, pallor, diarrhoea, etc.). Nicotine preparations are not capable of producing this "kick" because the delivery of nicotine from all formulations occurs more slowly than from a cigarette (see Figs. 4.5 and 4.9).

4.5.2
Molecular Biological Aspects of Dependence

The effects of nicotine have been frequently studied in self-administration ("self-reward") systems in rats and monkeys [70, 71]. Small multiple doses of nicotine, comparable with those delivered during cigarette smoking, have a locomotor stimulant effect similar to amphetamine or cocaine [127]. The locomotor stimulant and "self-rewarding" effects of nicotine are produced as a result of *increased release of dopamine from the nucleus accumbens* in the posterior region of the mesolimbic system [66, 72]. Neuronal nicotine receptors are found at various sites in the CNS, both at the terminal nerve endings and in the somato-dentritic dopamine-secreting neurons in the midbrain (nucleus accumbens) (Fig. 4.10). The increased secretion of dopamine occurs as a result of increased impulse density [74, 75]. Parallel with the stimulation of dopamine secretion, there is stimulation of the NMDA receptor, which is responsible for the binding of glycine and for potentiating the activity of glutamate [34, 76]. The increase in dopamine release is associated with a nicotine-preferring behaviour, which intensifies from "liking" to "craving." It is, therefore, highly probable

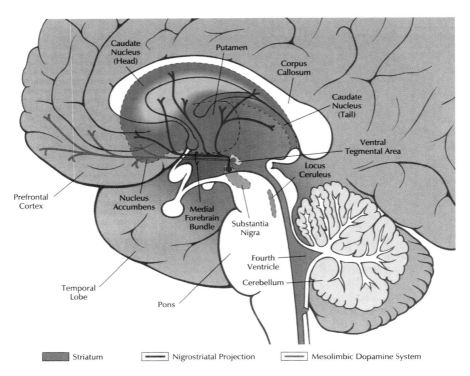

Fig. 4.10 Schematic illustration of the brain regions responsible for the development of dependence reactions and the sites of action of nicotine in the mesolimbic dopaminergic system [73]

that nicotine dependence unfolds via the same dopamine reactions as amphetamine and cocaine dependence [44]. However, since nicotine displays protracted activity via several receptors, these become desensitised in the course of long-term administration [6].

In addition, nicotine stimulates the release of NA from regions of the ventral hippocampus that are innervated from the locus coeruleus. Here, too, the nAChRs are isoforms that are desensitised by the permanent presence of nicotine [77].

The continuous delivery of nicotine leads to a regional reduction in 5-HT synthesis and concentration in the *hippocampus* [78]. Post-mortem studies in human brains (hippocampus) from heavy smokers also reveal reduced concentrations of 5-HT and its metabolite 5-hydroxyindoleacetic acid; however, this is not the case in the cerebral and cerebellar cortex or the medulla oblongata. The density of 5-HT_{1A} receptors, but not of 5-HT_2 receptors, was selectively increased in the hippocampal tissue of smokers [77]. Even though this situation has not been fully elucidated, anxiety stimuli in humans also lead to increased 5-HT release in the brain and conversely, anxiolytic agents can suppress this release [79]. Since nicotine also lowers 5-HT excess in the hippocampus, this might explain the anxiolytic effects of nicotine in some [80, 81], but not all experimental models [82]. Effective anxiolytic drugs act primarily on conduction pathways in the dorsal raphe nucleus, the connection to the frontal brain and the amygdala [75], whereas nicotine acts on the medial raphe nucleus, which radiates out to the dorsal hippocampus and stimulates the conduction pathways emanating from the dorsal raphe nucleus in the process [83]. The increased 5-HT release from neurons, which innervate the dorsal hippocampus from the medial raphe nucleus, may be responsible for a relative resistance to emotional and other stress reactions and may play an important role in the neuropathology of depression [84, 85]. In fact, depressive patients smoke more frequently than healthy individuals, suggesting an antidepressant effect in these patients (see Sect. 7.1.5 in Chap. 7) [86]. The inverse conclusion that antidepressants such as bupropion and nortriptyline might be useful in principle for smoking cessation therapy has been demonstrated in studies reported elsewhere in this book (see Chap. 11). It remains to be seen, however, whether these products will prove their usefulness in smoking cessation therapy.

Various studies indicate that nicotine also acts on opioid receptors. Endogenous opioids are released in response to nicotine absorption [87]. For example, nicotine produces an analgesic effect in the mouse that can be antagonised with naloxone [88]. In humans, opiate consumption and the craving to smoke are frequently associated, with each potentiating the other, and cigarette consumption increases during heroin or methadone self-administration [89, 90]. To date, however, a number of studies have failed to establish whether morphine antagonists might lead to more prolonged smoking cessation [91], a problem that awaits further investigation in the years to come (see Sect. 11.3.7 in Chap. 11).

Nicotine administration in animal studies leads to the release of GABA from the interneurons of hippocampal structures [92]. Vigabatrin administration increases GABA levels, whereas extracellular glutamate and dopamine overflow are decreased [93, 94].

4.5.3
Genetic Aspects

Genetic aspects appear to be less important than environmental factors (parents, school groups, education, religious involvement, attitude of society, advertising) in the development of nicotine dependence [95, 96]. By contrast, heavy smoking or the inability to stop smoking can no longer be explained in terms of environmental factors, with the result that biological (pharmacological factors, psychiatric disorders, neuroadaptation) and genetic effects [97, 98] are implicated, as is evident from research in twins.

Recent studies from molecular genetics have suggested an association between the tryptophan hydroxylase 1 (TPH1) gene and nicotine addiction, indicating a dysfunction of the serotonergic (5-HT) system in smoking behaviour. Reuter and Hennig published in 2004 that in a sample of 252 healthy subjects, a significant association between variations observed in nicotine dependence and the heterozygous AC-genotype of the TPH A779C polymorphism could be demonstrated. Moreover, the heterozygous genotype was significantly associated with a personality trait of neurotic aggression (indirect hostility, negativism), as measured by the Buss-Durkee-Hostility-Inventory (BDHI). The positive heterosis effects with respect to nicotine addiction and personality support the idea that the TPH1 gene exerts pleiotropic effects [99].

Dopamine is a key neurotransmitter of the mesolimbic reward pathway in the human brain, and tyrosine hydroxylase (TH) is the rate-limiting enzyme in dopamine biosynthesis. Consequently, Anney et al. postulated in 2004 that the gene encoding TH is a strong candidate for involvement in the genetic component of addiction. The importance of this gene in nicotine dependence is supported by many studies showing a link between nicotine administration and TH expression. A functional tetranucleotide repeat polymorphism within intron 1 of the TH gene (HUMTH01-VNTR) has been shown to modify tobacco use in two independent Caucasian samples from the USA and Australia. Using information drawn from an eight-wave Australian population-based longitudinal study of adolescent health, Anney et al. tested the effect of the HUMTH01-VNTR on nicotine dependence [100]. Comparisons were made between dependent smokers and non-dependent smokers. The results provided further support for a protective association between the K4 allele and dependent smoking (odds ratio 0.54, 95% confidence interval 0.28–1.0). No associations were observed at any of three other common TH polymorphisms (rs6356, rs6357 and HUMTH01-PstI). Including these data, three independent studies, two of which use identical phenotypes, have now identified a protective relationship between the K4 allele of the functional HUMTH01-VNTR polymorphism and high-level smoking [100].

In an investigation of personality factors and smoking behaviour in a total of 2,680 pairs of twins and 543 individual twins, it was found that phenotypic associations were more pronounced in monozygotic than in dizygotic twins [98]. While this finding underlines the genetic contribution to smoking behaviour, unequivocal statements on this issue are problematic because of the following potentially involved factors:

1. Enzyme CYP_{2A6} metabolises nicotine to cotinine. Smokers carrying a defective variant of CYP_{2A6} metabolise nicotine more slowly and exhibit reduced nicotine dependence [101]. Conversely, smokers with a normal CYP_{2A6} pattern may respond particularly well to nicotine replacement therapy. A defective allele frequency of 1–3% has been observed in Finnish, Spanish and Swedish populations, much lower than previously thought [102].

2. Dopamine has been increasingly incriminated in the production of dependence [103], and the reinforcing properties of nicotine have been linked to its effects on dopaminergic transmission [104, 105] and specifically, to its effects on the D2 receptor [106]. Subgroups of dopamine receptors (D1 and D2) exist in the CNS and genetic variations have been identified in the dopamine receptor (DRD2) gene and the dopamine transporter [DAT] gene (SLC6A3). The DAT influences concentrations of and responses to synaptic dopamine in these regions. There is experimental and epidemiological evidence to implicate these genes in a variety of disorders. The DRD2-A1 allele has been associated with a reduced density of dopamine receptors [107]. In comparison with people with DRD2-A2 genotypes, those with DRD2-A1 genotypes (A1/A1 or A1/A2) were found to be more likely to exhibit compulsive and addictive behaviours [108–111]. However, the data are inconsistent [112]. Also, according to investigations in patients with lung cancer, variant alleles in the D2 receptor may play a role in the development of nicotine dependence [71].

3. The two alleles TaqI-A1 and TaqI-A2Im are located in the genome fragment λhD2G1. While the A1 allele is found in about 20% of the population, 50–60% of alcoholics carry this allele [113, 114]. The children of alcoholics also have an increased prevalence of this A1 allele. One meta-analysis has reported an increased association of the DRD2-A1 allele with alcoholics (45%) compared with the general population (25%). By contrast, the rarer

A1 allele appears to occur in severe forms of alcoholism [114, 115]. This form of genetically-induced dependence also appears to apply in smokers [69–71, 109] in whom prevalence was increased (48.7%) compared with the "normal" population (25.9%) [109, 115]. People carrying this A1 allele start to smoke earlier and are also able to remain abstinent for short periods only [109]. It is thought that the A1 allele is associated with reduced D2 receptor activity due to lower receptor density, but not to altered structure or function [115].

4. The SLC6A3 gene regulates synaptic dopamine by coding for a reuptake protein known as the DAT [116]. This gene has also been implicated in Parkinson's disease [117], attention deficit disorder [118] and Tourette syndrome [119]. The SLC6A3 gene may display several single nucleotide polymorphisms (SNIPs) [120], with the 9-repeat allele being associated with cocaine-induced psychosis, a state attributed to diminished dopamine reuptake and greater availability of synaptic dopamine [121]. According to one study in twins, an altered dopamine transporter (SLC6A3) occurs in conjunction with the D2 dopamine receptor (DRD2) located on chromosome 11; it was found that individuals with the SLC6A3-9 genotype in conjunction with the DRD2-A2 genotype were less likely to be smokers [122]. Individuals with the SLC6A3 gene are more likely to be smokers and nicotine-dependent. In addition, an association has been reported between alcoholics and the presence of a D4 receptor [123].

5. Alcohol dependence and nicotine dependence share a considerable number of features in common, with heritability being 60.3% for nicotine dependence and 55.1% for alcohol dependence. A common genetic correlation has been demonstrated for the two dependence types [124]. Recent research indicates that fetal alcohol exposure may produce increased risk for later dependence on nicotine, alcohol and a variety of drugs [125].

Very rarely (<0.01% of cases), dependence may also develop during the course of smoking cessation therapy with nicotine preparations; in these circumstances, ex-smokers become fixated with nicotine preparations (for the most part nasal spray > chewing gum) and then frequently use these products over a period of months.

4.5.4
Withdrawal Symptoms

Withdrawal symptoms are encountered in heavy nicotine dependence (daily cigarette consumption >30–40 cigarettes, first morning cigarette smoked immediately upon waking, or the smoker even awakes during the night and then smokes one or two cigarettes). In addition, cigarette smoking influences mood and behaviour as well as appetite and fat metabolism (Table 4.4). The classic symptoms of withdrawal are:

- Mild agitation and restlessness
- Impaired ability to concentrate
- Anxiety feelings (relatively pronounced [126])
- Increased appetite and weight gain
- Sleep disturbances and drowsiness
- Strong craving for cigarettes

There are considerable variations in the degree to which individuals experience these withdrawal symptoms, which may last for several weeks to months. Like alcoholics, many ex-smokers are severely at risk because the least cause (going to a restaurant and having an alcoholic drink, meeting up with smokers) may trigger a return to smoking. With many smokers, however, it is "merely" the absence of the manual cues associated with the activity of smoking [120], which leads to a resumption of the habit and thus, undoes the initial success of smoking cessation therapy.

4.6
Concluding Remarks

- Nicotine is one of the most potent toxic alkaloids with a dependence-inducing effect, comparable to that of cocaine and heroin. Continued administration in the form of tobacco smoking (especially of cigarettes) may lead to dependence.
- Nicotine unfolds its effects by releasing CNS messenger substances, among which dopamine, NA and 5-HT are particularly important.
- Nicotine acts by stimulating nicotinic acetylcholine receptors (nAChRs): these are ion transporters that occur in the peripheral and CNS and are linked with various transmitter systems. The structure of nAChRs has been largely elucidated and the various subunits ($\alpha4\beta2$, $\alpha3\beta4$, $\alpha7$ etc.) can be assigned to different neural structures. The sites of action of agonists and competitive and non-competitive antagonists can be located in the receptor system.
- Unlike the absorption of nicotine from cigarettes, the nicotine available from pharmaceutical formulations is released very much more slowly and in smaller doses, and this is ultimately the reason for the products' lack of any dependence-inducing effect.
- In addition to external influences, the development of nicotine dependence can also be related to genetic factors. In this context, the cytochrome P450 subenzyme 2A6, the distribution of dopamine receptors (DRD1 vs. DRD2) and their alleles (A1 vs. A2), as well as the DAT gene SLC6A3 influence smoking initiation and nicotine dependence.
- The nAChR macromolecule is affected by several pathological conditions (congenital myasthenic syndromes, Alzheimer's and Parkinson's disease, schizophrenia, some forms of epilepsies, Gilles de la Tourette syndrome). A variety of strategies (e.g., synthesis of nAChR agonists and antagonists, subtle alterations to nAChR function or partial occlusion of the nAChR channel by blocking drugs) will result in new therapeutic modalities in the near future.

References

1. Langley JN, Anderson HK (1892) The actions of nicotine on the ciliary ganglion of the third cranial nerve. J Physiol (Lond) 13:460–468
2. Dale HH (1914) The action of certain esters and ethers of choline and their relation to muscarine. J Pharmacol Exp Ther 6:147–190

3. Karlin A (1993) Structure of nicotinic acetylcholine receptors. Curr Opin Neurobiol 3(3): 299–309

4. McGehee DS, Role LW (1995) Physiological diversity of nicotinic acetylcholine receptors expressed by vertebrate neurons. Annu Rev Physiol 57:521–546

5. Barrantes FJ (ed) (1998) Molecular pathology of the nicotinic acetylcholine receptor. In: The nicotine acetylcholine receptor. Current views and future trends. Springer, Berlin, pp 175–216

6. Wonnacott S (1990) Characterization of brain nicotinic receptor sites. In: Wonnacott S, MAH Russell (ed) Nicotine psychopharmacology: molecular, cellular and behavioural aspects. Oxford University Press, Oxford, London, pp 226–277

7. Flores CM, Rogers SW, Pabreza LA, Wolfe BB, Kellar KJ (1992) A subtype of nicotinic cholinergic receptor in rat brain is composed of alpha 4 and beta 2 subunits and is up-regulated by chronic nicotine treatment. Mol Pharmacol 41:31–37

8. Williams N, Sullivan JP, Arneric SP (1994) Neuronal nicotinic acetylcholine receptors. DN&P 7:205–223

9. Sharples CGV, Wonnacott S (2001) Neuronal nicotinic receptors. Tocris reviews no. 19. Tocris Cookson, Avonmouth

10. Wonnacott S (1990) The paradox of nicotinic acetylcholine receptor upregulation by nicotine. Trends Pharmacol Sci 11(6):216–219

11. Chen D, Patrick JW (1997) The alpha-bungarotoxin-binding nicotinic acetylcholine receptor from rat brain contains only the alpha7 subunit. J Biol Chem 272:24024–24029

12. Prince RJ, Sine SM (1998) The ligand binding domains of the nicotinic acetylcholine receptor. In: Barrantes FJ (ed) The nicotinic acetylcholine receptor: Current views and future trends. Springer, Berlin, pp 31–59

13. Grutter T, Changeux JP (2001) Nicotinic receptors in wonderland. Trends Biochem Sci 26(8): 459–463

14. Tapper AR, McKinney SL, Nashmi R, Schwarz J, Deshpande P, Labarca C, et al (2004) Nicotine activation of alpha4* receptors: sufficient for reward, tolerance, and sensitization. Science 306(5698):1029–1032

15. Corringer PJ, Le Novere N, Changeux JP (2000) Nicotinic receptors at the amino acid level. Annu Rev Pharmacol Toxicol 40:431–458

16. Lena C, Changeux JP (1993) Allosteric modulations of the nicotinic acetylcholine receptor. Trends Neurosci 16(5):181–186

17. Changeux JP, Edelstein SJ (1998) Allosteric receptors after 30 years. Neuron 21:959–980

18. McGehee DS, Role LW (1995) Physiological diversity of nicotinic acetylcholine receptors expressed by vertebrate neurons. Annu Rev Physiol 57:521–546

19. Kuryatov A, Olale FA, Choi C, Lindstrom J (2000) Acetylcholine receptor extracellular domain determines sensitivity to nicotine-induced inactivation. Eur J Pharmacol 393(1–3):11–21

20. McGehee DS, Heath MJ, Gelber S, Devay P, Role LW (1995) Nicotine enhancement of fast excitatory synaptic transmission in CNS by presynaptic receptors. Science 269(5231):1692–1696

21. Benwell ME, Balfour DJ, Anderson JM (1988) Evidence that tobacco smoking increases the density of (–)-[3H]nicotine binding sites in human brain. J Neurochem 50(4):1243–1247

22. Collins AC, Luo Y, Selvaag S, Marks MJ (1994) Sensitivity to nicotine and brain nicotinic receptors are altered by chronic nicotine and mecamylamine infusion. J Pharmacol Exp Ther 271(1):125–133

23. Gotti C, Moretti M, Maggi R, Longhi R, Hanke W, Klinke N, et al (1997) Alpha7 and alpha8 nicotinic receptor subtypes immunopurified from chick retina have different immunological, pharmacological and functional properties. Eur J Neurosci 9:1201–1211

24. Anderson DJ, Arneric SP (1994) Nicotinic receptor binding of [3H]cytisine, [3H]nicotine and [3H]methylcarbamylcholine in rat brain. Eur J Pharmacol 253:261–267

25. Chavez-Noriega LE, Crona JH, Washburn MS, Urrutia A, Elliott KJ, Johnson EC (1997) Pharmacological characterization of recombinant human neuronal nicotinic acetylcholine

receptors h alpha 2 beta 2, h alpha 2 beta 4, h alpha 3 beta 2, h alpha 3 beta 4, h alpha 4 beta 2, h alpha 4 beta 4 and h alpha 7 expressed in *Xenopus* oocytes. J Pharmacol Exp Ther 280: 346–356

26. Papke RL, Sanberg PR, Shytle RD (2001) Analysis of mecamylamine stereoisomers on human nicotinic receptor subtypes. J Pharmacol Exp Ther 297:646–656

27. Popik P, Layer RT, Fossom LH, Benveniste M, Geter-Douglass B, Witkin JM, et al (1995) NMDA antagonist properties of the putative antiaddictive drug, ibogaine. J Pharmacol Exp Ther 275:753–760

28. Slemmer JE, Martin BR, Damaj MI (2000) Bupropion is a nicotinic antagonist. J Pharmacol Exp Ther 295(1):321–327

29. Yamakura T, Chavez-Noriega LE, Harris RA (2000) Subunit-dependent inhibition of human neuronal nicotinic acetylcholine receptors and other ligand-gated ion channels by dissociative anesthetics ketamine and dizocilpine. Anesthesiology 92(4):1144–1153

30. Ke L, Lukas RJ (1996) Effects of steroid exposure on ligand binding and functional activities of diverse nicotinic acetylcholine receptor subtypes. J Neurochem 67:1100–1112

31. Paradiso K, Sabey K, Evers AS, Zorumski CF, Covey DF, Steinbach JH (2000) Steroid inhibition of rat neuronal nicotinic alpha4beta2 receptors expressed in HEK 293 cells. Mol Pharmacol 58(2):341–351

32. Valera S, Ballivet M, Bertrand D (1992) Progesterone modulates a neuronal nicotinic acetylcholine receptor. Proc Natl Acad Sci U S A 89:9949–9953

33. Wang HY, Lee DH, Davis CB, Shank RP (2000) Amyloid peptide Abeta(1–42) binds selectively and with picomolar affinity to alpha7 nicotinic acetylcholine receptors. J Neurochem 75:1155–1161

34. Balfour DJ (1994) Neural mechanisms underlying nicotine dependence. Addiction 89(11): 1419–1423

35. Benwell ME, Balfour JK (1985) Nicotine binding to brain tissue from drug-naive and nicotine-treated rats. J Pharm Pharmacol 37(6):405–409

36. Marks MJ, Burch JB, Collins AC (1983) Effects of chronic nicotine infusion on tolerance development and nicotinic receptors. J Pharmacol Exp Ther 226(3):817–825

37. Schwartz RD, Kellar KJ (1983) Nicotinic cholinergic receptor binding sites in the brain: regulation in vivo. Science 220(4593):214–216

38. Wonnacott S, Irons J, Rapier C, Thorne B, Lunt GG (1989) Presynaptic modulation of transmitter release by nicotinic receptors. Prog Brain Res 79:157–163

39. Marks MJ, Pauly JR, Gross SD, Deneris ES, Hermans-Borgmeyer I, Heinemann SF, et al (1992) Nicotine binding and nicotinic receptor subunit RNA after chronic nicotine treatment. J Neurosci 12(7):2765–2784

40. Clarke PB, Pert A (1985) Autoradiographic evidence for nicotine receptors on nigrostriatal and mesolimbic dopaminergic neurons. Brain Res 348(2):355–358

41. Corrigall WA, Franklin KB, Coen KM, Clarke PB (1992) The mesolimbic dopaminergic system is implicated in the reinforcing effects of nicotine. Psychopharmacology (Berl) 107(2–3): 285–289

42. Dani JA, Heinemann S (1996) Molecular and cellular aspects of nicotine abuse. Neuron 16(5): 905–908

43. Balfour DJ, Benwell ME, Birrell CE, Kelly RJ, Al Aloul M (1998) Sensitization of the mesoaccumbens dopamine response to nicotine. Pharmacol Biochem Behav 59:1021–1030

44. Wise RA, Bozarth MA (1987) A psychomotor stimulant theory of addiction. Psychol Rev 94(4):469–492

45. Joseph MH, Young AM, Gray JA (1996) Are neurochemistry and reinforcement enough – can the abuse potential of drugs be explained by common actions an a dopamine reward system in the brain? Hum Psychopharmacol 11:55–63

46. Henschler D. Tabak S (1992) In: Pharmakologie und Toxikologie, 6.Aufl. Hrsg. W. Forth, D. Henschler, W. Rummel, K. Starke. Wissenschaftsverlag, Mannheim pp 809–815

47. Roth L, Daunderer M, Korman K (Hrsg) (1984) Giftpflanzen-Pflanzengifte: Vorkommen-Wirkung-Therapie. Nicotin, S. IV-3-N, ecomed, Landsberg, pp 3–5

48. Quensel M, Agardh CD, Nilsson-Ehle P (1989) Nicotine does not affect plasma lipoprotein concentrations in healthy men. Scand J Clin Lab Invest 49(2):149–153

49. Warburton DM (1989) Nicotine: an addictive substance or a therapeutic agent? Prog Drug Res 33:9–41

50. Winternitz WW, Quillen D (1977) Acute hormonal response to cigarette smoking. J Clin Pharmacol 17(7):389–397

51. Targovnik JH (1989) Nicotine, corticotropin, and smoking withdrawal symptoms: literature review and implications for successful control of nicotine addiction. Clin Ther 11(6):846–853

52. Benowitz NL (1988) Pharmacologic aspects of cigarette smoking and nicotine addiction. N Engl J Med 319:1318–1330

53. Guthrie SK, Ni L, Zubieta JK, Teter CJ, Domino EF (2004) Changes in craving for a cigarette and arterial nicotine plasma concentrations in abstinent smokers. Prog Neuropsychopharmacol Biol Psychiatry 28(4):617–623

54. Jaffe JH (1985) Drug addiction and drug abuse: nicotine and tobacco. In: Gilman AG, Goldman LS, Rall TW, Murrad S (eds) Goodman and Gilman's the pharmacological basis of therapeutics. Macmillan, New York, pp 554–558

55. Benowitz NL, Porchet H, Jacob P (1990) Pharmacokinetics, metabolism and pharmacodynamics of nicotine. In: Wonnacott S, Russel MAH, Stolerman IP (eds) Nicotine psychopharmacology: molecular, cellular and behavioral aspects. Oxford University Press, New York, pp 112–157

56. Henningfield JE, Stapleton JM, Benowitz NL, Grayson RF, London ED (1993) Higher levels of nicotine in arterial than in venous blood after cigarette smoking. Drug Alcohol Depend 33(1):23–29

57. Benowitz NL, Jacob P III (1984) Nicotine and carbon monoxide intake from high- and low-yield cigarettes. Clin Pharmacol Ther 36:265–270

58. Zevin S, Gourlay SG, Benowitz NL (1998) Clinical pharmacology of nicotine. Clin Dermatol 16(5):557–564

59. Hoffmann D, Wynder EL (1994) Aktives und Passives Rauchen. In: Marquardt H, Schäfer SG (eds) Lehrbuch der Toxikologie. Wissenschaftsverlag, Mannheim, pp S.589–S.605

60. Acosta M, Buchhalter A, Breland A, Hamilton D, Eissenberg T (2004) Urine cotinine as an index of smoking status in smokers during 96-hr abstinence: comparison between gas chromatography/mass spectrometry and immunoassay test strips. Nicotine Tob Res 6(4):615–620

61. Schneider NG, Lunell E, Olmstead RE, Fagerstrom KO (1996) Clinical pharmacokinetics of nasal nicotine delivery. A review and comparison to other nicotine systems. Clin Pharmacokinet 31(1):65–80

62. Benowitz NL (1990) Pharmacokinetic considerations in understanding nicotine dependence. In: Bock G, Marsh J (eds) The biology of nicotine dependence. Ciba Foundation symposium 152. Wiley, Chichester, pp 186–209

63. Benowitz NL, Porchet H, Sheiner L, Jacob P (1988) Nicotine absorbtion and cardiovascular effects with smokeless tobacco use: comparison with cigarettes and nicotin gum. Clin Pharamcol Ther 5:23–28

64. Henningfield JE, Miyasato K, Jasinski DR (1985) Abuse liability and pharmacodynamic characteristics of intravenous and inhaled nicotine. J Pharmacol Exp Ther 234:1–12

65. Benowitz NL, Jaffe JH (1985) Drug addiction an drug abuse: nicotine and tobacco. In: Gilman AG, Goodman AS, Rall TW, Murrad F (eds) Goodman and Gilman's the pharmacological basis of therapeutics. Macmillan, New York, pp 554–558

66. Stein EA, Pankiewicz J, Harsch HH, Cho JK, Fuller SA, Hoffmann RG, et al (1998) Nicotine-induced limbic cortical activation in the human brain: a functional MRI study. Am J Psychiatry 155:1009–1015

67. Van Den Eijnden R., Spijkerman R, Fekkes D (2003) Craving for cigarettes among low and high dependent smokers: impact of norharman. Addict Biol 8(4):463–472

68. Fagerstrom KO, Kunze M, Schoberberger R, Breslau N, Hughes JR, Hurt RD, et al (1996) Nicotine dependence versus smoking prevalence: comparisons among countries and categories of smokers. Tob Control 5(1):52–56
69. American Psychiatric Association (1994) Diagnostic and statistical manual of mental disorder DSM-IV, 4th edn. American Psychatric Association, Washington
70. Goldberg SR, Spealman RD, Goldberg DM (1981) Persistent behavior at high rates maintained by intravenous self-administration of nicotine. Science 214(4520):573–575
71. Spitz MR, Shi H, Yang F, Hudmon KS, Jiang H, Chamberlain RM, et al (1998) Case-control study of the D2 dopamine receptor gene and smoking status in lung cancer patients. J Natl Cancer Inst 90(5):358–363
72. Clarke PB (1990) Dopaminergic mechanisms in the locomotor stimulant effects of nicotine. Biochem Pharmacol 40(7):1427–1432
73. Leshner AI (1996) Understanding drug addiction: implications for treatment. Hosp Pract 31: 47–49
74. Clarke PB (1998) Tobacco smoking, genes, and dopamine. Lancet 352(9122):84–85
75. Benwell ME, Balfour DJ, Lucchi HM (1993) Influence of tetrodotoxin and calcium on changes in extracellular dopamine levels evoked by systemic nicotine. Psychopharmacology (Berl) 112(4):467–474
76. Nisell M, Nomikos GG, Svensson TH (1994) Systemic nicotine-induced dopamine release in the rat nucleus accumbens is regulated by nicotinic receptors in the ventral tegmental area. Synapse 16(1):36–44
77. Shoaib M, Benwell ME, Akbar MT, Stolerman IP, Balfour DJ (1994) Behavioural and neurochemical adaptations to nicotine in rats: influence of NMDA antagonists. Br J Pharmacol 111(4): 1073–1080
78. Benwell MEM, Balfour DJK, Anderson JM (1990) Smoking associated changes in serotonergic systems of discrete regions of human brain. Psychopharmacology 102:68–72
79. Benwell MEM, Balfour DJK (1979) Effects of nicotine administration and its withdrawal an plasma corticosterone and brain 5-hydroxinidoles. Psychopharmacology 4:7–11
80. Graeff FG, Guimaraes FS, De Andrade TG, Deakin JF (1996) Role of 5-HT in stress, anxiety, and depression. Pharmacol Biochem Behav 54(1):129–141
81. Brioni JD, O'Neill AB, Kim DJ, Buckley MJ, Decker MW, Arneric SP (1994) Anxiolytic-like effects of the novel cholinergic channel activator ABT-418. J Pharmacol Exp Ther 271(1): 353–361
82. Costall B, Kelly ME, Naylor RJ, Onaivi ES (1989) The actions of nicotine and cocaine in a mouse model of anxiety. Pharmacol Biochem Behav 33(1):197–203
83. Morrison CF (1969) The effects of nicotine on punished behaviour. Psychopharmacologia 14(3):221–232
84. Ribeiro EB, Bettiker RL, Bogdanov M, Wurtman RJ (1993) Effects of systemic nicotine on serotonin release in rat brain. Brain Res 621(2):311–318
85. Deakin JFW, Graeff FG (1991) 5-HT and mechanisms of defence. J Psychopharmacol 5:305–315
86. Breslau N, Kilbey MM, Andreski P (1993) Nicotine dependence and major depression. New evidence from a prospective investigation. Arch Gen Psychiatry 50(1):31–35
87. Pomerleau OF, Pomerleau CS (1984) Neuroregulators and the reinforcement of smoking: towards a biobehavioral explanation. Neurosci Biobehav Rev 8:503–513
88. Aceto MD, Scates SM, Ji Z, Bowman ER (1993) Nicotine's opioid and anti-opioid interactions: proposed role in smoking behavior. Eur J Pharmacol 248:333–335
89. Chait LD, Griffiths RR (1984) Effects of methadone on human cigarette smoking and subjective ratings. J Pharmacol Exp Ther 229:636–640
90. Mello NK, Mendelson JH, Sellers ML, Kuehnle JC (1980) Effects of heroin self-administration on cigarette smoking. Psychopharmacology 67:45–52

91. Ismail Z, el Guebaly N (1998) Nicotine and endogenous opioids: toward specific pharmacotherapy. Can J Psychiatry 43:37–42

92. Albuquerque EX, Pereira EF, Mike A, Eisenberg HM, Maelicke A, Alkondon M (2000) Neuronal nicotinic receptors in synaptic functions in humans and rats: physiological and clinical relevance. Behav Brain Res 113(1–2):131–141

93. Kushner SA, Dewey SL, Kornetsky C (1997) Gamma-vinyl GABA attenuates cocaine-induced lowering of brain stimulation reward thresholds. Psychopharmacology 133(4):383–388

94. Smolders I, Khan GM, Lindekens H, Prikken S, Marvin CA, Manil J, et al (1997) Effectiveness of vigabatrin against focally evoked pilocarpine-induced seizures and concomitant changes in extracellular hippocampal and cerebellar glutamate, gamma-aminobutyric acid and dopamine levels, a microdialysis-electrocorticography study in freely moving rats. J Pharmacol Exp Ther 283(3):1239–1248

95. Bailey SL, Ennett ST, Ringwalt CL (1993) Potential mediators, moderators, or independent effects in the relationship between parents' former and current cigarette use and their children's cigarette use. Addict Behav 18(6):601–621

96. Koopmans JR, van Doornen LJ, Boomsma DI (1997) Association between alcohol use and smoking in adolescent and young adult twins: a bivariate genetic analysis. Alcohol Clin Exp Res 21(3):537–546

97. Hannah MC, Hopper JL, Mathews JD (1985) Twin concordance for a binary trait. II. Nested analysis of ever-smoking and ex-smoking traits and unnested analysis of a "committed-smoking" trait. Am J Hum Genet 37(1):153–165

98. Heath AC, Madden PA, Slutske WS, Martin NG (1995) Personality and the inheritance of smoking behavior: a genetic perspective. Behav Genet 25(2):103–117

99. Reuter M, Hennig J (2005) Pleiotropic effect of the TPH A779C polymorphism on nicotine dependence and personality. Am J Med Genet B Neuropsychiatr Genet 134(1):20–24

100. Anney RJ, Olsson CA, Lotfi-Miri M, Patton GC, Williamson R (2004) Nicotine dependence in a prospective population-based study of adolescents: the protective role of a functional tyrosine hydroxylase polymorphism. Pharmacogenetics 14(2):73–81

101. Pianezza ML, Sellers EM, Tyndale RF (1998) Nicotine metabolism defect reduces smoking. Nature 393(6687):750

102. Oscarson M, Gullsten H, Rautio A, Bernal ML, Sinues B, Dahl ML, et al (1998) Genotyping of human cytochrome P450 2A6 (CYP2A6), a nicotine C-oxidase. FEBS Lett 438(3):201–205

103. Carr LA, Basham JK, York BK, Rowell PP (1992) Inhibition of uptake of 1-methyl-4-phenylpyridinium ion and dopamine in striatal synaptosomes by tobacco smoke components. Eur J Pharmacol 215:285–287

104. Di Chiara G, Imperato A (1988) Drugs abused by humans preferentially increase synaptic dopamine concentrations in the mesolimbic system of freely moving rats. Proc Natl Acad Sci U S A 85:5274–5278

105. Henningfield JE, Schuh LM, Jarvik ME (1995) Pathophysiology of tobacco dependence. In: Bloom FE, Kupfer DJ (eds) Psychopharmacology: the fourth generation of progress. Raven, New York, pp 1715–1730

106. O'Neill MF, Dourish CT, Iversen SD (1991) Evidence for an involvement of D1 and D2 dopamine receptors in mediating nicotine-induced hyperactivity in rats. Psychopharmacology 104:343–350

107. Noble EP, Blum K, Ritchie T, Montgomery A, Sheridan PJ (1991) Allelic association of the D2 dopamine receptor gene with receptor-binding characteristics in alcoholism. Arch Gen Psychiatry 48:648–654

108. Blum K, Noble EP, Sheridan PJ, Montgomery A, Ritchie T, Jagadeeswaran P, et al (1990) Allelic association of human dopamine D2 receptor gene in alcoholism. JAMA 263(15):2055–2060

109. Comings DE, Muhleman D, Gysin R (1996) Dopamine D2 receptor (DRD2) gene and susceptibility to posttraumatic stress disorder: a study and replication. Biol Psychiatry 40(5):368–372

110. Comings DE, Ferry L, Bradshaw-Robinson S, Burchette R, Chiu C, Muhleman D (1996) The dopamine D2 receptor (DRD2) gene: a genetic risk factor in smoking. Pharmacogenetics 6:73–79
111. Noble EP, Noble RE, Ritchie T, Syndulko K, Bohlman MC, Noble LA, et al (1994) D2 dopamine receptor gene and obesity. Int J Eat Disord 15:205–217
112. Goldman D, Brown GL, Albaugh B, Goodson S, Trunzo M, Akhtar L, Wynne DK, et al (1994) D2 receptor genotype and linkage disequilibrium and function in Finnish, American Indian, and U. S. Caucasian patients. In: Gershon ES, Cloninger CR (eds) Genetic approaches to mental disorders. American Psychiatric Press, Washington, pp 327–344
113. Noble EP, Blum K, Khalsa ME, Ritchie T, Montgomery A, Wood RC, et al (1993) Allelic association of the D2 dopamine receptor gene with cocaine dependence. Drug Alcohol Depend 33(3):271–285
114. Blum K, Noble EP, Sheridan PJ, Montgomery A, Ritchie T, Ozkaragoz T, et al (1993) Genetic predisposition in alcoholism: association of the D2 dopamine receptor TaqI B1 RFLP with severe alcoholics. Alcohol 10(1):59–67
115. Noble EP (1993) The D2 dopamine receptor gene: a review of association studies in alcoholism. Behav Genet 23(2):119–129
116. Bannon MJ, Granneman JG, Kapatos G (1995) The dopamine transporter: potential involvement in neuropsychiatric disorders. In: Bloom FE, Kupfer DJ (eds) Psychopharmacology: the fourth generation of progress. Raven Press, New York, pp 179–188
117. Seeman P, Niznik HB (1990) Dopamine receptors and transporters in Parkinson's disease and schizophrenia. FASEB J 4:2737–2744
118. Cook EH Jr, Stein MA, Krasowski MD, Cox NJ, Olkon DM, Kieffer JE, et al (1995) Association of attention-deficit disorder and the dopamine transporter gene. Am J Hum Genet 56:993–998
119. Comings DE, Wu S, Chiu C, Ring RH, Gade R, Ahn C, et al (1996) Polygenic inheritance of Tourette syndrome, stuttering, attention deficit hyperactivity, conduct, and oppositional defiant disorder: the additive and subtractive effect of the three dopaminergic genes – DRD2, D beta H, and DAT1. Am J Med Genet 67:264–288
120. Vandenbergh DJ, Persico AM, Hawkins AL, Griffin CA, Li X, Jabs EW, et al (1992) Human dopamine transporter gene (DAT1) maps to chromosome 5p15.3 and displays a VNTR. Genomics 14:1104–1106
121. Gelernter J, O'Malley S, Risch N, Kranzler HR, Krystal J, Merikangas K, et al (1991) No association between an allele at the D2 dopamine receptor gene (DRD2) and alcoholism. JAMA 266:1801–1807
122. Lerman C, Caporaso NE, Audrain J, Main D, Bowman ED, Lockshin B, et al (1999) Evidence suggesting the role of specific genetic factors in cigarette smoking. Health Psychol 18(1):14–20
123. George SR, Cheng R, Nguyen T, Israel Y, O'Dowd BF (1993) Polymorphisms of the D4 dopamine receptor alleles in chronic alcoholism. Biochem Biophys Res Commun 196(1):107–114
124. True WR, Xian H, Scherrer JF, Madden PA, Bucholz KK, Heath AC, et al (1999) Common genetic vulnerability for nicotine and alcohol dependence in men. Arch Gen Psychiatry 56(7):655–661
125. Yates WR, Cadoret RJ, Troughton EP, Stewart M, Giunta TS (1998) Effect of fetal alcohol exposure on adult symptoms of nicotine, alcohol, and drug dependence. Alcohol Clin Exp Res 22(4):914–920
126. West R, Hajek P (1997) What happens to anxiety levels on giving up smoking? Am J Psychiatry 154(11):1589–1592
127. Clarke PB (1990) Dopaminergic mechanisms in the locomotor stimulant effects of nicotine. Biochem Pharmacol 40(7):1427–1432

Smoking and Lung Disease

5

Before affecting numerous other organs, smoking primarily causes damage to the respiratory tract, the arena where almost half of all smoking-related harmful effects unfold. A high proportion of these harmful effects – lung cancer and chronic obstructive pulmonary disease (COPD) – have a fatal outcome [1]. Lung cancer is the commonest form of cancer in the USA. Due to the increasing popularity of smoking among women, the prevalence of lung cancer in women has increased fourfold over the last 30 years and this figure will continue to rise [2]. Moreover, smokers die from COPD ten times more commonly than non-smokers, making COPD one of the leading causes of death in the USA [3].

Smoking must also be regarded as a principal cause of the increase in childhood disorders and diseases of the respiratory tract. New cases of bronchial asthma are reported in 8,000–26,000 children annually in the USA [4], not to mention other pulmonary diseases, including colds, bronchiolitis and a pulmonary haemorrhagic syndrome. Smoking affects the permeability of the lungs and has an impact on systemic immune mechanisms that are responsible for numerous reactions.

5.1
Immunological Reactions Caused by Cigarette Smoking

Unlike non-smokers, smokers suffer from inflammatory changes to cells in the bronchial tract, as has been demonstrated by bronchoalveolar lavage (BAL) [5]:

- The cell count in the lavage fluid is tripled
- There is a pro-rata increase in the macrophage count and a sixfold increase in the neutrophil count
- The eosinophil count is increased
- The percentage of lymphocytes is reduced (reduced proportion of T-helper cells, increased proportion of T-suppressor cells, reduced helper: suppressor ratio)
- IgM and IgG concentrations in the bronchial system are raised

Alveolar macrophages are immunologically active in that they form antigen-bearing cells and facilitate lymphocytic reactions [6]. The macrophages of smokers contain smoke residues

K.-O. Haustein, D. Groneberg, *Tobacco or Health?*
DOI: 10.1007/978-3-540-87577-2_5, © Springer Verlag Berlin Heidelberg 2010

and display an abnormal cell surface [7]. The alveolar macrophages of smokers exhibit abnormal cytokine reactions in response to a variety of stimuli [8–10]. Unlike lymphocytes from peripheral blood, lymphocytes from smokers' lungs display diminished proliferative responses to mitogens (polynuclear hydrocarbons and concanavalin A) [11]. In smokers, the total white cell count, including polymorphonuclear cells, eosinophils, monocytes and T-lymphocytes, is increased [12]: killer T-lymphocyte counts in smokers are reduced, but revert to normal levels within 1 month after smoking cessation [13]. Serum concentrations of IgG and IgE are elevated in smokers [14]. Some of the reactions described are probably promoted by immunological processes [15]. The increased permeability of pulmonary capillaries is also a consequence of inflammatory reactions.

5.2
Cigarette Smoking and Lung Cancer

For the most part a disease with a fatal outcome, lung cancer is on the increase and is caused primarily by cigarette smoking, as demonstrated by numerous studies from all over the world (Table 5.1). Lung cancer may be causally related to cigarette smoking in 90% of cases in men and in 79% of cases in women [17]. Conversely, 85% of all cases of lung cancer would be preventable if cigarette smoking were to be given up [18]. Likewise, there are established associations between passive smoking and susceptibility to lung cancer [19, 20]. Female smokers are at very much greater risk than male smokers for developing adenocarcinoma (AC) of the lung [21]. Age of smoking initiation and the number of cigarettes smoked daily are crucial determinants of the risk for bronchial carcinoma, with smoking initiation in early adolescence leading primarily to small cell bronchial carcinoma (odds ratio (OR) 3.0 [95% CI: 1.1–8.4]); furthermore, this risk is not abolished by smoking cessation [22]. An association has been demonstrated between disease prevalence

Table 5.1 Smokers' increased risk for developing lung cancer, based on data from prospective studies. The risk for non-smokers is 1.00 [16]

Population	Number	Deaths	Cigarette smokers
British doctors	34,000 (M)	441	14.0
	6,104 (F)	27	5.0
Swedish Study	27,000 (M)	55	7.0
	28,000 (F)	8	4.5
Japanese Study	122,000 (M)	940	3.76
	143,000 (F)	304	2.03
ACS "25 State Study"	358,000 (M)	2,018	8.53
	483,000 (F)	439	3.53
US Veterans Study	290,000 (M)	3,126	11.28
Canadian Veterans	78,000 (M)	331	14.20
ACS "9 State Study"	188,000 (M)	448	10.73
Californian men (nine occupational groups)	68,000 (M)	368	7.81

M male; *F* female

and sociological differences among smokers [23]. Smoking cessation can reduce the development of squamous cell carcinoma (SCC) or AC.

A survey of smoking behaviour comparing patients with bronchial carcinoma and controls revealed an increased risk (OR) of 14.9 for cigarette smokers, 9.0 for cigar and cigarillo smokers and 7.9 for pipe smokers. In all three groups, the duration and intensity of smoking were co-determinants of cancer development [24]. The risk of cancer has been shown to be increased by consumption of dark tobacco varieties [11, 25, 26]. Lifetime filter cigarette smoking in men and women reduces the frequency of SCC, but not of AC of the lung [27].

There has been a rapid rise in lung cancer in all countries of the world where cigarette consumption has increased. Lung cancer incidence in the USA has increased 2.5-fold since 1950 [28], reflecting the spiralling rise in cigarette consumption during the period after the First World War and continuing into the 1960s. The risk of death from lung cancer is 20 times higher among women who smoke two or more packs of cigarettes per day than women who do not smoke. Since 1950, there has been a 600% increase in death rates from lung cancer among women (Fig. 5.1), primarily caused by cigarette smoking [29]. Corresponding studies have confirmed similar increases for many countries [30–32]. A total of 590,000 smokers died of lung cancer in the developed countries in 1995 alone [31]. Rising lung cancer mortality should be viewed not only in terms of the increasing prevalence of the disease, but also of its extremely lethal nature; treatment successes have had only marginal impact on the 5-year survival rate when all tumour types are taken into account. According to one study conducted in 118,000 Californians, between 1960 and 1997, lung cancer deaths increased in men (from 1558 to 1728) and even more clearly in women (from 208 to 806) [29]. The number of cigarettes smoked correlates very closely with the increased lung cancer risk [33, 34].

The question as to whether women are more sensitive than men to the toxic products of smoke has been answered in the negative for the time being on the basis of the data from the Renfrew and Paisley study [35]. According to these results, all-cause mortality in men was slightly higher than in women where both men and women were light smokers

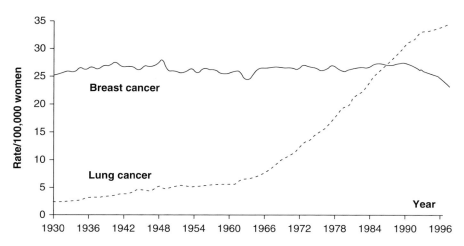

Fig. 5.1 Age-adjusted death rates for lung cancer and breast cancer among women in the United States from 1930 to 1996. Death rates were age-adjusted to the 1970 population [29]

(OR = 1.83 [1.61–2.07] vs. 1.41 [1.28–1.56]; p = −0.001). This difference was also reflected in the cause-specific mortality in men and women for neoplasms (OR = −2.57 [2.01–3.29] vs. 1.35 [1.14–1.61] and for lung cancer (OR = −11.10 [5.89–20.92] vs. 4.73 [2.99–7.50]; p = −0.03) [35]. No gender-specific sensitivity can be deduced from these data.

5.2.1
Association Between Smoking and Lung Cancer

In addition to cigarette smoking and the carcinogens inhaled in the process, (a) genetic disposition, (b) lifestyle and (c) environmental factors are important in the development of lung cancer.

Because activation of toxic (carcinogenic) substances depends on the inducibility of the cytochrome system, it is of interest that this enzyme inducibility is not limited to the liver, but it exists also in several other tissues [36]. The rat liver shows minimal or no reaction to the inducing activity of tobacco smoke [37]. Drug-metabolizing enzymes in other tissues of rats exposed to cigarette smoke were increased three- to tenfold, indicating the inducibility of these tissues [37–41]. On the basis of these experiments, it appears possible that carcinogenics are activated in several tissues, including the lung.

In the 1940s, German researchers had already produced scientific evidence to show an association between cigarette smoking and lung cancer development [28] (see Sect. 1.8 in Chap. 1). In the 1950s, a proven correlation was established in retrospective studies in which relative risks were calculated in comparison with patterns in non-smokers [42]. Prospective cohort studies in the 1950s and 1960s substantiated these findings, culminating in the Surgeon General's Advisory Committee report on Smoking and Health in the USA in 1964 [43]. This had been preceded by research in various countries in large numbers of smokers and non-smokers designed to calculate relative risks; also considering the plausibility of a causal association, these studies also investigated carcinogenesis and evidence for any dose–response relationship [44]. Other factors taken into consideration included age at smoking initiation [44–46], pack-years of smoking, depth of inhalation [45] and the tar and nicotine yields of the cigarettes smoked [42, 47–52]. Despite lower tar and nicotine yields, the prevalence of cancer in smokers is higher than in non-smokers. Lung cancer occurs chronologically and sequentially after smoking initiation (Table 5.1). Premalignant cells have been detected in the bronchial epithelium of smokers, but not of non-smokers [53, 54]; these cell alterations have been found to be reversed after smoking cessation. Figures 5.2 and 5.3 show illustrative cases of SCC and AC in patients who had smoked for decades and who subsequently died of their disease.

When DNA adducts in non-carcinomatous altered lung tissue and mononuclear cells from smokers were measured as risk factors for the development of bronchial carcinoma, significant correlations were found between the number of aromatic hydrophobic DNA adducts and pack-years of smoking. These adducts were more pronounced in current smokers than in ex-smokers (Fig. 5.4) [56]. Particular attention must be paid to changes occurring more commonly in adolescent smokers because these are also important for the premature development of tumours.

One study published only recently considered the influence of cigar smoking on disease prevalence: a population of 17,774 men (of whom 1,546 were cigar smokers) was

Fig. 5.2 Endoscopic view of an occluding bronchial carcinoma after laser coagulation has already been initiated in a 55-year-old patient with a 25-year history of smoking (by kind permission of Prof. Drings, Heidelberg)

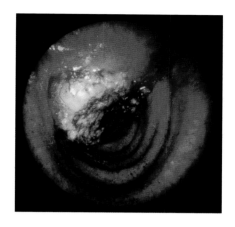

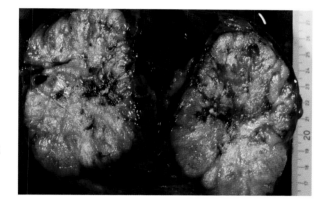

Fig. 5.3 Large adenocarcinoma of the right superior lobe following surgical resection from a 63-year-old smoker (surgery performed by Prof. Vogt-Moykopf, Heidelberg)

followed from 1971 to 1995. The risk (OR) for oropharyngeal cancer increased to 2.02 and for lung cancer to 2.14 [7]. Despite the fact that they continued smoking, cigarette smokers who switched to cigar or pipe had a somewhat reduced risk of lung cancer than would have been the case if they had continued smoking cigarettes, but switching tobacco products did not enable them to achieve the lower risk level of ex-smokers [57].

On the contrary, despite suspicions, mentholated cigarettes, which are smoked in preference in some countries, do not entail any additional risk for bronchial carcinoma [58].

Lung cancer is the most important risk factor for women, more so than for men. The risk increases in line with the dose (i.e., the number of cigarettes smoked) and is not lowered by dietary factors (β-carotene).

5.2.2
Types of Lung Cancer

Smoking encourages the development of all types of lung cancer: SCC, AC, small cell carcinoma and undifferentiated carcinoma. In this last category, the origin of the cells cannot

Fig. 5.4 Renal excretion of von 1-hydroxypyrene (**a**), benzo[*a*]pyrene adducts of haemoglobin (**b**) and of albumin (**c**) in 42 non-smokers and 27 smokers, classified by suburban or rural location of residence. The *vertical lines* show the standard error of the mean. $p = 0.056$ [55]

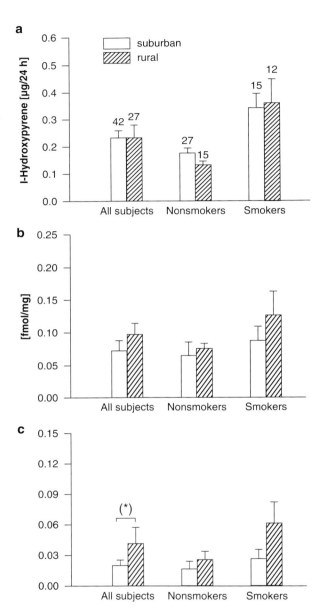

be identified [17, 59]. Whereas SCC used to be the predominant type, for about the last 10 years, it has been overtaken by AC, with small cell and undifferentiated carcinoma in third and fourth positions [60]. The change in incidence is thought to be due to the switch to low-tar and low-nicotine cigarette brands [61] where inhalation depth and frequency and nitro-samine exposure are increased [62]. As a result, smaller, less well-protected bronchial regions come into contact with smoke constituents, and this may be one reason for the change in predominant tumour type.

5.2.3
Genetic Factors That Increase the Risk for Bronchial Carcinoma

Shifts are plainly occurring in the presentation of different lung cancer types. While there has been a proportional decrease in SCC, AC has become more common, possibly due to the reduction in polynuclear aromatic hydrocarbons (PAH) in inhaled smoke from filtered low-yield cigarettes [27]. The enzymes CYP1A1 and GSTM1 play a major role in the metabolic activation and detoxification of PAH, while CYP2E1 is responsible more for the metabolic activation of nitrosamines. One case-control study conducted in 341 incident lung cancer cases compared with 456 healthy controls confirmed a 2.4-fold increase in the risk for SCC where the CYP1A1 MspI variant allele was present, and a 3.1-fold increase when this was combined with a GSTM1 deletion [63]. In contrast, CYP2E1 RsaI and DraI polymorphisms did not correlate with SCC risk; however, the presence of these enzyme variants was associated with a tenfold reduction in the risk for small cell lung cancer (SCLC), while AC development was encouraged by CYP2E1 mutants [63].

On stratified analysis, it is found that the polymorphic metabolic/oxidative enzyme myeloperoxidase (MPO) genotypes modified the effect of asbestos exposure on lung cancer risk. Specifically, G/G carriers who were exposed to asbestos had a higher risk, while A-allele carriers (G/A + A/A) showed a reduced OR of 0.89 (95% CI; 0.56–1.44). The A-allele genotypes, therefore, demonstrated protective effects on the development of lung cancer.

5.2.3.1
Tobacco-Specific Carcinogens

Several products have been implicated in the development of cancer in smokers: PAH, tobacco-specific nitrosamines (TSNA) und aromatic amines (AA). The metabolism of these toxic substances plays a crucial role, and this process may be influenced to a major extent by genetic differences in the metabolising cytochrome P450 (CYP) enzymes and by the glutathione S-transferase (GST) system.

Benzo[a]pyrene activates oncogenes and interacts with DNA; it also promotes the formation of diol-epoxides as key reactive substances. Benzo[a]pyrene undergoes transformation to phenol metabolites and benzo[a]pyrene-7,8-diole by the action of cytochrome enzymes such as epoxide hydrolases and other isoenzymes; the latter form the highly reactive (+)-anti-benzo[a]pyrene diol-epoxide (BPDE), which is a good substrate for GST M1, M2, M3 and an even better substrate for GSTPI [39]. These metabolic products have also been detected in lung tissue and in lymphocytes [36].

4-Methylnitrosoamino-1,3-pyridyl-1-butanone (NNK) and N'-nitrosonornicotine (NNN) (cf. Box 3.1in Chap. 3) are the most important TSNA; they are formed in unburned tobacco and during combustion. Smokers are principally confronted with both substances, though NNK in particular produces cancer in the upper respiratory tract. The metabolic pathways of NNK in humans and animals are identical. NNK doses absorbed by humans are definitely carcinogenic in animal experiments. Prior to binding to DNA, both nitrosamines require activation (α-methyl or α-methylene hydroxylation, pyridine-N-oxidation by CYP-mediated reactions and glucuronidation) [64, 65]. The alcohol from NNK is excreted in the urine and serves as an indicator for NNK exposure.

The AA, including 4-aminobiphenyl, are compounds that play a particular role in the development of carcinoma of the bladder [66] and therefore, will not be discussed further in the present context.

DNA damage is also produced as a result of oxidation processes and by lipid peroxidation. Inhaled material from tobacco contains oxygen and nitrogen groups, which react with the various body tissues in smokers. Consequently, oxidative DNA damage due to products formed by lipid peroxidation (malondialdehyde, crotonaldehyde, trans-4-OH-2-nonenal) is commonly found in the respiratory tract tissues of smokers. These metabolites are epoxidised by CYP-mediated reactions and form promutagenic DNA adducts in human tissue [40, 67, 68], leading to an increased cancer risk for the upper respiratory tract [41]. Chewing tobacco with or without betel produces cancers in the oral cavity [69].

5.2.3.2
The Cytochrome P450 and GST System and Carcinogenesis

Current epidemiological research into carcinogenesis in the lung indicates that several populations are at risk for the development of lung cancer, especially smokers and workers exposed to toxic substances. One genetic factor that deserves particular mention in this context is the induction of aryl hydrocarbon hydroxylase (CYP1A1; AHH). This enzyme transforms the PAH produced by cigarette smoke into compounds that are highly carcinogenic [70]. In addition, oxidation processes are catalysed by the CYP450 system and using debrisoquine-4-hydroxylation (CYP2D6) as a model reaction, a clear distinction can be drawn between lung cancer patients and matched controls [71–73]. Where there is extensive hydroxylation of the "model substance" debrisoquine, the risk for the development of lung cancer is simultaneously increased. To date, however, there are no routine tests for the prophylactic identification of such risk factors. As shown by the data summarised in Fig. 5.4, the renal excretion of carcinogens is higher in smokers than in non-smokers, with slight differences detected in terms of residential environment (suburban or rural) [56]. Several studies have been conducted in patients affected by these problems [66] and the key finding is that metabolites of these inhaled tobacco products form adducts with DNA (Fig. 5.4).

The CYP system plays a central role in the metabolism or activation of carcinogens [68, 74–77]. Case-control studies have revealed associations between tobacco smoke and cancer risks for the lungs, larynx, mouth, oesophagus, kidneys, urinary system and breasts.

CYP1A1: PAH and AA are activated by the enzyme. Approximately 10% of Caucasians have a highly inducible form of CYP1A1 (also known as B[a]P-hydroxylase), in conjunction with an increased risk for tumours of the bronchi, larynx and oral cavity [78]. Four different forms of the cytochrome enzyme 1A1 have been described to date (Table 5.2), though regrettably several nomenclatures are in use. The inducibility of CYP1A1 correlates with the occurrence of bronchial carcinoma [80], with the m2 mutant (Ile-$\rightarrow$-Val)

Table 5.2   Overview of CYP1A1 subforms [79]

Polymorphism	Point mutation	Systematic nomenclature for the mutation
Wild type allele, m1	None	wt
MspI allele, 3′, non-coding region, m2	6,235 T→C	m1
Ile→Val, exon 7, codon 462	4,889 A→G	m2
Afro-American-specific allele, intron 7	5,639 T→C	m3
Thr→Asn, exon 7, codon 461	4,887 C→A	m4

being twice as inducible as the m1 mutant [81]. Smokers with the m2 mutant have more DNA adducts in their leucocytes than smokers without this mutant [82]. These adducts are also increased in the cord venous blood of neonates with CYP1A1-MspI polymorphism [82]. B[a]PDE concentration and PAH-DNA adducts correlate positively with enzyme activity in the parenchymal lung tissue of smokers [36]. Homozygous CYP1A1-MspI alleles are observed more rarely in Caucasians than in Japanese [83].

Associations with CYP1A1 activity have been demonstrated in more than 20 studies in different ethnic populations (see Table 5.3). According to studies from Japan, the lung cancer risk was demonstrated with both m1 and m2 mutants [85]. The CYP1A1 phenotype was important in terms of the development of SCCs only in moderate smokers [88]. The results were not corroborated in Norwegian, Finnish, Swedish and US populations, a finding that was possibly attributable to the smaller occurrence of the m1 allele in Caucasians. Studies conducted in a mixed US population and in French patients showed no evidence of a preferred allele (m1 or m2) for increased cancer prevalence. In one study, individuals with the m3 mutation (m1/m1, m2) had an increased AC risk with an OR of 8.4 [97], whereas other cancer types did not occur with increased frequency (Table 5.3) [30, 97–100]. Where the m1 and m2 variants of CYP1A1 occurred in combination with the GSTM1 0/0 genotype, there was an increased incidence of SCC in Japanese subjects [63, 85, 101].

CYP1A2: This enzyme activates numerous procarcinogens from tobacco, preferentially aromatic and heterocyclic amines, and metabolises nicotine. The sequence of CYP1A2 is 72% identical with that of CYP1A1. However, it is formed principally in the liver and to a very much smaller extent in the lungs [102]. The enzyme is of marginal importance for an increased risk of lung cancer.

CYP2D6: This enzyme metabolises debrisoquine and poor metabolisers (PMs) have a lesser risk for the development of lung cancer than extensive metabolisers (EMs) [71]. However, the enzyme also activates NNK and metabolises nicotine [103]. Associations evidently exist between nicotine dependence and metaboliser status [104]. An increased lung cancer risk has been demonstrated in EMs [63, 93, 105–107], whereas two meta-analyses have rejected such an association on the basis of the data reviewed [22, 107, 108].

CYP2E1: CYP2E1, which is inducible by ethanol and numerous other agents, is capable of metabolising NNK, NNN and other soluble nitrosamines from tobacco smoke. Structural enzyme variants are less important for an increased lung cancer risk in Caucasians, with only 2 out of 11 studies showing such a finding [63, 109, 110]. RsaI and DraI polymorphisms of CYP2E1 have not been shown to correlate with the development of SCC; where these enzyme variants were present, there was a tenfold reduction in the

Table 5.3 CYP enzymes (1A1, 2D6 and 2E1) and the development of lung cancer

Gene, mutant	Cancer types	Cases/ controls	Genotype, frequency (%/%)	Significance (odds ratio; 95% CI)	References
1A1 m1	SCC, AC, SCLC, LCLC	68/104	m1/m1: 23.5/10.6; wt/wt: 35.3/49.0	LC: 3.1; SCC: 4.6	[84]
1A1 m2	SCC, AC	212/358	m2/m2: 12.3/4.7; wt/wt: 56.76/65.1	LC: 2.97 (1.59–5.57); SCC: 3.34 (1.49–7.52); AC: 2.54 (1.48–4.34)	[85]
1A1 m1,m2	SCC	85/170	m1/m1: 22.4/8.8; wt/wt: 38.8/48.2; m2/m2: 10.6/3.5; wt/wt: 58.8/64.7	m1/m1: sm+: 6.55 (2.49–17.24); sm++: 8.32 (2.34–29.62); m2/m2: sm+: 8.46 (2.48–28.85); sm++: 8.46 (1.68–42.73)	[86]
1A1 m1	SCC, AC, SCLC, LCLC	267/151	m1/m1: 16.9/10.6; wt/wt: 36.7/44.3	m1/m1 und m1/wt: 1.71 (1.07–2.69)	[87]
1A1 m1–4	LC	157/314	m3: 0/0; m4: 2.87/2.87	m2: 3.01 (1.29–7.26)	[88]
1A1 m1	AC, SCC	207/283	m1/m1: 1.0/0.7; m1/wt: 16.9/17.0; wt/wt: 82.1/82.3	m1/wt+m1/m1: LC 2.08 (1.15–3.73); AC sm +: 2.25 (1.13–4.48); m1/ wt: LC 1.15 (1.0–2.3)	[89]
1A1 m2	SCC, SCLC, AC	247/185	m2/m2: 11.3/3.8; m2/wt: 38.1/45.4; wt/wt: 50.6/50.8	m2/m2: LC 3.3 (1.3–8.6); SCC 4.9 (1.4–16.3); SCLC 9.4 (2.1–42.0)	[90]
1A1 m1, m2	SCC, AC, SCLC, LCLC	108/95	m1/m1: 22.2/10.5; wt/wt: 36.1/-; m2/ m2: 16.7/6.3; wt/wt: 53.7/–	m1/m1: LC 2.93 (1.26–6.84). m2/m2 LC: 3.45 (1.29–9.25)	[91]
1A1 m1, m2	SCC, SCLC, AC	85/63	m1/m1: 7/5; wt/wt: 40/46; m2/m2: ½; m2/wt: 80/95; wt/wt: 19/3	m2/m2 oder m2/wt: 0.14 (0.03–0.64)	[92]
2D6 *3, *4,*5	SCC, AC	106/122	PM: 0.9/5.7; HEM + EM: 99.1/94.3	EM: 6.4 (1.0–14.3)	[93, 94]
2E1 DraI	SCC, AC, SCLC	47/56	CC: 0/10.7; CD: 46.8/ 30.4; DD: 53.2/59.9	$p < 0.05$	[95, 96]
2E1 DraI	SCC, AC, SCLC, LCLC	91/76	CC: 2.2/14.5; CD: 46.2/ 28.9; 51.6/56.6	CC: 0.13 (0.04–0.51) aber CD: 2.1 (1.1–4.0)	[95, 96]
2E1 DraI, RsaI	SCC, AC, SCLC	341/456	DraI: CC 1.5/5.5; CD: 27.5/26.8; DD 71/ 67.7; RsaI: c2c2 0.6/ 3.1. c1c2: 19.6/22.5; c1c1 79.8/74.4	DraI allele LC: CC 0.2 (0.1–0.7); AC: CC 0.1 (0.0–0.5); RsaI: c2c2: 0.1 (0.0–0.5)	[63]

SCC squamous cell carcinoma; *AC* adenocarcinoma; *SCLC* small cell lung cancer; *LCLC* large cell lung cancer; *LC* lung cancer, *wt* wild type; *PM* poor metaboliser; *EM* extensive metaboliser; *HEM* heterozygous extensive metaboliser, m1 to m4: see Table 5.1, *C* minor Allele; *D* general allele, DraI, RsaI: see text risk for SCLC, while the development of AC was promoted by CYP2E1 mutants [63]. In one further study, the presence of a p53 mutation and a c2/c2 genotype was shown to correlate for the increased occurrence of SCC of the lung [111].

GST System: An unfavourable combination of CYP1A1 with a GSTM1 0/0 gene possibly leads to supra-additive DNA damage and to an increased cancer risk because detoxification may be delayed as a result of slower coupling of carcinogens to the GST system. Moreover, damaged GSTM1 activity is associated with a high inducibility of CYP1A1 by 2,3,7,8-tetrachlorodibenzo-p-dioxin [95], a phenomenon reflected in the detected presence of B[a]PDE adducts in the lung tissue of smokers and encountered primarily in Caucasians. High B[a]PDE-DNA adduct levels in lung tissue in Caucasians were associated with a GSTM1 phenotype defect due to high CYP1A1 inducibility or with a CYP1A1 allele [112, 113]. This constellation leads to tobacco-induced DNA damage and the increased occurrence of lung cancer. A weak correlation has even been found between the number of DNA adducts and the number of cigarettes smoked [20]. A Swedish study has now shown that heavy smokers with a GSTT1-positive genotype have a threefold increased risk for lung cancer with >23 pack-years of smoking (OR 2.6 [1.3–5.0], whereas the risk is increased ninefold (OR 9.3 [1.9–46.3) in smokers with the GSTT1-null genotype [114], a genuine risk constellation. Similar associations have also been reported with N-acetyl transferase (NAT2 genotype as PMs), particularly when combined with the GSTM1-null genotype [115].

These studies indicate that the highest-risk combination for increased susceptibility to lung cancer is the CYP1A1 genotype plus a GSTM1 defect because of the following:

- It results in more B[a]PDE adducts [112, 114–116]
- Approximately 100-fold higher B[a]PDE-DNA levels occur than with an active form of GSTM1 [112]

Carriers of homozygous CYP1A1 m1 have higher BPDE-DNA adduct levels than carriers of wild type CYP1A1 [114]. Thus, whatever their ethnic origin, carriers of the homozygous CYP1A1/GSTM1 0/0 trait are at increased risk for tobacco-induced cancer of the lungs, head and neck.

5.2.3.3
Peptide Receptors, α1-Antitrypsin and Carcinogenesis

Activation of gastrin-releasing peptide receptors (GRPR) in human airways has been associated with cigarette smoking. The GRPR gene is located on the X-chromosome and escapes inactivation, which occurs in females, with the result that women are more susceptible than men to carcinogens. GRPR-mRNA expression was detected in more female than male non-smokers (55 vs. 0%) and short-term smokers (1–25 pack-years: 75 vs. 20%). Female smokers exhibited GRPR-mRNA expression at a lower mean pack-year exposure than male smokers (37.4 vs. 56.3 pack-years; $p = -0.037$), permitting the conclusion that they have a higher susceptibility to tumour development [117].

Despite the known association between α_1-antitrypsin deficiency and COPD, investigations have also been conducted to establish whether heterozygous individuals who carry a deficient allele of the α_1-antitrypsin gene Pi (protease inhibitor) are at an increased risk of developing bronchial carcinoma. The Pi locus is polymorphic with more than 70 variants reported. There are at least ten alleles associated with α_1-antitrypsin deficiency [118]. Non-smokers carried a deficient allele three times more frequently (20.6%) than smokers. Nevertheless, patients with bronchial carcinoma or SCC had higher carrier rates than expected (15.9 and 23.8%, respectively). It may, therefore, be concluded that patients with an α_1-antitrypsin deficiency allele have an increased risk for lung cancer (specifically SCC) [118].

5.2.3.4
Exogenous Factors and Lung Cancer

Dietary factors may be important for the development of lung cancer, and the consumption of carotene-rich fruits and vegetables and high plasma levels of vitamin E and β-carotene are reported to reduce the risk [119]. β-carotene functions as an antioxidant and as a precursor for vitamin A or retinol. Retinoids are responsible for the differentiation of epithelial cells and they may suppress the malignant transformation of epithelial cells [120]. These findings, originally made in retrospective studies, have not been confirmed in prospective studies involving almost 30,000 smokers treated with vitamin E or β-carotene over a period of years. The incidence of cancer even increased (+18%) with β-carotene. The Beta-Carotene and Retinol Efficacy Trial (CARET) also concluded that mortality was increased in the active treatment group [79].

Several studies were also showing that smokers with a low body mass index have a higher risk for developing lung malignancies as compared with smokers of average weight. It is suggested that DNA adducts may play an important role in that mechanism. A current study could show that overweight subjects (BMI > 25) with little weight gain after smoking cessation (<median weight gain of 6%) had more persistent adduct levels as compared with those with lower BMI and higher weight gain ($p = 0.06$). Smokers with a low body mass index have a higher risk for developing lung malignancies as compared with smokers of average weight, but there is no mechanistic explanation for this observation. Carcinogens in cigarette smoke are thought to elicit cancer by the formation of DNA adducts, which give the opportunity to additionally investigate the biological link between BMI and lung cancer. Godschalk et al. published a study in 2002 in which DNA adduct levels in peripheral blood lymphocytes of 24 healthy smoking volunteers (0.76 ± 0.41 adducts per 10(8) nucleotides) positively correlated with cigarette consumption ($r = 0.51; p = 0.01$) and were inversely related with BMI ($r = -0.48; p = 0.02$) [121]. A significant overall relationship was observed when both parameters were included in multiple regression analysis ($r = 0.63; p = 0.007$). Moreover, body composition may affect DNA adduct persistence because lipophilic tobacco smoke-derived carcinogens accumulate in adipose tissue and can be mobilized once exposure ceases. Therefore, DNA adduct levels and BMI were reassessed in all of the subjects after a non-smoking period of 22 weeks. Adduct levels declined to 0.44 ± 0.23 per 10(8) nucleotides ($p = 0.002$) and the estimated half-life was 11 weeks on the basis of exponential decay to background levels in never-smoking controls (0.33 ± 0.18 per 10(8) nucleotides). Overweight subjects (BMI > 25) with little weight gain after smoking cessation (<median weight gain of 6%) had more persistent adduct levels as compared

with those with lower BMI and higher weight gain (p = 0.06). Overall, the authors concluded that leanness is a host susceptibility factor that affects DNA adduct formation, which could underlie the observed relationship between BMI and lung cancer risk [121].

Alcohol does not play a role in smokers in terms of the development of lung cancer. This was demonstrated in a study in 27,111 male smokers, 1,059 of whom developed lung cancer over a period of 7.7 years. Non-drinkers were at increased lung cancer risk compared with drinkers (relative risk = −1.2; 95% CI: 1.0–1.4) [122]. However, additional alcohol consumption is important for the development of cancers in the oral cavity, pharynx, larynx and oesophagus, the risk being twice as high as in patients with a current history of smoking, but without current daily drinking [123].

According to one study from Italy [122], patients with lung cancer and *HIV infection* were younger (38 vs. 53 years) and previously smoked more cigarettes per day (40 vs. 20) than the control group of patients with lung cancer, but without HIV infection. The main histological subtype was AC, with tumour stage TNM III–IV observed in the majority (53%) of patients. The median survival of the HIV patients was significantly shorter than that of the control group (5 vs. 10 months).

The development of lung cancer in smokers is supported by *exposure to asbestos* [124], with the risk being increased by many multiples (20-fold increase compared with non-smoking asbestos workers and 50-fold increase compared with non-smoking and non-asbestos-exposed persons) [25]. Other gaseous substances also encourage the development of bronchial carcinoma: arsenic compounds, chloromethyl ether, chromium, nickel and polynuclear aromatic compounds act synergistically with cigarette smoke [100]. Radon exposure is also associated with an increased risk of bronchial carcinoma due to its storage in lung tissue and high-energy α-radiation [64]. *Smokers employed in uranium mining* have a tenfold increased risk of bronchial carcinoma compared with non-smokers working in the same industry [64, 125, 126]. Even radiation from underground uranium can increase the lung cancer risk in cigarette smokers [64]. Radiation levels of 50 up to 140 Bq/m^3 are measured in various residential areas [127], leading to p53 mutations and increased cancer risk (OR = −1.4; CI: 0.7–2.6; OR for non-smokers = 3.2; CI: 0.7–15.5) [127].

Finally, the risk for bronchial carcinoma may be increased simply as a result of *urbanisation*, mainly due to air pollution [34]. However, this idea has not been confirmed by other studies [6, 18, 66].

Readers are referred to Chap. 3 for a discussion of bacterial endotoxins (lipopolysaccharides) contained in cigarettes and cigarette smoke.

5.3
Cigarette Smoking and COPD

COPD is the sixth most common disease worldwide, four places ahead of bronchial carcinoma (rank 10). In about 20 years' time, COPD, a condition that is smoking-related for the most part and is characterised by increasing exacerbations necessitating hospital intervention, will have risen to third place in the league table of diseases. In Germany, 3–4% of the population over the age of 18 years develop COPD and in 55-year-olds, prevalence is already 10–12%. For COPD alone, a disease that is chiefly encountered among smokers, the costs of treatment will continue to escalate.

Chronic bronchitis is characterised by chronic cough and excessive sputum secretion over a period of at least 3 months and up to several years. This form of bronchitis may occur both with and without accompanying ventilatory disorders arising primarily as a result of airspace dilatation distal to the terminal bronchiole without obvious fibrosis. COPD is said to be present where emphysema and airflow obstruction occur in addition to chronic bronchitis.

An epidemiological survey of COPD is problematic because the disease criteria are defined differently. In the USA, it is estimated that 14 million people suffer from the disease [128]. In recent decades, this figure has risen continuously, especially among women [128]. In 1992, more than 90,000 US Americans died from COPD, making it the fourth common-est cause of death. The disease is still contracted by more men than women, but the propor-tions are set to even out as a delayed response to the increasing number of female smokers. The COPD death rate for females increased by 382% from 1968 through 1999. In the same period, the rate for males increased by 27% [129]. COPD becomes more common with increasing age and smoking habits, and age-related lung changes have been identified.

5.3.1
Pathophysiology of COPD

Cigarette smoking triggers a wide range of harmful effects (see Table 5.4) as follows:

- Cilia loss and mucous gland hyperplasia in the main bronchi
- Inflammation, epithelial changes, fibrosis, secretory congestion in the more peripheral airways
- Hypertrophy of the bronchial musculature, vascular changes
- Alveolar destruction with loss of airways flexibility, elastic recoil and gas exchange surface area.

Table 5.4   Effects of smoking on the lung [130]

Changes in	Findings
Central airways	Cilia loss, mucous gland enlargement, goblet cell increase, regression of cilia pseudostratified epithelium to squamous metaplasia, carcinoma in situ and possibly bronchogenic carcinomas
Peripheral airways	Inflammation and atrophy, goblet cell metaplasia, squamous metaplasia, mucus congestion (blockade), smooth-muscle hypertrophy, peribronchial fibrosis
Alveoli and capillaries	Destruction of peribronchial alveoli, reduction in small arteries, pathological composition of bronchoalveolar lavage fluid, increased IgA and IgG, increase in activated macrophages and neutrophils
Immune system	Increased leucocyte count in periphery, eosinophilia, increased IgE levels, reduced responsiveness to allergy tests, reduced reactions to inhaled antigens

Smokers display inter-individual differences in terms of lung changes and functional lesions [131]. Changes in the terminal regions of the bronchial tree, the loss of bronchiolar consistency due to inflammatory processes and alveolar destruction lead to increasing functional impairment [128, 129, 131, 132]. Inflammatory processes sustain the progression of COPD [133]. Smoking-induced pulmonary emphysema is centrilobular and is principally restricted to the upper lung segments, where the attachment of the alveoli to the bronchioles becomes lost (see Table 5.4 for an overview of these changes) [128]. It is postulated that in COPD, a protease-antiprotease imbalance leads to accelerated destruction of lung tissue, with proteolytic activity being enhanced by cigarette smoke [134]. Neutrophils are encountered in larger numbers in the lower respiratory tract of smokers, especially in those with COPD. The concentration of inflammatory cells and their products in the lower respiratory tract correlates negatively with FEV_1 [135]. Moreover, smokers have higher elastase levels in BAL fluid than non-smokers [136], as well as a 50% reduction in α_1-antiprotease activity [76], probably as a result of oxidation processes caused by cigarette smoke. Biopsy studies indicate that in smokers with existing COPD, there is increased expression of the adhesion molecules E-selectin (on vessels) and ICAM-1 (on basal epithelial cells) [137]. The adhesion molecules are important in preparing cells for the inflammatory processes and hence, for the pathogenesis of airways obstruction in smokers.

Until a few years ago, emphysema was considered to be the decisive criterion for COPD; now, however, greater importance is assigned to the inflammatory and structural changes in the smaller airways [131]. CT scans of the lungs of patients with advanced COPD have revealed that detectable emphysema was also present in fewer than one third of patients with respiratory limitation [138]. Even in young smokers and the children of women who smoke, *respiratory bronchiolitis* is the first pathological sign of disturbed lung function and this occurs without obstruction (Fig. 5.4) [139]. In older smokers, the inflammatory changes are accompanied by connective tissue deposition [132]. Following thoracotomy, thickening of the bronchiolar membrane (<0.4 mm internal diameter) by 50% and of the bronchioles by 100% was detected only in smokers. These findings also correlated with the results of preoperative pulmonary function tests [132]. A reduction in wall thickness (bronchial atrophy and thinning of the bronchial wall) has also been detected in smokers, a possible indicator of airways collapse [51]. Hypertrophy of the bronchiolar musculature has been observed in smokers, possibly contributing to bronchial obstruction in COPD patients.

Thickening of the pulmonary muscular artery wall, particularly of the intimal layer, is seen in smokers with mild COPD [140]. These vascular changes are associated with disturbances of ventilation and perfusion and with a reduced vascular reaction in terms of pO_2 changes [140]. To date, it is unclear to what extent these findings contribute to the development of COPD. However, pulmonary vessel resistance at least is increased in patients with emphysema. These haemodynamic functional disturbances correlate with reduced diffusion capacity, but not with bronchial obstruction. The clinical correlate of these changes is increased cough and mucus secretion, reduced elastic recoil, increased expiratory obstruction, increased respiratory work, dyspnoea, wheezing and reduced gas exchange. These respiratory problems have been investigated in long-term studies [32]. Wheezing was the most common finding among smokers, being encountered in 11% of men and 9% of women.

5.3.2
Important Risk Factors for COPD

For more than 60 years now, COPD has been recognised as a consequence of cigarette smoking, especially since more than 80% of all COPD patients are smokers and also die as a result of this condition [17]. Mortality, morbidity and pulmonary function have been assessed in various retrospective and prospective studies in tens of thousands of patients [141, 142]. FEV_1 is already reduced in 25-year-old smokers and this effect increases over time. A close association exists between cumulative cigarette consumption and declining pulmonary function [116, 143]. In this context, the tar and nicotine yields of the cigarettes smoked, the use of filter tips and the method of smoking are important, but not crucial factors [144]. Initially, smokers have a normal forced expiratory volume; diminished FEV_1 with clinical signs of dyspnoea develops in only 15–30% of cases within a few years [128, 145].

The smoking-related changes co-exist alongside allergic processes, some of which are also genetically determined in the sense of an "asthmatic constitution" [146]. Methacholine as a bronchoconstrictor or β_1-mimetics as bronchodilators are important predictors for the smoking-related deterioration of pulmonary-function [147–149]. Bronchial hyperresponsiveness is an important risk factor for the development of COPD. In addition to decreases in pulmonary function indices, IgE levels and eosinophil and leucocyte counts have been shown to be increased in smokers; these variables returned to normal on smoking cessation [148]. In cases where smokers were aware that they had an allergic constitution, they were more often prepared to stop smoking than non-allergic individuals [150]. Overall, however, it is not clear whether eosinophilia or increased IgE levels in smokers are risk factors or markers for pulmonary obstruction [150, 151].

5.3.2.1
Genetic Factors

COPD is known to show familial clustering and genetic factors have been observed. This does not include α_1-antitrypsin deficiency, which leads to a clearly accelerated decline in pulmonary function more in smokers than in non-smokers [145]. Irrespective of smoking status, smokers with an antiprotease deficiency display considerable heterogeneity in terms of severity of bronchial obstruction [128, 152].

5.3.2.2
Occupational and Environmental Factors

A wide range of vapours, dusts and gases have a harmful effect on pulmonary function, leading to the increased occurrence of chronic bronchitis (cough and sputum). Bronchoobstructive reactions with a reduction in FEV_1 are also known to occur in response to exogenous factors. The severity of COPD is clearly intensified in cigarette smokers in developed countries [126]. Even severe air pollution or exposure to cement [153] may have an additive effect on the condition, irrespective of the harmful effects of cigarette smoke [147].

5.4
Cigarette Smoking and Bronchial Asthma

Cigarette smoking has a deleterious effect on physical performance in people with asthma [154]. Passive exposure to cigarette smoke (see Chap. 9) is also dangerous for children and leads to increased asthma morbidity [4]. Asthma sufferers should, therefore, be strongly advised not to start smoking or to stop smoking as quickly as possible.

5.4.1
Caveats Concerning the Informative Value of Studies

Prospective, randomised, double-blind and placebo-controlled studies to investigate a possible association between cigarette smoking and bronchial asthma are not acceptable on ethical grounds; consequently, only cohort and case-control studies are available. For the most part, such studies use extent of cigarette smoking as a parameter, but the information provided by patients frequently fails to reflect the true extent of consumption. Urinary and serum concentrations-of cotinine, exhaled CO and nicotine levels have also been used as aids to assessment [155]. One further source of bias is that asthmatic patients with severe symptoms possibly smoke less than those with no appreciable sense of being unwell. This already results in smoker selection in this disease group [156, 157].

Even the clinical diagnosis of bronchial asthma is problematic because rhonchi and wheezing may anticipate the diagnosis by several years [158] and furthermore, there is symptom overlap with COPD (e.g. wheezing, dyspnoea, emphysema). Reversible or irreversible bronchial obstruction may also occur in both conditions. β_1-adrenoceptor stimulants are neither sensitive nor specific enough to permit discrimination of the two diseases [159]. Likewise, the administration of histamine or methacholine to provoke a bronchial spasm is not specific for bronchial asthma because the response may also occur in chronic bronchitis, sarcoidosis, bronchiectasis or rhinitis [160, 161].

While an allergic disposition can be identified in asthmatics, the parameters used (skin testing, IgE levels and eosinophil count) are not reliable assessment criteria. Immediate-type skin reactions are linked with IgE antibodies [162] and are frequently positive in asthmatics [163]. However, IgE levels are neither sensitive nor specific for the diagnosis of asthma [160], even if associations with reduced pulmonary function have been detected specifically in asthmatics [164]. Eosinophils possibly play an important role in the inflammatory changes seen in asthmatics [165].

5.4.2
Cigarette Smoking and Bronchial Asthma in Adults

Despite various studies to investigate the possible association between bronchial asthma and cigarette smoking, such an association has not been demonstrated [158, 166, 167]. The NHANESI Study included patients from 100 different communities in 38 US

American states [52]. This primarily questionnaire-based study in smokers and non-smokers with a medical diagnosis of asthma came up with various conclusions: males and females had equal prevalence rates for asthma, but females had higher incidence rates [52]. Smoking prevalence was high and the diagnosis was made in all age groups (64.7%). In a Finnish cohort study [168], the prevalence of diagnosed asthma was higher among male smokers than among male non-smokers, whereas no significant difference was observed for women. Overall, the association between bronchial asthma and cigarette smoking is not clear-cut [169, 170].

Bronchial responsiveness to cigarette smoke was studied in 98 smokers by means of lung function measurements (FEV_1, $MEF_{75\%}$, $FEF_{\{25-75\%\}}$) in parallel with the methacholine challenge test. All lung function indices were decreased after just 12 cigarette smoke inhalations. FEV_1 fell by 10% and this effect correlated directly with vital capacity, pulmonary status (asthma, bronchitis) and cigarette consumption, but not with methacholine bronchial reactivity [171]. It is, therefore, clear that cigarette smoking is a major cause for the prognosis of bronchitis, bronchial asthma and COPD.

The comparison of increased bronchial responsiveness of smokers with that of non-smokers does not reveal consistent results without a simultaneously altered histamine response. Reduced pulmonary function was observed in male smokers who are older than 21 years of age [172]. Other studies have also yielded inconsistent results [170, 173]. One study conducted in Boston [174] in middle-aged and elderly patients revealed that current smoking status was associated with allergic disposition based on the determination of methacholine responsiveness. In addition, raised IgE levels and eosinophil counts have been detected in smokers [175]. The IgE concentration did not decline with age in smokers as compared to non-smokers.

Despite the numerous studies conducted, it is evident from the findings reported that no unequivocal association can yet be demonstrated between the development of bronchial asthma and cigarette smoking in adults because of the varied potential for bias. In children, numerous findings from more recent studies indicate that the risk for bronchial asthma is increased as a result of passive smoking.

5.4.3
Bronchial Asthma in Children

More than 50 epidemiology studies suggest that children who are exposed to tobacco smoke suffer increasingly from respiratory tract diseases [128]. The outcome variables studied in these children include respiratory tract symptoms such as cough and rhonchi, respiratory tract infections, new occurrence or deterioration of bronchial asthma, deterioration of pulmonary function, bronchial responsiveness, atopy and increased IgE levels. Passive smoking in childhood, particularly where the mother smokes, has been associated with some of these symptoms [154, 176–179] (see Figs. 5.5 and 5.6). However, the presence of external confounders (familial, socio-economic and environmental conditions) means that it is difficult to establish a definite causal relationship [177].

Passive smoking, particularly where both parents are smokers, is associated with bronchitic and asthmatic states in children and adolescents [182]. Several studies confirm an association between passive smoking and childhood obstructive and non-obstructive

Fig. 5.5 Maximum expiratory flow at functional residual capacity during the first year of life. ◆ Healthy control group; ■ children of women who smoked; ▲ total cohort [180]

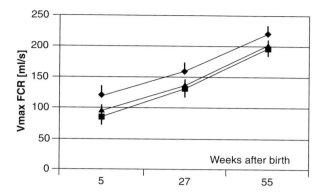

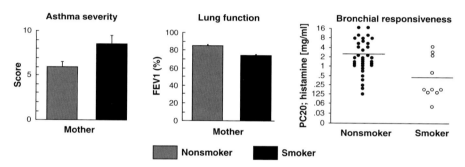

Fig. 5.6 Passive smoking and childhood bronchial asthma. The figure illustrates asthma severity, the extent of reduced pulmonary function and the increased bronchial responsiveness to histamine. Study conducted in 94 children aged between 7 and 17 years with a history of asthma. In each case, the pairs of columns represent non-smoking and smoking mothers (from [181])

airways disease; for the specific medical diagnosis of "asthma," this association is less clear [183]. The younger the children affected, the more definite the association of passive smoking with the bronchitic and asthmatic symptoms, as also reflected in hospital admissions [183–187]. In contrast to maternal smoking, paternal smoking was not found to exert any significant effect. A tendency for colds to go to the chest and for reduced FEV_{75} and FEV_{85} has been shown to correlate directly with salivary cotinine levels [185].

One sociomedical study showed an association between maternal smoking and a medical diagnosis of asthma in the child only where the mothers had 12 or fewer years of education [188].

The use of pulmonary function measurements, bronchial hyperresponsiveness measurements and skin prick tests as atopy markers to permit an objective diagnosis of asthma has yielded differing conclusions concerning the association between childhood asthma and passive smoking [155, 178, 179, 182, 185, 189, 190]. The majority of studies in which pulmonary function has been measured reveal a decrease in functional indices in passive smoking children. Two studies showed no association [178, 190]. The influence of passive smoking on skin prick test results is controversial [188, 191, 192].

Serum IgE levels and prevalence of eosinophilia were reported to be increased in one study in 9-year-old children of smoking parents [193]; likewise, elevated IgE levels have been detected in the cord serum in children of smoking mothers [77, 194]. Children whose parents smoked during pregnancy displayed more intense reactions following histamine challenge [195]. Bronchial responsiveness as tested by challenge methods was consistently increased in asthmatic, passively smoking children [188, 189, 196, 197].

Passive smoking also reflects the asthma of affected children (increased occurrence of exacerbations), but not the frequency of hospital admissions [198–200]. The association was clear between maternal smoking (number of cigarettes) and the deterioration of pulmonary function together with increased histamine responsiveness, with the effect on lung function occurring principally during cold wet weather [197]. When parental (maternal) cigarette consumption was restricted, childhood asthma status and lung function improved [181].

To summarise, it may be concluded that there is a clear association between passive smoking and childhood obstructive and non-obstructive airways disease, with smoke exposure apparently exacerbating pulmonary function and the course of asthma. However, there is as yet no convincing evidence that asthmatic diseases are directly caused by passive smoking.

5.5
Bronchitis and Pneumonia

Active smoking provokes acute respiratory tract diseases. While respiratory tract diseases are not found more commonly in smokers than in non-smokers, when they do occur, the lower respiratory tract is more often involved, leading to a more protracted duration of cough and more frequent pathological findings on auscultation [201, 202]. In one cohort study in male college students, smokers were found to have a significantly higher number of doctor visits and an even higher number of medical consultations for respiratory tract symptoms [203]. A clear dose–response relationship was found between smoking duration/consumption and the number of doctor visits for respiratory problems. In the smoker group, colds were more commonly associated with cough, mucus production, shortness of breath and rhonchi [204].

For children, passive smoking has long been regarded as a risk factor for the development of lower respiratory tract diseases. In the USA, each year, 150,000–300,000 children below the age of 18 months are reported to suffer from respiratory tract infections (bronchitis or pneumonia) as a result of passive smoking at home [4].

Active cigarette smoking is associated with a higher complication risk for pneumonia, especially influenza pneumonia: in one group of 250,000 veterans, mortality from influenza pneumonia was 1.78 times higher among smokers than among non-smokers [142]. The incidence and severity of influenza A (H1-N1) are also increased in smokers (50 vs. 30% for non-smokers) [46]. During a severe influenza epidemic, the incidence of clinical as well as subclinical infections (based on antibody titres) was increased among smokers [205]; while smoking exerted no effect on disease severity, the persistence of antibody titres in smokers was reduced. This may be one reason for increased susceptibility to influenza infections [206].

5.6
Other Lung Diseases Influenced by Cigarette Smoking

This category principally includes a respiratory bronchiolitis-associated interstitial lung disease [207] and pulmonary Langerhans cell granulomatosis [208, 209]. Pulmonary haemorrhage associated with Goodpasture's syndrome type is also significantly associated with cigarette smoking [50]. Women with breast cancer who smoke tend to develop lung metastases more frequently than non-smokers [210]. In contrast, sarcoidosis [211] and allergic pneumonitis occur more rarely in smokers than in non-smokers. Idiopathic pulmonary fibrosis is common among heavy smokers than former smokers (OR = −2.3; CI: 1.3–3.8 vs. 1.9 CI: 1.3–2.9), and the disease may even have its onset after sudden smoking cessation [73]. Obviously, explanations for the various diseases are to be sought in the effects of smoking on the inflammatory processes in the lung, on immune function and on vascular permeability.

Smokers are presumed to have a higher risk than non-smokers for developing-varicella pneumonia [110, 212]. Radiologically, pneumonia can be detected on the basis of diffuse interstitial or patchy infiltrates in up to 20% of adult cases [213], though often without clinical symptoms. The pulmonary symptoms usually set in during the first days after the onset of rash, and consist of cough, dyspnoea and varying degrees of hypoxaemia caused by inflammation and swelling of the bronchial epithelium [206, 214]. In untreated adults, the mortality rate from varicella pneumonia is approximately 10%, but may be as high as 50% where there is severe pulmonary involvement leading to pulmonary failure [206].

5.7
Concluding Remarks

- Current knowledge indicates that there is an established association between smoking and various forms of lung cancer. Exposure over months and years to the various inhalational products of tobacco, such as benzo[a]pyrene, nitrosamines (NNK, NNN), solvents (benzene, crotonaldehyde, formaldehyde) and [210]polonium, is an important aetiological factor. The organic compounds are metabolised (activated) by various enzymes in the CYP system and then form adducts with DNA in lung tissue and with leucocytes. In addition, the activity of the GST system plays an important role in the detoxification (elimination) of carcinogens.

- A significant risk for the development of lung cancer has been identified in individuals with high inducibility of CYP1A1 and reduced activity of glutathione S-reductase (GSTM1 0/0). The risk for bronchial carcinoma is particularly increased in carriers of the GSTM1 0/0 system. Bronchial carcinoma is commonly encountered and some 90% of cases are smoking-related; worldwide, its prevalence is increasing more among women than men.

- As the practice of smoking light cigarettes has become more widespread, there has been an increase in the prevalence of AC, a form of lung cancer that is less amenable to treatment than SCC.

- In addition, COPD (often sustained by years of smoking activity) is gaining importance because it is complex to treat and is even more common than bronchial carcinoma. In the near future, COPD will be the third most common disease worldwide.
- If they are exposed to environmental tobacco smoke (ETS), children are a target group for the development of lung diseases. Asthmatic diseases, especially among children, are not caused by passive smoking, but are sustained and accelerated in their progression by smoke inhalation.

References

1. U.S. Department of Health and Human Services; Public Health Services, Centres for Disease Control (1996) PHS document no.46-1123
2. Centres for Disease Control. (1993) Mortality trends for selected smoking-related cancers and breast cancer -- United States, 1550-1990. Morb Mortal Wkly Rep42: 857; 863–866
3. American Thoracic Society (1995) Standards for the diagnosis and care of patients with chronic obstructive pulmonary disease. Am Rev Respir Crit Care 152:77–121
4. Environmental Protection Agency (1992) Respiratory health effects of passive smoking: lung cancer and other disorders. Office of Research and Development, Office of Health and Environmental Assessment, Washington, DC. US_EPA, Report-No.EPA/600/6–90/006F
5. BAl Steering Committee (1990) Bronchoalveolar lavage constituents in healthy individuals, idiopathic pulmonary fibrosis, and selected comparison groups. The BAl Cooperative Group Steering Committee. Am Rev Respir Dis 141:169–202
6. Laughter AH, Martin RR, Twomey JJ (1977) Lymphoproliferative responses to antigens mediated by human pulmonary alveolar macrophages. J Lab Clin Med 89(6):1326–1332
7. Iribarren C, Tekawa IS, Sidney S, Friedman GD (1999) Effect of cigar smoking on the risk of cardiovascular disease, chronic obstructive pulmonary disease, and cancer in men. N Engl J Med 340(23):1773–1780
8. Brown GP, Iwamoto GK, Monick MM, Hunninghake GW (1989) Cigarette smoking decreases interleukin 1 release by human alveolar macrophages. Am J Physiol 256(2 Pt 1):C260–C264
9. Kline JN, Schwartz DA, Monick MM, Floerchinger CS, Hunninghake GW (1993) Relative release of interleukin-1 beta and interleukin-1 receptor antagonist by alveolar macrophages. A study in asbestos-induced lung disease, sarcoidosis, and idiopathic pulmonary fibrosis. Chest 104(1):47–53
10. Soliman DM, Twigg HL III (1992) Cigarette smoking decreases bioactive interleukin-6 secretion by alveolar macrophages. Am J Physiol 263(4 Pt 1):L471–L478
11. Daniele RP, Dauber JH, Altose MD, Rowlands DT, Gorenberg DJ (1977) Lymphocyte studies in asymptomatic cigarette smokers. A comparison between lung and peripheral blood. Am Rev Respir Dis 116(6):997–1005
12. Tollerud DJ, Clark JW, Brown LM, Neuland CY, Mann DL, Pankiw-Trost LK et al (1989) The effects of cigarette smoking on T cell subsets. A population-based survey of healthy Caucasians. Am Rev Respir Dis 139(6):1446–1451
13. Meliska CJ, Stunkard ME, Gilbert DG, Jensen RA, Martinko JM (1995) Immune function in cigarette smokers who quit smoking for 31 days. J Allergy Clin Immunol 95(4):901–910
14. U.S. Department Health Human Services; Public Health Services, Centres for Disease Control (1982) The Health benefits of smoking cessation. A report of the Surgeon General. PHS document no.90-8416

15. Burrows B, Hasan FM, Barbee RA, Halonen M, Lebowitz MD (1980) Epidemiologic observations on eosinophilia and its relation to respiratory disorders. Am Rev Respir Dis 122(5): 709–719

16. Murin S, Hilbert J, Reilly SJ (1997) Cigaret smoking and the lung. Clin Rev Allergy Immunol 15(3):307–361

17. U.S. Department Health Human Services PHSCfDC (1989) Reducing the health consequences of smoking: 25 years of progress. Report of the Surgeon General. PHS document no.89-8411

18. Doll R, Peto R (1981) The causes of cancer: quantitative estimates of avoidable risks of cancer in the United States today. J Natl Cancer Inst 66(6):1191–1308

19. Janerich DT, Thompson WD, Varela LR, Greenwald P, Chorost S, Tucci C et al (1990) Lung cancer and exposure to tobacco smoke in the household. N Engl J Med 323(10):632–636

20. Wang Y, Ichiba M, Iyadomi M, Zhang J, Tomokuni K (1998) Effects of genetic polymorphism of metabolic enzymes, nutrition, and lifestyle factors on DNA adduct formation in lymphocytes. Ind Health 36(4):337–346

21. Sekine I, Nagai K, Tsugane S, Yokose T, Kodama T, Nishiwaki Y et al (1999) Association between smoking and tumor progression in Japanese women with adenocarcinoma of the lung. Jpn J Cancer Res 90(2):129–135

22. Khuder SA, Dayal HH, Mutgi AB, Willey JC, Dayal G (1998) Effect of cigarette smoking on major histological types of lung cancer in men. Lung Cancer 22(1):15–21

23. Hart CL, Hole DJ, Gillis CR, Smith GD, Watt GC, Hawthorne VM (2001) Social class differences in lung cancer mortality: risk factor explanations using two Scottish cohort studies. Int J Epidemiol 30(2):268–274

24. Boffetta P, Pershagen G, Jockel KH, Forastiere F, Gaborieau V, Heinrich J et al (1999) Cigar and pipe smoking and lung cancer risk: a multicenter study from Europe. J Natl Cancer Inst 91(8):697–701

25. Becklake MR (1976) Asbestos-related diseases of the lung and other organs: their epidemiology and implications for clinical practice. Am Rev Respir Dis 114(1):187–227

26. Matos E, Vilensky M, Boffetta P, Kogevinas M (1998) Lung cancer and smoking: a case-control study in Buenos Aires, Argentina. Lung Cancer 21(3):155–163

27. Stellman SD, Muscat JE, Thompson S, Hoffmann D, Wynder EL (1997) Risk of squamous cell carcinoma and adenocarcinoma of the lung in relation to lifetime filter cigarette smoking. Cancer 80(3):382–388

28. Devesa SS, Silverman DT, Young JL, Pollack ES, Brown CC, Horm JW et al (1987) Cancer incidence and mortality trends among whites in the United States, 1947–84. J Natl Cancer Inst 79(4):701–770

29. Satcher D (2001) Women and smoking: a report of the Surgeon General 2001. US Department of Health and Human Services (ed). National Center for Chronic Disease Prevention and Health Promotion, Washington DC

30. Doll R, Peto R (1978) Cigarette smoking and bronchial carcinoma: dose and time relationships among regular smokers and lifelong non-smokers. J Epidemiol Community Health 32(4):303–313

31. Peto R, Lopez AD, Boreham J, Thun M, Heath C Jr (1992) Mortality from tobacco in developed countries: indirect estimation from national vital statistics. Lancet 339(8804): 1268–1278

32. Lebowitz MD, Burrows B (1977) Quantitative relationships between cigarette smoking and chronic productive cough. Int J Epidemiol 6(2):107–113

33. Armadans-Gil L, Vaque-Rafart J, Rossello J, Olona M, Alseda M (1999) Cigarette smoking and male lung cancer risk with special regard to type of tobacco. Int J Epidemiol 28(4):614–619

34. Sastre MT, Mullet E, Sorum PC (1999) Relationship between cigarette dose and perceived risk of lung cancer. Prev Med 28(6):566–571

35. Marang-van de Mheen PJ, Smith GD, Hart CL, Hole DJ (2001) Are women more sensitive to smoking than men? Findings from the Renfrew and Paisley study. Int J Epidemiol 30(4): 787–792
36. Pelkonen O, Pasanen M, Kuha H, Gachalyi B, Kairaluoma M, Sotaniemi EA et al (1986) The effect of cigarette smoking on 7-ethoxyresorufin O-deethylase and other monooxygenase activities in human liver: analyses with monoclonal antibodies. Br J Clin Pharmacol 22:125–134
37. Gielen JE, Goujon F, Sele J, Van Canfort J (1979) Organ specificity of induction of activating and inactivating enzymes by cigarette smoke and cigarette smoke condensate. Arch Toxicol 2(Suppl):239–251
38. Akin FJ, Benner JF (1976) Induction of aryl hydrocarbon hydroxylase in rodent lung by cigarette smoke: a potential short-term bioassay. Toxicol Appl Pharmacol 36:331–337
39. Down WH, Chasseaud LF, Sacharin RM (1981) Factors affecting induction of lung aryl hydrocarbon hydroxylase in rats exposed to cigarette smoke. Toxicology 19:255–262
40. Raunio H, Vahakangas K, Saarni H, Pelkonon O (1983) Effects of cigarette smoke on rat lung and liver ornithine decarboxylase and aryl hydrocarbon hydroxylase activities and lung benzo(a)pyrene metabolism. Acta Pharmacol Toxicol 52:168–174
41. Welch RM, Cavallito J, Loh A (1972) Effect of exposure to cigarette smoke on the metabolism of benzo(a)pyrene and acetophenetidin by lung and intestine of rats. Toxicol Appl Pharmacol 23:749–758
42. U.S. Department Health Human Services; Public Health Services, Centres for Disease Control (1982) The health consequences of smoking: cancer: a report of the Surgeon General. PHS document no. 82-50179
43. U.S. Department Health Human Services; Public Health Services, Centres for Disease Control (1964) Smoking and health: report of the Advisory Committee to the Surgeon General. PHS document no. 1103
44. Kahn HA (1966) The Dorn study of smoking and mortality among U.S. veterans: report on eight and one-half years of observation. Natl Cancer Inst Monogr 19:1–125
45. Hammond EC (1966) Smoking in relation to the death rates of one million men and women. Natl Cancer Inst Monogr 19:127–204
46. Kark JD, Lebiush M, Rannon L (1982) Cigarette smoking as a risk factor for epidemic a(h1n1) influenza in young men. N Engl J Med 307(17):1042–1046
47. Kunze MVC (1980) In: Banbury report 3: a safe cigarette? Gori G, Bock F (eds). Cold Spring Harbor Laboratory, Cold Spring Harbor, NY, pp 29–36
48. Rimington J (1981) The effect of filters on the incidence of lung cancer in cigarette smokers. Environ Res 24(1):162–166
49. Wynder EL, Stellman SD (1977) Comparative epidemiology of tobacco-related cancers. Cancer Res 37(12):4608–4622
50. Kelly PT, Haponik EF (1994) Goodpasture syndrome: molecular and clinical advances. Medicine (Baltimore) 73(4):171–185
51. Maisel JC, Silvers GW, George MS, Dart GA, Petty TL, Mitchell RS (1972) The significance of bronchial atrophy. Am J Pathol 67(2):371–386
52. McWhorter WP, Polis MA, Kaslow RA (1989) Occurrence, predictors, and consequences of adult asthma in NHANESI and follow-up survey. Am Rev Respir Dis 139(3):721–724
53. Auerbach O, Petrick TG, Stout AP, Statsinger AL, Muehsam GE, Formau JB et al (1956) The anatomical approach to the study of smoking and bronchogenic carcinoma. Cancer 9:76–83
54. Auerbach O, Gere JB, Formau JB, Petrick TG, Smolin HJ, Muehsam GE et al (1957) Changes in the bronchial epithelium in relation to smoking and cancer of the lung. N Engl J Med 256: 97–104
55. Scherer G, Frank S, Riedel K, Meger-Kossien I, Renner T (2000) Biomonitoring of exposure to polycyclic aromatic hydrocarbons of nonoccupationally exposed persons. Cancer Epidemiol Biomarkers Prev 9(4):373–380

56. Wiencke JK, Thurston SW, Kelsey KT, Varkonyi A, Wain JC, Mark EJ et al (1999) Early age at smoking initiation and tobacco carcinogen DNA damage in the lung. J Natl Cancer Inst 91(7):614–619

57. Wald NJ, Watt HC (1997) Prospective study of effect of switching from cigarettes to pipes or cigars on mortality from three smoking related diseases. BMJ 314(7098):1860–1863

58. Carpenter CL, Jarvik ME, Morgenstern H, McCarthy WJ, London SJ (1999) Mentholated cigarette smoking and lung-cancer risk. Ann Epidemiol 9(2):114–120

59. Lubin JH, Blot WJ (1984) Assessment of lung cancer risk factors by histologic category. J Natl Cancer Inst 73(2):383–389

60. Kreuzer M, Kreienbrock L, Muller KM, Gerken M, Wichmann E (1999) Histologic types of lung carcinoma and age at onset. Cancer 85(9):1958–1965

61. Wynder EL, Hoffmann D (1994) Smoking and lung cancer: scientific challenges and opportunities. Cancer Res 54(20):5284–5295

62. Herning RI, Jones RT, Bachman J, Mines AH (1981) Puff volume increases when low-nicotine cigarettes are smoked. Br Med J (Clin Res Ed) 283(6285):187–189

63. Le Marchand L, Sivaraman L, Pierce L, Seifried A, Lum A, Wilkens LR et al (1998) Associations of CYP1A1, GSTM1, and CYP2E1 polymorphisms with lung cancer suggest cell type specificities to tobacco carcinogens. Cancer Res 58(21):4858–4863

64. Harley N, Samet JM, Cross FT, Hess T, Muller J, Thomas D (1986) Contribution of radon and radon daughters to respiratory cancer. Environ Health Perspect 70:17–21

65. Hecht SS (1999) DNA adduct formation from tobacco-specific N-nitrosamines. Mutat Res 424:127–142

66. Brockmoller J, Cascorbi I, Kerb R, Sachse C, Roots I (1998) Polymorphisms in xenobiotic conjugation and disease predisposition. Toxicol Lett 102–103:173–183

67. Chung FL, Chen HJ, Nath RG (1996) Lipid peroxidation as a potential endogenous source for the formation of exocyclic DNA adducts. Carcinogenesis 17:2105–2111

68. Nair J, Barbin A, Velic I, Bartsch H (1999) Etheno DNA-base adducts from endogenous reactive species. Mutat Res 424:59–69

69. IARC Working Group, Lyon (1985) Tobacco habits other than smoking: betel-quid and area-nut chewing; and some related nitrosamines. IARC Monogr Eval Carcinog Risk Chem Hum 37:92–111

70. Kellermann G, Shaw CR, Luyten-Kellerman M (1973) Aryl hydrocarbon hydroxylase inducibility and bronchogenic carcinoma. N Engl J Med 289(18):934–937

71. Ayesh R, Idle JR, Ritchie JC, Crothers MJ, Hetzel MR (1984) Metabolic oxidation phenotypes as markers for susceptibility to lung cancer. Nature 312(5990):169–170

72. Bouchardy C, Benhamou S, Dayer P (1996) The effect of tobacco on lung cancer risk depends on CYP2D6 activity. Cancer Res 56(2):251–253

73. Baumgartner KB, Samet JM, Stidley CA, Colby TV, Waldron JA (1997) Cigarette smoking: a risk factor for idiopathic pulmonary fibrosis. Am J Respir Crit Care Med 155(1):242–248

74. Guengerich FP, Shimada T (1998) Activation of procarcinogens by human cytochrome P450 enzymes. Mutat Res 400:201–213

75. Puga A, Nebert DW, McKinnon RA, Menon AG (1997) Genetic polymorphisms in human drug-metabolizing enzymes: potential uses of reverse genetics to identify genes of toxicological relevance. Crit Rev Toxicol 27:199–222

76. Gadek JE, Fells GA, Crystal RG (1979) Cigarette smoking induces functional antiprotease deficiency in the lower respiratory tract of humans. Science 206(4424):1315–1316

77. Magnusson CG (1986) Maternal smoking influences cord serum IgE and IgD levels and increases the risk for subsequent infant allergy. J Allergy Clin Immunol 78(5 Pt 1): 898–904

78. Nebert DW, McKinnon RA, Puga A (1996) Human drug-metabolizing enzyme polymorphisms: effects on risk of toxicity and cancer. DNA Cell Biol 15:273–280

79. Omenn GS, Goodman GE, Thornquist MD, Balmes J, Cullen MR, Glass A et al (1996) Effects of a combination of beta carotene and vitamin A on lung cancer and cardiovascular disease. N Engl J Med 334(18):1150–1155

80. Peterson DD, McKinney CE, Ikeya K, Smith HH, Bale AE, McBride OW et al (1990) Human CYP1A1 gene: cosegregation of the enzyme inducibility phenotype and an RFLP. Ant J Hum Genet 48:720–725

81. Landi MT, Bertazzi PA, Shields PG, Clark G, Lucier GW, Garte SJ et al (1994) Association between CYP1A1 genotype, mRNA expression and enzymatic activity in humans. Pharmacogenetics 4:242–246

82. Whyatt RM, Bell DA, Jedrychowski W, Santella RM, Garte SJ, Cosma G et al (1998) Polycyclic aromatic hydrocarbon-DNA adducts in human placenta and modulation by CYP1A1 induction and genotype. Carcinogenesis 19:1389–1392

83. Cascorbi I, Brockmoller J, Roots I (1996) A C4887A polymorphism in exon 7 of human CYP1A1: population frequency, mutation linkages, and impact on lung cancer susceptibility. Cancer Res 56:4965–4969

84. Kawajiir K, Nakachi K, Intai K, Yoshii A, Shinoda N, Watanabe J (1990) Identification of genetically high rist individuals to lung cancer by DNA polymorphisms of the cytochrome P-7501A1 gene. FEBS Lett 263:131–133

85. Hayashi S, Watanabe J, Kawajiri K (1992) High susceptibility to lung cancer analyzed in terms of combined genotypes of P450IA1 and Mu-class glutathione S-transferase genes. Jpn J Cancer Res 83:866–870

86. Nakachi K, Imai K, Hayashi S, Kawajiri K (1993) Polymorphisms of the CYP1A1 and glutathione S-transferase genes associated with susceptibility to lung cancer in relation to cigarette dose in a Japanese population. Cancer Res 53:2994–2999

87. Okada T, Kawashima K, Fukushi S, Minakuchi T, Nishimura S (1994) Association between a cytochrome P450 CYPIA1 genotype and incidence of lung cancer. Pharmacogenetics 4:333–340

88. Nakachi K, Imai K, Hayashi S, Watanabe J, Kawajiri K (1991) Genetic susceptibility to squamous cell carcinoma of the lung in relation to cigarette smoking dose. Cancer Res 51:5177–5180

89. Garcia-Closas M, Kelsey KT, Wiencke JK, Xu X, Wain JC, Christiani DC (1997) A case-control study of cytochrome P450 1A1, glutathione S-transferase M1, cigarette smoking and lung cancer susceptibility (Massachusetts, United States). Cancer Causes Control 8:544–553

90. Sugimura H, Wakai K, Genka K, Nagura K, Igarashi H, Nagayama K et al (1998) Association of Ile462Val (Exon 7) polymorphism of cytochrome P450 IA1 with lung cancer in the Asian population: further evidence from a case-control study in Okinawa. Cancer Epidemiol Biomarkers Prev 7:413–417

91. Kiyohara C, Nakanishi Y, Inutsuka S, Takayama K, Hara N, Motohiro A et al (1998) The relationship between CYP1A1 aryl hydrocarbon hydroxylase activity and lung cancer in a Japanese population. Pharmacogenetics 8:315–323

92. Hong YS, Chang JH, Kwon OJ, Ham YA, Choi JH (1998) Polymorphism of the CYP1A1 and glutathione-S-transferase gene in Korean lung cancer patients. Exp Mol Med 30:192–198

93. Hirvonen A, Husgafvel-Pursiainen K, Anttila S, Karjalainen A, Vainio H (1993) Polymorphism in CYP1A1 and CYP2D6 genes: possible association with susceptibility to lung cancer. Environ Health Perspect 101(Suppl 3):109–112

94. Hirvonen A, Husgafvel-Pursiainen K, Anttila S, Karjalainen A, Pelkonen O, Vainio H (1993) PCR-based CYP2D6 genotyping for Finnish lung cancer patients. Pharmacogenetics 3:19–27

95. Vaury C, Laine R, Noguiez P, de Coppet P, Jaulin C, Praz F et al (1995) Human glutathione S-transferase M1 null genotype is associated with a high inducibility of cytochrome P450 1A1 gene transcription. Cancer Res 55:5520–5523

96. Uematsu F, Ikawa S, Kikuchi H, Sagami I, Kanamaru R, Abe T et al (1994) Restriction fragment length polymorphism of the human CYP2E1 (cytochrome P450IIE1) gene and susceptibility to lung cancer: possible relevance to low smoking exposure. Pharmacogenetics 4:58–63

97. Taioli E, Ford J, Trachman J, Li Y, Demopoulos R, Garte S (1998) Lung cancer risk and CYP1A1 genotype in African Americans. Carcinogenesis 19:813–817
98. Kelsey KT, Wiencke JK, Spitz MR (1994) A race-specific genetic polymorphism in the CYP1A1 gene is not associated with lung cancer in African Americans. Carcinogenesis 15:1121–1124
99. London SJ, Daly AK, Fairbrother KS, Holmes C, Carpenter CL, Navidi WC et al (1995) Lung cancer risk in African-Americans in relation to a race-specific CYP1A1 polymorphism. Cancer Res 55:6035–6037
100. Coultas DB, Samet JM (1992) Occupational lung cancer. Clin Chest Med 13(2):341–354
101. Centres of Disease Control (1993) Morb Mortal Wkly Rep 42:857–866
102. Mace K, Bowman ED, Vautravers P, Shields PG, Harris CC, Pfeifer AM (1998) Characterisation of xenobiotic-metabolising enzyme expression in human bronchial mucosa and peripheral lung tissues. Eur J Cancer 34:914–920
103. Raunio H, Hakkola J, Hukkanen J, Lassila A, Paivarinta K, Pelkonen O et al (1999) Expression of xenobiotic-metabolizing CYPs in human pulmonary tissue. Exp Toxicol Pathol 51:412–417
104. Saarikoski ST, Sata F, Husgafvel-Pursiainen K, Rautalahti M, Haukka J, Impivaara O et al (2000) CYP2D6 ultrarapid metabolizer genotype as a potential modifier of smoking behaviour. Pharmacogenetics 10(1):5–10
105. Agundez JA, Martinez C, Ladero JM, Ledesma MC, Ramos JM, Martin R et al (1994) Debrisoquin oxidation genotype and susceptibility to lung cancer. Clin Pharmacol Ther 55:10–14
106. Dolzan V, Rudolf Z, Breskvar K (1995) Human CYP2D6 gene polymorphism in Slovene cancer patients and healthy controls. Carcinogenesis 16:2675–2678
107. Christensen PM, Gotzsche PC, Brosen K (1997) The sparteine/debrisoquine (CYP2D6) oxidation polymorphism and the risk of lung cancer: a meta-analysis. Eur J Clin Pharmacol 51: 389–393
108. Rostami-Hodjegan A, Lennard MS, Woods HF, Tucker GT (1998) Meta-analysis of studies of the CYP2D6 polymorphism in relation to lung cancer and Parkinson's disease. Pharmacogenetics 8:227–238
109. Wu X, Shi H, Jiang H, Kemp B, Hong WK, Delclos GL et al (1997) Associations between cytochrome P4502E1 genotype, mutagen sensitivity, cigarette smoking and susceptibility to lung cancer. Carcinogenesis 18:967–973
110. Grayson ML, Newton-John H (1988) Smoking and varicella pneumonia. J Infect 16(3):312
111. Oyama T, Kawamoto T, Mizoue T, Sugio K, Kodama Y, Mitsudomi T et al (1997) Cytochrome P450 2E1 polymorphism as a risk factor for lung cancer: in relation to p53 gene mutation. Anticancer Res 17:583–587
112. Bartsch H (1996) DNA adducts in human carcinogenesis: etiological relevance and structure-activity relationship. Mutat Res 340:67–79
113. Rojas M, Alexandrov K, Cascorbi I, Brockmoller J, Likhachev A, Pozharisski K et al (1998) High benzo[a]pyrene diol-epoxide DNA adduct levels in lung and blood cells from individuals with combined CYP1A1 MspI/Msp-GSTM1*0/*0 genotypes. Pharmacogenetics 8:109–118
114. Hou SM, Falt S, Nyberg F (2001) Glutathione S-transferase T1-null genotype interacts synergistically with heavy smoking on lung cancer risk. Environ Mol Mutagen 38(1):83–86
115. Hou SM, Falt S, Yang K, Nyberg F, Pershagen G, Hemminki K et al (2001) Differential interactions between GSTM1 and NAT2 genotypes on aromatic DNA adduct level and HPRT mutant frequency in lung cancer patients and population controls. Cancer Epidemiol Biomarkers Prev 10(2):133–140
116. Higgins MW, Enright PL, Kronmal RA, Schenker MB, Anton-Culver H, Lyles M (1993) Smoking and lung function in elderly men and women. The Cardiovascular Health Study. JAMA 269(21):2741–2748
117. Shriver SP, Bourdeau HA, Gubish CT, Tirpak DL, Davis AL, Luketich JD et al (2000) Sex-specific expression of gastrin-releasing peptide receptor: relationship to smoking history and risk of lung cancer. J Natl Cancer Inst 92(1):24–33

118. Yang P, Wentzlaff KA, Katzmann JA, Marks RS, Allen MS, Lesnick TG et al (1999) Alpha1-antitrypsin deficiency allele carriers among lung cancer patients. Cancer Epidemiol Biomarkers Prev 8(5):461–465

119. Colditz GA, Stampfer MJ, Willett WC (1987) Diet and lung cancer. A review of the epidemiologic evidence in humans. Arch Intern Med 147(1):157–160

120. Peto R, Doll R, Buckley JD, Sporn MB (1981) Can dietary beta-carotene materially reduce human cancer rates? Nature 290(5803):201–208

121. Godschalk RW, Feldker DE, Borm PJ, Wouters EF, Van Schooten FJ (2002) Body mass index modulates aromatic DNA adduct levels and their persistence in smokers. Cancer Epidemiol Biomarkers Prev 11(8):790–793

122. Woodson K, Albanes D, Tangrea JA, Rautalahti M, Virtamo J, Taylor PR (1999) Association between alcohol and lung cancer in the alpha-tocopherol, beta-carotene cancer prevention study in Finland. Cancer Causes Control 10(3):219–226

123. Kinoshita N, Koyama Y, Yoshino K, Tanaka H, Ajiki W, Tukuma H et al (1997) [Second primary cancers occurring in patients with cancers of the mouth and meso-hypo pharynx in Japan]. Nippon Koshu Eisei Zasshi 44(3):201–206

124. Omenn GS, Merchant J, Boatman E, Dement JM, Kuschner M, Nicholson W et al (1986) Contribution of environmental fibers to respiratory cancer. Environ Health Perspect 70:51–56

125. Radford EP, Renard KG (1984) Lung cancer in Swedish iron miners exposed to low doses of radon daughters. N Engl J Med 310(23):1485–1494

126. Garshick E, Schenker MB, Dosman JA (1996) Occupationally induced airways obstruction. Med Clin North Am 80(4):851–878

127. Yngveson A, Williams C, Hjerpe A, Lundeberg J, Soderkvist P, Pershagen G (1999) p53 Mutations in lung cancer associated with residential radon exposure. Cancer Epidemiol Biomarkers Prev 8(5):433–438

128. American Thoracic Society (1996) Cigarette smoking and health. American Thoracic Society. Am J Respir Crit Care Med 153:861–865

129. Kazerouni N, Alverson CJ, Redd SC, Mott JA, Mannino DM (2004) Sex differences in COPD and lung cancer mortality trends – United States, 1968–1999. J Womens Health (Larchmt) 13(1):17–23

130. Sherman CB (1992) The health consequences of cigarette smoking. Pulmonary diseases. Med Clin North Am 76(2):355–375

131. Saetta M, Finkelstein R, Cosio MG (1994) Morphological and cellular basis for airflow limitation in smokers. Eur Respir J 7(8):1505–1515

132. Wright JL, Hobson J, Wiggs BR, Pare PD, Hogg JC (1987) Effect of cigarette smoking on structure of the small airways. Lung 165(2):91–100

133. Thurlbeck WM (1990) Pathophysiology of chronic obstructive pulmonary disease. Clin Chest Med 11(3):389–403

134. Welte T, Groneberg DA (2006) Asthma and COPD. Exp Toxicol Pathol 57(Suppl 2):35–40

135. Linden M, Rasmussen JB, Piitulainen E, Tunek A, Larson M, Tegner H et al (1993) Airway inflammation in smokers with nonobstructive and obstructive chronic bronchitis. Am Rev Respir Dis 148(5):1226–1232

136. Fera T, Abboud RT, Richter A, Johal SS (1986) Acute effect of smoking on elastaselike esterase activity and immunologic neutrophil elastase levels in bronchoalveolar lavage fluid. Am Rev Respir Dis 133(4):568–573

137. Di Stefano A, Maestrelli P, Roggeri A, Turato G, Calabro S, Potena A et al (1994) Upregulation of adhesion molecules in the bronchial mucosa of subjects with chronic obstructive bronchitis. Am J Respir Crit Care Med 149(3 Pt 1):803–810

138. Gelb AF, Schein M, Kuei J, Tashkin DP, Muller NL, Hogg JC et al (1993) Limited contribution of emphysema in advanced chronic obstructive pulmonary disease. Am Rev Respir Dis 147(5):1157–1161

139. Niewoehner DE, Kleinerman J, Rice DB (1974) Pathologic changes in the peripheral airways of young cigarette smokers. N Engl J Med 291(15):755–758

140. Barbera JA, Riverola A, Roca J, Ramirez J, Wagner PD, Ros D et al (1994) Pulmonary vascular abnormalities and ventilation-perfusion relationships in mild chronic obstructive pulmonary disease. Am J Respir Crit Care Med 149(2 Pt 1):423–429

141. Doll R, Peto R (1976) Mortality in relation to smoking: 20 years' observations on male British doctors. Br Med J 2(6051):1525–1536

142. Rogot E, Murray JL (1980) Smoking and causes of death among U.S. veterans: 16 years of observation. Public Health Rep 95(3):213–222

143. Lange P, Groth S, Nyboe GJ, Mortensen J, Appleyard M, Jensen G et al (1989) Effects of smoking and changes in smoking habits on the decline of FEV1. Eur Respir J 2(9):811–816

144. Buist AS, Vollmer W (1994) Smoking and other risk factors. In: Murray JR, Nadel JN (eds) Textbook of respirtory medicine, 2nd edn. W.B. Saunders, Philadelphia, pp 1259–1287

145. Speizer FE, Tager IB (1979) Epidemiology of chronic mucus hypersecretion and obstructive airways disease. Epidemiol Rev 1:124–142

146. Orie NGM, Sluiter HJ, De Vries K, Tammeling GH, Witkop J (1961) The host factor in bronchitis. In: Orie NGM, Sluiter HJ (eds) Bronchitis. Royal van Gorcum, Assen, pp 43–59

147. Tashkin DP, Altose MD, Connett JE, Kanner RE, Lee WW, Wise RA (1996) Methacholine reactivity predicts changes in lung function over time in smokers with early chronic obstructive pulmonary disease. The Lung Health Study Research Group. Am J Respir Crit Care Med 153(6 Pt 1):1802–1811

148. Taylor RG, Gross E, Joyce H, Holland F, Pride NB (1985) Smoking, allergy, and the differential white blood cell count. Thorax 40(1):17–22

149. Vollmer WM, Johnson LR, Buist AS (1985) Relationship of response to a bronchodilator and decline in forced expiratory volume in one second in population studies. Am Rev Respir Dis 132(6):1186–1193

150. Burrows B, Halonen M, Barbee RA, Lebowitz MD (1981) The relationship of serum immunoglobulin E to cigarette smoking. Am Rev Respir Dis 124(5):523–525

151. Dow L, Coggon D, Campbell MJ, Osmond C, Holgate ST (1992) The interaction between immunoglobulin E and smoking in airflow obstruction in the elderly. Am Rev Respir Dis 146 (2):402–407

152. Snider GL (1989) Pulmonary disease in alpha-1-antitrypsin deficiency. Ann Intern Med 111 (12):957–959

153. AbuDhaise BA, Rabi AZ, al Zwairy MA, el Hader AF, el Qaderi S (1997) Pulmonary manifestations in cement workers in Jordan. Int J Occup Med Environ Health 10(4):417–428

154. Althuis MD, Sexton M, Prybylski D (1999) Cigarette smoking and asthma symptom severity among adult asthmatics. J Asthma 36(3):257–264

155. Samet JM, Marbury MC, Spengler JD (1987) Health effects and sources of indoor air pollution. Part I. Am Rev Respir Dis 136(6):1486–1508

156. Sunyer J, Munoz A (1996) Concentrations of methacholine for bronchial responsiveness according to symptoms, smoking and immunoglobulin E in a population-based study in Spain. Spanish Group of the European Asthma Study. Am J Respir Crit Care Med 153(4 Pt 1): 1273–1279

157. Troisi RJ, Speizer FE, Rosner B, Trichopoulos D, Willett WC (1995) Cigarette smoking and incidence of chronic bronchitis and asthma in women. Chest 108(6):1557–1561

158. Dodge RR, Burrows B (1980) The prevalence and incidence of asthma and asthma-like symptoms in a general population sample. Am Rev Respir Dis 122(4):567–575

159. Kesten S, Rebuck AS (1994) Is the short-term response to inhaled beta-adrenergic agonist sensitive or specific for distinguishing between asthma and COPD? Chest 105(4):1042–1045

160. Britton J (1992) Airway hyperresponsiveness and the clinical diagnosis of asthma: histamine or history? J Allergy Clin Immunol 89:19–22

161. Rogers DF, O'Connor BJ (1993) Airway hyperresponsiveness: relation to asthma and inflammation? Thorax 48(11):1095–1096
162. Anonym (1995) JointTask Force an Practice Parameters. Practice parameters for the diagnoses and treatment of asthma. J Allergy Clin Immunol 96:707–870
163. Anonym (1991) Guidelines for the diagnosis and management of asthma. National Asthma Education Program. J Allergy Clin Immunol 88:425–534
164. Sherrill DL, Lebowitz MD, Halonen M, Barbee RA, Burrows B (1995) Longitudinal evaluation of the association between pulmonary function and total serum IgE. Am J Respir Crit Care Med 152(1):98–102
165. Kay AB (1991) Asthma and inflammation. J Allergy Clin Immunol 87(5):893–910
166. Dodge R, Cline MG, Lebowitz MD, Burrows B (1994) Findings before the diagnosis of asthma in young adults. J Allergy Clin Immunol 94(5):831–835
167. Schachter EN, Doyle CA, Beck GJ (1984) A prospective study of asthma in a rural community. Chest 85(5):623–630
168. Vesterinen E, Kaprio J, Koskenvuo M (1988) Prospective study of asthma in relation to smoking habits among 14,729 adults. Thorax 43(7):534–539
169. Flodin U, Jonsson P, Ziegler J, Axelson O (1995) An epidemiologic study of bronchial asthma and smoking. Epidemiology 6(5):503–505
170. Sunyer J, Anto JM, Sabria J, Rodrigo MJ, Roca J, Morell F et al (1992) Risk factors of soybean epidemic asthma. The role of smoking and atopy. Am Rev Respir Dis 145(5):1098–1102
171. Jensen EJ, Dahl R, Steffensen F (1998) Bronchial reactivity to cigarette smoke in smokers: repeatability, relationship to methacholine reactivity, smoking and atopy. Eur Respir J 11(3):670–676
172. Rijcken B, Schouten JP, Weiss ST, Speizer FE, van der LR (1988) The relationship between airway responsiveness to histamine and pulmonary function level in a random population sample. Am Rev Respir Dis 137(4):826–832
173. Vedal S, Enarson DA, Chan H, Ochnio J, Tse KS, Chan-Yeung M (1988) A longitudinal study of the occurrence of bronchial hyperresponsiveness in western red cedar workers. Am Rev Respir Dis 137(3):651–655
174. O'Connor GT, Sparrow D, Segal MR, Weiss ST (1989) Smoking, atopy, and methacholine airway responsiveness among middle-aged and elderly men. The Normative Aging Study. Am Rev Respir Dis 140(6):1520–1526
175. Sherrill DL, Halonen M, Burrows B (1994) Relationships between total serum IgE, atopy, and smoking: a twenty-year follow-up analysis. J Allergy Clin Immunol 94(6 Pt 1):954–962
176. Fielding JE, Phenow KJ (1988) Health effects of involuntary smoking. N Engl J Med 319(22):1452–1460
177. Guyatt GH, Newhouse MT (1985) Are active and passive smoking harmful? Determining causation. Chest 88(3):445–451
178. Sherman CB (1991) Health effects of cigarette smoking. Clin Chest Med 12(4):643–658
179. Tager IB (1988) Passive smoking – bronchial responsiveness and atopy. Am Rev Respir Dis 138(3):507–509
180. Young S, Sherrill DL, Arnott J, Diepeveen D, LeSouef PN, Landau LI (2000) Parental factors affecting respiratory function during the first year of life. Pediatr Pulmonol 29(5):331–340
181. Murray AB, Morrison BJ (1993) The decrease in severity of asthma in children of parents who smoke since the parents have been exposing them to less cigarette smoke. J Allergy Clin Immunol 91(1 Pt 1):102–110
182. Burchfiel CM, Higgins MW, Keller JB, Howatt WF, Butler WJ, Higgins IT (1986) Passive smoking in childhood. Respiratory conditions and pulmonary function in Tecumseh, Michigan. Am Rev Respir Dis 133(6):966–973
183. Cunningham J, O'Connor GT, Dockery DW, Speizer FE (1996) Environmental tobacco smoke, wheezing, and asthma in children in 24 communities. Am J Respir Crit Care Med 153(1):218–224

184. Stoddard JJ, Miller T (1995) Impact of parental smoking on the prevalence of wheezing respiratory illness in children. Am J Epidemiol 141(2):96–102

185. Strachan DP, Jarvis MJ, Feyerabend C (1990) The relationship of salivary cotinine to respiratory symptoms, spirometry, and exercise-induced bronchospasm in seven-year-old children. Am Rev Respir Dis 142(1):147–151

186. Taylor B, Wadsworth J (1987) Maternal smoking during pregnancy and lower respiratory tract illness in early life. Arch Dis Child 62(8):786–791

187. Wright AL, Holberg C, Martinez FD, Taussig LM (1991) Relationship of parental smoking to wheezing and nonwheezing lower respiratory tract illnesses in infancy. Group Health Medical Associates. J Pediatr 118(2):207–214

188. Martinez FD, Cline M, Burrows B (1992) Increased incidence of asthma in children of smoking mothers. Pediatrics 89(1):21–26

189. O'Connor GT, Weiss ST, Tager IB, Speizer FE (1987) The effect of passive smoking on pulmonary function and nonspecific bronchial responsiveness in a population-based sample of children and young adults. Am Rev Respir Dis 135(4):800–804

190. Tager IB, Weiss ST, Munoz A, Rosner B, Speizer FE (1983) Longitudinal study of the effects of maternal smoking on pulmonary function in children. N Engl J Med 309(12): 699–703

191. Kuehr J, Fischer T, Karmous W, Meinert R, Barth R, Hermann-Kunz E et al (1992) Relationship between low birth weight and symptoms in a cohort of primary school children. J Allergy Clin Immunol 90:358–363

192. Soyseth V, Kongerud J, Boe J (1995) Postnatal maternal smoking increases the prevalence of asthma but not of bronchial hyperresponsiveness or atopy in their children. Chest 107(2): 389–394

193. Ronchetti R, Macri F, Ciofetta G, Indinnimeo L, Cutrera R, Bonci E et al (1990) Increased serum IgE and increased prevalence of eosinophilia in 9-year-old children of smoking parents. J Allergy Clin Immunol 86(3 Pt 1):400–407

194. Ownby DR, Johnson CC, Peterson EL (1991) Maternal smoking does not influence cord serum IgE or IgD concentrations. J Allergy Clin Immunol 88(4):555–560

195. Young S, Le Souef PN, Geelhoed GC, Stick SM, Turner KJ, Landau LI (1991) The influence of a family history of asthma and parental smoking on airway responsiveness in early infancy. N Engl J Med 324(17):1168–1173

196. Frischer T, Kuehr J, Meinert R, Karmaus W, Barth R, Hermann-Kunz E et al (1992) Relationship between low birth weight and respiratory symptoms in a cohort of primary school children. Acta Paediatr 81(12):1040–1041

197. Murray AB, Morrison BJ (1988) Passive smoking and the seasonal difference of severity of asthma in children. Chest 94(4):701–708

198. Chilmonczyk BA, Salmun LM, Megathlin KN, Neveux LM, Palomaki GE, Knight GJ et al (1993) Association between exposure to environmental tobacco smoke and exacerbations of asthma in children. N Engl J Med 328(23):1665–1669

199. Evans D, Levison MJ, Feldman CH, Clark NM, Wasilewski Y, Levin B et al (1987) The impact of passive smoking on emergency room visits of urban children with asthma. Am Rev Respir Dis 135(3):567–572

200. Weitzman M, Gortmaker S, Walker DK, Sobol A (1990) Maternal smoking and childhood asthma. Pediatrics 85(4):505–511

201. Aronson MD, Weiss ST, Ben RL, Komaroff AL (1982) Association between cigarette smoking and acute respiratory tract illness in young adults. JAMA 248(2):181–183

202. Boake W (1959) A study of illnesses in a group of Cleveland families. N Engl J Med 259:1245–1249

203. Peters JM, Ferris BG Jr (1967) Smoking, pulmonary function, and respiratory symptoms in a college-age group. Am Rev Respir Dis 95(5):774–782

204. Peters JM, Ferris BG Jr (1967) Smoking and morbidity in a college-age group. Am Rev Respir Dis 95(5):783–789
205. Finklea JF, Sandifer SH, Smith DD (1969) Cigarette smoking and epidemic influenza. Am J Epidemiol 90(5):390–399
206. Feldman S (1994) Varicella-zoster virus pneumonitis. Chest 106(1 Suppl):22S–27S
207. Yousem SA, Colby TV, Gaensler EA (1989) Respiratory bronchiolitis-associated interstitial lung disease and its relationship to desquamative interstitial pneumonia. Mayo Clin Proc 64 (11):1373–1380
208. Tomashefski JF, Khiyami A, Kleinerman J (1991) Neoplasms associated with pulmonary eosinophilic granuloma. Arch Pathol Lab Med 115(5):499–506
209. Travis WD, Borok Z, Roum JH, Zhang J, Feuerstein I, Ferrans VJ et al (1993) Pulmonary Langerhans cell granulomatosis (histiocytosis X). A clinicopathologic study of 48 cases. Am J Surg Pathol 17(10):971–986
210. Scanlon EF, Suh O, Murthy SM, Mettlin C, Reid SE, Cummings KM (1995) Influence of smoking on the development of lung metastases from breast cancer. Cancer 75(11):2693–2699
211. Valeyre D, Soler P, Clerici C, Pre J, Battesti JP, Georges R et al (1988) Smoking and pulmonary sarcoidosis: effect of cigarette smoking on prevalence, clinical manifestations, alveolitis, and evolution of the disease. Thorax 43(7):516–524
212. Ellis ME, Neal KR, Webb AK (1987) Is smoking a risk factor for pneumonia in adults with chickenpox? Br Med J (Clin Res Ed) 294(6578):1002
213. Kaufman R (1983) Diagnosis and management. In: Pennington J (ed) Respiratory infections. Raven, New York, pp 317–328
214. Arvin AM (1996) Varicella-zoster virus. Clin Microbiol Rev 9(3):361–381
215. Hasday JD, Bascom R, Costa JJ, Fitzgerald T, Dubin W (1999) Bacterial endotoxin is an active component of cigarette smoke. Chest 115(3):829–835

Cardiovascular Disease, Disturbances of Blood Coagulation and Fibrinolysis

In numerous countries throughout the world active and passive tobacco smoking is an important factor in the development of cardiovascular disease and its associated mortality. In Germany, whereas 30,000 new cases of bronchial carcinoma are diagnosed in smokers every year, the corresponding annual figure for new cases of coronary heart disease (CHD), hypertension, peripheral arterial occlusive disease (PAOD), stroke etc. among smokers is 80,000–90,000. The first epidemiological studies to demonstrate an association between cigarette smoking and ischaemic heart disease were the Framingham Study and a study in male British doctors [1, 2]. The Framingham Study additionally showed that the incidence of stroke is increased by smoking [2, 3]. Smoking is further associated with an increased risk for arteriosclerotic vascular changes and with the occurrence of cerebral aneurysms [3, 4]. While other risk factors such as hyperlipidaemia, hyperfibrinogenaemia and hypertension are important in the context of CHD, the development of PAOD and of aortic aneurysm is largely smoking-related [2, 5–7].

As long ago as 1944, research was published indicating that the effects of nicotine on the blood vessels differ clearly in quantitative (and qualitative) terms from those of inhaled tobacco smoke (Fig. 6.1), a finding that is also important with regard to the use of nicotine products to achieve smoking cessation [8, 9].

6.1
Coronary Artery Disease and Myocardial Infarction

Epidemiological data from the USA demonstrate clearly that smoking cessation is beneficial for all age groups, including smokers over the age of 65 years [1, 10–12]. After smoking cessation, the cardiovascular risk falls more rapidly than the risk for lung cancer. For men and women the risk of myocardial infarction is halved within 1 year, attaining the risk levels of non-smokers within 2–3 years [13, 14]. For example, cardiovascular disease mortality was reduced by 24% in women who had quit smoking 2 years previously [15]. Smokers who have survived a myocardial infarction can expect a 25–50% risk reduction for reinfarction if they give up smoking [12, 16–19]. Similarly, continuing smokers' risk for restenosis after percutaneous transluminal coronary angioplasty (PTCA) is greater than in patients who have given up smoking [20]. Patients with coronary artery disease (CAD)

K.-O. Haustein, D. Groneberg, *Tobacco or Health?*
DOI: 10.1007/978-3-540-87577-2_6, © Springer Verlag Berlin Heidelberg 2010

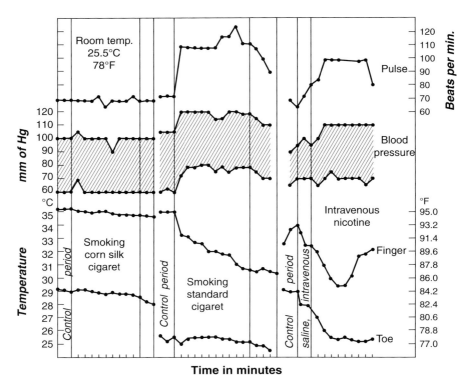

Fig. 6.1 Effect of smoking two corn silk or standard cigarettes and of intravenous injection of 2 mg nicotine on extremity skin temperature, blood pressure and heart rate (HR) of one normal person [152]

had reduced health-related quality of life (HRQoL) benefits after PTCA where they had not stopped smoking after the procedure [21].

In contrast to nicotine carbon monoxide (CO) is partially responsible for the development of arteriosclerosis in smokers. Additionally, other toxic agents included in cigarette smoke have a pronounced impact [22–24]. Experimental animal work indicates that such substances include formaldehyde, nitrosamines, acroleine, and NO_x. Several pathological processes are involved in the aorta of fowls treated with carcinogenic agents [25]. Smooth muscle cells proliferate and penetrate into the intima of larger vessels [25–28]. 3-Methylcholanthrene, benzo-[a]-pyrene (BP), and 7,12-dimethylbenz(a)anthracene (DMBA) initiate comparable intima lesions in the aorta of chickens and doves [25, 26, 29, 30]. Aortic tissue of chicken contains the subenzyme CYP_{1A1} which activates or detoxifies carcinogenic substances [31], and which can be induced by polycyclic aromatic hydrocarbons (PAH) [25, 27]. CYP_{1A1} is also present in human aortic smooth muscle cells, and the hydroxylation of BP and DMBA has also been described in cultured human foetal smooth muscle cells [32]. Thus, it seems highly likely that carcinogenic agents are partly responsible for lesions at the vessel wall and for activation of blood platelets [33].

Haematocrit is a decisive factor for the prognosis of CHD [34]: the association between haematocrit and CHD mortality was assessed in the large-scale NHANES II Mortality Study (1976–1992) in 8,896 patients aged 30–75 years, with smoking status as one of the covariates included. Women with haematocrit in the upper tertile were 1.3 times (CI 95%: 0.9–1.9) more likely to die from CHD than were women with haematocrit in the lowest tertile. Since similar associations could not be demonstrated for men, this must be a multifactorial phenomenon [34].

Among the 4,000 or more toxic substances absorbed during smoking, carbon monoxide (CO) and glycoproteins play a particularly important role in the development of smoking-related arteriosclerotic changes (see Sect. 6.4), and the severity of the changes produced is influenced by the cigarette dose and smoking duration [35, 36].

Smoking disturbs the O_2 supply/consumption ratio (up to 15% of haemoglobin is no longer available for O_2 transport), causing heart rate (HR) and blood pressure to increase slightly (see Fig. 6.1) [35, 37]. The nicotine absorbed with every cigarette puff (50–150 µg) may possibly not be entirely responsible for these changes, even though the alkaloid does produce measurable increments in plasma concentrations of adrenaline and noradrenaline [38]. These increases are very much smaller in habitual smokers than in occasional smokers. Also, while the occurrence of cardiac arrhythmias after smoking may be attributable to the effect of nicotine [39], this phenomenon is due more to the inhalation of other toxic substances (CO, formation of CO-haemoglobin) [16].

Years of habitual cigarette smoking lead to *coronary constriction* and *lower coronary reserve* on effort [40]. In habitual smokers simultaneously suffering from CHD, cigarette smoking lowers the angina threshold. Just 5 min after smoking one cigarette, coronary blood flow is reduced (7%) and coronary resistance is increased (21%), accompanied by a simultaneous rise in the rate-pressure product [41]. These changes are caused by coronary vessel constriction and by the very rapid onset of myocardial hypoxia. In angina patients, regardless of the number of cigarettes smoked, cigarette smoking produces narrowing of the coronary artery lumen detectable on angiography [42, 43], and this effect is particularly severe in patients with vasospastic angina [44].

Results confirm the minimal "harmfulness" of nicotine on the circulation (Fig. 6.2) [45]. This study compared cardiovascular risk factors in smokers, non-smokers and users of snuff and chewing tobacco (smokeless tobacco). Smokeless tobacco consumption over a period of years does not produce a significant increase in risk factors for the development of CHD or in the atherogenic index (Fig. 6.2) [45]. These data also point to the harmful effects of the combustion products of tobacco smoke in the development of cardiovascular disease.

In the Trial on Reversing Endothelial Dysfunction (TREND Study) 54 patients (smokers and non-smokers) each underwent quantitative coronary angiography at baseline and again after 6-month follow-up to measure coronary artery diameter responses to acetylcholine [46, 47]. Impairment of endothelium-dependent vasodilatation by chronic smoking is clearly caused by tobacco smoke and not by nicotine [48–51]. One study involving angiographic assessments over a 2-year period demonstrated progression of coronary atherosclerosis and the development of numerous new coronary lesions in smokers [52]. The reduced vascular response (e.g. measured at the brachial artery) is reversible after smoking cessation [48], and a correlation has been found between the CO content of expired air [53] and the ischaemia threshold [54]. If this response also applies for the coronary arteries, it

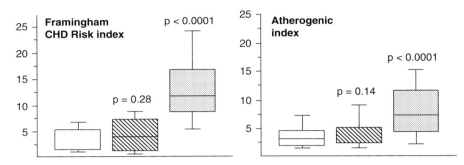

Fig. 6.2 Box plots showing the 10th, 25th, 50th, 75th and 90th percentiles of the indices for cardiovascular risk factors (Framingham CHD Risk Index and Atherogenic Index). ANOVA and Fisher's test for the comparison of different tobacco users (smokeless tobacco users: *cross-hatched boxes*; smokers: *stippled boxes*) with non-smokers (*white boxes*) were statistically significant ($p < 0.05$) [45]

probably explains the lower incidence of reinfarction among men who stopped smoking after a first myocardial infarction compared with those who continued to smoke [55].

Cigarette smoking appreciably increases the risk of myocardial infarction. In the multi-centre GISSI-2 Trial [56] risk factors were determined in 916 patients with acute myocardial infarction: by comparison with lifelong non-smokers, the relative risk (RR) was 1.3 for ex-smokers, 2.0 for current smokers of less than 15 cigarettes/day, 3.1 for current smokers of 15–24 cigarettes/day, and 4.9 for current smokers of more than 25 cigarettes/day. The duration of smoking was less important than the age of the smoker: below the age of 45 years, smokers of 25 or more cigarettes/day had a 33-fold higher risk compared with non-smokers, whereas older smokers had smaller risks (45–54 years: 7.5-fold; 55–64 years: 4.4-fold; >65 years: 2.5-fold) [56]. In Italy about 50% of all acute myocardial infarctions could be directly attributable to smoking.

According to the Rochester CHD Project, a study conducted in 40–59-year-old women, cigarette smoking increases the risk for CHD or sudden cardiac death. The odds ratio for the association between steroidal oestrogen use in non-smokers and CHD was 0.6 and rose to 5.1 in smokers, with 64% of all cases of myocardial infarction and sudden cardiac death occurring in smokers [57, 58]. A cardiac catheterisation study in 8,705 smokers also revealed an association between the location of coronary sclerosis and smoking behaviour: stenoses occurred more commonly in the right coronary artery than in the left circumflex artery or left anterior descending artery [59].

According to one case-control study in 555 women below the age of 50 years, the risk of myocardial infarction increased with the number of cigarettes smoked, regardless of whether other predisposing factors (total cholesterol, HDL, oral contraceptive use, hypertension, diabetes mellitus) were present [60]. The risk to women is underscored by a further study, according to which the risk of myocardial infarction was increased 2.47-fold in smokers of just 1–5 cigarettes daily [61]. The risk was increased 74.6-fold in women who were heavy smokers (≥40 cigarettes daily); oral contraceptive use did not entail any increased risk, whereas there were additive risks with hypertension and diabetes mellitus [61].

In one study in 5,572 patients at risk compared with 6,268 controls, the coronary risk fell from 3.5 to 1.5 for men and from 4.8 to 1.6 for women who had quit smoking for

1–3 years [62]. After 4–6 years of smoking cessation, the risk was comparable with that of never-smokers [62]. Also, compared with non-smokers, the first myocardial infarction has been shown to occur 13.8 years earlier in male smokers and 3.6 years earlier in female smokers [63].

The data presented in the literature indicate that nicotine itself exerts no appreciable deleterious effects on myocardial perfusion or in terms of increasing risk factors for CHD [55]. While nicotine administration to rats during the post-infarction period does lead to delayed regression of left-ventricular changes [64], it would be premature to draw far-reaching conclusions from these findings.

6.2
Systemic Vascular Changes

Cigarette smoking is associated with a sevenfold increase in the risk for PAOD [65, 66], whereas the risk for CHD is merely doubled [67, 68]. The vascular changes caused by smoking differ, depending on location: for example, heavy smoking produces more severe damage in the vessels of the leg than in the coronary vessels [69, 70].

No reliable epidemiological studies have been performed concerning the development of *hypertension* in cigarette smokers. On average, in fact, lower blood pressure values are measured in smokers than in non-smokers, and blood pressure in ex-smokers is comparable with that in non-smokers [13, 71], apart from nocturnal diastolic measurements which are elevated compared with those of non-smokers [72]. In habitual smokers, smoking a single cigarette produces increases in blood pressure (6%), HR (14%) and cardiac index (16%), whereas stroke volume and total peripheral resistance are not significantly altered. After wrist occlusion, only muscle blood flow and not skin blood flow is increased [73]. Cigarette smoking leads to disturbances of left-ventricular diastolic function regardless of whether coronary sclerotic changes are present or not [74–76]. Administration of nicotine in a transdermal patch produced a minimal increase in diastolic blood pressure in normotensive but not in hypertensive smokers 2–4 h post-dose. Simultaneously measured thromboxane B_2 levels were increased in response to nicotine in non-smokers but not in normotensive or hypertensive smokers where thromboxane B_2 was already elevated [77].

Smokers with hypertension are less likely to be aware of their high blood pressure or to be treated than non-smokers (ex-smokers) with hypertension (OR 1.25; 1.06–1.47; $p = 0.009$) [78].

In one study, 1,016 professional athletes using smokeless tobacco were compared with a control group without tobacco consumption in terms of cardiovascular risk factors. Over a 1-year period there were no changes in systolic blood pressure, HR and total or HDL cholesterol in the tobacco users or in the controls. Only diastolic blood pressure correlated with the plasma nicotine level. Overall, the influence of smokeless tobacco on cardiovascular risk factors was classified as minimal [79]. According to one Danish study, blood pressure is slightly lower in smokers than in non-smokers, indicating that the "white coat" effect during ambulatory blood pressure measurements was less pronounced in smokers than in non-smokers [80].

Kidney disease is associated with an increased risk for the development of cardiovascular disease and end-stage renal disease; however, risk factors for kidney disease have not been well studied and smoking is a candidate factor [81]. Fox et al. identified predictors of the development of new-onset kidney disease in 2004. A community-based, longitudinal cohort study of 2,585 participants who attended both a baseline examination in 1978–1982 and a follow-up examination in 1998–2001, and who were free of kidney disease at baseline. The researchers showed that after a mean follow-up of 18.5 years, 244 participants (9.4%) had developed kidney disease. In multivariable models, baseline age (odds ratio [OR], 2.36 per 10-year increment; 95% confidence interval [CI], 2.00–2.78), GFR (< 90 mL/min per 1.73 m^2: OR, 3.01; 95% CI, 1.98–4.58; 90–119 mL/min per 1.73 m^2: OR, 1.84; 95% CI, 1.16–2.93), body mass index (OR, 1.23 per 1 SD; 95% CI, 1.08–1.41), diabetes (OR, 2.60; 95% CI, 1.44–4.70), and smoking (OR, 1.42; 95% CI, 1.06–1.91) were related to the development of kidney disease [81].

In the *cerebral vessels* smoking causes acute vasodilatation and increased blood flow in the grey matter (+15.7%). This increase in blood flow was detected without any change in O$_2$ metabolism and, following consumption of a single cigarette, was most pronounced in non-smokers, less pronounced in ex-smokers and least pronounced in smokers [82]. Cerebral blood flow was measured by ^{133}Xe inhalation in a population of 192 volunteers, including 84 patients with risk factors for stroke. The study population included 75 habitual smokers (0.5–3.5 packs per day for 25 years). Grey matter blood flow was clearly more impaired in the smokers than in the non-smokers [83], and the arteriosclerotic vascular changes also appear to be the decisive factor in terms of a subsequent stroke. The incidence of stroke in relation to cigarette smoking was investigated over an 8-year period in a cohort study of 118,539 women between the ages of 30 and 55 and free from CHD, stroke and cancer. In the 274 patients with stroke, compared with women who had never smoked, those who smoked 1–14 cigarettes/day had a relative stroke risk of 2.2, whereas those who smoked 25 or more cigarettes/day had a relative risk of 3.7. The 71 observed cases of subarachnoid haemorrhage mainly included smokers, whose relative risk for such an event was 9.8, as compared with women who had never smoked [84]. These data support the association between cigarette smoking and stroke among young and middle-aged women.

According to newer research, a correlation exists between increased serum thiocyanate levels and stroke risk, as shown by investigations in 67 stroke patients (OR 3.00; 1.06–8.48; $p < 0.05$), prompting the recommendation that serum thiocyanate levels should be measured as an indicator of smoking status in stroke patients [85].

Aortic aneurysms occurring predominantly in the abdominal region are a common cause of death among elderly men [86]. In one study in 73,451 veterans aged 50–79 years, most of whom were smokers, vascular changes were detected by ultrasound screening. A larger proportion of abdominal aortic aneurysms (AAA) (*n* = 1,917; 3.6%) were ≤3 cm in diameter, and only 613 aneurysms (1.2%) were 4-cm or larger. The respective odds ratios for smoking were 4.45 (CI: 3.27–6.05) and 5.07 (CI: 4.24–7.31), whereas a raised cholesterol level yielded odds ratios of only 1.29 (1.06–1.58) and 1.54 (CI: 1.31–1.80). The excess prevalence associated with smoking accounted for 75% of all AAA of 4 cm or larger in diameter in the total population of 126,196 persons studied by this research group [87]. One noteworthy and as yet unanswered question is why patients with diabetes mellitus have aortic aneurysms more rarely (*OR* = 0.50; CI: 0.39–0.65 and 0.54; CI: 0.44–0.65)

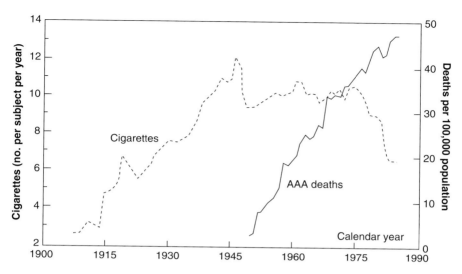

Fig. 6.3 Cigarette consumption and mortality from abdominal aortic aneurysm (AAA). There is a lag intervals of about 40 years between increasing consumption of cigarettes and increasing mortality from AAA in England and Wales [94]. Data for cigarette consumption were taken from UK Tobacco Advisory Board

than other patients [87–89]. In smokers, the risk of developing an AAA increases with increasing mean arterial (≥100 mmHg) and diastolic blood pressure (≥90 mmHg) and the number of cigarettes currently smoked and the depth of inhalation [90]. Similar associations between the development of aortic aneurysms and smoking have also been demonstrated in smaller studies [91, 92], and in one study women were found to have a threefold higher risk of aneurysm rupture than men [93]. In any event, smoking cessation is regarded as an important strategy to delay progression. According to the results shown in Fig. 6.3, there is a lag interval of about 40 years between increasing consumption of cigarettes and increasing mortality from AAA in England and Wales [94]. Stop smoking and an improved treatment of hypertension are essential if mortality from AAA is to be reduced.

6.2.1
Regulation of Vascular Tone

Tobacco smoking stimulates adrenergic mechanisms in the heart and circulation, although these mechanisms are triggered more by smoking than by nicotine per se (Table 6.2) [95], and cause an increase in the lactate/pyruvate ratio and in urinary excretion of adrenaline. These mechanisms can be suppressed by adrenergic blockade [38] and arise as a result of noradrenaline release from the terminal axon. Acetylcholine (ACh) can be used to measure vascular responsiveness or blood flow (vasodilatation with NO release) in individual vessels: these variables are clearly diminished in smokers, as is the angiotensin I-mediated vasoconstrictor response [96]. Lisinopril, an angiotensin-converting enzyme (ACE) inhibitor, has been shown to improve endothelial function in chronic cigarette smokers, as demonstrated by an increased forearm blood flow response to acetylcholine, whereas there was no effect on the response to sodium nitroprusside [97]. Bradykinin-mediated NO release induced by lisinopril has been suggested as the possible mechanism responsible [96]. In contrast to smoking, nicotine (e.g. when administered as a patch) does not reduce the surface area of coronary segments and also does not additively enhance the vasoconstrictor effect of sympathetic stimulation produced by the cold pressor test [98]. Differences between cigarette smoke and nicotine were also seen in changes of the flow-mediated dilatation (FMD) which declined in 16 healthy smokers: this variable declined to a greater extent after smoking one cigarette (1 mg nicotine) than after administration of nasal spray (1 mg nicotine) (means: -3.6 vs. -5.1%; smoke vs. nicotine). Nitroglycerine-induced dilatation remained similar under both experimental conditions [99]. Irrespective of differences in nicotine kinetics after the two methods of administration, the mechanism of action of nicotine on the endothelium remains unclear.

In terms of nitric oxide (NO) release, endothelial NO synthase (NOS) gene polymorphism (a/b polymorphism) plays a decisive role in the occurrence of acute myocardial infarction. This risk is increased particularly in younger smokers (aged < 51 years) with a/a polymorphism, irrespective of the additional presence of diabetes mellitus or hypertension [100].

The vasoconstrictor effect on coronary vessels may be caused by reduced prostacyclin (PGI_2) levels in the coronary endothelial cells. In comparison with non-smokers, smokers have reduced blood levels of PGI_2 and increased blood levels of 11-dehydro-TXB_2 [101, 102]. Nevertheless, the reactions produced by cigarette smoking in terms of adrenaline, noradrenaline and dopamine release are different from those produced by nicotine administration, as shown by the data presented in Table 6.1. Catecholamine release due to nicotine administration is quantitatively smaller than that due to cigarette smoke [95, 103].

During cigarette smoking, nicotine is absorbed very rapidly, leading to varying degrees of adrenaline- and noradrenaline-induced vasoconstriction via α_1-adreno-ceptor stimulation. Occasional smokers compensate for this vasoconstrictor effect by releasing NO and prostacyclin from endothelium, whereas in heavy smokers this mechanism no longer operates. In this context it should be pointed out that vascular tone is regulated by two vasoactive substances with opposing effects: $NO^{\cdot}$ and $O_2^{-\cdot}$. NO has a pivotal role here, particularly

Table 6.1 Catecholamine release associated with cigarette smoking [38] (mean, mean standard error) and urinary catecholamine excretion in smokers and following nicotine administration (patch) [171]

		Noradrenaline [pg/ml]	Adrenaline [pg/ml]	
Control patients		227 (23)	44 (4)	
Smokers		324 (39)	113 (27)	
	Plasma nicotine AUC [ng/ml·h]	Noradrenaline [µg/g creatinine]	Adrenaline [µg/g creatinine]	Dopamine [µg/g creatinine]
Cigarette smoking	451 ± 62	176 ± 23	28 ± 3	$1,099 \pm 86$
Nicotine patch	356 ± 30	166 ± 25	21 ± 3	$1,051 \pm 87$
Placebo patch	–	172 ± 20	22 ± 2	950 ± 65
p-value	n.s	<0.06	<0.05	<0.05

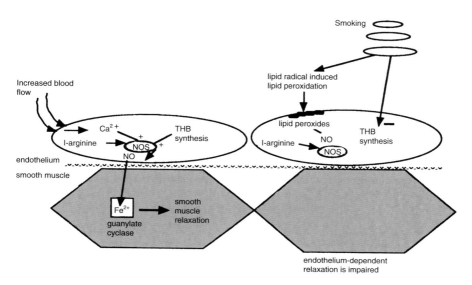

Fig. 6.4 Harmful effects of smoking on vascular relaxation. A rise in Ca^{2+} causes an increase in NO synthesis from L-arginine by NOS. Tetrahydrobiopterin (THB) is an important co-factor. NO penetrates the vascular cell and stimulates guanylate cyclase; this in turn forms cGMP which has a vasodilator action. Smoking limits the synthesis of cGMP. In addition, the radicals formed in the blood promote oxo-LDL formation. A fall in THB also reduces NO synthesis [209]

since post-occlusive vasodilatation (in the forearm, for example) is associated with NO production and release from endothelium. NO is formed from L-arginine by NOS, which is dependent on NADPH, flavin adenine nucleotides and tetrahydrobiopterin (THB). Atherogenic activity has been attributed to the toxic substance (ONOO⁻), in conjunction with activation of the renin-angiotensin system [104]. NO is able to form free radicals, and to activate guanylate cyclase in endothelial cells and platelets (Fig. 6.4).

Acute cigarette smoking leads to temporary endothelial dysfunction, which is an early event in atherogenesis. Sufficient data concerning the effect of cigarettes with low tar and nicotine yield are lacking. Therefore, Papamichael et al. studied seventeen healthy individuals (nine women, eight men, aged 27.8 ± 3.6 years) who were subjected to evaluation of endothelial function by means of endothelium-dependent, FMD of the brachial artery, before, immediately after and 30, 60 and 90 min after smoking a regular cigarette (nicotine 0.9 mg, tar 12 mg) or the corresponding "light" cigarette (nicotine 0.6 mg, tar 8 mg) [105]. The following day, measurements were repeated after smoking the opposite kind of cigarette. Baseline FMD was $6.1 \pm 1.6\%$ and $7.2 \pm 2.0\%$ in the light and regular cigarette groups, respectively ($p = NS$). The overall effect of the regular cigarette over time on FMD compared with the light cigarette was significantly different ($F = 3.039$, $p = 0.023$). FMD was significantly depressed after smoking both types (light: $F = 8.192$, $p < 0.001$; regular: $F = 16.698$, $p < 0.001$). Immediately after smoking, FMD declined in both groups (light: 3.0 $\pm 2.4\%$ and regular: $1.6 \pm 3.2\%$, $p < 0.001$ and $p < 0.001$, respectively), and it remained significantly depressed in the regular cigarette group at 30 min ($0.75 \pm 1.5\%$, $p < 0.001$) and 60 min ($3.5 \pm 3.1\%$, $p = 0.024$), while in the light cigarette group FMD differences were abolished at 30, 60 and 90 min after smoking. The authors concluded that acute smoking of both regular and light cigarettes leads to temporary vasomotor dysfunction; its duration is shorter after smoking a "light" cigarette [105].

Vasodilatation and inhibition of platelet aggregation is achieved as a result of cGMP release. NO is therefore of major pathogenetic importance in that it prevents platelet aggregation, monocyte adhesion and vascular smooth muscle cell proliferation. By reducing NO formation, smoking counteracts these preventive processes [106]. Where dysfunctional NOS III activity is associated with inhibition of NO production, supplementary administration of THB improves endothelium-dependent vasodilatation in chronic smokers [107]. Glyceryl trinitrate or sodium nitroprusside influence these processes because they have a vasodilator action in response to NO production. The interplay of LDL oxidation and NOS dysfunction is supported by in-vitro experiments in saphenous vein rings and platelets [108, 109], showing that impaired endothelium-dependent relaxation is attributable to inadequate THB synthesis resulting from the harmful effects of cigarette smoke constituents (Fig. 6.5) [108, 110]. In hypercholesterolaemia the adverse effect on vascular function results from the oxidation of LDL to oxo-LDL [111]. As an antioxidant, ascorbic acid is reported to improve smoking-induced vascular responses [112]. Smoking-related endothelial damage

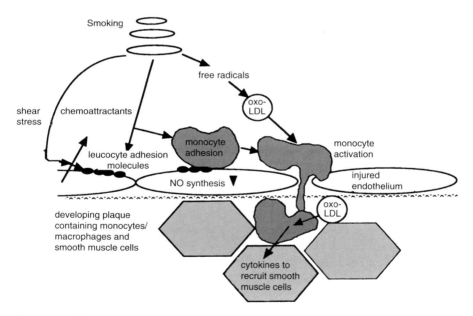

Fig. 6.5 Smoking stimulates monocyte adhesion, migration and activation. Increased shear forces alter the endothelial surface and increase the production of the adhesion molecules ICAM-1 and VCAM-1 on vascular endothelium. In addition, chemical adhesives are released from monocytes, and the reduction in NO synthesis increases monocyte adhesion to the endothelial cells. The endothelium becomes porous, with the result that oxo-LDL molecules are able to pass through. These in turn activate monocytes/macrophages which release cytokines and growth factors – a starting point for atherosclerotic changes in the vessel [209]

is partially reversible if smoking cessation is maintained for at least 12 months [113, 114]. Disturbed prostacyclin synthesis is associated with the increased production of vasoconstrictor thromboxanes [115].

6.2.2
Changes in Endothelial Function and Microcirculation

The basis for the evolution of *arteriosclerosis* with subsequent cardiac events is formed by smoking-induced changes in coronary vascular tone, increased platelet aggregation and altered endothelial integrity, even in younger adults [102, 113]. Cigarette smoking produces *endothelial changes* with detectable ultrastructural damage to the aorta and pulmonary vessels [116–118]. The tobacco constituent NNK (see Table 3.6, Box 3.1 in Chap. 3) causes considerable endothelial damage. Its binding to β_1- and β_2-adrenoceptors is followed by activation of arachidonic acid, associated with endothelial damage and apoptosis of endothelial cells. These effects of NNK can be prevented by β-receptor blockers (atenolol) [119].

Bernhard et al. demonstrated in 2003 that tobacco smoke dramatically changes vascular endothelial cell and tissue morphology, leading to a loss of endothelial barrier function within minutes. In these experiments long-term exposure of endothelial cells to tobacco smoke extracts induced necrosis that may trigger a pro-inflammatory status of the vessel wall [120]. Pre-incubation of the extracts without cells for 6 h at 37°C led to a complete loss of activity. Furthermore, the endothelium could be rescued by changing to fresh medium even at times when the extracts had lost their activity. It was also shown that N-acetyl cysteine and statins inhibit the adverse tobacco smoke effects [120].

The regulation of vascular tone is disturbed when NO production is diminished. Based on the damage to endothelial function outlined above, short periods of smoking potentiate the vasoconstrictor effect of endothelin-1 [121]. It has long been known that endothelium-dependent coronary dilatation is disturbed in the presence of hypercholesterolaemia, the premature onset of arteriosclerosis and/or hypertension [122–124]. In addition, habitual smoking diminishes the vasodilator reserve of the tiniest vessels and thus encourages the harmful hypoxic effects which are detectable in habitual smokers long before the appearance of recognisable cardiovascular disease [125, 126]. Bradykinin-induced venous dilatation in the dorsal veins of the hand is suppressed both in non-smokers and in smokers by transdermal administration of nicotine, with the result that a pivotal role in endothelial dysfunction must be conceded for the alkaloid [127]. These studies have also shown a slight rise in blood pressure in response to nicotine.

Alongside endothelial damage, the flow properties of the blood and blood coagulation processes are also influenced by cigarette smoking but not by nicotine (Table 6.2). It is generally accepted that *plasma fibrinogen levels are increased* in smokers, due to reduced plasminogen activity in the blood [128, 129], and that increasing age leads to a further rise in fibrinogen. As a result, the fluidity of the blood is lowered and the viscosity of whole blood and plasma is increased [38, 71, 128, 130]. The haemorheological properties of the blood are further exacerbated by the increase in haematocrit [130, 131] – evidently in compensation for the transformation of up to 15% of haemoglobin into CO-haemoglobin

Table 6.2   Differences between cigarette smoking and nicotine administration on haemorheological variables [8]

Variables	Smoking	Nicotine	Reference nos
Plasma fibrinogen concentration	⇑	⇔	[71, 128–130, 136, 137, 157, 203–205]
Platelet aggregation (CO-induced)	⇑	⇔	[41]
Haematocrit	⇑	⇔	[71, 130, 131]
Leucocyte count	⇑	⇔	[135–137]
von Willebrand factor	⇑	⇔	[136, 137]
Factor XIIa	⇑	⇔	[141]
Plasminogen	⇓	⇔	[128, 129]
Vascular permeability for fibrinogen	⇑	⇔	[206–208]
Red cell deformability	⇓	⇔	[132, 133, 173]
Viscosity (plasma, blood)	⇑	⇔	[71, 128, 130, 131]
CO-haemoglobin	⇑	⇔	[95]
Catecholamines in blood and urine	⇑	⇑, ⇔	[179, 195]

Results from clinical studies. ⇑: elevated, ⇓: low or reduced, ⇔: unchanged or normal

– and by the progressive decline in red cell deformability [132, 133]. The supply of O_2 to the tissues is thus also reduced. In addition, the following variables are elevated in smokers: leucocyte count [134–136], CO-induced platelet aggregability [41], and factor XIII and von Willebrand factor activity [136–138]. All these smoking-induced reactions tend to normalise following smoking cessation and/or nicotine substitution (Table 6.2).

Previous thinking concerning the important vasoconstrictor effect of nicotine in terms of the evolution of vascular disease should be revised to take account of the very much greater part played by CO and CO-haemoglobin and by glycoproteins in bringing about changes in the vessels and the microcirculation (Fig. 6.1, Table 6.2 [8]).

Based on experimental animal work, it has been reported that nicotine stimulates new blood vessel formation (angiogenesis), and this is associated with endothelial proliferation [139]. Overall, this study attributes tumorigenic activity to nicotine [139].

Further research is required to confirm whether these results can be transposed to the situation in man. To date, at least, there is no evidence to show that nicotine displays such properties in humans.

6.2.3
Microcirculation and O_2 Supply

Smoking-induced damage to the microcirculation, including the skin and O_2 supply, has been studied in humans and in experimental animals [140–143]. In particular, dramatic reactions have been demonstrated in smokers undergoing revascularisation procedures [144, 145]. Likewise, skin necroses have been described in smokers following cosmetic facial surgery [141, 146, 147]. These harmful effects were elicited by the toxic constituents of cigarette smoke and by CO, and to a very much smaller extent by nicotine [9]. In smokers, skin flaps also show delayed healing or fail to survive at all (see Chap. 7.8) [144, 148, 149].

Dalla et al studies in 2004 the effects of acute and chronic smoking on skin microvascular properties of young healthy subjects. In this observational study, using a totally non-invasive approach, employing continuous palmar microvascular flow (laser Doppler) and arterial pressure measurements, a total of 20 healthy male subjects (nine habitual smokers and 11 non-smokers; aged 27 ± 1 and 29 ± 2 years, respectively) were examined [150]. Measures were obtained at baseline and after iontophoretic administration of acetylcholine (ACh), an endothelium-dependent vasodilator and of sodium nitroprusside (NP), an endothelium-independent vasodilator. The study showed that smokers showed significant lower baseline microvascular resistive (Z0) and oscillatory (impedance, i.e. ZC) properties than non-smokers. In the non-smokers group, ACh and NP iontophoresis induced a significant decrease of both Z0 and ZC, before and after smoking one cigarette ($p < 0.02$). Conversely, in the smokers group, both Z0 and ZC were not affected by ACh iontophoresis before acute smoking, while, after smoking, a significant decrease of both Z0 and ZC ($p < 0.02$) was detected after ACh challenge. The study indicates that smokers have a complex disruption of peripheral microcirculatory regulation, including inappropriate resting vasodilation, impaired endothelium-dependent and independent vasodilation, paradoxical recovery of endothelium-dependent vasodilation in response to acute smoking [151].

In a further study, the acute effects of smoking on microvascular function in healthy smokers was studied using measures of HR, blood pressure, capillary recruitment during peak reactive hyperaemia and endothelium-dependent and endothelium-independent vasodilatation of the skin microcirculation with iontophoresis of acetylcholine and sodium nitroprusside respectively combined with laser Doppler fluxmetry [151] It was found that in comparison with sham smoking, acute smoking caused increases in HR (smoking, 9.3 ± 4.1 beats/min; sham, −1.3 ± 3.0 beats/min; $p < 0.001$) and systolic blood pressure (smoking, 6.3 ± 8.8 mmHg; sham, 0.8 ± 4.4 mmHg; $p < 0.05$). Also, decreases in absolute (smoking, −4.9 ± 6.9 per mm²; sham, 0.8 ± 2.1 per mm(2); $p = 0.01$) and relative (smoking, −13.8 ± 21.4%; sham, 1.9 ± 6.9%; $p = 0.02$) capillary recruitment during peak reactive hyperaemia; and decreases in absolute [smoking, -62.4 ± 47.7 perfusion units (PU); sham, −30.8 ± 32.6 PU; $p = 0.04$] and relative (smoking, −147 ± 163%; sham, 32 ± 225%; $p = 0.07$) vasodilatation caused by acetylcholine were demonstrated. From this study it can be concluded that acute smoking is associated with impaired capillary recruitment during peak reactive hyperaemia and impaired microvascular endothelium-dependent vasodilatation. These findings may also explain the increased blood pressure and decreased insulin sensitivity that have been observed after acute smoking [151].

Vascular response and O_2 supply of the skin and deeper tissue layers can be measured by *laser Doppler flowmetry* and by determining *transcutaneous partial O2 pressure* with *platinum electrodes*, as our own research has demonstrated [9]. Attention was drawn long ago to the differences between the reactions produced by cigarette smoke and by nicotine [152]. Reactive hyperaemia occurring after 1–3 min occlusion of the upper arm with a *blood pressure cuff* and its normalisation have been found to differ between smokers and non-smokers [9, 153, 154], with reactive hyperaemia in smokers being less than that in non-smokers (see Fig. 6.6): the reasons for this are certainly to be sought in vasoresponsiveness (NO production) and in the viscosity of the blood, which influences its flow properties [9]. The differences in vasoreactivity were still detectable even after a 6-month observation period (Fig. 6.7) [8]. For a summary of the findings on this topic, readers are

Fig. 6.6 Post-ischaemic reactive hyperaemia on the skin, measured by laser Doppler flowmetry in 16 smokers before (straight line) and after (dashed line) smoking. The *vertical bars* indicate ± standard error of the mean [210]

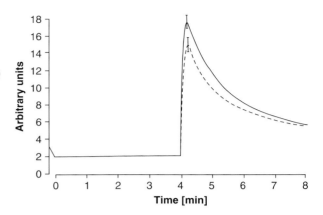

Fig. 6.7 Changes in maximal rate of increase (t-p$_{max}$ in s) in intracapillary flow of red cells after 3 min of forearm ischaemia. Ex-smokers, relapsers and smokers over the 26-week study period. The vertical bars indicate the standard deviations at each measuring time [9]

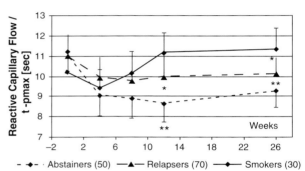

referred to [155]. Simultaneous photoplethysmographic recordings of blood flow at different tissue sites revealed a considerable vasocontrictive response in the fingers and a more modest response in the toes; the response was absent in the forehead and ear recordings [154]. The magnitude of the vascular response in the fingers did not correlate with the nicotine yield of the cigarettes.

O$_2$ supply is associated with tissue perfusion. After smoking or chewing nicotine-containing gum, digital blood flow was reduced, and this effect occurred earlier after smoking (after 5 min) than after chewing nicotine gum (after 45 min) [137]. By contrast, no changes in tcpO$_2$ were measured either after smoking or after nicotine [156, 157]. These findings stand in contrast to our own long-term results from the NiveS Study (Fig. 6.8) where a change in tcpO$_2$ could still be detected even after 6 months' smoking cessation, in comparison with smokers [8]. Investigation of tcpO$_2$ in smoking and non-smoking mothers has revealed a less pronounced hyperaemic reaction in smoking mothers than in non-smoking mothers (see Chap. 8). When an invasive method was used to measure O$_2$, a reduction in O$_2$ supply lasting for 30–50 min was detected after a single cigarette had been smoked [158]. In overall terms, according to the results of the 6-month NiveS Study [9], the inhaled combustion products of tobacco have greater significance for the pathogenesis than nicotine. While nicotine does possess vasoconstrictor properties of its own, these are not responsible for the hypoxaemic reactions, as also confirmed by clinical trials in angina patients

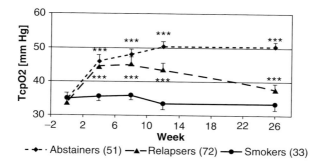

Fig. 6.8 Changes in transcutaneous partial oxygen pressure base value (mean ± standard deviation; 95% CI) between baseline and 26 weeks. *** $p < 0.001$ between baseline and the various time points in abstainers and relapsers. Significance ($p = 0.0339$ to $p < 0.001$) also between smokers vs. abstainers or relapsers at all time points [9]

Table 6.3 Effect of nicotine patches on perfusion in the damaged myocardium of patients with CAD [55]

	Controls ($n = 36$)	14 mg nicotine patch ($n = 36$)	21 mg nicotine patch ($n = 36$)	p-value
Perfusion defect (% LV)				
– Total	17.5 ± 10.6	12.6 ± 10.1	11.8 ± 9.9	<0.001
– Ischaemia	10.1 ± 8.5	7.2 ± 6.7	6.7 ± 6.3	0.036
CO (ppm)	23.3 ± 10.5	13.8 ± 9.6	12.4 ± 8.8	<0.001
Nicotine (ng/ml)	15.8 ± 8.3	24.2 ± 12.0	30.4 ± 10.8	<0.001
Cotinine (ng/ml)	290 ± 137	338 ± 186	422 ± 224	<0.002
Cigarette consumption (daily)	31 ± 11	11 ± 10	8 ± 7	<0.001

Measurements by 201Tl-SPECT 3 and 6 days after daily application of a nicotine patch

(see Table 6.3) [55]. Ultimately, the facial colouring of a person who has smoked for decades speaks for itself [159].

Blood flow defects were recorded by [82]rubidium emission tomography in 8 out of 13 patients with CHD undergoing bicycle ergometer exercise; in 6 of these 8 patients the blood flow defects were also recorded at the same sites when a single cigarette was smoked. A causal relationship with smoking may be assumed, with reduced O_2 availability [95, 103], increased platelet aggregation together with raised plasma fibrinogen concentrations [5, 109, 160], reduced NO and EDRF [49, 50, 113] and increased blood CO levels [161, 162] contributing to myocardial ischaemia. In 63 patients (non-smokers) with stable angina and with proven 70% stenosis for at least one coronary artery, ergometer exercise produced ST-segment depression after exposure to 2 or 4% carbon monoxide (see Fig. 6.9). Simultaneously, the time to onset of angina, time to ST-segment depression as well as exercise time were recorded as endpoints (Fig. 6.9) [162]. The effects were very much more pronounced after exposure to 4% CO than to 2% CO. Smokers with CO-Hb levels >5% should give up smoking because of the danger associated with the consequences of existing ischaemic heart disease.

Fig. 6.9 Consequences of CO exposure in patients with coronary artery disease (CAD). Exercise time, time to onset of angina and time to ST-segment depression were reduced overall after changing from room air to air with an increased CO content, resulting in COHb values of 2 and 4% respectively [162]

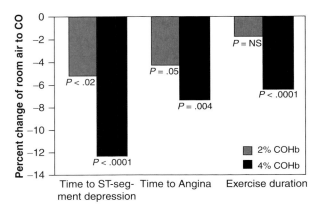

6.2.4
Arteriosclerotic and Inflammatory Vascular Reactions

Disturbed NO production and prostacyclin synthesis are just one aspect of the vascular changes initiated by smoking. In addition, the increased adhesion and migration of monocytes into the subendothelial space are important, and these phenomena are intensified by cytokines and LDL oxidation [163]. Leucocytes come into contact with the endothelium where they deposit proteins and glycoproteins on to endothelial cells and monocytes (Fig. 6.6). The adhesion of the cells is facilitated by adhesion proteins (intercellular adhesion molecule: ICAM-1 and vascular cell adhesion molecule: VCAM-1) and by integrins, and NO plays an important regulatory role in adhesion [164].

A study conducted in 2004 evaluated the effects of cigarette smoking on the plasma concentrations of VCAM-1 in patients with CAD. The soluble VCAM-1 level was quantified in smoking CHD patients in comparison to those from patients with CAD alone. It was found that soluble VCAM-1 levels were significantly higher in smokers than in non-smokers (32.1279 ± 21.6421 vs. 9.4570 ± 7.8138 ng/mL, $p < 0.01$) [165].

Anti-adhesive properties become lost as a result of smoking. Ibuprofen has been shown to reduce the adhesion of monocytes to TNFα-stimulated human umbilical vein endothelial cells, accompanied by reduced radical generation [166]. It has been demonstrated in human umbilical vein endothelial cells that smoke condensate causes a very rapid rise in the expression of both adhesion proteins on the surface of cultured cells [167]. Ascorbic acid is reported to counteract the increased adhesiveness of monocytes in smokers [168]. On the biochemical level, it has also been shown that Nicotine could augment adhesion molecule expression in human endothelial cells through macrophages secreting the immunomediators TNF-α, IL-1β [169].

Smoking also alters the haemodynamic forces at the blood-endothelium interface [170, 171]; likewise the concentration of adhesion molecules on the endothelial surface is regulated by haemodynamic forces [172]. In addition, the concentration of the monocyte adhesion protein MCP-1 (together with VCAM-1) is increased by the shear forces in smokers, and this is important for the adhesion of monocytes and macrophages to the endothelium (Fig. 6.6).

The vessels gradually become "denuded" of endothelial cells, which in turn disappear in the flowing blood [173]. The collagen of the subendothelial matrix supports platelet adhesion and aggregation, resulting in the increased production of platelet-derived growth factor (PDGF) which acts as a mitogen for the vascular muscle cells, the true starting point for arteriosclerotic changes [163]. Having undergone these changes, the vascular cells take up oxo-LDL molecules in large numbers, and this leads in turn to the release of inflammatory cytokines with the likelihood of cell death.

An insertion/deletion (I/D) polymorphism of the ACE gene has been associated with increased risk for acute myocardial infarction, cardiomyopathy, cardiac hypertrophy and carotid thickening. The DD genotype in particular should be considered as a risk factor for early arteriosclerosis, even controlling other potential confounding factors such as smoking [174, 175].

Smoking is the most powerful risk factor for the development of atherosclerosis, even ahead of hypertension, diabetes mellitus, and male gender. Pack-years smoked correlate with the extent of arteriosclerotic changes in the common carotid artery [176]. The risk of having severe atherosclerosis for a person who has smoked for 40 years is increased 3.5-fold compared with that for someone who has never smoked.

6.3
Blood Coagulation and Fibrinolysis

Critical events (myocardial infarction, stroke) due to arteriosclerotic changes are triggered by unstable arteriosclerotic plaques: acutely formed thrombi occlude vessels of varying calibre. Smokers have a shortened platelet survival half-life [177], a situation in which thromboxane A_2 synthesis is increased [178].

Smokers live permanently at risk because their platelets react very much more rapidly to form aggregates than those of non-smokers.

- Activation of the blood coagulation system (thrombosis) is important for the occurrence of acute and chronic coronary events, and in this context the effect of smoking on platelets has been studied most extensively: smoking two cigarettes increases platelet activation 100-fold [41].
- Smoking increases the production of PDGF, a key factor in the atherogenic growth of vascular cells [14].
- Smoking (but not nicotine) stimulates pro-aggregatory prostanoids, thromboxane B_2 and A_2, prostaglandin $F_1\alpha$, platelet factor 4 and β-thromboglobulin [178, 179].
- Plasma fibrinogen levels [35, 129, 179] and factor VII activity [35] are elevated in smokers, and the increase in the fibrinogen level depends on the number of cigarettes smoked [129]. Raised fibrinogen is a risk factor for venous bypass graft patency and for restenosis after PTCA [180, 181]. Normalisation after smoking cessation takes a few months [8], if not several years [35]. The RIVAGE Study has clearly shown that the plasma fibrinogen level is the only independent variable associated with increased risk for a cardiovascular event [182].

Although some studies have found the fibrinolytic activity of the blood to be unaltered [129], the data summarised in Table 6.2 point to a reduction in such activity. Nicotine itself induces substance P-mediated release of tissue plasminogen activator (t-PA) without any effect on endothelium-dependent or -independent vasodilatation [183]. One recently published study points to reduced fibrinolytic potential in the myocardium of smokers. An inverse correlation was found between plaque burden in the left anterior descending coronary artery and the release of t-PA ($r = -0.61$; $p = 0.003$). Cigarette smoking is associated with considerably impaired coronary release of active t-PA [184]. After smoking cessation fibrinogen levels fall by about 5% within 5 years [160]. Fibrinogen should also be regarded as important firstly as a haemorheological factor because blood viscosity rises when fibrinogen levels increase [8], and secondly as a mediator of inflammation because leucocyte adhesion to activated endothelium and cytokine release (IL-8 and MCP-1) are increased at a time [185] when plaque formation is still not at all important [186]. Consequently, even before plaque formation occurs, the correlation between fibrinogen concentration and carotid wall thickness seems to be plausible [187].

6.3.1
Genetic Factors

Interactions appear to exist between smoking and genotype. Apolipoprotein polymorphism and the cholesteryl ester transfer protein gene display interactions [39, 188, 189]. In individuals with specific genotypes smoking produces an increase in LDL cholesterol and a reduction in HDL cholesterol, with both processes occurring as a part of a proatherogenic effect. Likewise, there are smokers in whom plasma fibrinogen levels are clearly increased [190, 191]. Smokers with a rare variant of the NOS gene (ecNOS4α) are found in increased numbers among patients with severely stenosed coronary arteries verified by angiography [192]. These findings appear to indicate the potential for considerable interactions between smoking and genetic factors.

6.3.2
Nicotine and Ischaemic Heart Disease

The findings presented suggest that *nicotine itself is of only secondary importance as a harmful agent in the context of CHD*. Instead, the inhaled combustion products of tobacco smoke should be viewed as the culprits in this respect. Nicotine replacement therapy as opposed to cigarette smoking produces no harmful cardiac effects [55, 193]. When nicotine is administered therapeutically after smoking cessation, toxic substances are no longer inhaled [194]. According to existing data, nicotine replacement therapy should be implemented with caution in patients with cardiac arrhythmias, CHD and recently completed stroke [126, 195–197], and further investigations would appear useful to establish the contraindications. The consequences of a smoking-induced increase in CO-haemoglobin are similar to those of chronic CO poisoning [198], and may lead to an increased incidence of cardiovascular complications.

In smokers (>20 cigarettes daily) with existing CAD, perfusion in several myocardial regions was improved when cigarette consumption was replaced in part by nicotine patches (14 and 21 mg) (Table 6.3). Perfusion defects were improved significantly even within this short period (Table 6.3). There was a reduction in perfusion defect size as exhaled CO levels fell; this reduction occurred despite an increase in patients' treadmill exercise duration and higher serum nicotine levels (compared with controls) although cigarette consumption had fallen [55]! Another study in 156 smokers (>20 cigarettes daily) with CAD confirmed the reduction in angina frequency during nicotine replacement therapy after they had stopped smoking [199].

6.4
Concluding Remarks

The smoking-induced changes in the cardiovascular system described in this chapter should suffice to ensure that smoking is viewed very much more critically in future.

- In particular, extensive findings indicate that the combustion products of tobacco in mainstream and side-stream smoke are primarily responsible for the harmful effects repeatedly ascribed to nicotine. While numerous authors have implicated nicotine in terms of vasoconstrictor effects, the large body of evidence accumulated following administration of nicotine for smoking cessation or at least for smoking reduction now militates against the theory that nicotine might trigger a myocardial infarction or stroke or promote PAOD. Experimental animal work appears to indicate that the toxic products of tobacco smoke may also undergo bioactivation in the tissues of the blood vessels.
- The interrelationships depicted in Fig. 6.10 are intended to illustrate these concepts once again. Smokers rarely perceive themselves to be at increased risk in terms of myocardial infarction or bronchial carcinoma. In a comprehensive survey of both diseases, these risks were acknowledged by only 39 and 49% of respondents respectively, and less educated smokers were definitely less likely to perceive any increased personal risk [200]. Comprehensive analysis of the effects of nicotine on the development of arteriosclerosis continues to be controversial and unclear, even though the alkaloid is known to activate the sympathetic nervous system. In experimental animal studies nicotine has been suspected of accelerating the progression of arteriosclerosis (activation of fatty acid metabolism, reduced HDL turnover); on the other hand, however, there are no findings to support an increase in hypertension or activation of platelet aggregation [201].
- Short-term interventions involving primary prevention programmes over several weeks (physical exercise, temporary smoking cessation) do not improve vascular endothelial function in adults with increased coronary risk factors [202].
- Furthermore, the level of smoking-related information available in some countries is truly deplorable. Even smokers who have survived an acute myocardial infarction receive only inadequate advice from the physicians treating them. According to one study conducted in Israel, only 62% of such patients reported receiving anti-smoking advice [63].

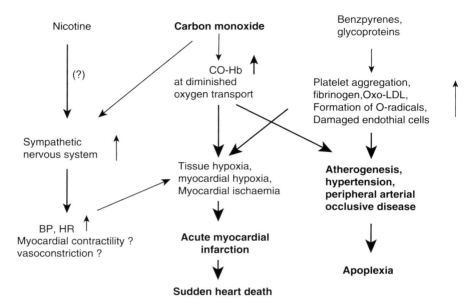

Fig. 6.10   Effects of nicotine and the combustion products of cigarette smoke. *BP* blood pressure, *HR* heart rate

Reference

1. Doll R, Peto R, Wheatley K, Gray R, Sutherland I (1994) Mortality in relation to smoking: 40 years' observations on male British doctors. BMJ 309(6959):901–911
2. Hammond EC, Garfinkel L (1969) Coronary heart disease, roke, and aortic aneurysm. Factors in the etiology. Arch Environ Health 19(2):167–182
3. Abbott RD, Yin Y, Reed DM, Yano K (1986) Risk of stroke in male cigarette smokers. N Engl J Med 315(12):717–720
4. Adamson J, Humphries SE, Ostergaard JR, Voldby B, Richards P, Powell JT (1994) Are cerebral aneurysms atherosclerotic? Stroke 25(5):963–966
5. Fitzgerald GA, Oates JA, Nowak J (1988) Cigarette smoking and hemostatic function. Am Heart J 115(1 Pt 2):267–271
6. Fowkes FG (1988) Epidemiology of atherosclerotic arterial disease in the lower limbs. Eur J Vasc Surg 2(5):283–291
7. Kannel WB, Shurtleff D (1973) The Framingham study. Cigarettes and the development of intermittent claudication. Geriatrics 28(2):61–68
8. Haustein KO (1999) Smoking, cardiovascular diseases and possibilities for treating nicotine dependence. Wien Med Wochenschr 149(1):19–24
9. Haustein KO, Krause J, Haustein H, Rasmussen T, Cort N (2002) Effects of cigarette smoking or nicotine replacement on cardiovascular risk factors and parameters of haemorheology. J Intern Med 252(2):130–139
10. LaCroix AZ, Lang J, Scherr P, Wallace RB, Cornoni-Huntley J, Berkman L, et al (1991) Smoking and mortality among older men and women in three communities. N Engl J Med 324(23):1619–1625

11. Rosenberg L, Kaufman DW, Helmrich SP, Shapiro S (1985) The risk of myocardial infarction after quitting smoking in men under 55 years of age. N Engl J Med 313(24):1511–1514

12. US Department of Health and Human Services (1990). The Health Benefits of Smoking Cessation: A Report of the Surgeon General. US Department of Health and Human Services, Public Health Service, Center for Disease Control, Office on Smoking and Health. DHHS Publication No. (CDC) 908416

13. Seltzer CC (1974) Effect of smoking on blood pressure Am Heart J 87(5):558–564

14. Shah PK, Helfant RH (1988) Smoking and coronary artery disease. Chest 94(3):449–452

15. Kawachi I, Colditz GA, Stampfer MJ, Willett WC, Manson JE, Rosner B, et al (1993) Smoking cessation in relation to total mortality rates in women. A prospective cohort study. Ann Intern Med 119(10):992–1000

16. Aberg A, Bergstrand R, Johansson S, Ulvenstam G, Vedin A, Wedel H, et al (1983) Cessation of smoking after myocardial infarction. Effects on mortality after 10 years. Br Heart J 49(5):416–422

17. Daly LE, Mulcahy R, Graham IM, Hickey N (1983) Long term effect on mortality of stopping smoking after unstable angina and myocardial infarction. Br Med J (Clin Res Ed) 287(6388): 324–326

18. Hallstrom AP, Cobb LA, Ray R (1986) Smoking as a risk factor for recurrence of sudden cardiac arrest. N Engl J Med 314(5):271–275

19. Sparrow D, Dawber TR (1978) The influence of cigarette smoking on prognosis after a first myocardial infarction. A report from the Framingham study. J Chronic Dis 31(6–7):425–432

20. Galan KM, Deligonul U, Kern MJ, Chaitman BR, Vandormael MG (1988) Increased frequency of restenosis in patients continuing to smoke cigarettes after percutaneous transluminal coronary angioplasty. Am J Cardiol 61(4):260–263

21. Taira DA, Seto TB, Ho KK, Krumholz HM, Cutlip DE, Berezin R, et al (2000) Impact of smoking on health-related quality of life after percutaneous coronary revascularization. Circulation 102:1369–1374

22. Kannel WB (1981) Update on the role of cigarette smoking in coronary artery disease. Am Heart J 101:319–328

23. Schievelbein H, Londong V, Londong W, Grumbach H, Remplik V (1970) Nicotine and arteriosclerosis. An experimental contribution to the influence of nicotine on fat metabolism. Z Klin Chem Klin Biochem 8:190–196

24. Schievelbein H, Richter F (1984) The influence of passive smoking on the cardiovascular system. Prev Med 13:626–644

25. Majesky MW, Reidy MA, Benditt EP, Juchau MR (1985) Focal smooth muscle proliferation in the aortic intima produced by an initiation-promotion sequence. Proc Natl Acad Sci USA 82:3450–3454

26. Bond JA, Gown AM, Yang HL, Benditt EP, Juchau MR (1981) Further investigations of the capacity of polynuclear aromatic hydrocarbons to elicit atherosclerotic lesions. J Toxicol Environ Health 7:327–335

27. Ross R, Glomset J, Harker L (1978). The response to injury and atherogenesis: The role of endothelium and smooth muscle. In: Paoletti R, Gotto AM (eds) Atherosclerosis Reviews, vol 3. New York, Raven Press, pp 69–76

28. Ross R (1986) The pathogenesis of atherosclerosis – an update. N Engl J Med 314:488–500

29. Majesky MW, Yang HY, Benditt EP, Juchau MR (1983) Carcinogenesis and atherogenesis: differences in monooxygenase inducibility and bioactivation of benzo[a]pyrene in aortic and hepatic tissues of atherosclerosis-susceptible versus resistant pigeons. Carcinogenesis 4:647–652

30. Penn A, Batastini G, Soloman J, Burns F, Albert R (1981) Dose-dependent size increases of aortic lesions following chronic exposure to 7,12-dimethylbenz(a)anthracene. Cancer Res 41:588–592

31. Bond JA, Yang HY, Majesky MW, Benditt EP, Juchau MR (1980) Metabolism of benzo[a] pyrene and 7,12-dimethylbenz[a]anthracene in chicken aortas: monooxygenation, bioactivation to mutagens, and covalent binding to DNA in vitro. Toxicol Appl Pharmacol 52:323–335

32. Bond JA, Kocan RM, Benditt EP, Juchau MR (1979) Metabolism of benzo[a]pyrene and 7,12-dimethylbenz[a]anthracene in cultured human fetal aortic smooth muscle cells. Life Sci 25:425–430

33. Davis JW, Shelton L, Eigenberg DA, Hignite CE, Watanabe IS (1985) Effects of tobacco and non-tobacco cigarette smoking on endothelium and platelets. Clin Pharmacol Ther 37:529–533

34. Brown DW, Giles WH, Croft JB (2001) Hematocrit and the risk of coronary heart disease mortality. Am Heart J 142(4):657–663

35. McBride PE (1992) The health consequences of smoking. Cardiovascular diseases. Med Clin North Am 76(2):333–353

36. McGill HC Jr (1988) The cardiovascular pathology of smoking. Am Heart J 115(1 Pt 2): 250–257

37. Quillen JE, Rossen JD, Oskarsson HJ, Minor RL Jr, Lopez AG, Winniford MD (1993) Acute effect of cigarette smoking on the coronary circulation: constriction of epicardial and resistance vessels. J Am Coll Cardiol 22(3):642–647

38. Cryer PE, Haymond MW, Santiago JV, Shah SD (1976) Norepinephrine and epinephrine release and adrenergic mediation of smoking-associated hemodynamic and metabolic events. N Engl J Med 295(11):573–577

39. Glisic S, Savic I, Alavantic D (1995) Apolipoprotein B gene DNA polymorphisms (EcoRI and MspI) and serum lipid levels in the Serbian healthy population: interaction of rare alleles and smoking and cholesterol levels. Genet Epidemiol 12(5):499–508

40. Klein LW, Pichard AD, Holt J, Smith H, Gorlin R, Teichholz LE (1983) Effects of chronic tobacco smoking on the coronary circulation. J Am Coll Cardiol 1(2 Pt 1):421–426

41. Pittilo RM, Clarke JM, Harris D, Mackie IJ, Rowles PM, Machin SJ, et al (1984) Cigarette smoking and platelet adhesion. Br J Haematol 58(4):627–632

42. Maouad J, Fernandez F, Barrillon A, Gerbaux A, Gay J (1984) Diffuse or segmental narrowing (spasm) of the coronary arteries during smoking demonstrated on angiography. Am J Cardiol 53(2):354–355

43. Maouad J, Fernandez F, Hebert JL, Zamani K, Barrillon A, Gay J (1986) Cigarette smoking during coronary angiography: diffuse or focal narrowing (spasm) of the coronary arteries in 13 patients with angina at rest and normal coronary angiograms. Cathet Cardiovasc Diagn 12(6):366–375

44. Sugiishi M, Takatsu F (1993) Cigarette smoking is a major risk factor for coronary spasm. Circulation 87(1):76–79

45. Bolinder G (1997) Smokeless tobacco – a less harmful alternative? In: Bollinger CT, Fagerstrom KO (eds) The Tobacco Epidemic. S. Karger, Basel, pp 199–212

46. Mancini GB, Henry GC, Macaya C, O'Neill BJ, Pucillo AL, Carere RG, et al (1996) Angiotensin-converting enzyme inhibition with quinapril improves endothelial vasomotor dysfunction in patients with coronary artery disease. The TREND (trial on reversing endothelial dysfunction) study. Circulation 94(3):258–265

47. Pepine CJ, Schlaifer JD, Mancini GB, Pitt B, O'Neill BJ, Haber HE (1998) Influence of smoking status on progression of endothelial dysfunction. TREND Investigators. Trial on reversing endothelial dysfunction. Clin Cardiol 21(5):331–334

48. Celermajer DS, Adams MR, Clarkson P, Robinson J, McCredie R, Donald A, et al (1996) Passive smoking and impaired endothelium-dependent arterial dilatation in healthy young adults. N Engl J Med 334(3):150–154

49. Nitenberg A, Benvenuti C, Aptecar E, Antony I, Deleuze P, Loisance D et al (1993) Acetylcholine-induced constriction of angiographically normal coronary arteries is not time dependent in transplant recipients. Effects of stepwise infusion at 1, 6, 12 and more than 24 months after transplantation. J Am Coll Cardiol 22(1):151–158

50. Zeiher AM, Schachinger V, Minners J (1995) Long-term cigarette smoking impairs endothelium-dependent coronary arterial vasodilator function. Circulation 92(5):1094–1100

51. Voors AA, Oosterga M, Buikema H (1997) Dose-response relation between cigarette consumption and endothelial function (Abstr.). J Am Coll Cardiol 29(Suppl A):263A–264A

52. Waters D, Lesperance J, Gladstone P, Boccuzzi SJ, Cook T, Hudgin R, et al (1996) Effects of cigarette smoking on the angiographic evolution of coronary atherosclerosis. A Canadian Coronary Atherosclerosis Intervention Trial (CCAIT) Substudy. CCAIT Study Group. Circulation 94(4):614–621

53. Jarvis MJ, Belcher M, Vesey C, Hutchison DC (1986) Low cost carbon monoxide monitors in smoking assessment. Thorax 41(11):886–887

54. Anderson EW, Andelman RJ, Strauch JM, Fortuin NJ, Knelson JH (1973) Effect of low-level carbon monoxide exposure on onset and duration of angina pectoris. A study in ten patients with ischemic heart disease. Ann Intern Med 79(1):46–50

55. Mahmarian JJ, Moye LA, Nasser GA, Nagueh SF, Bloom MF, Benowitz NL, et al (1997) Nicotine patch therapy in smoking cessation reduces the extent of exercise-induced myocardial ischemia. J Am Coll Cardiol 30(1):125–130

56. Negri E, La Vecchia C, Nobili A, D'Avanzo B, Bechi S (1994) Cigarette smoking and acute myocardial infarction. A case-control study from the GISSI-2 trial. GISSI-EFRIM Investigators. Gruppo Italiano per lo Studio della Sopravvivenza nell'Infarto - Epidemiologia dei Fattori di Rischio dell'infarto Miocardioco. Eur J Epidemiol 10(4):361–366

57. Beard CM, Kottke TE, Annegers JF, Ballard DJ (1989) The Rochester Coronary Heart Disease Project: effect of cigarette smoking, hypertension, diabetes, and steroidal estrogen use on coronary heart disease among 40- to 59-year-old women, 1960 through 1982. Mayo Clin Proc 64 (12):1471–1480

58. Rosenberg L, Palmer JR, Shapiro S (1990) Decline in the risk of myocardial infarction among women who stop smoking. N Engl J Med 322(4):213–217

59. Vander ZR, Lemp GF, Hughes JP, Ramanathan KB, Sullivan JM, Schick EC et al (1988) The effect of cigarette smoking on the pattern of coronary atherosclerosis. A case-control study. Chest 94(2):290–295

60. Rosenberg L, Kaufman DW, Helmrich SP, Miller DR, Stolley PD, Shapiro S (1985) Myocardial infarction and cigarette smoking in women younger than 50 years of age. JAMA 253(20):2965–2969

61. Dunn NR, Faragher B, Thorogood M, de Caestecker L, MacDonald TM, McCollum C, et al (1999) Risk of myocardial infarction in young female smokers. Heart 82(5):581–583

62. McElduff P, Dobson A, Beaglehole R, Jackson R (1998) Rapid reduction in coronary risk for those who quit cigarette smoking. Aust N Z J Public Health 22(7):787–791

63. Weiner P, Waizman J, Weiner M, Rabner M, Magadle R, Zamir D (2000) Smoking and first acute myocardial infarction: age, mortality and smoking cessation rate. Isr Med Assoc J 2(6): 446–449

64. Villarreal FJ, Hong D, Omens J (1999) Nicotine-modified postinfarction left ventricular remodeling. Am J Physiol 276(3 Pt 2):H1103–H1106

65. Heliovaara M, Karvonen MJ, Vilhunen R, Punsar S (1978) Smoking, carbon monoxide, and atherosclerotic diseases. Br Med J 1:268–270

66. Hughson WG, Mann JI, Tibbs DJ, Woods HF, Walton I (1978) Intermittent claudication: factors determining outcome. Br Med J 1:1377–1379

67. Doll R, Peto R (1976) Mortality in relation to smoking: 20 years' observations on male British doctors. Br Med J 2:1525–1536

68. Doll R, Gray R, Hafner B, Peto R (1980) Mortality in relation to smoking: 22 years' observations on female British doctors. Br Med J 280:967–971

69. Fowkes FG, Housley E, Riemersma RA, Macintyre CC, Cawood EH, Prescott RJ, et al (1992) Smoking, lipids, glucose intolerance, and blood pressure as risk factors for peripheral atherosclerosis compared with ischemic heart disease in the Edinburgh artery study. Am J Epidemiol 135(4):331–340

70. Price JF, Mowbray PI, Lee AJ, Rumley A, Lowe GD, Fowkes FG (1999) Relationship between smoking and cardiovascular risk factors in the development of peripheral arterial disease and coronary artery disease: Edinburgh artery study. Eur Heart J 20:344–353

71. Gudmundsson M, Bjelle A (1993) Plasma, serum and whole-blood viscosity variations with age, sex, and smoking habits. Angiology 44(5):384–391

72. Green MS, Jucha E, Luz Y (1986) Blood pressure in smokers and nonsmokers: epidemiologic findings. Am Heart J 111(5):932–940

73. Kool MJ, Hoeks AP, Struijker Boudier HA, Reneman RS, Van Bortel LM (1993) Short- and long-term effects of smoking on arterial wall properties in habitual smokers. J Am Coll Cardiol 22(7):1881–1886

74. Berlin I, Cournot A, Renout P, Duchier J, Safar M (1990) Peripheral haemodynamic effects of smoking in habitual smokers. A methodological study. Eur J Clin Pharmacol 38(1):57–60

75. Kyriakides ZS, Kremastinos DT, Rentoukas E, Mavrogheni S, Kremastinos DI, Toutouzas P (1992) Acute effects of cigarette smoking on left ventricular diastolic function. Eur Heart J 13(6):743–748

76. Stork T, Eichstadt H, Mockel M, Bortfeldt R, Muller R, Hochrein H (1992) Changes of diastolic function induced by cigarette smoking: an echocardiographic study in patients with coronary artery disease. Clin Cardiol 15(2):80–86

77. Tanus-Santos JE, Toledo JC, Cittadino M, Sabha M, Rocha JC, Moreno H Jr (2001) Cardiovascular effects of transdermal nicotine in mildly hypertensive smokers. Am J Hypertens 14(7 Pt 1):610–614

78. Gulliford MC (2001) Low rates of detection and treatment of hypertension among current cigarette smokers. J Hum Hypertens 15(11):771–773

79. Siegel D, Benowitz N, Ernster VL, Grady DG, Hauck WW (1992) Smokeless tobacco, cardiovascular risk factors, and nicotine and cotinine levels in professional baseball players. Am J Public Health 82(3):417–421

80. Mikkelsen KL, Wiinberg N, Hoegholm A, Christensen HR, Bang LE, Nielsen PE, et al (1997) Smoking related to 24-h ambulatory blood pressure and heart rate: a study in 352 normotensive Danish subjects. Am J Hypertens 10(5 Pt 1):483–491

81. Fox CS, Larson MG, Leip EP, Culleton B, Wilson PW, Levy D (2004) Predictors of new-onset kidney disease in a community-based population. JAMA 291(7):844–850

82. Mathew RJ, Wilson WH (1991) Substance abuse and cerebral blood flow. Am J Psychiatry 148(3):292–305

83. Rogers RL, Meyer JS, Shaw TG, Mortel KF, Hardenberg JP, Zaid RR (1983) Cigarette smoking decreases cerebral blood flow suggesting increased risk for stroke. JAMA 250(20):2796–2800

84. Colditz GA, Bonita R, Stampfer MJ, Willett WC, Rosner B, Speizer FE, et al (1988) Cigarette smoking and risk of stroke in middle-aged women. N Engl J Med 318(15):937–941

85. Wang H, Sekine M, Yokokawa H, Hamanishi S, Chen X, Sayama M, et al (2001) The relationship between new stroke onset and serum thiocyanate as an indicator to cigarette smoking. J Epidemiol 11(5):233–237

86. Silverberg E, Boring CC, Squires TS (1990) Cancer statistics, 1990. CA Cancer J Clin 40:9–26

87. Lederle FA, Johnson GR, Wilson SE, Chute EP, Hye RJ, Makaroun MS, et al (2000) The aneurysm detection and management study screening program: validation cohort and final results. Aneurysm detection and management veterans affairs cooperative study investigators. Arch Intern Med 160:1425–1430

88. Kanagasabay R, Gajraj H, Pointon L, Scott RA (1996) Co-morbidity in patients with abdominal aortic aneurysm. J Med Screen 3:208–210

89. Mattes E, Davis TM, Yang D, Ridley D, Lund H, Norman PE (1997) Prevalence of abdominal aortic aneurysms in men with diabetes. Med J Aust 166:630–633

90. Franks PJ, Edwards RJ, Greenhalgh RM, Powell JT (1996) Risk factors for abdominal aortic aneurysms in smokers. Eur J Vasc Endovasc Surg 11:487–492

91. Powell JT, Brown LC (2001) The natural history of abdominal aortic aneurysms and their risk of rupture. Acta Chir Belg 101:11–16

92. Vardulaki KA, Walker NM, Day NE, Duffy SW, Ashton HA, Scott RA (2000) Quantifying the risks of hypertension, age, sex and smoking in patients with abdominal aortic aneurysm. Br J Surg 87:195–200

93. Brown LC, Powell JT (1999) Risk factors for aneurysm rupture in patients kept under ultrasound surveillance. UK small aneurysm trial participants. Ann Surg 230:289–296

94. Fowkes FG, Macintyre CC, Ruckley CV (1989) Increasing incidence of aortic aneurysms in England and Wales. BMJ 298:33–35

95. Benowitz NL (1988) Drug therapy. Pharmacologic aspects of cigarette smoking and nicotine addition. N Engl J Med 319(20):1318–1330

96. Butler R, Morris AD, Struthers AD (2001) Cigarette smoking in men and vascular responsiveness. Br J Clin Pharmacol 52(2):145–149

97. Butler R, Morris AD, Struthers AD (2001) Lisinopril improves endothelial function in chronic cigarette smokers. Clin Sci (Lond) 101(1):53–58

98. Nitenberg A, Antony I (1999) Effects of nicotine gum on coronary vasomotor responses during sympathetic stimulation in patients with coronary artery stenosis. J Cardiovasc Pharmacol 34:694–699

99. Neunteufl T, Heher S, Kostner K, Mitulovic G, Lehr S, Khoschsorur G, et al (2002) Contribution of nicotine to acute endothelial dysfunction in long-term smokers. J Am Coll Cardiol 39:251–256

100. Park JE, Lee WH, Hwang TH, Chu JA, Kim S, Choi YH, et al (2000) Aging affects the association between endothelial nitric oxide synthase gene polymorphism and acute myocardial infarction in the Korean male population. Korean J Intern Med 15(1):65–70

101. Benowitz NL (1993) Smoking-induced coronary vasoconstriction: implications for therapeutic use of nicotine. J Am Coll Cardiol 22(3):648–649

102. Klein LW (1984) Cigarette smoking, atherosclerosis and the coronary hemodynamic response: a unifying hypothesis. J Am Coll Cardiol 4(5):972–974

103. Benowitz NL (1991) Nicotine and coronary heart disease. Trends Cardiovasc Med 1: 315–321

104. Munzel T, Hink U, Heitzer T, Meinertz T (1999) Role for NADPH/NADH oxidase in the modulation of vascular tone. Ann N Y Acad Sci 874:386–400

105. Papamichael CM, Aznaouridis KA, Stamatelopoulos KS, Karatzis EN, Protogerou AD, Papaioannou TG, et al (2004) Endothelial dysfunction and type of cigarette smoked: the impact of 'light' versus regular cigarette smoking. Vasc Med 9(2):103–105

106. Celermajer DS, Sorensen KE, Gooch VM, Spiegelhalter DJ, Miller OI, Sullivan ID, et al (1992) Non-invasive detection of endothelial dysfunction in children and adults at risk of atherosclerosis. Lancet 340(8828):1111–1115

107. Heitzer T, Brockhoff C, Mayer B, Warnholtz A, Mollnau H, Henne S, et al (2000) Tetrahydrobiopterin improves endothelium-dependent vasodilation in chronic smokers: evidence for a dysfunctional nitric oxide synthase. Circ Res 86(2):E36–E41

108. Higman DJ, Strachan AM, Buttery L, Hicks RC, Springall DR, Greenhalgh RM, et al (1996) Smoking impairs the activity of endothelial nitric oxide synthase in saphenous vein. Arterioscler Thromb Vasc Biol 16(4):546–552

109. Ichiki K, Ikeda H, Haramaki N, Ueno T, Imaizumi T (1996) Long-term smoking impairs platelet-derived nitric oxide release. Circulation 94(12):3109–3114

110. Cosentino F, Katusic ZS (1995) Tetrahydrobiopterin and dysfunction of endothelial nitric oxide synthase in coronary arteries. Circulation 91(1):139–144

111. Heitzer T, Yla-Herttuala S, Luoma J, Kurz S, Munzel T, Just H, et al (1996) Cigarette smoking potentiates endothelial dysfunction of forearm resistance vessels in patients with hypercholesterolemia. Role of oxidized LDL. Circulation 93(7):1346–1353

112. Heitzer T, Just H, Munzel T (1996) Antioxidant vitamin C improves endothelial dysfunction in chronic smokers. Circulation 94(1):6–9

113. Celermajer DS, Sorensen KE, Georgakopoulos D, Bull C, Thomas O, Robinson J, et al (1993) Cigarette smoking is associated with dose-related and potentially reversible impairment of endothelium-dependent dilation in healthy young adults. Circulation 88(5 Pt 1): 2149–2155

114. Higman DJ, Strachan AM, Powell JT (1994) Reversibility of smoking-induced endothelial dysfunction. Br J Surg 81(7):977–978

115. Lassila R, Seyberth HW, Haapanen A, Schweer H, Koskenvuo M, Laustiola KE (1988) Vasoactive and atherogenic effects of cigarette smoking: a study of monozygotic twins discordant for smoking. BMJ 297(6654):955–957

116. He JF (1991) Morphologic and morphometric studies of pulmonary artery endothelial abnormalities in rats induced by smoking. Zhonghua Bing Li Xue Za Zhi 20(3):165–168

117. Lin SJ, Hong CY, Chang MS, Chiang BN, Chien S (1992) Long-term nicotine exposure increases aortic endothelial cell death and enhances transendothelial macromolecular transport in rats. Arterioscler Thromb 12(11):1305–1312

118. Zimmerman M, McGeachie J (1987) The effect of nicotine on aortic endothelium. A quantitative ultrastructural study. Atherosclerosis 63(1):33–41

119. Tithof PK, Elgayyar M, Schuller HM, Barnhill M, Andrews R (2001) 4-(methylnitrosamino)-1-(3-pyridyl)-1-butanone, a nicotine derivative, induces apoptosis of endothelial cells. Am J Physiol Heart Circ Physiol 281(5):H1946–H1954

120. Bernhard D, Pfister G, Huck CW, Kind M, Salvenmoser W, Bonn GK, et al (2003) Disruption of vascular endothelial homeostasis by tobacco smoke: impact on atherosclerosis. FASEB J 17(15):2302–2304

121. Kiowski W, Linder L, Stoschitzky K, Pfisterer M, Burckhardt D, Burkart F, et al (1994) Diminished vascular response to inhibition of endothelium-derived nitric oxide and enhanced vasoconstriction to exogenously administered endothelin-1 in clinically healthy smokers. Circulation 90(1):27–34

122. Brush JE Jr, Faxon DP, Salmon S, Jacobs AK, Ryan TJ (1992) Abnormal endothelium-dependent coronary vasomotion in hypertensive patients. J Am Coll Cardiol 19(4): 809–815

123. Drexler H, Zeiher AM (1991) Endothelial function in human coronary arteries in vivo. Focus-on hypercholesterolemia. Hypertension 18(Suppl 4):II90–II99

124. Seiler C, Hess OM, Buechi M, Suter TM, Krayenbuehl HP (1993) Influence of serum cholesterol and other coronary risk factors on vasomotion of angiographically normal coronary arteries. Circulation 88(5 Pt 1):2139–2148

125. Hashimoto H (1994) Impaired microvascular vasodilator reserve in chronic cigarette smokers – a study of post-occlusive reactive hyperemia in the human finger. Jpn Circ J 58(1):29–33

126. Ottervanger JP, Festen JM, de Vries AG, Stricker BH (1995) Acute myocardial infarction while using the nicotine patch. Chest 107(6):1765–1766

127. Sabha M, Tanus-Santos JE, Toledo JC, Cittadino M, Rocha JC, Moreno H Jr (2000) Transdermal nicotine mimics the smoking-induced endothelial dysfunction. Clin Pharmacol Ther 68(2):167–174

128. Belch JJ, McArdle BM, Burns P, Lowe GD, Forbes CD (1984) The effects of acute smoking on platelet behaviour, fibrinolysis and haemorheology in habitual smokers. Thromb Haemost 51(1):6–8

129. Eliasson M, Asplund K, Evrin PE, Lundblad D (1995) Relationship of cigarette smoking and snuff dipping to plasma fibrinogen, fibrinolytic variables and serum insulin. The Northern Sweden MONICA Study. Atherosclerosis 113(1):41–53

130. Feher MD, Rampling MW, Brown J, Robinson R, Richmond W, Cholerton S ,et al (1990) Acute changes in atherogenic and thrombogenic factors with cessation of smoking. J R Soc Med 83(3):146–148

131. Dal Bianco P, Zeiler K, Baumgartner C, Kollegger H, Oder W Deecke L (1989) Use of nicotine – a risk factor for stroke? Wien Klin Wochenschr 101(20):687–694

132. Salbas K (1994) Effect of acute smoking on red blood cell deformability in healthy young and elderly non-smokers, and effect of verapamil on age- and acute smoking-induced change in red blood cell deformability. Scand J Clin Lab Invest 54(6):411–416

133. Salbas K, Gurlek A, Akyol T (1994) In vitro effect of nicotine on red blood cell deformability in untreated and treated essential hypertension. Scand J Clin Lab Invest 54(8):659–663

134. Blann AD (1992) The acute influence of smoking on the endothelium. Atherosclerosis 96(2–3):249–250

135. Calori G, D'Angelo A, Della VP, Ruotolo G, Ferini-Strambi L, Giusti C, et al (1996) The effect of cigarette-smoking on cardiovascular risk factors: a study of monozygotic twins discordant for smoking. Thromb Haemost 75(1):14–18

136. Thomas GA, Davies SV, Rhodes J, Russell MA, Feyerabend C, Sawe U (1995) Is transdermal nicotine associated with cardiovascular risk? J R Coll Physicians Lond 29(5):392–396

137. Blann AD, Steele C, McCollum CN (1997) The influence of smoking and of oral and transdermal nicotine on blood pressure, and haematology and coagulation indices. Thromb Haemost 78(3):1093–1096

138. Miller GJ, Esnouf MP, Burgess AI, Cooper JA, Mitchell JP (1997) Risk of coronary heart disease and activation of factor XII in middle-aged men. Arterioscler Thromb Vasc Biol 17 (10):2103–2106

139. Heeschen C, Jang JJ, Weis M, Pathak A, Kaji S, Hu RS, et al (2001) Nicotine stimulates angiogenesis and promotes tumor growth and atherosclerosis. Nat Med 7:833–839

140. Mosely LH, Finseth F (1977) Cigarette smoking: impairment of digital blood flow and wound healing in the hand. Hand 9(2):97–101

141. Mosely LH, Finseth F, Goody M (1978) Nicotine and its effect on wound healing. Plast Reconstr Surg 61(4):570–575

142. Nolan J, Jenkins RA, Kurihara K, Schultz RC (1985) The acute effects of cigarette smoke exposure on experimental skin flaps. Plast Reconstr Surg 75(4):544–551

143. Riefkohl R, Wolfe JA, Cox EB, McCarty KS Jr (1986) Association between cutaneous occlusive vascular disease, cigarette smoking, and skin slough after rhytidectomy. Plast Reconstr Surg 77(4):592–595

144. Harris GD, Finseth F, Buncke HJ (1980) The hazard of cigarette smoking following digital replantation. J Microsurg 1(5):403–404

145. Wilson GR, Jones BM (1984) The damaging effect of smoking on digital revascularisation: two further case reports. Br J Plast Surg 37(4):613–614

146. Dardour JC, Pugash E, Aziza R (1988) The one-stage preauricular flap for male pattern baldness: long-term results and risk factors. Plast Reconstr Surg 81(6):907–912

147. Rees TD, Liverett DM, Guy CL (1984) The effect of cigarette smoking on skin-flap survival in the face lift patient. Plast Reconstr Surg 73(6):911–915

148. Craig S, Rees TD (1985) The effects of smoking on experimental skin flaps in hamsters. Plast Reconstr Surg 75(6):842–846

149. Lawrence WT, Murphy RC, Robson MC, Heggers JP (1984) The detrimental effect of cigarette smoking on flap survival: an experimental study in the rat. Br J Plast Surg 37(2):216–219

150. Dalla VL, Palombo C, Ciardetti M, Porta A, Milani O, Kozakova M, et al (2004) Contrasting effects of acute and chronic cigarette smoking on skin microcirculation in young healthy subjects. J Hypertens 22(1):129–135

151. Ijzerman RG, Serne EH, van Weissenbruch MM, de Jongh RT, Stehouwer CD (2003) Cigarette smoking is associated with an acute impairment of microvascular function in humans. Clin Sci (Lond) 104(3):247–252

152. Roth GM, McDonald JB, Sheard C (1944) The effect of smoking cigarettes and of intravenous administration of nicotine on the eletrocardiogram, banal metabolic rate, cutaneous temperature, blood pressure and pulse rate of normale persons. J Am med Ass 125:761–767

153. Richardson DR (1985) Effects of habitual tobacco smoking on reactive hyperemia in the human hand. Arch Environ Health 40(2):114–119
154. Suter TW, Buzzi R, Battig K (1983) Cardiovascular effects of smoking cigarettes with different nicotine deliveries. A study using multilead plethysmography. Psychopharmacology (Berl) 80(2):106–112
155. Leow YH, Maibach HI (1998) Cigarette smoking, cutaneous vasculature, and tissue oxygen. Clin Dermatol 16(5):579–584
156. Bounameaux H, Griessen M, Benedet P, Krahenbuhl B, Deom A (1988) Nicotine induced haemodynamic changes during cigarette smoking and nicotine gum chewing: a placebo controlled study in young healthy volunteers. Cardiovasc Res 22(2):154–158
157. Netscher DT, Wigoda P, Thornby J, Yip B, Rappaport NH (1995) The hemodynamic and hematologic effects of cigarette smoking versus a nicotine patch. Plast Reconstr Surg 96(3):681–688
158. Jensen JA, Goodson WH, Hopf HW, Hunt TK (1991) Cigarette smoking decreases tissue oxygen. Arch Surg 126(9):1131–1134
159. Model D (1985) Smoker's face: an underrated clinical sign? Br Med J (Clin Res Ed) 291 (6511):1760–1762
160. Meade TW, Imeson J, Stirling Y (1987) Effects of changes in smoking and other characteristics on clotting factors and the risk of ischaemic heart disease. Lancet 2(8566):986–988
161. Adams KF, Koch G, Chatterjee B, Goldstein GM, O'Neil JJ, Bromberg PA, et al (1988) Acute elevation of blood carboxyhemoglobin to 6% impairs exercise performance and aggravates symptoms in patients with ischemic heart disease. J Am Coll Cardiol 12(4):900–909
162. Allred EN, Bleecker ER, Chaitman BR, Dahms TE, Gottlieb SO, Hackney JD, et al (1989) Short-term effects of carbon monoxide exposure on the exercise performance of subjects with coronary artery disease. N Engl J Med 321(21):1426–1432
163. Davies MJ, Woolf N (1993) Atherosclerosis: what is it and why does it occur? Br Heart J 69(Suppl 1):S3–S11
164. Tsao PS, Lewis NP, Alpert S, Cooke JP (1995) Exposure to shear stress alters endothelial adhesiveness. Role of nitric oxide. Circulation 92(12):3513–3519
165. Cavusoglu Y, Timuralp B, Us T, Akgun Y, Kudaiberdieva G, Gorenek B, et al (2004) Cigarette smoking increases plasma concentrations of vascular cell adhesion molecule-1 in patients with coronary artery disease. Angiology 55(4):397–402
166. Zapolska-Downar D, Naruszewicz M, Zapolski-Downar A, Markiewski M, Bukowska H, Millo B (2000) Ibuprofen inhibits adhesiveness of monocytes to endothelium and reduces cellular oxidative stress in smokers and non-smokers. Eur J Clin Invest 30(11):1002–1010
167. Shen Y, Rattan V, Sultana C, Kalra VK (1996) Cigarette smoke condensate-induced adhesion molecule expression and transendothelial migration of monocytes. Am J Physiol 270(5 Pt 2):H1624–H1633
168. Weber C, Erl W, Weber K, Weber PC (1996) Increased adhesiveness of isolated monocytes to endothelium is prevented by vitamin C intake in smokers. Circulation 93(8):1488–1492
169. Wang Y, Wang L, Ai X, Zhao J, Hao X, Lu Y, et al (2004) Nicotine could augment adhesion molecule expression in human endothelial cells through macrophages secreting TNF-alpha, IL-1beta. Int Immunopharmacol 4(13):1675–1686
170. Caro CG, Lever MJ, Parker KH, Fish PJ (1987) Effect of cigarette smoking on the pattern of arterial blood flow: possible insight into mechanisms underlying the development of arteriosclerosis. Lancet 2(8549):11–13
171. Ernst E, Matrai A, Schmolzl C, Magyarosy I (1987) Dose-effect relationship between smoking and blood rheology. Br J Haematol 65(4):485–487
172. Resnick N, Gimbrone MA Jr (1995) Hemodynamic forces are complex regulators of endothelial gene expression. FASEB J 9(10):874–882
173. Sbarbati R, de Boer M, Marzilli M, Scarlattini M, Rossi G, van Mourik JA (1991) Immunologic-detection of endothelial cells in human whole blood. Blood 77(4):764–769

174. Jeng JR (2000) Carotid thickening, cardiac hypertrophy, and angiotensin converting enzyme gene polymorphism in patients with hypertension. Am J Hypertens 13(1 Pt 1):111–119

175. Schut AF, Sayed-Tabatabaei FA, Witteman JC, Avella AM, Vergeer JM, Pols HA, et al (2004) Smoking-dependent effects of the angiotensin-converting enzyme gene insertion/deletion polymorphism on blood pressure. J Hypertens 22(2):313–319

176. Whisnant JP, Homer D, Ingall TJ, Baker HL Jr, O'Fallon WM, Wievers DO (1990) Duration of cigarette smoking is the strongest predictor of severe extracranial carotid artery atherosclerosis. Stroke 21(5):707–714

177. Fuster V, Chesebro JH, Frye RL, Elveback LR (1981) Platelet survival and the development of coronary artery disease in the young adult: effects of cigarette smoking, strong family history and medical therapy. Circulation 63(3):546–551

178. Nowak J, Murray JJ, Oates JA, Fitzgerald GA (1987) Biochemical evidence of a chronic abnormality in platelet and vascular function in healthy individuals who smoke cigarettes. Circulation 76(1):6–14

179. Benowitz NL, Fitzgerald GA, Wilson M, Zhang Q (1993) Nicotine effects on eicosanoid formation and hemostatic function: comparison of transdermal nicotine and cigarette smoking. J Am Coll Cardiol 22(4):1159–1167

180. Montalescot G, Ankri A, Vicaut E, Drobinski G, Grosgogeat Y, Thomas D (1995) Fibrinogen after coronary angioplasty as a risk factor for restenosis. Circulation 92(1):31–38

181. Wiseman S, Kenchington G, Dain R, Marshall CE, McCollum CN, Greenhalgh RM, et al (1989) Influence of smoking and plasma factors on patency of femoropopliteal vein grafts. BMJ 299(6700):643–646

182. Mazoyer E, Drouet L, Soria C, Fruchard JC, Pellerin A, Arcan JC, et al (1999) Risk factors and outcomes for atherothrombotic disease in French patients: the RIVAGE study. RIsque VAsculaire Group d'Etude. Thromb Res 95:163–176

183. Pellegrini MP, Newby DE, Maxwell S, Webb DJ (2001) Short-term effects of transdermal nicotine on acute tissue plasminogen activator release in vivo in man. Cardiovasc Res 52(2):3 21–327

184. Newby DE, McLeod AL, Uren NG, Flint L, Ludlam CA, Webb DJ, et al (2001) Impaired coronary tissue plasminogen activator release is associated with coronary atherosclerosis and cigarette smoking: direct link between endothelial dysfunction and atherothrombosis. Circulation 103(15):1936–1941

185. Languino LR, Plescia J, Duperray A, Brian AA, Plow EF, Geltosky JE, et al (1993) Fibrinogen mediates leukocyte adhesion to vascular endothelium through an ICAM-1-dependent pathway. Cell 73(7):1423–1434

186. Qi J, Kreutzer DL (1995) Fibrin activation of vascular endothelial cells. Induction of IL-8 expression. J Immunol 155(2):867–876

187. Joensuu T, Salonen R, Winblad I, Korpela H, Salonen JT (1994) Determinants of femoral and carotid artery atherosclerosis. J Intern Med 236(1):79–84

188. Freeman DJ, Griffin BA, Holmes AP, Lindsay GM, Gaffney D, Packard CJ, et al (1994) Regulation of plasma HDL cholesterol and subfraction distribution by genetic and environmental factors. Associations between the TaqI B RFLP in the CETP gene and smoking and obesity. Arterioscler Thromb 14(3):336–344

189. Reilly SL, Ferrell RE, Kottke BA, Sing CF (1992) The gender-specific apolipoprotein E genotype influence on the distribution of plasma lipids and apolipoproteins in the population of Rochester, Minnesota. II. Regression relationships with concomitants. Am J Hum Genet 51(6):1311–1324

190. Behague I, Poirier O, Nicaud V, Evans A, Arveiler D, Luc G, et al (1996) Beta fibrinogen gene polymorphisms are associated with plasma fibrinogen and coronary artery disease in patients with myocardial infarction. The ECTIM Study. Etude Cas-Temoins sur l'Infarctus du Myocarde. Circulation 93(3):440–449

191. Thomas AE, Green FR, Kelleher CH, Wilkes HC, Brennan PJ, Meade TW, et al (1991) Variation in the promoter region of the beta fibrinogen gene is associated with plasma fibrinogen levels in smokers and non-smokers. Thromb Haemost 65(5):487–490

192. Wang XL, Sim AS, Badenhop RF, McCredie RM, Wilcken DE (1996) A smoking-dependent risk of coronary artery disease associated with a polymorphism of the endothelial nitric oxide synthase gene. Nat Med 2(1):41–45

193. Joseph AM, Norman SM, Ferry LH, Prochazka AV, Westman EC, Steele BG, et al (1996) The safety of transdermal nicotine as an aid to smoking cessation in patients with cardiac disease. N Engl J Med 335(24):1792–1798

194. Murray RP, Bailey WC, Daniels K, Bjornson WM, Kurnow K, Connett JE, et al (1996) Safety of nicotine polacrilex gum used by 3,094 participants in the Lung Health Study. Lung Health Study Research Group. Chest 109(2):438–445

195. Dacosta A, Guy JM, Tardy B, Gonthier R, Denis L, Lamaud M, et al (1993) Myocardial infarction and nicotine patch: a contributing or causative factor? Eur Heart J 14(12):1709–1711

196. Fredrickson PA, Hurt RD, Lee GM, Wingender L, Croghan IT, Lauger G, et al (1995) High dose transdermal nicotine therapy for heavy smokers: safety, tolerability and measurement of nicotine and cotinine levels. Psychopharmacology (Berl) 122(3):215–222

197. Jackson M (1993) Cerebral arterial narrowing with nicotine patch. Lancet 342(8865):236–237

198. Stewart RD, Stewart RS, Stamm W, Seelen RP (1976) Rapid estimation of carboxyhemoglobin level in fire fighters. JAMA 235(4):390–392

199. Anon (1994) Nicotine replacement therapy for patients with coronary artery disease. Working group for the study of transdermal nicotine in patients with coronary artery disease. Arch Intern Med 154(9):989–995

200. Ayanian JZ, Cleary PD (1999) Perceived risks of heart disease and cancer among cigarette smokers. JAMA 281(11):1019–1021

201. Kilaru S, Frangos SG, Chen AH, Gortler D, Dhadwal AK, Araim O, et al (2001) Nicotine: a review of its role in atherosclerosis. J Am Coll Surg 193(5):538–546

202. Jodoin I, Bussieres LM, Tardif JC, Juneau M (1999) Effect of a short-term primary prevention program on endothelium-dependent vasodilation in adults at risk for atherosclerosis. Can J Cardiol 15:83–88

203. Iso H, Shimamoto T, Sato S, Koike K, Iida M, Komachi Y (1996) Passive smoking and plasma fibrinogen concentrations. Am J Epidemiol 144(12):1151–1154

204. Kannel WB, D'Agostino RB, Belanger AJ (1987) Fibrinogen, cigarette smoking, and risk of cardiovascular disease: insights from the Framingham study. Am Heart J 113(4): 1006–1010

205. Lowe GD, Fowkes FG, Dawes J, Donnan PT, Lennie SE, Housley E (1993) Blood viscosity, fibrinogen, and activation of coagulation and leukocytes in peripheral arterial disease and the normal population in the Edinburgh artery study. Circulation 87(6):1915–1920

206. Allen DR, Browse NL, Rutt DL (1989) Effects of cigarette smoke, carbon monoxide and nicotine on the uptake of fibrinogen by the canine arterial wall. Atherosclerosis 77(1):83–88

207. Allen DR, Browse NL, Rutt DL, Butler L, Fletcher C (1988) The effect of cigarette smoke, nicotine, and carbon monoxide on the permeability of the arterial wall. J Vasc Surg 7(1):139–152

208. Marshall M, Hess H (1981) Acute effects of low carbon monoxide concentrations on blood rheology, platelet fuction, and the arterial wall in the minipig (author's transl). Res Exp Med (Berl) 178(3):201–210

209. Powell JT (1998) Vascular damage from smoking: disease mechanisms at the arterial wall. Vasc Med 3(1):21–28

210. Tur E, Yosipovitch G, Oren-Vulfs S (1992) Chronic and acute effects of cigarette smoking on skin blood flow. Angiology 43(4):328–335

Other Organ Systems

7

7.1
Central Nervous System

In many countries, smoking is the foremost health threat to the populace. The current mortality rate in the EU resulting from the direct effects of tobacco smoking is one million deaths a year [1]. Recent data reveal that a disproportionately large number of psychiatric patients are smokers compared with other demographic groups [2–4]. In the US, cigarette consumption is twice as high among these patients (Table 7.1) [5]. A number of research teams have found raised cigarette consumption rates in specific mental patient groups and cohorts with, for instance, bipolar disorder, depression, schizophrenia and panic attacks [6–11]. On the whole, it appears that smoking cessation is more difficult for mentally ill patients than for persons not suffering from such illnesses [3, 12, 13]. Smoking has no beneficial effects on the prognosis for depression and schizophrenic disorders.

A secret paper written for the R. J. Reynolds Tobacco Company in 1981 [14] clearly states that smokers smoke because of a "mood-enhancing" effect and "positive stimulation", from which it was concluded that smokers use cigarettes to treat depressive symptoms and cigarettes help them to "perk up" and "think out problems". This document also describes cigarettes as "anxiety relief", helping people to "gain self-control", "calm down" and making them more able "to cope with stress". Although tobacco product advertising has been shown to increase smoking behaviour in adolescents and adults [15], no large set of data has yet been collected on the influence of tobacco advertising on the mentally ill. However, there are numerous studies on the influence of nicotine dependence, i.e. on diurnal variations of subjective activation and mood in smokers. Adan et al. published a study in 2004 in which they analysed the influence of nicotine dependence on the post-lunch phenomenon, a semi-circadian rhythm overlapped with diurnal variations [16]. It was shown that at 0800 h smokers were in a state of nicotine deprivation. Subjective activation and mood of smokers improved after they smoked their first morning cigarette, and this effect was greater for high-dependent subjects. Mood scores were lower in high-dependent smokers throughout the day, intermediate in low-dependent smokers and greater in non-smokers. The study confirmed that differences exist in the circadian rhythmicity between non-smokers and smokers, and that the level of nicotine dependence in smokers is a relevant factor for the interpretation of the diurnal variations [16].

K.-O. Haustein, D. Groneberg, *Tobacco or Health?*   149
DOI: 10.1007/978-3-540-87577-2_7, © Springer Verlag Berlin Heidelberg 2010

Table 7.1 Smoker status of patients with manifestation of mental illness (defined according to DSM-III-R[137]) in the past month and differences in terms of smoking cessation. Comparison with a population without mental illness

Diagnosis (4 weeks previously)	US population (%)	Current smokers (%)	Have smoked at some time (%)	Smoking cessation (%)
No mental illness	50.7	22.5	39.1	42.5
Agoraphobia	1.3	48.1*	63.2*	23.2**
Panic syndrome	1.4	42.6***	63.5*	32.9
Depression	4.9	44.7*	60.4*	26.0***
Panic attacks	2.0	46.4*	66.1*	29.8**
Alcohol abuse, dependence	2.6	56.1*	67.5*	16.9*
Drug abuse, dependence	1.0	67.9*	87.5*	22.4****
Manic-depressive disease	0.9	60.6*	81.8*	25.9
Non-affective psychosis	0.2	45.3	45.3	0

Significance of difference compared with persons without mental illness: $^*p \leq 0.0001$; $^{**}p \leq 0.05$; $^{***}p \leq 0.01$; $^{****}\chi^2, p \leq 0.01$

7.1.1
Cognitive Impairment

Longitudinal studies indicate that smoking increases the risk for cognitive impairment whereas moderate alcohol intake may be a preventive factor. Cognitive impairment was assessed in 889 subjects at baseline and 1 year later using an organic brain syndrome (OBS) scale [17]. Unlike alcohol and in contrast with earlier results, smoking was associated with an increased risk of cognitive impairment (relative risk (RR) 3.7; 95% CI: 1.1–12.3) independently of age, sex, alcohol intake, educational level, occupational class, depression and baseline cognitive function. Older people, in particular, should therefore be encouraged to stop smoking in view of the increased associated risk of cognitive impairment [16]. Word recognition in elderly smokers receiving nicotine tended to be delayed by comparison with young and elderly non-smokers [18]. Shorter reaction times indicative of speedier information processing have been measured in healthy non-smokers following subcutaneous injection of 0.8 mg nicotine, compared with placebo [19]. Furthermore, compared with non-smokers, memory test reaction times in smokers and in smokers during enforced 12 h abstention (deprived smokers) were faster, supporting the hypothesis that nicotine has distinct effects in improving memory-related perceptual and motor aspects of working memory, and this may also be linked with the cholinergic activity of nicotine [20, 21]. In a functional magnetic resonance imaging (MRI) study, the effects of nicotine (0.75–2.25 mg/70 kg body weight i.v.) were studied in 16 active cigarette smokers. The nicotine injections produced dose-dependent increases in behavioural parameters, including feelings of "rush" and "high", and nicotine was found to increase neuron activity in the nucleus accumbens, amygdala, cingulate and frontal lobes. Activation in these structures is consistent with nicotine's behaviour-arousing and behaviour-reinforcing properties [22]. Cognitive performance in smokers was monitored in 3,429 Japanese-American participants in a long-term study [23]. On the basis of the Cognitive Abilities Screening Instrument (CASI) score, a significantly higher risk of cognitive impairment was associated with long-term smoking (OR = 1.36; CI: 1.03–1.80); smoking cessation had a discernible influence, but did not abolish the effect in comparison with non-smokers. To date, a direct correlation has been observed overall between smoking and cognitive information processing, with smoking postulated to have a negative effect [23].

However, this association is contested by the findings from a 4 year population-based study [24].

In a study of 131 children aged 9–12 years, postnatal secondhand smoke exposure has been reported to be associated with reduced language ability (measured using a language score) [25].

There may also be negative effects on certain occupations with a high level of responsibility, e.g. pilots. In this respect, pilots who smoke, if obliged to abstain from nicotine intake during flight, may exhibit certain symptoms leading to performance decrement. Giannakoulas et al. studied 20 healthy male aviators, who were regular smokers, (mean age 33.7 ± 1.4 year) operating military fixed- and rotary-wing aircrafts (C-47 Dakota, F-16, A. Bell 205) [26]. The pilots were subjected to a 12-h abstinence from cigarette smoking, during which time they performed flight duties. After landing, the intensity of the nicotine withdrawal syndrome, as well as its effect on physiological parameters, psychological functions and cognitive tasks were studied. The researches reported that the most frequent symptoms reported during nicotine deprivation were nervousness, craving for tobacco, tension-anxiety, fatigue, difficulty in concentration, decrease in alertness, disorders of fine adjustments, prolonged reaction times, anger-irritability, drowsiness, increase in appetite and impairment of judgement. It was concluded that an abrupt cessation of smoking may be detrimental to flight safety and the smoking withdrawal syndrome may influence flying parameters [26].

7.1.2
Influence on Cognitive Performance

Nicotine has been reported to enhance performance in tasks of selective attention [27]. In this context, efficient attentional filtering obviously depends on the successful inhibition of distracting information. A larger negative priming effect was found in participants who had smoked in comparison with those who sham-smoked. It is suspected that nicotine promotes the filtering of distracting information, thus enhancing selective attention [27]. Transdermal nicotine patches have some of the same effects on performance and mood as cigarette smoking in that they produce a calming effect and a feeling of happiness, as well as improving attentional processing and memory functions (repetition of word lists) [28]. Nicotine improves cognitive performance not only after smoking cessation, but also apparently in normal non-smoking subjects and in people with a variety of disease states (e.g. Alzheimer's disease, children and adolescents with attention deficit hyperactivity disorder (ADHD)) [29, 30].

According to other investigators, learning processes and attention are adversely affected, although it is unclear whether these changes are due to perceptual or impaired motor aspects of the tasks involved. Event-related potentials, reaction times and tests of working memory (word recognition) were assessed in one study in order to elucidate this question. The smokers were tested in a "smoking" and a 12 h "deprived" condition. Smokers exhibited faster reaction times for words occurring new in the tests, together with effects suggesting that smoking facilitates processes related to the motor output aspects of working memory. During the 12 h enforced abstention from smoking, reaction times were delayed (as also found for non-smokers), with the result that nicotine may ultimately be assumed to promote working memory [20].

In contrast to smoking, nicotine (4 mg nicotine chewing gum) influences various EEG components (increased theta and alpha frequency, decreased delta power). However, neither reaction times nor event-related brain potentials were changed, as has been reported after cigarette smoking [31].

The *anxiolytic effects* induced by *smoking* depend on the benign distraction of the smoker [32]. Only those who smoked a cigarette with a high nicotine yield, paired with participation in a distracting activity, experienced a reduction in anxiety. Those who smoked in the absence of distraction even experienced an exacerbation of anxiety [32]. These findings suggest that nicotine – rather than the behavioural or sensory aspects of smoking – interacts with distraction and leads to the alleviation of anxiety or apprehension [32]. Under laboratory conditions, in contrast, nicotine tends to display anxiogenic activity [33].

Smokers' reactions to a lexical decision-making test (decision as to whether or not a sequence of letters represents a word) were also faster and more complete than those of placebo cigarette smokers [34]. According to other data, while cigarette smoking has no negative effect upon performance for simple perceptual tasks smoking was found to exert measurable negative effects upon performance for more complex information processing tasks [35]. The residual effects of smoking consist primarily of retardation of cognitive processes in older adults [36], whereas this negative effect is not observed in ex-smokers and non-smokers. In a comparison with placebo, visual information processing was also increased under 4 mg nicotine gum and cigarette smoking, whereas self-reported feelings of alertness and energy were assessed as higher while cigarette smoking than under 4 mg nicotine gum [37].

Memory (list of 20 words) was tested in smokers of cigarettes with different nicotine yields. Smokers of higher-yield cigarette brands were found to have better recall than smokers of lower-yield brands [38]. When performing more difficult tasks, adolescent smokers altered their smoking behaviour by taking more puffs per cigarette and inhaling more deeply. Women responded more than men to the concentration task [39]. The effects of smoking a low (0.7 mg) and a middle nicotine yield (1.3 mg) cigarette on learning and retention were tested in undergraduate smokers [40]. Both nicotine levels had an effect on retention only, with task difficulty appearing to be of secondary relevance. Serial learning data suggested that the effect is shown more on long-term than on short-term memory.

7.1.3
Intellectual Impairment in Childhood

Several studies indicate that intellectual development is impaired in children whose mothers actively smoke during pregnancy and that this harmful effect is less pronounced in the children of passive smokers [41, 42]. Other confounding variables were also eliminated from the psychological tests employed. Contradictory results have been found for cognitive and language ability [43–45]. Children exposed to the harmful effects of tobacco smoke were found to have more behavioural abnormalities [43, 46–50], namely, heightened aggressiveness [21, 46–49, 51], and an increased tendency to drug and nicotine dependence [47, 50]. Secondly, depressive and anxious reactions have been described, and this finding applies more to boys than to girls [41, 48, 51]. Naturally, the value of any conclusion regarding childhood behaviour depends on the test selected (Child Behaviour Check-List, Child Problem Behaviour Index, Home Observation for Measurement of the Environment etc.) [50, 51, 54]. Two studies have shown an increased frequency of ADHD in children whose mothers smoked during pregnancy [45, 55]. Similarly, an increased prevalence of idiopathic mental retardation was detected in children passively exposed to cigarette smoke during pregnancy and postnatally (OR = 1.9; CI: 1.0–3.4), compared with a non-exposed control group [56].

According to a study published in 1999, long-term nicotine consumption has been linked with self-medicating efforts to cope with the effects of adverse childhood experiences; people exposed to highly adverse experiences in childhood will also be under increased stress in adulthood [57]. In a retrospective cohort study, a total of 9,215 adults with mean ages of 55.3 years (women) and. 58.1 years (men) responded to a survey questionnaire to identify the adverse experiences to which they had been exposed in childhood: emotional, physical and sexual abuse; a battered mother; parental separation or divorce; and growing up with a substance-abusing, mentally ill or incarcerated household member. In persons reporting five or more categories of adverse childhood experiences, the association with cigarette consumption was unequivocal: they had a 5.4-fold higher risk of smoking initiation by the age of 14 years; a 3.1-fold higher risk of ever smoking at a later time; and a 2.8-fold higher risk of still being a smoker at the time of the survey [57]. Primary prevention of these adverse childhood experiences and specific treatment for those affected could help to reduce smoking.

Trinidad et al. examined interactions between emotional intelligence (EI) and smoking risk factors on smoking intentions in adolescents [58]. They defined EI as the ability to: accurately perceive, appraise and express emotion; access and/or generate feelings in facilitating thought; understand emotion and emotional knowledge; and regulate emotions. EI of 416 sixth graders (53% girls) from middle schools in the Los Angeles area (mean age = 11.3 years; 32% Latino, 29% Asian/Pacific Islander, 13% white, 19% Multiethnic, 6% Others) was assessed with an abbreviated version of the Multifactor Emotional Intelligence Scale, Adolescent Version (MEIS). This was a competence-based measure assessing an individual's ability to perceive, understand and manage emotion. Logistic regression models were fit to test interactions between EI and ever trying cigarettes, hostility and perceived ability to refuse a cigarette from someone just met, on intentions to smoke in the next year. The scientists found that high EI adolescents were more likely to intend to smoke in the next year if they had previously experimented with smoking. Those with low EI were more likely to intend to smoke if their perceived ability to refuse a cigarette offer from a person they just met was low or hostility level was high. In conclusion, the study indicated that EI interacts with risk factors to reduce smoking intentions, and contributes evidence to a link between EI and smoking in adolescents [58].

In examining the criminal behaviour of children whose mothers smoked during pregnancy [59, 60], two large-scale studies have revealed a higher rate of criminal offences in adulthood among such offsprings [55]. In a cohort of 5,636 men, compared with the sons of mothers who did not smoke, the sons of mothers who smoked during pregnancy had a more than twofold risk of having committed a violent crime or having repeatedly offended [55].

When maternal smoking during pregnancy was combined with predisposing factors such as maternal age <20 years, a single-parent family, an unwanted pregnancy, and a developmental lag in walking and talking, the odds ratios increased ninefold for violent crimes and 14-fold for persistent offences. Non-violent crimes were not associated with maternal smoking. A second study in 4,169 men [58] revealed associations between violent crimes and maternal smoking, particularly in the third trimester of pregnancy. This study took account of additional data such as maternal rejection, socio-economic status, maternal age, pregnancy and delivery complications, paternal criminal record and parental psychiatric hospitalisation.

Although plausible explanations have not yet been found for an association between violent crime and maternal smoking, the social and educational level of the parents is particularly important because in some countries (Great Britain, Norway) smoking is primarily an activity of people who leave school at an early age (see Sect. 2.7 in Chap. 2). In these terms, it is essential that assessments of such findings in future should also take account of all the socio-demographic factors pertinent to the child. Failure to do so could lead to rash and unwarranted conclusions with considerable social and political impact.

7.1.4
Smoker Personality Profiles and Genetic Inheritance of Smoking

In a study carried out from 1991 to 1995 and involving 12,057 subjects, it was demonstrated that increases in the number of cigarettes smoked are seen to occur in very young and old patients and particularly those who have suffered psychiatric disturbances (16–21- and 51–75-year-olds, OR = 1.5 and 1.57; χ^2 = 6.8; p = 0.078) [58]. This is especially problematic for smokers who are virtually still adolescents, since they go on to become heavily dependent. One year after a psychiatric disturbance, these persons smoked increasing numbers of cigarettes [61]. The genetic inheritance of smoking was seen by analysing smoking behaviour in three successive generations. The results revealed evidence of Mendelian inheritance ratios modified by familial factors [62].

A common interpretation of why mentally ill people smoke larger numbers of cigarettes than people without any mental illness is that smoking provides a kind of "self-treatment" of their symptoms [63, 64]. Such diseases might encourage smoking, revealing a causality between the two factors. A causal relationship is assumed [8, 11, 65] in depressive adolescents and adults in whom a significantly raised level of cigarette consumption correlated with a high risk of developing a depressed mood syndrome [65]. Smokers also show a higher level of risk for first occurrence of panic attacks, and severe anxiety disorders in late adolescence and early adulthood than non-smokers or ex-smokers [8, 66]. Cigarette smoking by schizophrenic patients also encourages the induction of new episodes [11].

More pronounced extraversion has been observed in smokers than in non-smokers [67]. Tobacco dependence and withdrawal symptoms were more frequently associated with neurotic disturbances and these phenomena have also been described in a review article: neurotic personality traits (depression, anxiety, irritability) and disturbed social reactions (impulsive reactions, search for asocial stimuli, low level of conscientiousness, a limited ability to compromise) and lower socio-economic status [68] were found in connection with smoking.

Psychosocial characteristics that predispose adolescents to take up smoking were investigated in a sixth grade class and again 2 years later in the eighth grade in Canada [69]. The significant factors were found to include attitudes and behaviour relative to smoking, smoking by others in the children's environment, gender and stress. The gender difference in the sixth grade lay in the fact that boys were more influenced than girls by people smoking in their environment. In the eighth grade, on the other hand, boys tended to start smoking for reasons related to personal abilities (coping with life, self-respect, social integration, acquisition of skills), conformist tendencies and rebellion. The main reasons why girls took up smoking at this age were related to people in their environment who smoked and rebellion. Regular smoking often begins as experimental smoking within one's peer group, especially in children of a depressive or anxious nature [70]. In female teenagers, regular smoking correlates with a tendency to depression and anxiety reactions [71]. Other depressive symptoms that predispose to adolescent smoking include unhappiness, despondency, hopelessness about the future and difficulty in falling asleep [71].

According to the findings from twins research, the comorbidity of organic depression and nicotine dependence results from general familial factors that may be of a genetic nature [72]. A genetic study revealed relationships between neuroses and smoking behaviour (nicotine volume uptake, dependence, motivation to smoke) and the polymorphic region (5-HTT-LPR: s or l allele, short or long allele, s/s or s/l) linked to the 5-HT transporter gene. A predominance of functional polymorphism of the serotonin transporter gene was posited, as was domination of the genotype 5-HTTLPR-s over 5-HTTLPR-l. Apparently, the neurosis and the 5-HTTLPR-s constellation interact in their influence on nicotine dependence [73, 74]. Another study involving 72 autistic subjects revealed variances in the distribution of the two phenotypes s/s and s/l [75].

7.1.5
Depression

7.1.5.1
Smoking Prevalence

The prevalence of smoking among those who suffer from depression is higher than in the normal population [5] but lower than among people with schizophrenia. In recent years, there has been growing interest in the thesis of comorbidity of depressive conditions and raised cigarette consumption, already pronounced in adolescence (Table 7.2) [4, 6, 72, 76, 77]. Depressive symptoms and clinical pictures with depressive content are more common among people who

Table 7.2 Nicotine dependence among 1,265 adolescents with or without concurrent depression. Frequency figures, absolute and percentage (%), as well as odds ratios with a 95% confidence interval [52]

Variable	Depressive illness	No depressive illness	OR (95% CI)
Whole group	90 (20.0)	857 (5.1)	4.6 (2.5–8.4)
Men	26 (23.1)	447 (5.2)	5.5 (2.0–15.1)
Women	64 (18.9)	410 (5.1)	4.3 (2.0–9.2)

also smoke (OR between 2.1 and 5.7) [6, 72, 78–80]. Women who smoke are more likely to have a history of depression [81]. Among depressive patients, however, there are no gender differences in terms of smoking prevalence [6]. Among 272 New Zealand women smokers (>20 years of age), 63.2% had concurrent psychiatric disease and only 22.7% were psychiatrically normal. A study involving over 3,200 patients demonstrated that all of the 74% who had experienced a depressive episode in their lives had also been smokers, whereas only 53% of the psychologically healthy patients had smoked and that too only once [6].

7.1.5.2
Peculiarities of the Smoker's Personality

The motives for smoking [82], expressed by both sexes suffering from a depressive state more frequently than by non-depressives, are the hoped for stimulation (correlating positively with the degree of dependence), sedation (irrespective of the degree of dependence) and mastery of negative emotional situations. Depressive patients showed a higher rate of dependence and, in connection with this, reduced *joie de vivre* (anhedonia). An increased frequency of depressive episodes in the spring occurs only in smokers, i.e. it is not seen in non-smokers [83]. Smokers of both sexes in a psychiatric clinic had a higher suicide rate than a corresponding group of non-smoking clinic patients. A previous suicide attempt was found twice as often in the medical histories of smokers than in non-smokers, and moderate to severe suicide fixations were expressed 1.43 times more frequently among the smokers than among the non-smoking group [84]. Therefore an interactive relationship appears to exist between smoking and depression: smoking leads to a higher rate of depression and depression predisposes people to smoke [85, 86]. These interactions also apply to adolescents [87].

Both those predisposed to depression and depressive smokers displayed less-effective "cognitive coping strategies" than non-smokers and non-depressives in terms of Ways of Responding (WOR) tests, leading to an attempt at additional "cognitive behavioural therapy" as part of withdrawal therapy for smokers at high risk of depression [88]. Any connection between a disposition to psychiatrically relevant disturbances (mood, anxiety or substance-abuse disorders) and therapeutic success was rejected on the basis of combined withdrawal therapy with fluoxetine plus behavioural therapy, so that a connection between mood and unsatisfactory treatment outcome was only detected in smokers without any previous psychiatric disease [89].

7.1.5.3
Reasons for Increased Cigarette Consumption

In view of the fact that tobacco smoke contains a number of psychoactive substances in addition to nicotine, it is conceivable that these substances interact with the nicotine receptor to increase the release of neurotransmitters. The secretion of many neurotransmitters (noradrenaline, serotonin, dopamine, acetylcholine, γ-amino-butyric acid and glutamate) is increased by the binding of nicotine to central nicotine receptors. Changes in serotonin (5-HT) formation and secretion caused by chronic smoking are also under discussion [90].

Cigarette smoke inhibits the activity of monoamine oxidase (MAO) B, which is partly responsible for the catabolism of serotonin (5-HT), dopamine and noradrenaline in the brain. Inhibition of MAO B, causing up to 40% loss of activity, probably does not occur until heavy smoking has taken place for months or even years [91, 92]. It is probable that MAO B reacts sensitively to peroxidation processes, and thus to oxidative stress, with neurodegenerative manifestations [93]. MAO A inhibition has also been observed after many years of smoking [94]. Suppression and inhibition of both forms of MAO apparently contribute to the tendency of smokers to react depressively [95, 96]. Smokers with a depressive disease reportedly show lower noradrenaline levels at rest than smokers with no depressive tendency [81]. The effect of tobacco smoke can be interpreted as analogous to an MAO inhibitor. In contrast to earlier assumptions, MAO activity itself is unchanged in people at high risk of depression or with a history of depression, and is therefore not a marker for a depressive tendency [81]. The action of antidepressants is also similar to that of an MAO inhibitor, suggesting that various antidepressants could also be supportive in smoking cessation, especially in depressive patients.

7.1.5.4
Comorbidity Between Depression and Smoking

A frequently described comorbidity might result from social, familial and individual risk factors, finally manifesting in the form of depression and nicotine dependence, a hypothesis that is supported by numerous study findings [55, 76, 89, 97–100].

Another hypothesis is derived from the self-medication theory of increased substance use [2, 7, 101, 102]. Raised cigarette consumption could be a way of easing depressive symptoms and the accompanying stress symptoms. The adolescent age range up to 20 years in which these symptoms occur is particularly interesting [72, 87, 103, 104]. Another documented fact is that cigarette consumption increases significantly between the ages of 14 and 18 [80, 88] and there is also a greater frequency of depressive disturbances in this age group [89, 100, 105, 106]. These results were confirmed in investigations involving 1,265 16-year-olds within the framework of a longitudinal study. Here, as well, an odds ratio of 4.6 (95% CI: 2.5–8.4) was determined for additional nicotine dependence with concomitant depression [107].

Yet, a third hypothesis assumes that nicotine or one of the other inhaled substances induces a depressive reaction by way of toxic effects [108], as reflected in a longitudinal study involving a thousand subjects aged between 21 and 30: only 4.8% of the non-smokers, but 12% of the heavy smokers (20 cigarettes a day), developed depressive symptoms [108, 109].

7.1.6
Schizophrenia

7.1.6.1
Prevalence

The "normal" population has 30–40% smokers. The risk of heavy smoking is increased significantly in cases of schizophrenia [2]. The prevalence of smoking among schizophrenics is estimated at 62–81% [12, 105, 110] and the correlation with the paranoid form of schizophrenia is particularly noticeable [7, 101, 105, 110]. Schizophrenic smokers, frequently young men, are more likely to have the most severe forms, with earlier onset and more frequent hospitalisation [101].

7.1.6.2
Reasons for Increased Cigarette Consumption

Although the changes to the α_7-ACh_N receptor are clearly psychosis-associated (most clearly with schizoaffective types, moderately with bipolar types, and least of all with schizophrenic disorders) and smoking is particularly widespread among schizophrenics, the craving to smoke cannot be seen as directly related to the receptor change since no such links exist in healthy smokers and non-smokers [111]. Reversible changes in event-evoked potentials also raise the question of whether brain function is altered by smoking [112]. The following three observations are made in connection with the smoking behaviour of schizophrenics: (1) they have greater difficulty in quitting smoking; (2) smoking is often taken up after the psychosis breaks out; (3) in many cases, however, these people tend to start smoking earlier in youth than the average age in the normal population, i.e. before any outbreak of a psychosis, leading to the hypothesis that starting smoking early in adolescents might be a marker for a later schizophrenic outbreak where there is a familial disposition to schizophrenia [108]. As is the case with depression, alcoholism and phobias, reduced MAO activity in the thrombocytes of schizophrenics was found to be tobacco-induced and not to be a marker for a disposition to develop the disease [109]. One change seen in schizophrenics that may be significant in a pathogenic sense, an abnormal expression and function of the gene family for the neuronal α_7-ACh_N receptor, appears to be compensated for by nicotine use: a deficit in acoustically evoked potentials recognised in schizophrenics is not seen during nicotine use [113].

Another indication of an altered α_7-ACh_N receptor in schizophrenics is the fact that the use of nicotine by this group does not stimulate the proliferation of pulmonary neuroendocrine tissue, which is mediated by this receptor, as strongly as in healthy subjects (measured in terms of the secretion of bombesin-like peptides by the neuroendocrine tissue) [114]. This could also be one of the reasons for the lower incidence of lung cancer among schizophrenics.

7.1.6.3
Extent of Cigarette Consumption

The severity of the smoking habit correlates with the severity of impairment of cognitive functions caused by the schizophrenia, so that smoking is in some cases considered self-treatment in that it increases dopaminergic neurotransmission in prefrontal areas [102]. According to other findings, the number of cigarettes smoked does not correlate with the severity of psychotic symptoms, but rather with non-specific neurotic and anxiety-related symptoms [105]. The "self-therapy" smoking hypothesis is supported by a New Zealand study in women. These women smokers showed a better improvement rate in various psychiatric categories than the other women patients who did not smoke [80], while smoking was considered a mood elevator and a supportive element in resolving daily tasks. Tobacco consumption is seen to correlate with the extent of dyskinesias, commonly affecting the neck and upper body and possibly triggered by the nicotine-induced dopamine secretion [115]. In more severe, therapy-resistant forms of schizophrenia, which were treated episode-wise with antipsychotics, smoking appears to be associated with more pronounced psychopathological symptoms (as shown by scores for "Verbal Positive", "Paranoia" and "Loss of Function") than non-smoking is [104]. However, this effect is no longer detectable 30 days after discontinuation of treatment with antipsychotics. On the other hand, neuroleptic-induced parkinsonism is seen less frequently in schizophrenic smokers and can also be rendered milder by high-level tobacco consumption [7, 13].

Schizophrenic patients have deficits in neuropsychological performance. These patients also have high rates of smoking and resistance to smoking cessation interventions. Therefore, Dolan et al. examined whether the presence of neuropsychological deficits prior to smoking cessation treatment was associated with smoking cessation treatment failure in schizophrenic as compared to non-psychiatric control smokers. They used neuropsychological assessments which were performed prior to treatment with pharmacological agents during the course of placebo-controlled trials in schizophrenic and non-psychiatric control smokers, and included the Wisconsin Card Sorting Test (WCST), a Visuospatial Working Memory (VSWM) task, the Stroop Color-Word Test (SCWT) and the Continuous Performance Test (CPT) [116]. They found that in schizophrenics ($n = 32$), subjects who had greater deficits in VSWM and WCST performance were significantly less likely to quit smoking, but this association was not observed in controls ($n = 40$). Differences between quitters and non-quitters were not likely related to atypical antipsychotic treatment or differences in depressive symptoms. No associations between baseline performance on CPT or SCWT and quit status were found in either group. The data indicate that in schizophrenics, neuropsychological deficits are associated with smoking cessation treatment failure [116].

7.1.7
Effects of Smoking in Forms of Dementia

Findings regarding the effects of nicotine on the central nervous system (CNS) are in some cases contradictory, with smoking (nicotine) acting as both an anxiolytic and a psychostimulant. Nicotine improves the number of words recalled from a 32-item list, a result which is consistent with the hypothesis that the alkaloid was supplying additional processing resources and that deployment of these is under the strategic control of the subject [117]. Additionally, nicotine may improve the intensity feature of attention and the cognitive and psychomotor function [118, 119]. These speculations are supported by the proven fact that Alzheimer's patients show a loss of ACh_N receptors as well as, albeit post mortem, reduction of nicotine binding to cortical ACh_N receptors [120–122]. Loss of cortical α4-subunit appears to be a characteristic feature of neurodegenerative dementia but not

Table 7.3 Smoking and influences on dementia: results of four studies

Smoking habits	Years of observation [n]	Alzheimer's disease Cases (n)	Alzheimer's disease OR (95%, CI)	Different forms of dementia Cases (n)	Different forms of dementia OR (95%, CI)	References
S[a] vs. NS	3	34	1.1 (0.5–2.4)	46	1.4 (0.8–2.7)	[26]
S vs. NS	3	76	0.7 (0.3–1.4)	–	–	[138]
S vs. NS	2	277	1.74 (1.21–2.50)	400	1.39 (1.03–1.89)	[51]
Curr S vs. NS	47	370	0.99 (0.78–1.25)	473	0.96 (0.78–1.18)	[125][b]

[a]Not including smokers who smoked <5 cigarettes a day and who quit 1–2 decades ago
[b]Study involving British physicians and based on smoker status during the last 10–15 years of life
Curr current

dementia of vascular origin [123]. The cholinergic effects of nicotine would lead one to expect an effect in Alzheimer's disease. The assumption that smoking has an Alzheimer-protective effect received due attention from the tobacco industry. These results were not confirmed by other groups [17, 124]. A study published several years ago revealed only negative effects, so that the question of whether nicotine has an effect on Alzheimer's disease remains unanswered [125–127]. Also, in a study in 238 Alzheimer's disease patients, no significant association was found between smoker status and cognitive status [128]. A small number of retrospective studies have reported an inverse relationship between Alzheimer's disease and smoking, although artefacts may have influenced these evaluations [129]. The neuroprotective effects of smoking recorded in animal experiments are thus not transferable to humans [130].

Smoking (nicotine) is also claimed to have an anti-dementia effect, although no evidence has been found to support this claim [28, 131]. Conversely, smoking increases the risk of stroke based on microcirculatory and vasoactive reactions [132], so that dementia from vascular aetiologies may also result from long-term smoking [129, 133]. The prospective EURODEM study involving male British doctors over the age of 65 is based on this thesis and early results are available [53, 129]. It can be assumed that smoking tends to lead to premature rather than late-onset dementia, thus exacerbating and complicating a primary psychotic illness. According to the Doll study [129], there is no significant relationship between smoking and any form of dementia (RR 0.86; 95% CI: 0.55–1.34). The prospective studies summarised in Table 7.3 clearly show that no protective effects of smoking against developing dementia have been demonstrated, to date, in humans. Instead, it must be assumed that smoking leads to the accelerated outbreak of dementia.

7.1.8
Smoking and Parkinson's Disease

Various epidemiological studies have suggested a negative association between cigarette smoking and the risk of Parkinson's disease [134-137]. In one study conducted over a total 30-year period, the rate ratios (95% confidence intervals) for Parkinson's disease relative to never-smokers was 0.4 (0.2–0.7) for current female smokers and 0.3 (0.1–0.8) for current male smokers. For both sexes, the strength of the association decreased with time since quitting, but increased with the number of cigarettes per day and pack-years of smoking [131]. An inverse association between smoking and the incidence of Parkinson's disease therefore exists in both men and women [137]. These data were confirmed in a meta-analysis [136]. According to the EUROPARKINSON Study Group, a family history and smoking, especially in the elderly (>75 years old), interact synergistically to increase the risk for the development of Parkinson's disease (OR = 17.6; CI: 1.9–160.5) [137]. At the same time, on the basis of the dopaminergic action of nicotine, experimental animal work tends to support the theory that cigarette smoking confers a protective effect in terms of Parkinson's disease. Recent experiments in mice and rats indicate that the L-form of nicotine exerts a neuroprotective effect in animal models of parkinsonism (induced by diethyldithiocarbamate or methamphetamine) [138]. Initial studies in humans also confirm that nicotine administration (slow intravenous infusion followed by transdermal nicotine patch application) leads to improvements in extrapyramidal functioning and reaction time, and to decreased tracking errors [139].

Neuroleptic-induced parkinsonism in smokers is associated with higher neuroleptic doses [140]. Evidently, by increasing the induction of drug-metabolising enzymes in the liver, the smoker attempts to reduce the unwanted effects of neuroleptics.

7.2
Ocular Diseases

Unlike the ears, eyes are very much more at risk from the effects smoking than was previously assumed. When the increased level of risk associated with smoking is present in conjunction with other risk factors, numerous ocular diseases may occur in intensified form. Pupil diameter in smokers, immediately after smoking one tobacco cigarette, is slightly smaller than that of non-smokers after sham-smoking [141].

This is another field in which hardly any publication differentiates the effects of nicotine from those of inhaled smoke. Chronic hypoxaemia over a period of decades clearly also plays a pivotal role in the context of eye disease. It is therefore unsurprising that the number of ocular diseases in cigarette smokers has not only undergone a quantitative increase, but also that more ocular diseases are thought to be associated with smoking [142]. Aside from diabetic retinopathy and open-angle glaucoma, macular degeneration (often leading to blindness), Graves' ophthalmopathy, and lens opacity (cataract development) have recently been linked with smoking.

7.2.1
Diabetic Retinopathy

As with other complications of type I or II diabetes mellitus, a special role in the pathogenesis is played by glycated proteins, including haemoglobin, which are deposited in various organs, including the vascular wall, kidneys and retina [143]. Recent research indicates that smoking influences these glycation processes [143].

An older study in a sample of 181 diabetic patients with diabetic retinopathy already showed that the progression of the disease in smokers increases as a function of pack-years of smoking and the duration of diabetes [144, 145], with prevalence among men reportedly being higher than among women [145, 146]. This association has not been confirmed in studies involving larger number of patients [147–149]. Instead, it is believed that the formation of glycohaemoglobin as a result of smoking tends to encourage nephropathy rather than retinopathy [148, 150]. Elsewhere, an association was suspected only in men with a younger onset of disease [151], or the relations between cigarette smoking and retinopathy or nephropathy were variable depending on the statistical models used [152]. The recently published EURODIAB IDDM Complications Study also found an increased risk for the development of diabetic retinopathy in smokers only where there was an early onset of IDDM together with a genetic component for hypertension [153].

7.2.2
Cataract and Lens Opacity

The [86]rubidium efflux technique (rubidium is a mimic of potassium) has been used in animal experiments to study the influence of tobacco smoke on cultured rat lenses, which are metabolically active and have functional defence systems. It was found that the smoke particles are actively transported into the lens and are not absorbed as a result of increased permeability; histologically, the lenses also exhibited morphological changes such as hyperplasia, hypertrophy and multi-layering of epithelial cells [154]. In addition, the heavy metals copper, lead and cadmium inhaled from cigarette smoke accumulate in the lens and are possibly involved in cataract development [155]. Moreover, the inhaled nitrous gases and NO, which accumulate in the anterior chamber during ocular inflammation, lead to changes in α-crystallin indicative of oxidative damage which show up as increased fluorescence (L-kynurenine may be an intermediate causative agent) [156].

A clinical study in 838 watermen investigated the occurrence of nuclear or cortical lens opacities, and a dose-dependent association was found in smokers between nuclear opacity and pack-years of smoking [157], a finding that has been confirmed in other studies [149, 158–160]. These lens opacities regressed partially on smoking cessation [157]. A 10-year prospective study in 17,824 physicians, in whom 557 incident cataracts were confirmed during 5 years of follow-up, demonstrated that the risk of cataract in heavy smokers (>20 cigarettes/day) was doubled compared with never-smokers (RR = 2.16; CI: 1.46–3.20), with nuclear sclerotic changes being observed in particular (RR = 2.24; CI: 1.47–3.41) [161]. Past smokers had an elevated risk of posterior subcapsular cataract (RR = 1.44), whereas current smokers of <20 cigarettes/day did not have an increased cataract risk [161]. The association between pipe smoking and nuclear cataract (OR = 3.1; CI: 1.5–8.2) was stronger than the association with cigarette smoking [162].

Additional moderate alcohol intake ($\leq$4 drinks/day) lowered cataract prevalence, whereas heavy alcohol consumption potentiated the effects of cigarette smoking (OR compared with non-drinkers = 3.9; CI: 0.9–16.6) [162, 163]. The incidence of cataracts in diabetic patients was not significantly affected by additional smoking [164]. Cataract operations (lens nucleus extraction) in female smokers were associated with a risk of more frequent complications [165].

7.2.3
Graves' Ophthalmopathy

Graves' ophthalmopathy, a condition commonly encountered in hyperthyroidism, is critically influenced by the release of interleukin-1 (IL-1) [166], and smoking is known to increase the production of IL-1, and of IFN-γ and TNF-α [166, 167].

The increased risk for Graves' ophthalmopathy associated with cigarette smoking is 2.4 (CI: 1.12–5.18), and Europeans have a substantially greater risk of developing this complication than have Asians [168]. These results are confirmed by a study conducted in Taiwan [169]. Cigarette smoking also encourages the progression of the disease, and the effectiveness of radiotherapy and of glucocorticoids is reduced [170].

7.2.4
Macular Degeneration

Age-related macular degeneration causes blindness in thousands of patients, particularly in the USA, and the medical treatment options are limited at best [171].

It is therefore understandable that several studies have attempted to establish an association with cigarette smoking. One meta-analysis assessed data from three studies conducted in 14,752 patients with age-related macular degeneration. Since the population originated from three continents, there were geographical differences but no gender differences in disease prevalence [172]. This study also clearly showed the harmful effects of smoking in terms of the development of macular degeneration [172].

The risk for macular degeneration has been shown to be associated with cigarette smoking and raised serum cholesterol levels [173]. Compared with ex-smokers or never-smokers, the relative odds for age-related macular degeneration in females who were current smokers has been reported as 2.50 (95% CI: 1.01–6.20); for males it was 3.29 (95% CI: 1.03–10.50). In both cases, the exudative form predominated [174]. Macular pigment density in smokers was substantially reduced compared with that in non-smokers (0.16 vs. 0.34; $p < 0.0001$); an inverse correlation was identified between macular pigment density and pack-years of smoking [175]. Investigations in 6,174 persons, 55 years and older, have also shown that, compared with non-smokers, the risk for age-related macular degeneration is increased 6.6-fold in current smokers (>10 pack-years of smoking) and 3.2-fold in ex-smokers. Arteriosclerotic changes did not alter the association between smoking and macular degeneration [176]. Among women who currently smoked the relative risk for macular degeneration was 2.4 compared with women who had never smoked [177], although the association was less strong than in men [178]. It should be emphasised that the risk for macular degeneration increases dramatically above a consumption of 20 cigarettes/day [179] and that neovascularisation has been detected in addition [180].

Recently, smoking has also been reported to be associated with hereditary optic neuropathy, a rare disease with higher penetrance in men than in women [181].

7.2.5
Glaucoma

In a comparison of 83 patients with definite glaucoma, 121 suspected cases and 237 healthy controls, the risk for glaucoma was found to be increased in current smokers (OR compared with non-smokers = 2.9; CI: 1.3–6.6). However, this increased risk was smaller than that accounted for by untreated hypertension (OR = 5.8; CI: 2.2–15) [182]. Suggestive associations were also found with family history of glaucoma, definite or borderline diabetes and myopia. The vascular effects of nicotine were studied in a comparison of 11 glaucoma patients and 8 controls: although flow velocities were slightly reduced, no significant differences were detected [183].

Bonovas et al. performed a detailed meta-analysis of studies published in peer-reviewed literature on the role of cigarette smoking as a risk factor for primary open-angle glaucoma (POAG). They analysed seven studies and reported summary odds ratios from a fixed-effects model which were 1.37 (95% CI: 1.00–1.87) for current smokers and 1.03 (95% CI: 0.77–1.38) for past smokers. The authors concluded that current smokers are at significantly increased risk of developing POAG. Efforts should be directed towards augmenting the campaign against smoking by adding the increased risk of POAG to the better-known arguments against smoking [184].

7.2.6
Strabismus

A multicentre case-control study was conducted in 377 children born to mothers who smoked. Examination of these children revealed that cigarette smoking was associated with an increased risk for esotropia (OR compared with controls = 1.8; 95% CI: 1.1–2.8) but not for exotropia. The association of maternal smoking throughout pregnancy and esotropia was strongest for children who weighed less than 2,500 g (OR = 8.2; CI: 1.1–62.7) or 3,500 g or more at birth (OR = 5.6; CI: 2.1–15.4). The risk was increased when the mother also smoked after pregnancy in the presence of the child [185].

7.2.7
Ocular Tumours

While it is uncertain whether any causal relationship exists at all, an association has been reported between cigarette smoking and basal cell carcinoma of the eyelids in women but not in men (OR = 2.87 vs. 1.30; not statistically significant) [186]. The question as to whether uveal melanomas are encouraged by smoking remains to be clarified. However, no differences were reported between non-smokers and smokers in terms of progression within 3 years following irradiation [187].

7.2.8
Retinal Detachment

The question of an association with smoking was pursued in a study in 198 patients with retinal detachment. It was found that the relative risk for retinal detachment was increased age-dependently by the presence of myopia, but was decreased by current smoking (RR = 0.5; 95% CI: 0.3–0.8) [188].

7.3
Ears, Oral Cavity and Larynx

7.3.1
Harmful Effects on the Ears

The literature contains only a small number of publications on the effects of smoking on hearing, although it can probably be assumed that blood flow in the middle and inner ear is comparable with that in the CNS and that hypoxaemic states together with microcirculatory changes (raised fibrinogen, etc.) are causally linked with the harmful effects of smoking [189]. According to a study in 163 patients with sudden deafness, smokers also had significantly more risk factors for coronary heart disease compared with a healthy control group [190]. Similarly, in 2,348 patients with noise-induced hearing loss, the relative risks for smokers were significantly elevated (ever-smoker: OR = 1.27, $p = 0.02$; current smoker: OR = 1.39, $p = 0.002$) compared with never-smokers, and associations were even detected with the number of pack-years of smoking [191]. In a further experimental series, the hearing of smokers and non-smokers was compared, following adjustment for other factors: current smokers were 1.69 times as likely to have hearing loss as non-smokers [192]. Compared with non-exposed persons, passive smokers who lived with a smoker were also found to be at increased risk for hearing loss (OR = 1.94; CI: 1.01–3.74) [192]. It has not yet been fully established whether auditory damage occurs primarily in the high-frequency range [193].

7.3.2
Changes in the Oral Cavity

All tobacco consumption (i.e. including chewing tobacco) and especially cigarette smoking produces changes in the oral cavity, for example, mucosal changes in the form of gingivitis [194], [195] and increased tooth loss [194, 196–198]. Periodontal diseases are disproportionately prevalent in smokers [199–202]. In the USA, 80% of all adult cases of periodontal disease can be associated with smoking [203]. Acute ulcerative gingivitis as a consequence of smoking has been known for more than 50 years [194]: firstly, local lesions are produced on the mucosal surface by the tar and other smoke products; and secondly, plaque formation with bacterial colonisation is encouraged [204]. Many of the processes involved have still to be elucidated. However, it has been demonstrated that smokers have reduced salivary IgA and

IgG antibody levels, indicative of an immunosuppressive effect [205]. In addition, nicotine has been reported to inhibit the proliferation of osteoblasts in vitro [206] and to reduce the gingival circulation [207], although these findings need to be confirmed in further investigations.

Increased plaque formation is a proven finding among smokers [208], and this leads to increased bacterial colonisation of the oral cavity and gingival region [209] with all the attendant consequences. Furthermore, melanosis of the tongue (black hairy tongue) and of the oral mucosa may result from the pigmentation of basal keratinocytes [210]. These changes are reversible on smoking cessation. As a result of the thermal insult of smoke, pipe smokers often display stomatitis or smoker's palate [211], a condition that may undergo transformation to a precancerous lesion in rare cases.

With a consumption of 20 cigars/day for 13 years, Sigmund Freud may serve as a typical example: he developed leukoplakia with recurring oral cancers, for which he had to undergo surgery on numerous occasions. Despite having to wear a prosthetic plate in his upper and lower jaw, he continued to smoke persistently until his death.

Smoking encourages discolouration of the teeth and abrasion (especially in pipe smokers or users of chewing tobacco). In association with tooth loss, these changes ultimately lead to occlusive disturbances [211]. Such findings are encountered more frequently in the USA than in Europe, particularly since 10–16 million US Americans use smokeless tobacco as an alternative to smoking cigarettes [212].

Compared with non-exposed children, children passively exposed to maternal smoking are found to be at increased risk for the development of caries (OR = 1.54 vs. 1.06; $p < 0.05$) [213].

7.3.3
Oral and Laryngeal Cancer

More than 9 out of 10 oral cavity cancers in men and 6 out of 10 in women are caused by smoking, while alcohol has been identified as the strongest additional risk factor [214]. Compared with non-smokers, the relative risk in smokers is increased by 2- to 18-fold [215], the increase being dependent on the number of cigarettes smoked daily [216]. The risk of cancer development declines just a few years after smoking cessation [217], in one study by 50% after 3–5 years of smoking abstinence [216]. The efficacy of radiation therapy in such tumours is considerably reduced where patients continue to smoke [218]. Likewise, 8 out of 10 cases of laryngeal cancer are caused by cigarette smoking [219], and the causal relationship has been confirmed by numerous epidemiological and clinical studies [220]. The risk of laryngeal cancer is also associated with the number of cigarettes smoked [220]. For every incremental increase in pack-years of smoking, there is a small but measurable increase in the odds that a patient's laryngeal cancer will already be stage III or IV at initial diagnosis [221]. The bidi cigarettes commonly smoked in India constitute a particular danger: compared with non-smokers, smokers of >20 bidi cigarettes/day have a 12.68-fold higher relative risk for laryngeal cancer [222].

It has been suggested that the mechanisms underlying carcinogenesis are mediated by acetaldehyde formed by alcohol and cigarette smoke, a process that is also encouraged by microbial oxidation of ethanol by the oral microflora [223]. The implications are especially

Table 7.4 Frequency distribution, by socio-demographic variables, of patients with cancers of the oral cavity, pharynx and larynx compared with controls [224]

Variables	Manufactured cigarettes		Hand-rolled cigarettes	
	Patients (%)	Controls (%)	Patients (%)	Controls (%)
Age (years)				
40–49	5 (14.3)	16 (22.2)	8 (4.8)	10 (6.2)
50–59	11 (31.4)	15 (20.8)	48 (28.9)	36 (22.2)
60–69	15 (42.9)	28 (38.9)	80 (48.2)	65 (40.1)
70–79	4 (11.4)	13 (18.1)	30 (18.1)	51 (31.5)
Place of residence				
Rural	33 (94.3)	67 (93.1)	119 (71.7)	97 (59.9)
Urban	2 (5.7)	5 (6.9)	47 (28.3)	65 (40.1)
Education (years)				
0–4	16 (45.7)	41 (56.9)	129 (77.7)	124 (76.5)
≥5	19 (54.3)	31 (43.1)	37 (22.3)	38 (23.5)
Total number of patients	35	72	166	162

serious where smokers hand-roll their own cigarettes – a practice that is still customary in some parts of the world (see Table 7.4) and is also becoming increasingly common again for financial reasons in Germany. Contact with the unfiltered smoke and its constituents damages both the oral mucosa as well as that of the pharynx and larynx [224].

The increased risk for laryngeal cancer associated with excessive alcohol intake has been demonstrated in heavy drinkers and binge drinkers (207 ml pure alcohol or more daily): the relative risks in these categories were 9.6 and 28.4, respectively, compared with 2.6 in non-drinking smokers [225].

7.4
Disorders of Lipid and Glucose Metabolism

7.4.1
Lipid and Cholesterol Metabolism

Serum concentrations of triglycerides and total cholesterol are dependent in particular on dietary habits, but also on genetic factors, body weight and alcohol consumption. Ex-smokers often revise their diet to include more vegetable protein, and these new dietary habits restore serum cholesterol and lipids to normal levels [226]. When patients at increased risk of coronary heart disease were given brief behavioural counselling to implement lifestyle changes, their odds of moving to action/maintenance of behavioural intervention were improved, compared with control patients: for example, fat reduction (OR = 2.15; CI: 1.30–3.56), increased physical activity (OR = 1.89; CI: 1.07–3.36) and smoking cessation (OR = 1.77; CI: 0.76–4.14) [227].

Most epidemiological studies [228] indicate that smokers have raised triglyceride concentrations compared with non-smokers, a finding that has not been confirmed in long-term studies [229–232]. Smoking increases circulating levels of atherogenic LDL cholesterol by accelerating the lipid conversion of HDL cholesterol and delaying the clearance of LDL cholesterol from the plasma compartment [233].

According to a more recent study in which energy intake and basal metabolic rate were calculated in 205 women and 141 men, cigarette smokers had a higher energy intake from fat than non-smokers (29 vs. 26%), a lower intake from carbohydrates (50 vs. 54%) and a lower intake of vitamin C (11 vs. 16 mg) [234].

An epidemiological study conducted in Westphalia in several thousand men and women showed that the frequency of subjects with low plasma HDL cholesterol values (<0.907 mmole/l in men, <1.166 mmole/l in women) was about 10% higher in smokers than in ex-smokers or non-smokers [235]. A study of cardiovascular risk factors in 166 cigarette smokers revealed lower serum HDL cholesterol (0.76 vs. 0.81 mmole/l) and higher serum triglycerides (1.92 vs. 1.71 mmole/l) in comparison with values measured in 312 non-smokers [236]. Higher triglyceride and total cholesterol levels have also been reported in other studies of smokers compared with non-smokers and ex-smokers [237–245]. A meta-analysis of data obtained in children and adolescents aged 8–19 years revealed associations between smoking (or non-smoking) status, and blood lipids and cholesterol fractions; the findings were analogous to those obtained in adults [228]. Plasma thiocyanate levels, measured as an indicator of the extent of tobacco exposure during a smoking reduction programme, correlated significantly and inversely with HDL cholesterol and skinfold thickness, but not with LDL cholesterol or triglycerides [230]. The less an individual smoked, the greater was the increase in HDL cholesterol.

Smoking during pregnancy has been found to produce significant differences in various lipid parameters in the newborns of smoker mothers compared with the newborns of non-smoker mothers:

- Lower HDL cholesterol (21 vs. 26 mg/dl)
- Higher total cholesterol/HDL cholesterol ratio (4.7 vs. 3.7)
- Lower apolipoprotein A-1 (105 vs. 129 mg/dl)
- Higher apolipoprotein B/ apolipoprotein A-1 ratio (0.44 vs. 0.3)

Similar differences were also detected in the smoker and non-smoker mothers [246]. In adult smokers, the deleterious consequences for the coronaries are attributable to the changes in HDL cholesterol and apolipoprotein A-1 levels [226].

Attempts to use antioxidants (vitamin C, α-tocopherol) to reduce LDL oxidisability due to smoking or to block superoxide anion production by leucocytes have been largely unsuccessful in various studies [247], as have been the efforts to reduce raised plasma levels of soluble intercellular adhesion molecule-1 (sICAM-1) or antibodies against oxidised LDL [248].

During smoking cessation therapy with nicotine products in smokers attempting to quit, triglycerides and HDL cholesterol are increased whereas LDL cholesterol is lowered [249–251]. Plasma triglyceride levels after smoking cessation have shown varying responses: unchanged values have been found in some studies [229, 232, 252, 253] whereas a 17.2% reduction has been reported after 6 weeks of smoking cessation [231]. Total cholesterol rises minimally (2.2%) [254], and HDL cholesterol more markedly (20–30%)

[231, 254]. The extent of the rise in HDL cholesterol correlated with the type of diet, with HDL cholesterol being increased more rapidly by a high-fat than a low-fat diet [254].

7.4.2
Diabetes and Smoking

People with diabetes have a tendency to develop complications simply because of their underlying disease. The extensive body of smoking-related findings published during the past two decades should make diabetic patients (and the physicians who treat them) ponder seriously the implications of failing to quit smoking. Specific complications said to be "supported" by smoking include:

- Increasing insulin resistance
- Renal microangiopathy with increasing albuminuria
- Progression of atherosclerosis in the coronary arteries (coronary heart disease, myocardial infarction, stroke) [255] and the peripheral blood vessels (peripheral arterial occlusive disease) [256]

Research conducted in the Netherlands, USA and Japan suggests that cigarette smoking should also be regarded as a risk factor in its own right for the development of type 2 diabetes [257–261]; however, a cohort study in Great Britain has not corroborated this theory [262]. It remains open to speculation whether ethnic or methodological differences (in characterising a person with diabetes) might be responsible for these discrepant findings. As demonstrated by the results from a large Japanese patient population (Table 7.5), a statistically significant association exists between pack-years of cigarette smoking and the risk for acquiring type 2 diabetes.

The association between diabetic neuropathy and cigarette smoking has not been studied extensively. However, diabetic patients with autonomic neuropathy have been shown to have more profound vasoconstrictor responses to cigarette smoking than diabetic patients without neuropathy or healthy controls [263], assuming that the measured reductions in skin temperature are acceptable correlates of blood flow.

Table 7.5 Data on the relative risk for the development of non-insulin-dependent diabetes mellitus as function of pack-years of smoking [261]

Pack-years	Total person-years	Cases of type 2 diabetes	Age-adjusted relative risk (95% CI)	Relative risk, multi-variate[a] (95% CI)
0	13,266	79	1.00	1.00
0.1–20.0	15,132	93	1.12 (0.82–1.69)	1.22 (0.89–1.67)
20.1–30.0	12,980	120	1.56 (1.17–1.81)	1.57 (1.16–2.11)
30.1–40.0	5,332	47	1.44 (1.00–2.64)	1.55 (1.06–2.26)
>40.0	3,854	42	1.69 (1.15–2.49)	1.73 (1.15–2.60)
p for trend			0.0007	0.001

[a]Covariates: age, body mass index, alcohol consumption, physical activity, family history of diabetes, fasting glucose level, total cholesterol, triglycerides, HDL cholesterol and haematocrit

Arteriosclerotic changes in the major vessels occur at an early stage in type 1 diabetic patients who die early from smoking [264]. Levels of circulating adhesion molecules (cAM) are increased, and these ultimately influence endothelial function and hence promote the risk of cardiovascular disease [265–267]. A study of the levels of circulating intercellular adhesion molecule (cICAM) in type 1 diabetic patients without clinical macroangiopathy, in comparison with healthy controls, revealed raised plasma cICAM concentrations in type 1 diabetic smokers, with the highest plasma levels (+25%) being recorded in individuals smoking more than 10 cigarettes/day [268].

7.4.2.1
Insulin Resistance

According to recently published findings, smoking may have a deleterious effect on insulin activity both in healthy subjects [269, 270] and in non-insulin-dependent diabetic (NIDDM) patients [271]. In addition, compared with non-smokers, non-diabetic smokers are insulin-resistant and exhibit hyperinsulinaemia [272–275]. Furthermore, smokers display typical signs of an insulin resistance syndrome. The deviations from normal metabolism are related to smoking habits [272]. The progression of arteriosclerosis is directly and indirectly fostered by compensatory hyperinsulinaemia [276]. In a study of 28 non-obese NIDDM smokers compared with 12 otherwise similar non-smokers, plasma insulin and C-peptide responses to oral glucose load after fasting were significantly higher in smokers than non-smokers, whereas glucose levels were not substantially different (see Fig. 7.1). In addition, the rate of total insulin-mediated glucose disposal depends on the number of cigarettes smoked (Fig. 7.2). Fasting glucose levels and HbA_{1c} were also higher in smokers than in non-smokers [276], as reflected in the propensity of these patients to develop diabetic complications more often [277].

7.4.2.2
Diabetic Nephropathy

The effect of smoking in accelerating the progression of diabetic nephropathy has been demonstrated in numerous studies [278–284]. As illustrated by the data presented in Fig. 7.3, the effect on shortening survival is particularly evident in diabetic patients in end-stage nephropathy where the patient requires haemodialysis [285].

Diabetic nephropathy is characterised primarily by a decline in excretory function because of vascular damage caused by diabetes. In patients with type 2 diabetes, renal damage additionally accelerates the progression of arteriosclerosis, as assessed in terms of carotid artery intima-media thickness (IMT) [286]. Whereas age and impaired creatinine clearance lead to thickening of the carotid artery wall ($p \leq 0.001$), the duration of diabetes and smoking status were found to affect the femoral artery ($p < 0.0001$) [286].

An early sign of nephropathy is the onset of microalbuminuria [287–289], accompanied in addition by increased numbers of free radicals in plasma. In insulin-treated diabetic patients, albumin excretion is already triggered by smoking-related glomerular

Fig. 7.1 Plasma insulin and C-peptide concentrations in fasting NIDDM patients and effect of oral glucose loading with 75 g [276]. *Open circle* non-smokers; *filled circle* smokers

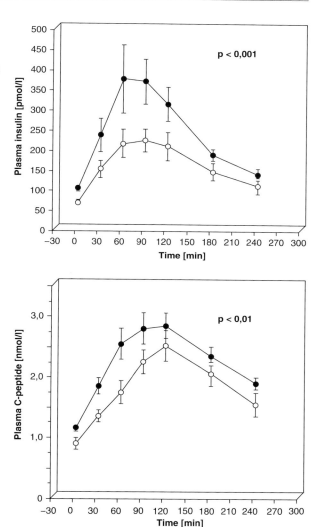

hyperfiltration [282], a phenomenon that has been shown to correlate with the number of cigarettes smoked (Fig. 7.4). Nowadays, therefore, alongside the coronary system, the kidneys should be viewed as the second organ system endangered by the harmful effects of smoking. Cigarette smoking encourages the progression of nephropathy in both type 1 and type 2 diabetes [290]. In contrast – although a subject of controversy in the past – associations have not necessarily been found between diabetic retinopathy and cigarette smoking (see Sect. 7.2.1). In a 1-year prospective study, nephropathy progression was detected in 53% of smokers and 33% of ex-smokers, compared with only 11% of non-smokers [291]. Similar results have been obtained in smokers, based on self-reported smoking behaviour [279]. An investigation conducted in 574 type 2 diabetic patients, aged 40–60

Fig. 7.2 The rate of total
insulin-mediated glucose
disposal in relation to the
number of cigarettes smoked
per day [276]

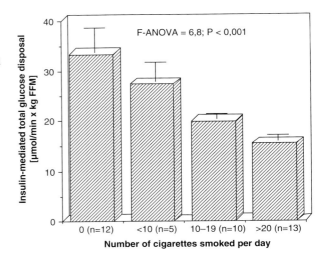

Fig. 7.3 Five-year survival rate
of diabetic non-smokers and
smokers requiring dialysis
therapy for advanced
nephropathy [293]

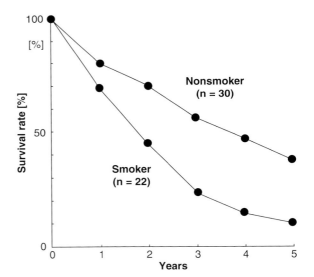

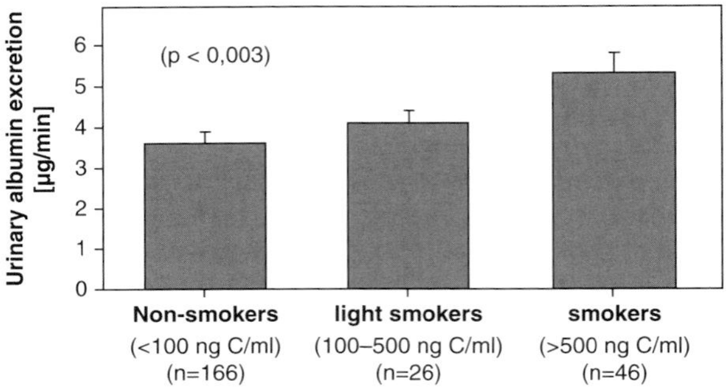

Fig. 7.4 Mean nocturnal
urinary albumin excretion in
patients with type 1 diabetes,
classified on the basis of
smoking habit [285]. The
vertical bars show the
standard error

years, identified slightly raised blood pressure, slightly raised total cholesterol and HbA_{1c} as risk factors for the development of diabetic nephropathy [292].

Smoking among adolescents with type 1 diabetes is associated with an increase in mortality and hospital admissions, including number of treatment days, and these patients feel "unwell". Since details on smoking behaviour provided by diabetic patients are known to be imprecise and unreliable, urinary cotinine measurements have proved useful for monitoring cigarette consumption [293]. According to the results summarised in Fig. 7.3, following assignment to groups on the basis of urinary cotinine excretion the smoking status of type 1 diabetic patients correlated with the extent of renal albumin excretion [293].

Blood pressure in type 1 diabetics is increased, depending on the number of cigarettes smoked [281, 294]; however, these findings have been contested [293]. In contrast, passive smoking by children and adults has been shown to have adverse implications for the progression of diabetes (e.g. based on HbA_{1c} measurements) [295].

Overall, the medical profession should seriously urge men and women with diabetes to give up smoking, particularly since the progression of the disease has been shown to be accelerated by smoking, as confirmed by major national studies [259, 296].

7.5
Gastrointestinal Tract

According to one older study in 456 patients, associations were found between gastrointestinal disease and ingestion of aspirin or non-steroidal anti-inflammatory drugs (NSAIDs), but no correlations were detected with smoking or alcohol [297]. Smoking is known to modify the blood glucose response to an oral glucose load, possibly by altering gastrointestinal tract motility: this is reflected in higher serum motilin (a hormone secreted by the stomach) in smokers than in non-smokers [298].

7.5.1
Oesophageal Cancer

After lung cancer, cancers of the oesophagus are the commonest smoking-related tumours [299, 300]. One possible cause is thought to be the UDP-glucuronyltransferase 1A7 (UGT1A7) system which detoxifies tobacco carcinogens; this is genetically altered in various individuals, and the risk for orolaryngeal cancers is increased in subjects with low-activity UGT1A7 genotypes who are heavy smokers (OR = 6.1; CI: 1.5–25) or light smokers (OR = 3.7; CI: 1.1–12) [301]. In addition, tobacco smoke is regarded as the target for the p53 gene [302]. These tumours are caused by contact carcinogens, particularly since these are condensed in the pharynx, then cleared by the lungs and transported to the oesophageal mucosa where they produce neoplasia [303].

The risk of oesophageal cancer increases with duration of smoking and falls following smoking cessation, as has been confirmed in a US study (OR = 2.1), and the risk is somewhat reduced by filter cigarettes compared with non-filter cigarettes [304]. In a multi-ethnic study, current cigarette smoking was a significant risk factor for oesophageal cancers: the association was strongest for oesophageal adenocarcinomas (OR = 2.80; CI: 1.8–4.3), intermediate for gastric cardia adenocarcinomas (OR = 2.12; CI: 1.5–3.1), and weaker for distal gastric adenocarcinomas (OR = 1.50; CI: 1.1–2.1) [305]. In the USA, 80% of cases of oesophageal cancer observed in the 1990s were related to smoking. Alcohol intake potentiates the carcinogenic effect of smoking [306, 307]. The odds ratio for adenocarcinoma of the distal oesophagus for current smokers has been reported at 2.3 (CI: 1.4–3.9) compared with 1.9 for ex-smokers (CI: 1.2–3.0). Drinkers (four or more glasses of whisky/day) also have an odds ratio of 2.3 (CI: 1.3–4.3), and an additive effect of alcohol and smoking is likely [308].

7.5.2
Gastrointestinal Ulcers

Peptic ulcers show a particular association with smoking, as demonstrated by a wealth of publications in the literature from the 1950s to the 1980s. According to one meta-analysis, 24% of all peptic ulcers are attributable to NSAIDs, 48% to *Helicobacter pylori* and 23% to cigarette smoking [309]. Women who smoke are twice as likely as non-smokers to develop peptic ulcers, and it is estimated that approximately 20% of incident peptic ulcer cases among US women are attributable to cigarette smoking [310]. A larger Polish study conducted in eight different regions underlines these findings [311], although other authors consider smoking (unlike *Helicobacter pylori* infection) not to be an independent factor for ulcer development [312].

On the basis of endoscopy findings, an association has been reported between cigarette smoking and *Helicobacter pylori* infection [313], with the result that increased susceptibility to *Helicobacter pylori* may be assumed. Gastritis caused by *Helicobacter pylori* or by smoking is associated with reduced concentrations of the intragastric epidermal growth factor (EGF), a substance found in the mucosa and produced in increased quantities when ulcers develop; however, this growth factor did not play a role in the pathogenesis of duodenal ulcer [314]. Experimental animal work indicates that smoking reduces EGF-induced angiogenesis and delays ulcer healing [315]. In addition, smoking depresses gastric mucosal blood flow as well as the production of NO by inhibiting NO synthase [316].

One study from Spain in *Helicobacter pylori*-positive patients did not reveal any association between *Helicobacter pylori* infection and alcohol consumption or smoking [317]. Smoking was also not an additional risk factor for dyspepsia [318]. Where smokers had successfully undergone therapy to eradicate *Helicobacter pylori*, cigarette smoking did not increase the recurrence of peptic ulcers [319].

Duodenal ulcers are also provoked by smoking, and smokers have been reported to have more relapses and bleeding episodes than ex-smokers or non-smokers (63.3 vs. 31.2 vs. 34.5% for relapses). Ulcer bleeding occurred in smokers, but not in response to nicotine intake [320]. It has been established that smoking encourages the development of duodenal ulcers by inhibiting duodenal mucosal bicarbonate secretion, an important defence mechanism against acid and peptic damage [321]. Moreover, serum pepsinogen I levels are elevated in smokers because of augmented pepsin secretory capacity [322].

Experimental animal work has shown that simultaneous cigarette smoking markedly impairs the absorption of cimetidine, thus attenuating its efficacy [323]. The smoking status of patients was found to be unimportant for treatment with omeprazole [324]. This finding has been confirmed in clinical trials in patients with duodenal ulcers [325, 326].

7.5.3
Cancers of the Gastrointestinal Tract

According to a Polish study in 741 gastric cancer patients, smokers of non-filter cigarettes had an increased risk for gastric cardia cancers (OR = 3.72; CI: 1.35–10.23), compared with controls [327]. Other authors have also reported that smokers are at increased risk, particularly for tumours in the lower oesophagus/gastric cardia [308, 328–331], and the number of cigarettes smoked daily is also important for the increased level of risk [330]. Compared with non-smokers, current smokers of 80 or more pack-years were at substantially higher risk for squamous cell cancer (OR = 16.9; CI: 4.1–69.1) [332], and the risk was consistent with body mass index (BMI): the more pack-years of smoking and the higher the BMI, the greater the risk. However, smoking is also regarded as a risk factor for adenocarcinomas in the distal gastric region and for diffuse gastric cancers [331]. Among patients with adenocarcinomas and malignant carcinoids of the small intestine who had already experienced ulcer disease ($n = 36$), compared with 52-healthy controls, the odds ratio for cigarette smoking was 4.6 (CI: 1.0–20.7) [333], with the result that a causal relationship may be assumed. In most of the studies the risk was further increased by simultaneous alcohol (spirits) intake [328]. In one study from Russia, for example, heavy vodka consumption had a potentiating effect for the development of cancer of the cardia in men (OR = 3.4; CI: 1.2–10.2) and for cancer of sites other than the gastric cardia in women (OR = 1.5; CI: 1.0–2.3) [334]. While carcinomas of lower sections of the small intestine have been linked with smoking, no studies have been conducted to support this [335].

7.5.4
Pancreatic Cancer

According to several prospective studies, smoking doubles the risk for the development of pancreatic cancer in both men and women [336]. K-ras mutations, associated with alcohol consumption, organochlorines and smoking, have been implicated in pancreatic carcinogenesis [337].

The risk is increased fivefold in people smoking >40 cigarettes daily. In terms of tumour development, smokers do not attain the risk level of non-smokers until 10–15 years after smoking cessation [336]. As also with urinary tract cancer, cadmium has recently been suggested as a factor involved in the development of pancreatic cancer: during smoking, this non-essential metal is absorbed in trace amounts and is known to accumulate particularly in the pancreas [338]. An Italian study has now shown that compared with non-smokers, cigarette smokers are 17.3 times more likely to be found in the group with chronic pancreatitis and 5.3 times more likely to be found in those with pancreatic cancer [339].

Similar results have been obtained in further studies [340–344]. Smoking cessation could eliminate 25% of deaths from pancreatic cancer in the United States [343]. Current cigar smoking, especially when the smoke is inhaled, is also associated with an increased risk for pancreatic cancer (RR = 2.7; CI: 1.5–4.8) [345].

7.6
Urinary Tract Diseases

Along with the lungs and heart, kidneys are among the most important target organs for the harmful effects of smoking. In terms of preserving renal function in an older population, smoking is counterproductive because pre-existing hypertension and vascular disease, in tandem with smoking, will damage small and large renal vessels, even in patients without diabetes [346]. As long ago as 1907, the German physician Hesse advised his patients with nephrosclerosis to give up smoking [347].

Sections of myocardium and kidney from autopsied subjects display parallel smoking-related changes in terms of increased intima thickness of small vessels; while the degree of increase did not correlate with pack-years, it did show a positive correlation with age in the kidney [348]. Within-subject variability has so far limited the usefulness of biomarker determinations – e.g. microalbumin, N-acetyl-β-D-glucosaminidase (NAG) and alanine aminopeptidase (AAP) – for the diagnosis of renal function [349]. Whereas acute smoking has been reported to have no influence on renal albumin excretion [350], microalbuminuria is already increased in the presence of diabetic changes (see Sect. 7.4.2.2).

Smoking-induced elevations in blood pressure and heart rate result from increased secretion of arginine vasopressin and adrenaline, whereas glomerular filtration rate (GFR) falls with a simultaneous increase in renal vascular resistance (Fig. 7.5) [351]. Overall, non-smokers

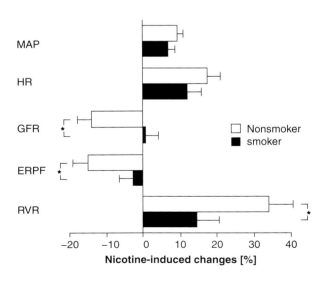

Fig. 7.5 Mean percentage changes in mean arterial pressure (MAP), heart rate (HR), glomerular filtration rate (GFR), effective renal plasma flow (ERPF) and renal vascular resistance (RVR) in 9 smokers and 10 non-smokers following administration of 4-mg nicotine chewing gum for 30 min [351]

respond more intensively than smokers to the administration of nicotine, suggesting that years of smoking produce a diminished response or tachyphylaxis [351, 352].

Stress-related urinary incontinence develops primarily in smokers despite their higher urethral sphincter tone; it is concluded that the simultaneous and persistent presence of violent coughing in smokers overcomes the advantage of a stronger urethral sphincter [353].

The development of renal and lower urinary tract tumours is associated with genetic defects in detoxifying enzymes (e.g. the cytochrome P450 system, and the aromatic amine acetyltransferases NAT-1 and NAT-2) [354] and with the accumulation of heavy metals, such as cadmium. In men particularly, but also in women, the incidence of cancers of the kidneys, bladder and genitalia increases as a function of pack-years of smoking, as shown by one study from Finland [355] and a 26-year follow-up study from Sweden [356].

7.6.1
Toxic Substances and Inducers

Cadmium: Differences in total body cadmium burden were identified years ago between non-smokers (19.3 mg) and smokers (35.5 mg; average 38.7 pack-year smoking history) at age 50, and cadmium is also known to be nephrotoxic [357]. The renal cadmium burden increases with age [358], only to decline again after the age of 60. Cigarette smoking results in the absorption of 1.9 µg of cadmium per pack of. The elimination half-life of cadmium is 15.7 years [359]. In renal cancer patients from Finland, the mean concentrations of cadmium were 9.43 mg/kg renal tissue for women and 14.70 mg/kg renal tissue for men. These levels are not regarded as very high [360], but they are also associated with reduced environmental exposure to heavy metals in Scandinavian countries over the last 20 or 30 years [361, 362], whereas higher levels have been measured in Japan [363].

In explant cultures of human bladder, *benzo[a]pyrene* undergoes transformation to reactive metabolites which form adducts with DNA [364]: these adducts are encountered 2–20 times more commonly in the bladder (biopsy specimens) of smokers than of non-smokers [365, 366]. The relevance of this finding to human bladder cancer is unknown. Aryl hydrocarbon hydroxylase (AHH) activity was measured in kidney cortex biopsy specimens: AHH activity was found to be slightly higher in cancer tissue compared with healthy tissue [367].

Nitrosamines: Tobacco contains procarcinogenic nitrosamines: in the urine of animals as well as in that of infants (see Chap. 8), nitrosamines undergo transformation to 4-(methylnitrosamino)-1-(3-pyridyl)-1-butanone (NNK) and its butanol analogue (NNAL; cf. Box 3.1 in Chap. 3). NNK and NNAL are also formed in increased quantities by various bacterial strains responsible for bladder infections, leading to an increased carcinogen burden [368]. There is evidence to indicate that smoking produces alterations in chromosome 9 and in p53 and c-met which encourage bladder cancer [369–372]. According to a further study in 89 renal tumours, the frequency and pattern of p53 mutations were similar in transitional cell carcinomas of the bladder and the renal pelvis, and no influence of smoking or of phenacetin abuse could be identified [373].

4-Aminobiphenyl adducts: At low nicotine-cotinine levels, *N*-acetyltransferase polymorphism leads to high 4-aminobiphenyl adduct levels in slow acetylators [374]. These findings indicate that carcinogen clearance is decreased in slow acetylators, with the result that these individuals are at greater risk for tumour development [375]. Also, as a result of genetic polymorphism, aromatic amine acetyltransferase (NAT-1) activity in the urinary bladder mucosa causes increased bioactivation of N-hydroxy arylamines into reactive N-acetoxy esters that form DNA adducts [376]. Tobacco smoke is reported to induce the CYP2E1 enzyme in renal tissue, leading to DNA strand breaks [377].

Infections with the human papilloma virus (HPV) are reported to encourage the development of cancer of the cervix in female smokers because HPV promotes the breakdown of tobacco constituents such as benzo[a]pyrene, giving rise to highly reactive products (e.g. [3H]B[a]P-9,10-diol or [3H]trans-anti-B[a]P-tetraol) which form increased levels of DNA adducts, a prerequisite for malignant cell growth [378].

In addition, smoking causes a fourfold increase in micronucleated cells in urothelial tissue; no difference was observed between micronucleated cell rates of smokers and ex-smokers, suggesting that smoking may generate clones of these cells [379]. Little is known concerning the causation of urothelial cancer. In one study conducted in West Berlin between 1990 and 1995, it was shown that the risk for such cancer is increased more by current smoking (OR = 3.46; CI: 2.50–4.78) than by previous but now abandoned smoking (OR = 1.51; CI: 1.09–2.81) [380].

Tissue factor (TF) encrypted in the plasma membrane of renal cells is a physiological initiator of blood coagulation and is thought to be important in a variety of solid malignancies, particularly where angiogenesis is a critical factor. TF is also excreted in the urine, but excreted levels are not affected either by age or by smoking [381].

Smokers who consume more than 10 g tobacco daily excrete more β-hexosaminidase (a marker of renal injury) than non-smokers [382].

7.6.2
Kidney Cancer

According to an analysis of the incidence of kidney cancer in Central Europe, the highest observed rate was recorded in the former Czechoslovakia with 8.37 cases/100,000 population (1990–1994): this figure is expected to rise to 10.38 cases/100,000 for the period 2000–2004. Alcohol and cigarette consumption are cited as the most important determining factors [383]. In a study of 133 histologically confirmed cases of kidney cancer, multivariate analysis revealed that smoking habits accounted for 26% of cases, while genetic factors accounted for only 3% [384].

Concurrent presence of β-carotene deficiency was associated with an additional increase in the risk of kidney cancer. Adolescents who start to smoke before the age of 18 double their risk of developing cancer of the renal pelvis, whereas renal cell cancer was observed only after 25 years of smoking [385]. According to one recent study, cigarette smoking was found to increase the risk of kidney cancer among males (OR = 1.8; CI: 1.3–2.7) more than among females (OR = 1.2; CI: 0.8–1.8) [386]. A case of papillary kidney cancer has been reported in a young man who had smoked marijuana heavily for years [387].

7.6.3
Bladder Cancer

The causes of bladder cancer are to be sought in genetic changes in various key enzymes (see Sects. 7.6.1 and 7.6.4) and in the renal excretion of the combustion products of smoking.

Chromosome 9 alterations have been described in smoking-related bladder cancer [388]. Half of all kidney and bladder cancers in men are related to smoking. According to an Italian study, 46% of bladder cancers are attributable to smoking [389]. In male smokers, the risk of bladder cancer is 3–7 times higher than in non-smokers [390–392]. Among women 37% of bladder cancers and 12% of kidney cancers are smoking-related [393, 394], and odds ratios of 2.4 (CI: 1.5–4.0) and 2.8 (CI: 1.2–6.3) have been reported [391]. Frequent coffee consumption has been cited as an additional risk factor for bladder cancer. Twenty years ago, a case–control study detected an increased smoking-related risk for bladder cancer in men (RR = 4.8; CI: 2.4–9.3) and women (1.7; CI: 1.0–2.7), with the extent of smoking influencing the risk of cancer [395, 396]. In particular, heavy cigarette smokers (≥ 2 pack-years) who inhaled deeply increased their risk sevenfold whereas cigar smoking had no effect on the development of bladder cancer [397]. Transitional cell carcinomas also occurred primarily in smokers, with military personnel being at greater risk than other population groups [398]. The results of treatment for bladder cancer also depend on smoking cessation [399]. Differences in terms of increased risk have been shown between smokers of cigarettes (OR = 3.5; CI: 2.9–4.2), pipes (OR = 1.9; CI: 1.2–3.1) and cigars (OR = 2.3; CI: 1.6–3.5), but the duration of cigar or cigarette smoking had no effect on the incidence of carcinoma [400]. Non-transitional-cell carcinoma(s) are reported principally in smokers (OR = 3.61; CI: 2.08–6.28), with extremely heavy smokers being at even greater risk (OR = 7.01; CI: 3.60–13.66) [401].

7.6.4
Cancer of the Cervix

A high proportion of cervical cancers and of cases of cervical intraepithelial neoplasia (stage III) may be regarded as smoking-related [402–408], as shown by the studies from countries all over the world. Genetic polymorphism at detoxifying enzyme loci such as CYP2D6 and glutathione S-transferase (GSTM1) may determine susceptibility to these cancers [408, 409]. Smoking is an independent risk factor [410] which also correlates with pack-years of smoking, causing the risk to increase by as much as 12-fold [411]. In one case–control study conducted in a relatively large population in Utah/USA, the risk of cervical cancer was increased depending on pack-years of smoking (ever-smokers vs. smokers >5 pack-years: OR = 2.21; CI: 1.44–3.39 vs. 3.42; CI: 2.10–5.57) [412]. One-third of all 1,993 newly diagnosed cases of cervical cancer were attributable to smoking [412, 413], and in these tumours too the breakdown products of smoke excreted via the cervical epithelium act as inducers of carcinogenesis [413, 414]. Nicotine and cotinine have been detected in the cervical mucus (their levels correlate with the number of cigarettes smoked) [415], and passive smokers are also affected. In particular, one carcinogenic tobacco-specific nitrosamine, NNK (see Sect. 7.6.1), has been detected in the cervical mucus of current smokers in concentrations that were three times higher than those in non-smokers [416]. NNK

Table 7.6 Relative risks (RR) with 95% confidence intervals (CI) for cancer incidence in the period 1964–1989: ex-smokers and current smokers were compared with non-smokers (at the start of the study). The data were adjusted for age and place of residence [356]

Site of neoplasm (ICD–7)	Number (n)	Ex-smokers RR (95% CI)	Current smokers RR (95% CI)
Total (140-209)	4,023	1.14 (0.95–1.35)	1.20 (1.09–1.31)
Oral cavity (140-4)	46	–	1.60 (0.74–3.45)
Pharynx (145–8)	17	–	2.87 (0.85–9.69)
Oesophagus (150)	25	3.60 (0.81–15.96)	1.68 (0.53–5.25)
Upper respiratory tract (140-8, 150, 161)	94	0.93 (0.23–3.83)	2.14 (1.27–3.61)
Stomach (151)	226	0.18 (0.02–1.26)	1.25 (0.84–1.86)
Colon-rectum (153-4)	559	1.16 (0.72–1.86)	0.88 (0.67–1.16)
Liver (155.0)	41	–	0.70 (0.24–2.05)
Gallbladder (155.1-155.9)	110	0.32 (0.04–2.33)	0.66 (0.33–1.34)
Pancreas (157)	144	2.47 (1.14–5.34)	1.77 (1.09–2.87)
Lung (162.0, 162.1, 163)	153	1.08 (0.34–3.44)	4.82 (3.38–6.88)
Breast (170)	996	1.21 (0.88–1.67)	0.95 (0.79–1.14)
Cervix uteri (171)	138	1.01 (0.37–2.78)	2.54 (1.74–3.70)
Endometrium (172)	248	1.02 (0.52–2.01)	0.81 (0.55–1.18)
Ovaries (175)	216	1.14 (0.56–2.34)	0.93 (0.62–1.39)
Kidneys (180.0)	94	1.86 (0.75–4.65)	1.09 (0.59–2.01)
Bladder (181.0)	102	2.51 (1.08–5.86)	2.34 (1.43–3.83)
Other urinary organs (180.1, 181.1-9)	23	–	5.17 (2.03–13.2)
Malignant melanoma (190)	101	0.89 (0.28–2.85)	1.15 (0.68–1.95)
Skin (191)	124	1.27 (0.46–3.47)	1.14 (0.64–2.00)
Brain (193)	122	1.53 (0.66–3.52)	1.04 (0.63–1.73)
Thyroid (194)	50	0.55 (0.07–4.00)	0.98 (0.45–2.17)
Non-Hodgkin's lymphoma (200)	94	0.66 (0.16–2.69)	0.87 (0.43–1.64)
Hodgkin's lymphoma (201)	18	–	1.92 (0.56–6.51)
Myelomas (203)	71	2.38 (0.85–6.63)	1.24 (0.60–2.57)
Leukaemias (204-9)	110	1.03 (0.32–3.29)	1.24 (0.71–2.18)
All other organs	432	0.87 (0.47–1.59)	1.06 (0.80–1.41)

has also been detected in non-smokers, probably because of environmental exposure [416]. Smoking cessation should reduce lesion size in cervical cancer [417]. The increased risk for cervical cancer is evident from the data presented in Table 7.6 summarising cancer incidence statistics from a follow-up study conducted over 26 years [356].

7.6.5
Prostatic Hyperplasia and Prostatic Cancer

Lower urinary tract symptoms have been reported to occur equally in various age categories in smokers and non-smokers. In men aged 40–49 years, the symptom score correlated with pack-years, with urinary tract infections being noted more commonly [418]. Alcohol consumption correlates more clearly than current cigarette smoking with the development of benign prostatic hyperplasia (BPH); however, at 35 or more cigarettes/day the risk for BPH was found to be increased (OR = 1.45; CI: 1.07–1.97). Moderate alcohol consumption and avoidance of smoking may benefit BPH [419].

Prostatic cancers are not among the neoplasias primarily caused by smoking. However, a few follow-up studies [420–422] indicate that smoking may increase the risk slightly by 18%. In heavy smokers (40 or more cigarettes/day), the relative risk rises to 51 or 80% [422]. One study performed in more than 340,000 men revealed risk increases of 21% ($\leq$25 cigarettes/day) and of 45% ($\geq$26 cigarettes/day), indicating that cigarette smoking should also be viewed as a risk factor for prostatic cancer [423]. A Canadian study has confirmed an increased risk for prostatic cancer among smokers (OR = 2.31; CI: 1.09–4.89), with a high BMI increasing the risk still further [424].

A raised leptin level may be important for prostatic growth and angiogenesis, especially since prostatic tissue contains leptin receptors [425]. An association between smoking habits and the development of prostatic cancer was not confirmed in 22,071 men participating in the Physicians' Health Study: the relative risks for prostate cancer were 1.14 (CI: 1.00–1.30) for past smokers and 1.10 (CI: 0.84–1.44) for current smokers (20 or more cigarettes/day) [426].

7.6.6
Fertility Disorders

The literature contains growing evidence to indicate that smoking is harmful to both male and female fertility because the carcinogens and mutagens present in cigarette smoke reach the germline cells [427]. In men, smoking diminishes semen quality, including sperm concentration, motility and morphology. The associations between male smoking and semen quality can be demonstrated more clearly in "healthy" men than in men from infertility-clinic populations [428]. The changes in semen quality were already evident in men above the age of 22 years [428]. However, these results have not been confirmed in a clinical trial in married couples [429]. In a study conducted in young soldiers from the Czech Republic, smoking was found to produce changes in sperm, including X and Y chromosome aggregation, reduced-linearity of sperm motion, and more "round-headed" sperm (see Fig. 7.6) [430].

In women, cigarette smoking has been associated with an increase in the average time to conception – 5.1 months for current smokers compared with 4.3 months for women who never smoked [431]. Since cotinine enters the follicular fluid, the likelihood that the nicotine metabolite has a tubal effect in normal ovulatory cycles is considered minimal and has been rejected [432, 433].

Ovarian function and fertility were assessed in a cohort of 499 women, and gonadotrophin-stimulated ovarian function was found to be reduced in smokers compared with non-smokers [434]. A history of increasing tobacco exposure was associated with decreasing serum oestradiol levels, number of retrieved oocytes and number of embryos, with the result that smoking adversely affected the implantation rate and ongoing pregnancy rate [434]. The increased miscarriage rate in smokers is also evidently attributable to cadmium and polyaromatic hydrocarbons, which influence trophoblast differentiation [435]. It is currently under discussion whether nicotine also has such effects (see Chap. 8).

Fig. 7.6 Sperm analysis of smokers (S; $n = 10$) and non-smokers (NS; $n = 15$) [430]. *AI* abstinence interval in days, ($p < 0.02$); *SV* semen volume (ml); *SZ* semen cells (10^7/ml); *TSZ* total sperm count per sample (10^7/ml; $p < 0.001$); *MS* motile sperm (%); *TMS* total motile sperm (10^6/ml; $p < 0.02$). The p-values indicate significance for the comparison S vs. NS

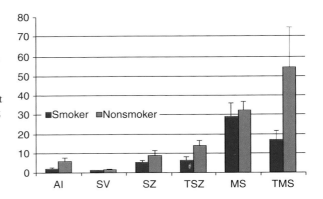

Investigations in 11,888 women have failed to establish unequivocally whether simultaneous smoking and coffee intake influence fecundity [436]. Another study of this question concluded that moderate smoking, coffee drinking and alcohol consumption do not have a deleterious effect on fecundity [437], but only 259 women were included in this study.

7.7
Disorders of Mineral Metabolism and Bone

For several years, an association has been suspected between smoking and disorders of mineral metabolism, and studies have recently been published which demonstrate a significant effect of decades of smoking on calcium metabolism and hence on bone density. In this context, the key hormones are 25-hydroxyvitamin D (25-OH-D) and parathyroid hormone (PTH) [438–443]. Adrenocortical, anterior pituitary and thyroid hormones are also adversely affected [444–446].

Clinical studies in recent years have focussed on the harmful effects of smoking in women. Investigations in rats indicate that nicotine has no adverse consequences in terms of bone mineral density or fracture tendency [447]. When rats were treated with extremely high-dose nicotine infusions (2.5-fold higher concentrations than the average in smokers), no changes were produced in serum concentrations of calcium, 25-OH-D and 1,25-dihydroxyvitamin D (1,25-$(OH)_2$-D); however, serum phosphorus and PTH concentrations were increased [448]. It is further conceivable that various tobacco smoke constituents, such as cadmium, hydroquinone, thiocyanate and nitrosamines, exert an influence on calcium metabolism [449–451].

7.7.1
Vitamin D and Oestrogen Metabolism

Smoking causes reductions in 25-OH-D, osteocalcin [452] and PTH which cannot be explained in terms of other lifestyle factors [453]. The decline in PTH levels is evidently not influenced by differing serum levels of calcium or phosphorus (for review, see [454]). Smokers and non-smokers may behave very differently in terms of coffee, alcohol and vitamin D intake and physical activity [455], and reduced calcium intake may also lead to an increase in $1,25\text{-}(OH)_2\text{-}D$ via a reduction in oestrogen levels [453, 456]. Oestrogen metabolism is increased by the induction of 2-hydroxylation of oestradiol in the liver (increased production of 2-OH-oestrogens) [457], and smoking has a more pronounced effect on the activity of orally than parenterally administered oestrogens [458]. Oestrogens are metabolised more rapidly in the liver of smokers, and this in turn may lead to reduced PTH levels. Similarly, the raised cadmium burden in the kidneys may contribute to the reduction in $1,25\text{-}(OH)_2\text{-}D$ [459, 460]. Owing to this reduction in $1,25\text{-}(OH)_2\text{-}D$, less calcium would be absorbed [461, 462] and taken up into bone. Reduced osteocalcin levels in smokers diminish osteoblast activity, as has also been demonstrated in in vitro experiments [463]. Calculated in terms of decades, bone density naturally declines significantly, even without smoking, and 25-OH-D levels correlate with bone density [464, 465]. According to a study from Denmark, 25-OH-D and $1,25\text{-}(OH)_2\text{-}D$ levels in smokers are reduced by 10% and PTH levels by about 20% [453]. These reduced levels were detected in 50% of smokers [453], as also confirmed in another recently published study [452]. Continued smoking does not alter bone alkaline phosphatase and urinary hydroxyproline excretion [452].

7.7.2
Osteoporosis

Osteoporosis is assessed in terms of bone mineral density, and the common occurrence of femoral neck fractures is important in this context [466]. The influence of smoking has been a topic of controversial discussion in the past [467], and research has focussed particularly on postmenopausal women. An association between bone mineral density and smoking was already demonstrated in the 1980s [467–470]. In summary, a moderate effect of cigarette smoking was identified on the reduction in bone mineral density of pre- and post-menopausal women. The number of cigarettes smoked daily correlated approximately with bone mineral density [471]. This correlation was independent of body weight. A relatively large study (in 544 men and 822 women) detected decreases in hip bone mineral density in smokers compared with non-smokers [472], reflecting the positive association between smoking and decreased bone mineral density in old age.

The anti-osteoporotic effect of hormone replacement therapy (HRT) with oestrogens is attenuated by smoking whereas the anti-osteoporotic effect of raloxifene remains unchanged [473]. Female smokers with a low BMI have an increased risk for bone loss, even during HRT [474]. The ageing-related rise in IL-6 levels is important for the pathogenesis, and IL-6 is further increased by smoking [475].

Men and women aged 61–73 years, born and residing in a rural area of England and at risk for cardiovascular disease and osteoporosis, were compared with a control group in terms of smoking habits [476]. The data revealed reduced bone mineral density in men and women who smoked (see Fig. 7.7), with greater decreases detected in the spine than in the femoral neck. The subjects' build, drinking habits and physical activity were not associated with the reduction in bone mineral density (Fig. 7.8) [476].

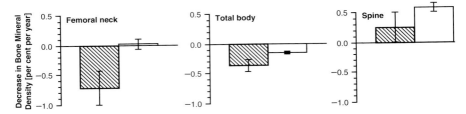

Fig. 7.7 Adjusted mean change in bone mineral density in the femoral neck, whole body and spine in smokers ($n = 31$; *hatched bars*) and non-smokers ($n = 354$; *white bars*). Bone mineral density was corrected for body weight, age, sex, nutritional status (calcium + vitamin D or placebo) and for calcium intake. Statistically significant differences between smokers and non-smokers were detected for the femoral neck ($p < 0.02$) and whole body ($p < 0.05$) [461]

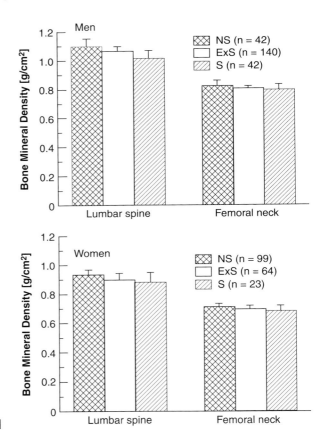

Fig. 7.8 Cigarette smoking and bone mineral density in men and women. Mean values and 95% confidence interval, halved. *NS* non-smokers; *ExS* ex-smokers; *S* smokers [476]

A low BMI consistent with extreme thinness is a risk factor for reduced bone mineral density: thin women have a very much lower bone mineral density than women who are more corpulent [477], and this adverse situation is further compounded by cigarette smoking [469, 478, 479]. A recently published study has confirmed the potentiating effect of thinness and smoking together [480], but these factors can be counteracted by HRT.

7.7.3
Hip Fractures

Smoking has been reported to increase the likelihood of osteoporotic hip fractures [467, 481]; while some investigators have affirmed this association [482–488], others have argued against it [489, 490]. A dose-dependent effect (number of cigarettes smoked) has so far proved difficult to verify. In particular, the increasing cigarette consumption among younger women is problematic [491].

In a cohort study conducted in 116,229 female nurses aged 34–59 years at baseline, information on smoking habits, postmenopausal oestrogen consumption and diseases was collected on biennial questionnaires over a total period of 12 years [478]. Current smokers and ex-smokers accounted respectively for 31 and 26% of the survey sample. A total of 377 incident hip fractures were recorded in women with a mean age of 60 years. The relative risks for hip fracture were 1.3 (CI: 1.0–1.7) for all current smokers and 1.6 (CI: 1.1–2.3) for current smokers of 25 or more cigarettes/day. After adjustment for menopausal status, the relative risks in the two groups fell to 1.2 and 1.4, respectively. The risk in ex-smokers was not higher than that in non-smokers, but the benefit was not observed until 10 years after cessation. Both the increased risk among current smokers and the decline in risk after smoking cessation are in part accounted for by the differences in body weight [478].

According to a study from Denmark in 13,393 women and 17,379 men, the risk of hip fracture in smokers compared with non-smokers is increased 1.36-fold (CI: 1.12–1.65) in women and 1.59-fold (CI: 1.04–2.43) in men. There appears to be no gender difference is smoking-related risk. After 5 years of smoking cessation, the fracture risk was already found to be clearly reduced in men but not in women [492, 493]. Similar results have been reported in a study from Lebanon indicating that postmenopausal women who smoke are particularly at risk [494]. Differences in risk factor patterns have been reported between cervical and trochanteric hip fractures: compared with never-smokers, current smokers have a higher risk for trochanteric fractures (OR = 1.48; CI: 1.12–1.95) than for cervical fractures (OR = 1.22; CI: 0.98–1.52). In women, HRT reduced the risk for trochanteric fractures (OR = 0.55; CI: 0.33–0.92) more than for cervical fractures (OR = 1.00; CI: 0.71–1.39) [495].

Associations between low body weight and smoking have been repeatedly reported [471, 483, 496], and this was also the case in the Danish study cited above [478]. Since women, in particular, are taking up smoking at an ever younger age, the problem of osteoporotic fractures demands increasingly serious attention [497].

7.8
Skin and Mucosa

The skin changes produced by smoking are many and varied, ranging from inflammatory, allergic reactions through to the development of malignant anomalies. Of particular importance in this context are the carcinogenic and mitogenic properties of tobacco smoke and its capacity for radical formation.

Nicotine displays a variety of reactions with mucocutaneous tissue, in particular because different nAChR subtypes (see Sect. 4.1 in Chap. 4) located there are formed by keratinocytes

[498–500], fibroblasts, endothelial cells [501], melanocytes [502] and lymphocytes [503]. Filaggrin, a humectant which improves skin texture, is formed in this way in keratinocytes by Ca^{2+}-mediated secretion [504]. Nicotine disturbs the equilibrium between cell proliferation, growth arrest and apoptosis, but this need not be connected with tumour growth-promoting activity (cf. the findings reported by Heeschen [505]).

A suggested role for nicotine in the pathogenesis of palmoplantar pustulosis (PPP) was investigated but the observed alteration in the nAChR subtypes (α_7- and α_3-subtype) was not clearly demonstrated because ex-smokers were used in the ex vivo experiments [506] and differentiation between the causes (nicotine or tobacco smoke) was impossible. The enhanced occurrence of PPP in smokers seems to be conclusive [507].

The constituents of tobacco and the toxic substances formed during the process of combustion (see Sect. 3.1 in Chap. 3) are capable primarily of forming haemoglobin adducts. Polynuclear aromatic hydrocarbons pose a particular danger to the skin and mucosa, in addition to the lungs. The most noticeable findings in smokers are:

- Yellow staining of the fingers
- Wrinkling, especially on the facial skin of women
- Precancerous lesions and squamous cell carcinomas of the lips and buccal mucosa
- Delayed wound healing [508]
- Frequent and premature necrosis of skin grafts [509–511]

7.8.1
Skin Changes

As long ago as the 1850s, during the assessments for insurance purposes, it was remarked that smokers' skin was pale yellow and wrinkled [512]. Around the same time, in contrast with non-smokers, similar symptoms were noted in smokers among British army officers who had served in colonial India [513]. Skin ageing is encouraged by smoking and exposure to sunlight [514]. The skin of cigarette smokers has been characterised as pale and thickened, with a greyish hue but without any change in pigmentation. In some cases, evidence of wrinkling of the entire skin surface is visible in the cheeks. This skin type is encountered in 79% of female smokers and only 19% of female non-smokers [514]. In this context, cigarette smoking is a factor that operates independently of other noxious agents [515, 516]. Heavy smokers (>50 pack-years) are affected more than less-intensive smokers. The increased risk for facial wrinkling has been reported as dose-dependent (pack-years), but BMI, alcohol consumption and sun exposure (total >50,000 h) are also important, as well as age and gender [515].

The development of these changes can be attributed to the effects of combustion products of tobacco on the epidermis and dermis via the blood supply. In the facial region, the reduced moisture of the stratum corneum is a major factor [517]. Changes involving the lips may be related to mechanical factors due to pursing of the lips and contact with combustion products during smoking. Smokers have also been reported to exhibit elastosis independently of sun exposure, as demonstrated by skin biopsies [518]. Both the number and thickness of the elastic fibres are increased, as also in smokers who are simultaneously suffering from smoking-related lung diseases. Cigarette smoking increases neutrophil elastase activity in plasma [519, 520] and α_1-proteinase inhibitor is inactivated in the process [521]. This imbalance is possibly not only responsible for lung changes in smokers, but also has implications for the skin. In addition, tobacco smoke inhibits lysyl oxidase, an enzyme necessary for the cross-linking of elastin [522], resulting in the production of subfunctional elastin. Radical formation also inactivates this enzyme and the α_1-proteinase inhibitor [523, 524]. Only passing reference will be made here to the fact that smokers have reduced plasma concentrations of retinol, and α- and β-carotene [525]. Microcirculatory alterations in smokers (see Chap. 6) are an additional adverse component.

Tobacco smoke condensate alters the function of human skin fibroblasts and affects extracellular matric turnover in vitro. The biosynthesis of type I and III collagens is decreased [526] and fibroblast-mediated gel contraction is reduced [527]. This effect appears in parallel with wound healing. As compared with non-smokers, the synthesis rates of type I and III collagens were lower by 18 and 22%, respectively, while matrix metalloproteinase-8 was increased by 100% [528]. Thus, the balance of extracellular matrix turnover in skin is also altered, possibly leading to skin deterioration in the long term.

According one publication from the early 1990s, smoking exerts hardly any effect on acne vulgaris [529]. It was even suspected that nicotine or some other constituent of tobacco smoke might display anti-inflammatory activity. Only recently has a published study in 896 patients shown that acne prevalence is clearly higher among smokers (40.8%, OR = 2.04; 95% CI: 1.40–2.99) as compared with non-smokers (25.2%). A dose-dependent correlation was also reported between acne severity and daily cigarette consumption ($p = 0.001$) [530]. By contrast, no association has been shown between atopic dermatitis and cigarette smoking (OR = 1.1; CI: 0.65–1.86; $p = 0.8$) [531].

7.8.2
Psoriasis

While an association between psoriasis and smoking is controversially debated, an association does exist with kidney cancer [532–534]. The authors of one epidemiological study from Norway have reported an association between psoriasis and smoking [535]. However, as with all epidemiological studies, it is problematic to separate cleanly the chronic course of psoriasis from smoking habits that extend over a period of decades. Case–control and cohort studies have shown that smoking is associated with an increased risk for psoriasis (OR = 2.7; CI: 1.44–5.42; 2.1; CI: 1.1–4.0; 3.3; CI: 1.4–7.9) [536–539] and only one study has shown no risk increase [540]. Smoking among patients with psoriasis is strongly associated with pustular lesions (OR = 10.5; CI: 3.3–33.5) [541]. Since the predisposition for psoriasis may be inherited, an additive risk increase has been demonstrated where psoriasis patients still smoke (OR = 18.8; CI: 6.4–54.8) [542]. Psoriasis is sustained by smoking, with the result that smoking cessation should be an urgent goal for these patients. Transdermal nicotine therapy has little or no effect on the skin lesions [543].

7.8.3
Skin Tumours

The development of squamous cell carcinoma of the skin as a result of smoking has not been proven. PPP, a condition associated with immunological changes, was found to be associated with smoking in 56 out of 59 patients, all of whom had started smoking before the onset of PPP [507].

The development of squamous cell carcinoma of the skin in smokers is controversial, with a causal relationship being supported by some published evidence [544–546] and refuted elsewhere [545–551]. The risk of squamous cell carcinoma is possibly increased in men over the age of 60 years (RR = 2.01; CI: 1.21–3.34), with daily cigarette consumption, duration of smoking and exposure to intense sunlight being crucial for the development of the condition [546]. The opposite view is presented in a study of 73,366 female nurses: basal cell carcinoma was more likely to develop in women with red, blonde or light-brown hair, and very much less likely to occur in women with naturally dark-brown hair. Risk was positively associated with tendency to sunburn as a child or adolescent and with the lifetime number of severe episodes of sunburn, but not at all with cigarette smoking [547]. One case-control study from 1992 in 88 men did not find evidence to support an association between smoking and the development of skin cancer [548]. Similarly, no association has been detected between cigarette smoking and melanoma [549]; however, smoking has been linked with forms of anogenital skin cancer (vulva, vagina, cervix, anus, penis) [547]. The risk for the development of carcinoma of the penis is reported to be increased in cigarette smokers (>10 cigarettes/day) twofold [552] or threefold (>45 pack-years) [553]. More than 50% of women with cancer in the anal region are smokers [554], and smokers have a 7.7-fold increased risk for anal cancer compared with non-smokers [555]. Cancer of the vulva was detected when 10–20 cigarettes/day were smoked for more than 20 years [556–558].

Cancer of the lip occurs in smokers generally in conjunction with exposure to strong sunlight [559, 560]; however, other authors have found no such association [561]. Heavy cigarette smoking (>15 pack-years) and 13 other variables were tested by Cox multivariate analysis for their ability to predict death in 196 patients with clinical Stage I melanoma. Smoking may be regarded as an adverse prognostic marker ($p = 0.0065$), and melanoma lesion thickness was clearly greater in smokers than in non-smokers [562].

7.8.4
Breast Cancer

Where they have been made at all, assessments of changes in the female breast in association with smoking vary widely. According to one Canadian study in women with biopsy-confirmed fibroadenoma, cigarette smoking was associated with a reduced risk of fibroadenoma (RR = 0.66; CI: 0.40–1.10). An inverse correlation was even found in as much as the risk was slightly higher where smoking habits were lighter (RR = 0.49; CI: 0.24–0.98) [563]. Unequivocal evidence has not been found for the development of breast cancer in female smokers. Among 2,569 women with histologically confirmed breast cancer, the odds ratios (compared with women who had never smoked) were 0.84 (CI: 0.7–1.0) for current smokers and 1.14 (CI: 0.9–1.4) for ex-smokers. There was also no increase in cancer risk as a function of cigarettes smoked [564]. Similar findings had already been reported in an older US study in 4,720 women with breast cancer (OR = 1.2; CI: 1.1–1.3) [565]. Comparison of the incidence of breast cancer as compared with that of lung cancer over more than 50 years, the incidence of lung cancer was increased by multiples over the same period (cf. Fig. 5.1 in Chap. 5).

The California Environmental Protection Agency (Cal/EPA) completed a health effects assessment of exposure to environmental tobacco smoke (ETS) which resulted in California listing ETS as a toxic air contaminant in January 2006. As part of the assessment, studies on the association between exposure to ETS and breast cancer were reviewed. Miller et al. analysed 26 published reports (including three meta-analyses) evaluating the data and reviewd the association between ETS exposure and breast cancer. A weight-of-evidence approach was applied to evaluate the data and draw conclusions about the association between breast cancer and ETS exposure. The published data indicate an association between ETS and breast cancer in younger primarily premenopausal women. Thirteen of the 14 studies (ten case-control and four cohort) that allowed analysis by menopausal status reported elevated risk estimates for breast cancer in premenopausal women, seven of which were statistically significant. Our meta-analyses indicated elevated summary relative risks ranging from OR 1.68 (95% C.I. 1.31, 2.15) for all 14 studies to 2.20 (95% C.I. 1.69, 2.87) for those with the best exposure assessment. The Cal/EPA with its experts concluded that regular ETS exposure is causally related to breast cancer diagnosed in younger, primarily premenopausal women and that the association is not likely explained by bias or confounding [566].

7.9
Haematopoietic System

Evidence indicating a possible association between smoking and the development of leukaemia was not published until 1986 [567], and subsequently this has been demonstrated not only for leukaemias in children but also in adults [568, 569]. Several cohort studies [570–572] and case–control studies [568, 573] focussing on this issue have been published.

Genetic defects in NAT2 acetylation [574] or in the cytochrome system (CYP1A1, CYP2D6 or CYP2C19) [575] has no influence on the development of acute myeloid or lymphoblastic forms of leukaemia.

Results published, to date, are highly contradictory, particularly because several studies have reported no association between smoking and leukaemia [576–583]. In a 20-year follow-up of more than 17,500 white males, compared with non-smokers, seasoned smokers had an increased relative risk for lymphoblastic leukaemia (RR = 2.7) and other unspecified leukaemia (RR = 1.5) [584]. Further studies have confirmed that smoking confers an increased risk for various forms of leukaemia in adult men and women (OR = 1.5; CI: 1.1–2.0 and 1.4;

CI: 1.0–1.9) [568]. The well-known Seventh Day Adventist study was conducted in a cohort of 34,000 subjects known to be non-smokers on religious grounds. Ex-smokers (i.e. converts who smoked prior to their baptism into the church) had a relative risk of 2.00 for leukaemia and 3.01 for myeloma, and risk increased dose-dependently with increasing numbers of cigarettes smoked. The cigarette smoking–leukaemia relationship was strongest for myeloid leukaemia (RR = 2.24; CI: 0.91–5.53) [572]. A Norwegian study in 26,000 men and women identified an association with smoking for numerous cancer types, but not for leukaemia [585]. According to other studies, drinking habits play a far larger role than smoking; for example, in the development of acute myeloid leukaemia [586].

In China, smoking is many times more prevalent among men than women (<1% of young women smoke [587, 588]); paternal smoking during the preconceptional period was therefore studied [589] because the role of maternal smoking during pregnancy had already been investigated [590–594]. Controversy also surrounds this aspect: while some studies have accepted that an association exists [586, 589, 594–599], others have found no causal association between maternal smoking during pregnancy and the development of childhood leukaemias [593, 597, 598, 600–609]. According to Ji et al. [589], a definite association exists between paternal smoking habits (>5 pack-years) before conception and the subsequent development of cancer in offspring before the age of 5 years. Compared with children whose fathers had never smoked, the children of fathers who smoked had increased odds ratios for the following cancers:

- Acute lymphoblastic leukaemia (OR = 3.8; CI: 1.3–12.3)
- Acute myeloid leukaemia (OR = 2.3)
- Lymphoma (OR = 4.5; CI: 1.2–16.8)
- Non-Hodgkin's lymphomas (OR = 1.2; CI: 1.0–1.4) [578]
- Brain tumours (OR = 2.7; CI: 0.8–9.9)
- All cancers combined (OR = 1.7; CI: 1.2–2.5)

These results are underlined by those from a recently published study in which children with low birth weight and whose mothers smoked during pregnancy were found to have an increased risk for the development of brain tumours [610] and acute leukaemia [611]. The causes are postulated to be the harmful effects of smoking (DNA adduct formation [612]) on sperm cells [595, 597, 613] but also the transplacental passage of smoke constituents to reach the foetus [614–616] (cf. Table 7.7). Following investigations in 2,359 cases of acute lymphoblastic leukaemia or acute myeloid leukaemia, other workers have rejected an association between the development of acute leukaemia and parental smoking history during pregnancy (OR = 1.04; CI: 0.91–1.19 for paternal and/or maternal smoking) [617].

On the basis of model calculations and life tables, an association has been established between benzene inhalation by cigarette smokers and leukaemia: it is estimated that benzene is responsible for one-tenth to one-half of smoking-induced leukaemia mortality [618]. Earlier studies have confirmed that urinary levels of benzene-related compounds (e.g. catechol, hydroquinone and trans-trans-muconic acid) are higher in smokers than in non-smokers [619].

Overall, evidence is accumulating to support the association between smoking habits and the development of cancers of the haematopoietic system.

Table 7.7 Age-dependent odds ratios and 95% confidence intervals for childhood cancers as a function of paternal smoking habits prior to conception (Shanghai Study) [589]

Smoking habits	Time of cancer diagnosis (age)	
	0–4 years	5–9 years
Cigarettes/day		
<10	2.1 (1.2–3.5)	1.0 (0.5–2.1)
10–14	1.6 (0.9–2.7)	0.8 (0.4–1.6)
≥15	2.5 (1.4–4.5)	0.7 (0.3–1.6)
p (trend)	0.004	0.38
Duration (years)		
<5	1.7 (0.9–3.2)	0.8 (0.3–1.7)
5–9	1.5 (0.9–2.6)	1.1 (0.5–2.1)
≥10	2.3 (1.4–3.8)	0.9 (0.4–2.0)
p (trend)	0.0002	0.92
Pack-years		
≤2	1.6 (1.0–2.7)	0.7 (0.3–1.7)
>2 to <5	1.8 (1.8–3.1)	1.0 (0.5–2.1)
≥5	3.5 (1.8–6.6)	0.7 (0.3–1.6)
p (trend)	0.0002	0.71

7.10
Concluding Remarks

- In addition to the harm caused by smoking principally to the cardiovascular system and respiratory tract, renal changes also constitute a serious health problem, especially in patients with diabetes.
- Even adolescent smokers already display fertility disturbances, the implications of which (including childhood cancers in offspring) are difficult to gauge at present.
- Osteoporosis and cancer of the oropharynx seen in alcoholics who smoke are known sequelae of tobacco consumption, whereas no definite association exists between breast cancer and smoking.

References

1. Peto R, Lopez AD, Boreham J, Thun M, Heath C, Doll R (1996) Mortality from smoking worldwide. Br Med Bull 52(1):12–21
2. de Leon J, Dadvand M, Canuso C, White AO, Stanilla JK, Simpson GM (1995) Schizophrenia and smoking: an epidemiological survey in a state hospital. Am J Psychiatry 152(3):453–455
3. Hughes JR, Hatsukami DK, Mitchell JE, Dahlgren LA (1986) Prevalence of smoking among psychiatric outpatients. Am J Psychiatry 143(8):993–997
4. Hughes JR (1986) Genetics of smoking: a brief review. Behav Ther 17:335–345
5. Lasser K, Boyd JW, Woolhandler S, Himmelstein DU, McCormick D, Bor DH (2000) Smoking and mental illness: a population-based prevalence study. JAMA 284(20):2606–2610

6. Glassman AH, Helzer JE, Covey LS, Cottler LB, Stetner F, Tipp JE, et al (1990) Smoking, smoking cessation, and major depression. JAMA 264(12):1546–1549
7. Goff DC, Henderson DC, Amico E (1992) Cigarette smoking in schizophrenia: relationship to psychopathology and medication side effects. Am J Psychiatry 149(9):1189–1194
8. Breslau N, Klein DF (1999) Smoking and panic attacks: an epidemiologic investigation. Arch Gen Psychiatry 56(12):1141–1147
9. Breslau N (1995) Psychiatric comorbidity of smoking and nicotine dependence. Behav Genet 25(2):95–101
10. Gonzalez-Pinto A, Gutierrez M, Ezcurra J, Aizpuru F, Mosquera F, Lopez P, et al (1998) Tobacco smoking and bipolar disorder. J Clin Psychiatry 59(5):225–228
11. Kelly C, McCreadie RG (1999) Smoking habits, current symptoms, and premorbid characteristics of schizophrenic patients in Nithsdale, Scotland. Am J Psychiatry 156(11): 1751–1757
12. Addington J, el Guebaly N, Campbell W, Hodgins DC, Addington D (1998) Smoking cessation treatment for patients with schizophrenia. Am J Psychiatry 155(7):974–976
13. Ziedonis DM, George TP (1997) Schizophrenia and nicotine use: report of a pilot smoking cessation program and review of neurobiological and clinical issues. Schizophr Bull 23(2): 247–254
14. Nordine R (1981) Segmentation study: overview. http://galen.library.ucsf.edu/tobacco/angini/html/c/039/otherpages/index.html
15. Siegel M (1998) Mass media antismoking campaigns: a powerful tool for health promotion. Ann Intern Med 129(2):128–132
16. Adan A, Prat G, Sanchez-Turet M (2004) Effects of nicotine dependence on diurnal variations of subjective activation and mood. Addiction 99(12):1599–1607
17. Cervilla JA, Prince M, Mann A (2000) Smoking, drinking, and incident cognitive impairment: a cohort community based study included in the Gospel Oak project. J Neurol Neurosurg Psychiatry 68(5):622–626
18. Knott VJ, Harr A, Mahoney C (1999) Smoking history and aging-associated cognitive decline: an event-related brain potential study. Neuropsychobiology 40(2):95–106
19. Le Houezec J, Halliday R, Benowitz NL, Callaway E, Naylor H, Herzig K (1994) A low dose of subcutaneous nicotine improves information processing in non-smokers. Psychopharmacology (Berl) 114(4):628–634
20. Pineda JA, Herrera C, Kang C, Sandler A (1998) Effects of cigarette smoking and 12-h abstention on working memory during a serial-probe recognition task. Psychopharmacology (Berl) 139(4):311–321
21. Witte EA, Davidson MC, Marrocco RT (1997) Effects of altering brain cholinergic activity on covert orienting of attention: comparison of monkey and human performance. Psychopharmacology (Berl) 132(4):324–334
22. Stein EA, Pankiewicz J, Harsch HH, Cho JK, Fuller SA, Hoffmann RG, et al (1998) Nicotine-induced limbic cortical activation in the human brain: a functional MRI study. Am J Psychiatry 155(8):1009–1015
23. Galanis DJ, Petrovitch H, Launer LJ, Harris TB, Foley DJ, White LR (1997) Smoking history in middle age and subsequent cognitive performance in elderly Japanese-American men. The Honolulu-Asia Aging Study. Am J Epidemiol 145(6):507–515
24. Ford AB, Mefrouche Z, Friedland RP, Debanne SM (1996) Smoking and cognitive impairment: a population-based study. J Am Geriatr Soc 44(8):905–909
25. Fried PA, Watkinson B, Siegel LS (1997) Reading and language in 9- to 12-year olds prenatally exposed to cigarettes and marijuana. Neurotoxicol Teratol 19(3):171–183
26. Giannakoulas G, Katramados A, Melas N, Diamantopoulos I, Chimonas E (2003) Acute effects of nicotine withdrawal syndrome in pilots during flight. Aviat Space Environ Med 74 (3):247–251

27. Rodway P, Dienes Z, Schepman A (2000) The effects of cigarette smoking on negative priming. Exp Clin Psychopharmacol 8(1):104–111

28. Wang HX, Fratiglioni L, Frisoni GB, Viitanen M, Winblad B (1999) Smoking and the occurrence of Alzheimer's disease: cross-sectional and longitudinal data in a population-based study. Am J Epidemiol 149(7):640–644

29. Levin ED, Conners CK, Silva D, Hinton SC, Meck WH, March J, et al (1998) Transdermal nicotine effects on attention. Psychopharmacology (Berl) 140(2):135–141

30. Levin ED, Rezvani AH (2000) Development of nicotinic drug therapy for cognitive disorders. Eur J Pharmacol 393(1–3):141–146

31. Michel C, Hasenfratz M, Nil R, Battig K (1988) Cardiovascular, electrocortical, and behavioral effects of nicotine chewing gum. Klin Wochenschr 66(Suppl 11):72–79

32. Kassel JD, Unrod M (2000) Smoking, anxiety, and attention: support for the role of nicotine in attentionally mediated anxiolysis. J Abnorm Psychol 109(1):161–166

33. West R, Hajek P (1997) What happens to anxiety levels on giving up smoking? Am J Psychiatry 154(11):1589–1592

34. Hale CR, Gentry MV, Meliska CJ (1999) Effects of cigarette smoking on lexical decision-making. Psychol Rep 84(1):117–120

35. Spilich GJ, June L, Renner J (1992) Cigarette smoking and cognitive performance. Br J Addict 87(9):1313–1326

36. Hill RD (1989) Residual effects of cigarette smoking on cognitive performance in normal aging. Psychol Aging 4(2):251–254

37. Parrott AC, Winder G (1989) Nicotine chewing gum (2 mg, 4 mg) and cigarette smoking: comparative effects upon vigilance and heart rate. Psychopharmacology (Berl) 97(2):257–261

38. Peeke SC, Peeke HV (1984) Attention, memory, and cigarette smoking. Psychopharmacology (Berl) 84(2):205–216

39. Rose JE, Ananda S, Jarvik ME (1983) Cigarette smoking during anxiety-provoking and monotonous tasks. Addict Behav 8(4):353–359

40. Mangan GL (1983) The effects of cigarette smoking on verbal learning and retention. J Gen Psychol 108:203–210

41. Makin J, Fried PA, Watkinson B (1991) A comparison of active and passive smoking during pregnancy: long-term effects. Neurotoxicol Teratol 13(1):5–12

42. Olds DL, Henderson CR Jr, Tatelbaum R (1994) Intellectual impairment in children of women who smoke cigarettes during pregnancy. Pediatrics 93(2):221–227

43. Fergusson DM, Lloyd M (1991) Smoking during pregnancy and its effects on child cognitive ability from the ages of 8 to 12 years. Paediatr Perinat Epidemiol 5(2):189–200

44. Fogelman KR, Manor O (1988) Smoking in pregnancy and development into early adulthood. BMJ 297(6658):1233–1236

45. Naeye RL, Peters EC (1984) Mental development of children whose mothers smoked during pregnancy. Obstet Gynecol 64(5):601–607

46. Fergusson DM, Horwood LJ, Lynskey MT (1993) Maternal smoking before and after pregnancy: effects on behavioral outcomes in middle childhood. Pediatrics 92(6):815–822

47. McGee R, Stanton WR (1994) Smoking in pregnancy and child development to age 9 years. J Paediatr Child Health 30(3):263–268

48. Orlebeke JF, Knol DL, Verhulst FC (1997) Increase in child behavior problems resulting from maternal smoking during pregnancy. Arch Environ Health 52(4):317–321

49. Weissman MM, Warner V, Wickramaratne PJ, Kandel DB (1999) Maternal smoking during pregnancy and psychopathology in offspring followed to adulthood. J Am Acad Child Adolesc Psychiatry 38(7):892–899

50. Williams GM, O'Callaghan M, Najman JM, Bor W, Andersen MJ, Richards D, et al (1998) Maternal cigarette smoking and child psychiatric morbidity: a longitudinal study. Pediatrics 102(1):e11

51. Weitzman M, Gortmaker S, Sobol A (1992) Maternal smoking and behavior problems of children. Pediatrics 90(3):342–349
52. Kandel DB, Wu P, Davies M (1994) Maternal smoking during pregnancy and smoking by adolescent daughters. Am J Public Health 84(9):1407–1413
53. Launer LJ, Andersen K, Dewey ME, Letenneur L, Ott A, Amaducci LA, et al (1999) Rates and risk factors for dementia and Alzheimer's disease: results from EURODEM pooled analyses. EURODEM Incidence Research Group and Work Groups. European Studies of Dementia. Neurology 52(1):78–84
54. Fergusson DM, Lynskey MT, Horwood LJ (1996) Comorbidity between depressive disorders and nicotine dependence in a cohort of 16-year-olds. Arch Gen Psychiatry 53(11):1043–1047
55. Milberger S, Biederman J, Faraone SV, Jones J (1998) Further evidence of an association between maternal smoking during pregnancy and attention deficit hyperactivity disorder: findings from a high-risk sample of siblings. J Clin Child Psychol 27(3):352–358
56. Drews CD, Murphy CC, Yeargin-Allsopp M, Decoufle P (1996) The relationship between idiopathic mental retardation and maternal smoking during pregnancy. Pediatrics 97(4):547–553
57. Anda RF, Croft JB, Felitti VJ, Nordenberg D, Giles WH, Williamson DF, et al (1999) Adverse childhood experiences and smoking during adolescence and adulthood. JAMA 282(17): 1652–1658
58. Trinidad DR, Unger JB, Chou CP, Azen SP, Johnson CA (2004) Emotional intelligence and smoking risk factors in adolescents: interactions on smoking intentions. J Adolesc Health 34 (1):46–55
59. Miller SK, Slap GB (1989) Adolescent smoking. A review of prevalence and prevention. J Adolesc Health Care 10(2):129–135
60. Rasanen P, Hakko H, Isohanni M, Hodgins S, Jarvelin MR, Tiihonen J (1999) Maternal smoking during pregnancy and risk of criminal behavior among adult male offspring in the Northern Finland 1966 Birth Cohort. Am J Psychiatry 156(6):857–862
61. Ismail K, Sloggett A, De Stavola B (2000) Do common mental disorders increase cigarette smoking? Results from five waves of a population-based panel cohort study. Am J Epidemiol 152(7):651–657
62. Cheng LS, Swan GE, Carmelli D (2000) A genetic analysis of smoking behavior in family members of older adult males. Addiction 95(3):427–435
63. Addington J (1998) Group treatment for smoking cessation among persons with schizophrenia. Psychiatr Serv 49(7):925–928
64. Carmody TP (1989) Affect regulation, nicotine addiction, and smoking cessation. J Psychoactive Drugs 21(3):331–342
65. Wu LT, Anthony JC (1999) Tobacco smoking and depressed mood in late childhood and early adolescence. Am J Public Health 89(12):1837–1840
66. Johnson JG, Cohen P, Pine DS, Klein DF, Kasen S, Brook JS (2000) Association between cigarette smoking and anxiety disorders during adolescence and early adulthood. JAMA 284(18):2348–2351
67. Yoshimura K (2000) The psychological characteristics of tobacco dependence in a rural area of Japan. J Epidemiol 10(4):271–279
68. Batra A (2000) [Tobacco use and smoking cessation in the psychiatric patient]. Fortschr Neurol Psychiatr 68(2):80–92
69. Koval JJ, Pederson LL, Mills CA, McGrady GA, Carvajal SC (2000) Models of the relationship of stress, depression, and other psychosocial factors to smoking behavior: a comparison of a cohort of students in grades 6 and 8. Prev Med 30(6):463–477
70. Patton GC, Carlin JB, Coffey C, Wolfe R, Hibbert M, Bowes G (1998) Depression, anxiety, and smoking initiation: a prospective study over 3 years. Am J Public Health 88(10):1518–1522
71. Wang MQ, Fitzhugh EC, Westerfield RC, Eddy JM (1994) Predicting smoking status by symptoms of depression for U.S. adolescents. Psychol Rep 75(2):911–914

72. Kendler KS, Neale MC, MacLean CJ, Heath AC, Eaves LJ, Kessler RC (1993) Smoking and major depression. A causal analysis. Arch Gen Psychiatry 50(1):36–43

73. Hu S, Brody CL, Fisher C, Gunzerath L, Nelson ML, Sabol SZ, et al (2000) Interaction between the serotonin transporter gene and neuroticism in cigarette smoking behavior. Mol Psychiatry 5(2):181–188

74. Lerman C, Caporaso NE, Audrain J, Main D, Boyd NR, Shields PG (2000) Interacting effects of the serotonin transporter gene and neuroticism in smoking practices and nicotine dependence. Mol Psychiatry 5(2):189–192

75. Zhong N, Ye L, Ju W, Brown WT, Tsiouris J (1999) Cohen I. 5-HTTLPR variants not associated with autistic spectrum disorders. Neurogenetics 2(2):129–131

76. Breslau N, Kilbey MM, Andreski P (1993) Nicotine dependence and major depression. New evidence from a prospective investigation. Arch Gen Psychiatry 50(1):31–35

77. Glassman AH (1993) Cigarette smoking: implications for psychiatric illness. Am J Psychiatry 150(4):546–553

78. Anda RF, Williamson DF, Escobedo LG, Mast EE, Giovino GA, Remington PL (1990) Depression and the dynamics of smoking. A national perspective. JAMA 264(12):1541–1545

79. Breslau N, Kilbey M, Andreski P (1991) Nicotine dependence, major depression, and anxiety in young adults. Arch Gen Psychiatry 48(12):1069–1074

80. Romans SE, McNoe BM, Herbison GP, Walton VA, Mullen PE (1993) Cigarette smoking and psychiatric morbidity in women. Aust N Z J Psychiatry 27(3):399–404

81. Berlin I, Spreux-Varoquaux O, Said S, Launay JM (1997) Effects of past history of major depression on smoking characteristics, monoamine oxidase-A and -B activities and withdrawal symptoms in dependent smokers. Drug Alcohol Depend 45(1–2):31–37

82. Carton S, Jouvent R, Widlocher D (1994) Nicotine dependence and motives for smoking in depression. J Subst Abuse 6(1):67–76

83. D'Mello DA, Flanagan C (1996) Seasons and depression: the influence of cigarette smoking. Addict Behav 21(5):671–674

84. Black DW, Zimmerman M, Coryell WH (1999) Cigarette smoking and psychiatric disorder in a community sample. Ann Clin Psychiatry 11(3):129–136

85. Breslau N, Peterson EL, Schultz LR, Chilcoat HD, Andreski P (1998) Major depression and stages of smoking. A longitudinal investigation. Arch Gen Psychiatry 55(2):161–166

86. Covey LS, Glassman AH, Stetner F (1998) Cigarette smoking and major depression. J Addict Dis 17(1):35–46

87. Brown RA, Lewinsohn PM, Seeley JR, Wagner EF (1996) Cigarette smoking, major depression, and other psychiatric disorders among adolescents. J Am Acad Child Adolesc Psychiatry 35(12):1602–1610

88. Rabois D, Haaga DA (1997) Cognitive coping, history of depression, and cigarette smoking. Addict Behav 22(6):789–796

89. Keuthen NJ, Niaura RS, Borrelli B, Goldstein M, DePue J, Murphy C, et al (2000) Comorbidity, smoking behavior and treatment outcome. Psychother Psychosom 69(5):244–250

90. Balfour DJ, Ridleyl DL (2000) The effects of nicotine on neural pathways implicated in depression: a factor in nicotine addiction? Pharmacol Biochem Behav 66(1):79–85

91. Quattrocki E, Baird A, Yurgelun-Todd D (2000) Biological aspects of the link between smoking and depression. Harv Rev Psychiatry 8(3):99–110

92. Fowler JS, Volkow ND, Wang GJ, Pappas N, Logan J, MacGregor R, et al (1998) Neuropharmacological actions of cigarette smoke: brain monoamine oxidase B (MAO B) inhibition. J Addict Dis 17(1):23–34

93. Fowler JS, Volkow ND, Logan J, Pappas N, King P, MacGregor R, et al (1998) An acute dose of nicotine does not inhibit MAO B in baboon brain in vivo. Life Sci 63(2):L19–L23

94. Fowler JS, Volkow ND, Wang GJ, Pappas N, Logan J, Shea C, et al (1996) Brain monoamine oxidase A inhibition in cigarette smokers. Proc Natl Acad Sci U S A 93(24):14065–14069

95. Berlin I, Said S, Spreux-Varoquaux O, Launay JM, Olivares R, Millet V, et al (1995) A reversible monoamine oxidase A inhibitor (moclobemide) facilitates smoking cessation and abstinence in heavy, dependent smokers. Clin Pharmacol Ther 58(4):444–452

96. Berlin I, Said S, Spreux-Varoquaux O, Olivares R, Launay JM, Puech AJ (1995) Monoamine oxidase A and B activities in heavy smokers. Biol Psychiatry 38(11):756–761

97. Angold A (1988) Childhood and adolescent depression. I. Epidemiological and aetiological aspects. Br J Psychiatry 152:601–617

98. Conrad KM, Flay BR, Hill D (1992) Why children start smoking cigarettes: predictors of onset. Br J Addict 87(12):1711–1724

99. Fleming JE, Offord DR (1990) Epidemiology of childhood depressive disorders: a critical review. J Am Acad Child Adolesc Psychiatry 29(4):571–580

100. Rutter M, Izard CE, Read PB (1986) Depression in young people. Developmental and clinical perspectives. Guildford, New York

101. Ebeling H, Moilanen I, Linna SL, Tirkkonen T, Ebeling T, Piha J, et al (1999) Smoking and drinking habits in adolescence – links with psychiatric disturbance at the age of 8 years. Eur Child Adolesc Psychiatry 8(Suppl 4):68–76

102. Taiminen TJ, Salokangas RK, Saarijarvi S, Niemi H, Lehto H, Ahola V, et al (1998) Smoking and cognitive deficits in schizophrenia: a pilot study. Addict Behav 23(2):263–266

103. Breslau N, Johnson EO (2000) Predicting smoking cessation and major depression in nicotine-dependent smokers. Am J Public Health 90(7):1122–1127

104. Curtin L, Brown RA, Sales SD (2000) Determinants of attrition from cessation treatment in smokers with a history of major depressive disorder. Psychol Addict Behav 14(2):134–142

105. Herran A, de Santiago A, Sandoya M, Fernandez MJ, Diez-Manrique JF, Vazquez-Barquero JL (2000) Determinants of smoking behaviour in outpatients with schizophrenia. Schizophr Res 41(2):373–381

106. Gilbert DG, Crauthers DM, Mooney DK, McClernon FJ, Jensen RA (1999) Effects of monetary contingencies on smoking relapse: influences of trait depression, personality, and habitual nicotine intake. Exp Clin Psychopharmacol 7(2):174–181

107. Apud JA, Egan MF, Wyatt RJ (2000) Effects of smoking during antipsychotic withdrawal in patients with chronic schizophrenia. Schizophr Res 46(2–3):119–127

108. de Leon J (1996) Smoking and vulnerability for schizophrenia. Schizophr Bull 22(3): 405–409

109. Pomerleau CS, Marks JL, Pomerleau OF (2000) Who gets what symptom? Effects of psychiatric cofactors and nicotine dependence on patterns of smoking withdrawal symptomatology. Nicotine Tob Res 2(3):275–280

110. Combs DR, Advokat C (2000) Antipsychotic medication and smoking prevalence in acutely hospitalized patients with chronic schizophrenia. Schizophr Res 46(2–3):129–137

111. Stassen HH, Bridler R, Hagele S, Hergersberg M, Mehmann B, Schinzel A, et al (1996) Schizophrenia and smoking: evidence for a common neurobiological basis? Am J Med Genet 173–177

112. Anokhin AP, Vedeniapin AB, Sirevaag EJ, Bauer LO, O'Connor SJ, Kuperman S, et al (2000) The P300 brain potential is reduced in smokers. Psychopharmacology (Berl) 149(4):409–413

113. Leonard S, Breese C, Adams C, Benhammou K, Gault J, Stevens K, et al (2000) Smoking and schizophrenia: abnormal nicotinic receptor expression. Eur J Pharmacol 393(1–3):237–242

114. Olincy A, Leonard S, Young DA, Sullivan B, Freedman R (1999) Decreased bombesin peptide response to cigarette smoking in schizophrenia. Neuropsychopharmacology 20(1):52–59

115. Yassa R, Lal S, Korpassy A, Ally J (1987) Nicotine exposure and tardive dyskinesia. Biol Psychiatry 22(1):67–72

116. Dolan SL, Sacco KA, Termine A, Seyal AA, Dudas MM, Vessicchio JC, Wexler BE, George TP (2004) Neuropsychological deficits are associated with smoking cessation treatment failure in patients with schizophrenia. Schizophr Res 70(2–3):263–275

117. Warburton DM, Mancuso G (1998) Evaluation of the information processing and mood effects of a transdermal nicotine patch. Psychopharmacology (Berl) 135(3):305–310

118. Sherwood N (1995) Effects of cigarette smoking on performance in a simulated driving task. Neuropsychobiology 32:161–165

119. Mancuso G, Warburton DM, Melen M, Sherwood N, Tirelli E (1999) Selective effects of nicotine on attentional processes. Psychopharmacology (Berl) 146:199–204

120. Giacobini E (1990) Cholinergic receptors in human brain: effects of aging and Alzheimer disease. J Neurosci Res 27(4):548–560

121. Whitehouse PJ, Martino AM, Antuono PG, Lowenstein PR, Coyle JT, Price DL, et al (1986) Nicotinic acetylcholine binding sites in Alzheimer's disease. Brain Res 371(1):146–151

122. Nordberg A, Hartvig P, Lilja A, Viitanen M, Amberla K, Lundqvist H, et al (1990) Decreased uptake and binding of 11C-nicotine in brain of Alzheimer patients as visualized by positron emission tomography. J Neural Transm Park Dis Dement Sect 2(3):215–224

123. Martin-Ruiz C, Court J, Lee M, Piggott M, Johnson M, Ballard C, et al (2000) Nicotinic receptors in dementia of Alzheimer, Lewy body and vascular types. Acta Neurol Scand Suppl 176:34–41

124. Lopez-Arrieta JM, Rodriguez JL, Sanz F (2001) Efficacy and safety of nicotine on Alzheimer's disease patients. Cochrane Database Syst Rev (2):CD001749

125. Ott A, Slooter AJ, Hofman A, van Harskamp F, Witteman JC, Van Broeckhoven C, et al (1998) Smoking and risk of dementia and Alzheimer's disease in a population-based cohort study: the Rotterdam Study. Lancet 351(9119):1840–1843

126. Kukull WA (2001) The association between smoking and Alzheimer's disease: effects of study design and bias. Biol Psychiatry 49(3):194–199

127. Tyas SL, Pederson LL, Koval JJ (2000) Is smoking associated with the risk of developing Alzheimer's disease? Results from three Canadian data sets. Ann Epidemiol 10(7):409–416

128. Debanne SM, Rowland DY, Riedel TM, Cleves MA (2000) Association of Alzheimer's disease and smoking: the case for sibling controls. J Am Geriatr Soc 48:800–806

129. Doll R, Peto R, Boreham J, Sutherland I (2000) Smoking and dementia in male British doctors: prospective study. BMJ 320(7242):1097–1102

130. Perry E, Martin-Ruiz C, Lee M, Griffiths M, Johnson M, Piggott M, et al (2000) Nicotinic receptor subtypes in human brain ageing, Alzheimer and Lewy body diseases. Eur J Pharmacol 393(1–3):215–222

131. Brayne C (2000) Smoking and the brain. BMJ 320(7242):1087–1088

132. Gorelick PB, Sacco RL, Smith DB, Alberts M, Mustone-Alexander L, Rader D, et al (1999) Prevention of a first stroke: a review of guidelines and a multidisciplinary consensus statement from the National Stroke Association. JAMA 281(12):1112–1120

133. Skoog I (1994) Risk factors for vascular dementia: a review. Dementia 5(3–4):137–144

134. Baron JA (1986) Cigarette smoking and Parkinson's disease. Neurology 36(11):1490–1496

135. Hernan MA, Zhang SM, Rueda-deCastro AM, Colditz GA, Speizer FE, Ascherio A (2001) Cigarette smoking and the incidence of Parkinson's disease in two prospective studies. Ann Neurol 50(6):780–786

136. Sugita M, Izuno T, Tatemichi M, Otahara Y (2001) Meta-analysis for epidemiologic studies on the relationship between smoking and Parkinson's disease. J Epidemiol 11(2):87–94

137. Elbaz A, Manubens-Bertran JM, Baldereschi M, Breteler MM, Grigoletto F, Lopez-Pousa S, et al (2000) Parkinson's disease, smoking, and family history. EUROPARKINSON Study Group. J Neurol 247(10):793–798

138. Maggio R, Riva M, Vaglini F, Fornai F, Molteni R, Armogida M, et al (1998) Nicotine prevents experimental parkinsonism in rodents and induces striatal increase of neurotrophic factors. J Neurochem 71(6):2439–2446

139. Kelton MC, Kahn HJ, Conrath CL, Newhouse PA (2000) The effects of nicotine on Parkinson's disease. Brain Cogn 43(1–3):274–282

140. Decina P, Caracci G, Sandik R, Berman W, Mukherjee S, Scapicchio P (1990) Cigarette smoking and neuroleptic-induced parkinsonism. Biol Psychiatry 28(6):502–508

141. Lie TC, Domino EF (1999) Effects of tobacco smoking on the human pupil. Int J Clin Pharmacol Ther 37:184–188

142. Solberg Y, Rosner M, Belkin M (1998) The association between cigarette smoking and ocular diseases. Surv Ophthalmol 42(6):535–547

143. Nicholl ID, Bucala R (1998) Advanced glycation endproducts and cigarette smoking. Cell Mol Biol (Noisy -le-grand) 44(7):1025–1033

144. Paetkau ME, Boyd TA, Winship B, Grace M (1977) Cigarette smoking and diabetic retinopathy. Diabetes 26(1):46–49

145. Walker JM, Cove DH, Beevers DG, Dodson PM, Leatherdale BA, Fletcher RF, et al (1985) Cigarette smoking, blood pressure and the control of blood glucose in the development of diabetic retinopathy. Diabetes Res 2(4):183–186

146. Eadington DW, Patrick AW, Collier A, Frier BM (1989) Limited joint mobility, Dupuytren's contracture and retinopathy in type 1 diabetes: association with cigarette smoking. Diabet Med 6(2):152–157

147. Klein R, Klein BE, Davis MD (1983) Is cigarette smoking associated with diabetic retinopathy? Am J Epidemiol 118(2):228–238

148. Telmer S, Christiansen JS, Andersen AR, Nerup J, Deckert T (1984) Smoking habits and prevalence of clinical diabetic microangiopathy in insulin-dependent diabetics. Acta Med Scand 215(1):63–68

149. West S, Munoz B, Schein OD, Vitale S, Maguire M, Taylor HR, et al (1995) Cigarette smoking and risk for progression of nuclear opacities. Arch Ophthalmol 113(11):1377–1380

150. Chase HP, Garg SK, Marshall G, Berg CL, Harris S, Jackson WE, et al (1991) Cigarette smoking increases the risk of albuminuria among subjects with type I diabetes. JAMA 265(5):614–617

151. Moss SE, Klein R, Klein BE (1996) Cigarette smoking and ten-year progression of diabetic retinopathy. Ophthalmology 103(9):1438–1442

152. Muhlhauser I, Bender R, Bott U, Jorgens V, Grusser M, Wagener W, et al (1996) Cigarette smoking and progression of retinopathy and nephropathy in type 1 diabetes. Diabet Med 13 (6):536–543

153. Karamanos B, Porta M, Songini M, Metelko Z, Kerenyi Z, Tamas G, et al (2000) Different risk factors of microangiopathy in patients with type I diabetes mellitus of short versus long duration. The EURODIAB IDDM Complications Study. Diabetologia 43(3):348–355

154. Rao CM, Qin C, Robison WG Jr, Zigler JS Jr (1995) Effect of smoke condensate on the physiological integrity and morphology of organ cultured rat lenses. Curr Eye Res 14(4): 295–301

155. Cekic O (1998) Effect of cigarette smoking on copper, lead, and cadmium accumulation in human lens. Br J Ophthalmol 82(2):186–188

156. Paik DC, Dillon J (2000) The Nitrite/alpha crystallin reaction: a possible mechanism in lens matrix damage. Exp Eye Res 70(1):73–80

157. West S, Munoz B, Emmett EA, Taylor HR (1989) Cigarette smoking and risk of nuclear cataracts. Arch Ophthalmol 107(8):1166–1169

158. Flaye DE, Sullivan KN, Cullinan TR, Silver JH, Whitelocke RA (1989) Cataracts and cigarette smoking. The City Eye Study. Eye 3(Pt 4):379–384

159. Hiller R, Sperduto RD, Podgor MJ, Wilson PW, Ferris FL III, Colton T, et al (1997) Cigarette smoking and the risk of development of lens opacities. The Framingham studies. Arch Ophthalmol 115(9):1113–1118

160. Klein BE, Klein R, Linton KL, Franke T (1993) Cigarette smoking and lens opacities: the Beaver Dam Eye Study. Am J Prev Med 9(1):27–30

161. Christen WG, Manson JE, Seddon JM, Glynn RJ, Buring JE, Rosner B, et al (1992) A prospective study of cigarette smoking and risk of cataract in men. JAMA 268(8):989–993

162. Cumming RG, Mitchell P (1997) Alcohol, smoking, and cataracts: the Blue Mountains Eye Study. Arch Ophthalmol 115(10):1296–1303

163. Klein BE, Klein RE, Lee KE (1999) Incident cataract after a five-year interval and lifestyle factors: the Beaver Dam eye study. Ophthalmic Epidemiol 6(4):247–255

164. Janghorbani MB, Jones RB, Allison SP (2000) Incidence of and risk factors for cataract among diabetes clinic attenders. Ophthalmic Epidemiol 7(1):13–25

165. Hankinson SE, Willett WC, Colditz GA, Seddon JM, Rosner B, Speizer FE, et al (1992) A prospective study of cigarette smoking and risk of cataract surgery in women. JAMA 268(8):994–998

166. Hofbauer LC, Muhlberg T, Konig A, Heufelder G, Schworm HD, Heufelder AE (1997) Soluble interleukin-1 receptor antagonist serum levels in smokers and nonsmokers with Graves' ophthalmopathy undergoing orbital radiotherapy. J Clin Endocrinol Metab 82(7):2244–2247

167. Mann K (1999) Risk of smoking in thyroid-associated orbitopathy. Exp Clin Endocrinol Diabetes 107(Suppl 5):S164–S167

168. Tellez M, Cooper J, Edmonds C (1992) Graves' ophthalmopathy in relation to cigarette smoking and ethnic origin. Clin Endocrinol (Oxf) 36(3):291–294

169. Chen YL, Chang TC, Chen CJ (1994) Influence of smoking on Graves' disease with or without ophthalmopathy and nontoxic nodular goiter in Taiwan. J Formos Med Assoc 93(1):40–44

170. Bartalena L, Martino E, Marcocci C, Bogazzi F, Panicucci M, Velluzzi F, et al (1989) More on smoking habits and Graves' ophthalmopathy. J Endocrinol Invest 12(10):733–737

171. Chan D (1998) Cigarette smoking and age-related macular degeneration. Optom Vis Sci 75(7):476–484

172. Smith W, Assink J, Klein R, Mitchell P, Klaver CC, Klein BE, et al (2001) Risk factors for age-related macular degeneration: pooled findings from three continents. Ophthalmology 108(4):697–704

173. The Eye Disease Case-Control Study Group (1992) Risk factors for neovascular age-related macular degeneration. Arch Ophthalmol 110(12):1701–1708

174. Klein R, Klein BE, Linton KL, DeMets DL (1993) The Beaver Dam Eye Study: the relation of age-related maculopathy to smoking. Am J Epidemiol 137(2):190–200

175. Hammond BR Jr, Wooten BR, Snodderly DM (1996) Cigarette smoking and retinal carotenoids: implications for age-related macular degeneration. Vision Res 36(18):3003–3009

176. Vingerling JR, Hofman A, Grobbee DE, de Jong PT (1996) Age-related macular degeneration and smoking. The Rotterdam Study. Arch Ophthalmol 114(10):1193–1196

177. Seddon JM, Willett WC, Speizer FE, Hankinson SE (1996) A prospective study of cigarette smoking and age-related macular degeneration in women. JAMA 276(14):1141–1146

178. Klein R, Klein BE, Moss SE (1998) Relation of smoking to the incidence of age-related maculopathy. The Beaver Dam Eye Study. Am J Epidemiol 147(2):103–110

179. Christen WG, Glynn RJ, Manson JE, Ajani UA, Buring JE (1996) A prospective study of cigarette smoking and risk of age-related macular degeneration in men. JAMA 276(14):1147–1151

180. Tamakoshi A, Yuzawa M, Matsui M, Uyama M, Fujiwara NK, Ohno Y (1997) Smoking and neovascular form of age related macular degeneration in late middle aged males: findings from a case-control study in Japan. Research Committee on Chorioretinal Degenerations. Br J Ophthalmol 81(10):901–904

181. Tsao K, Aitken PA, Johns DR (1999) Smoking as an aetiological factor in a pedigree with Leber's hereditary optic neuropathy. Br J Ophthalmol 83(5):577–581

182. Wilson MR, Hertzmark E, Walker AM, Childs-Shaw K, Epstein DL (1987) A case-control study of risk factors in open angle glaucoma. Arch Ophthalmol 105(8):1066–1071

183. Rojanapongpun P, Drance SM (1993) The effects of nicotine on the blood flow of the ophthalmic artery and the finger circulation. Graefes Arch Clin Exp Ophthalmol 231(7):371–374

184. Bonovas S, Filioussi K, Tsantes A, Peponis V (2004) Epidemiological association between cigarette smoking and primary open-angle glaucoma: a meta-analysis. Public Health 118(4): 256–61
185. Hakim RB, Tielsch JM (1992) Maternal cigarette smoking during pregnancy. A risk factor for childhood strabismus. Arch Ophthalmol 110(10):1459–1462
186. Wojno TH (1999) The association between cigarette smoking and basal cell carcinoma of the eyelids in women. Ophthal Plast Reconstr Surg 15(6):390–392
187. Egan KM, Gragoudas ES, Seddon JM, Walsh SM (1992) Smoking and the risk of early metastases from uveal melanoma. Ophthalmology 99(4):537–541
188. Austin KL, Palmer JR, Seddon JM, Glynn RJ, Rosenberg L, Gragoudas ES, et al (1990) Case-control study of idiopathic retinal detachment. Int J Epidemiol 19(4):1045–1050
189. Hesch RD (1982) [Therapeutic considerations in vascular diseases of the inner ear]. HNO 30(10):365–374
190. Friedrich G (1985) [Etiology and pathogenesis of sudden deafness]. Laryngol Rhinol Otol (Stuttg) 64(2):62–66
191. Barone JA, Peters JM, Garabrant DH, Bernstein L, Krebsbach R (1987) Smoking as a risk factor in noise-induced hearing loss. J Occup Med 29(9):741–745
192. Cruickshanks KJ, Klein R, Klein BE, Wiley TL, Nondahl DM, Tweed TS (1998) Cigarette smoking and hearing loss: the epidemiology of hearing loss study. JAMA 279(21):1715–1719
193. Cunningham DR, Vise LK, Jones LA (1983) Influence of cigarette smoking on extra-high-frequency auditory thresholds. Ear Hear 4(3):162–165
194. Ragnarsson E, Eliasson ST, Olafsson SH (1992) Tobacco smoking, a factor in tooth loss in Reykjavik, Iceland. Scand J Dent Res 100(6):322–326
195. Pindborg J (1949) Tobacco and gingivitis:II. Correlation between consumption of tobacco, ulceromembranous gingivitis and calculus. J Dent Res 28:460–463
196. Ahlqwist M, Bengtsson C, Hollender L, Lapidus L, Osterberg T (1989) Smoking habits and tooth loss in Swedish women. Community Dent Oral Epidemiol 17(3):144–147
197. Holm G (1994) Smoking as an additional risk for tooth loss. J Periodontol 65(11):996–1001
198. Osterberg T, Mellstrom D (1986) Tobacco smoking: a major risk factor for loss of teeth in three 70-year-old cohorts. Community Dent Oral Epidemiol 14(6):367–370
199. Bartecchi CE, MacKenzie TD, Schrier RW (1994) The human costs of tobacco use (1). N Engl J Med 330(13):907–912
200. Grossi SG, Genco RJ, Machtei EE, Ho AW, Koch G, Dunford R, et al (1995) Assessment of risk for periodontal disease. II. Risk indicators for alveolar bone loss. J Periodontol 66(1):23–29
201. Grossi SG, Zambon JJ, Ho AW, Koch G, Dunford RG, Machtei EE, et al (1994) Assessment of risk for periodontal disease. I. Risk indicators for attachment loss. J Periodontol 65(3):260–267
202. Locker D, Leake JL (1993) Risk indicators and risk markers for periodontal disease experience in older adults living independently in Ontario, Canada. J Dent Res 72(1):9–17
203. U.S. Public Health Service NIoDR (1987) Oral health of United States adults: National findings. NIDR, Bethesda, MD. NIH Publication No. 87-2868
204. Kenney EB, Kraal JH, Saxe SR, Jones J (1977) The effect of cigarette smoke on human oral polymorphonuclear leukocytes. J Periodontal Res 12(4):227–234
205. Bennet KR, Reade PC (1982) Salivary immunoglobulin A levels in normal subjects, tobacco smokers, and patients with minor aphthous ulceration. Oral Surg Oral Med Oral Pathol 53(5): 461–465
206. Fang MA, Frost PJ, Iida-Klein A, Hahn TJ (1991) Effects of nicotine on cellular function in UMR 106–01 osteoblast-like cells. Bone 12(4):283–286
207. Clarke NG, Shephard BC, Hirsch RS (1981) The effects of intra-arterial epinephrine and nicotine on gingival circulation. Oral Surg Oral Med Oral Pathol 52(6):577–582
208. The Research, Science and Therapy Committee of The American Academy of Periodontology (1996) Tobacco use and the periodontal patient. J Periodontol 67(1):51–56

209. Solomon HA, Priore RL, Bross ID (1968) Cigarette smoking and periodontal disease. J Am Dent Assoc 77(5):1081–1084
210. Regazi J, Scuibba J (1993) Oral pathology: clinical-pathologic correlations, 2nd edn. W.B. Saunders, Philadelphia, pp 162–163
211. Regazi J, Scuibba J (1993) Oral pathology: clinical-pathologic correlations, 2nd edn. W.B.Saunders, Philadelphia, pp 500–501
212. McGowan J, Ship J (1996) Fighting the use of smokeless tobacco. J Pract Hygiene 5:29–32
213. Williams SA, Kwan SY, Parsons S (2000) Parental smoking practices and caries experience in pre-school children. Caries Res 34(2):117–122
214. Mecklenburg RE, Greenspan D, Kleinuran DV (1992) Tobacco effects in the mouth: A National Cancer Institute and National Institute of Dental Research Guide for Health Professionals. National Cancer Institute, Washington. NIH Publ No. 92-3330
215. US Department of Health and Human Services (1982) The health consequences of smoking: cancer. A report of the Surgeon General. US Department of Health and Human Services, Public Health Service, Assistant Secretary for Health, Office an Smoking and Health. DHHS Publ No (PHS) 82-50179
216. Blot WJ, McLaughlin JK, Winn DM, Austin DF, Greenberg RS, Preston-Martin S, et al (1988) Smoking and drinking in relation to oral and pharyngeal cancer. Cancer Res 48(11):3282–3287
217. Fletcher C, Peto R, Tinker C (1976) The natural history of chronic bronchitis and emphesema. Oxford University Press, Oxford
218. Browman GP, Wong G, Hodson I, Sathya J, Russell R, McAlpine L, et al (1993) Influence of cigarette smoking on the efficacy of radiation therapy in head and neck cancer. N Engl J Med 328(3):159–163
219. Department of Health and Human Services (1989) Reducing the health consequences of smoking: 25 years of progress: a report of the Surgeon General: executive summary. Department of Health and Human Services, Rockwille. DHHS Publ No (CDC) 89-8411
220. US Department of Health and Human Services (1990) The health benefits of smoking cessation: a report of the Surgeon General. US Department of Health and Human Services, Rockwille. DHHS Publ No (CDC) 90-8416
221. Trigg DJ, Lait M, Wenig BL (2000) Influence of tobacco and alcohol on the stage of laryngeal cancer at diagnosis. Laryngoscope 110(3 Pt 1):408–411
222. Sankaranarayanan R, Duffy SW, Nair MK, Padmakumary G, Day NE (1990) Tobacco and alcohol as risk factors in cancer of the larynx in Kerala, India. Int J Cancer 45(5):879–882
223. Homann N, Tillonen J, Meurman JH, Rintamaki H, Lindqvist C, Rautio M,, et al (2000) Increased salivary acetaldehyde levels in heavy drinkers and smokers: a microbiological approach to oral cavity cancer. Carcinogenesis 21(4):663–668
224. De Stefani E, Oreggia F, Rivero S, Fierro L (1992) Hand-rolled cigarette smoking and risk of cancer of the mouth, pharynx, and larynx. Cancer 70(3):679–682
225. Muscat JE, Wynder EL (1992) Tobacco, alcohol, asbestos, and occupational risk factors for laryngeal cancer. Cancer 69(9):2244–2251
226. Richard F, Marecaux N, Dallongeville J, Devienne M, Tiem N, Fruchart JC,, et al (1997) Effect of smoking cessation on lipoprotein A-I and lipoprotein A-I: A-II levels. Metabolism 46(6):711–715
227. Steptoe A, Kerry S, Rink E, Hilton S (2001) The impact of behavioral counseling on stage of change in fat intake, physical activity, and cigarette smoking in adults at increased risk of coronary heart disease. Am J Public Health 91(2):265–269
228. Craig WY, Palomaki GE, Haddow JE (1989) Cigarette smoking and serum lipid and lipoprotein concentrations: an analysis of published data. BMJ 298(6676):784–788
229. Prieme H, Nyyssonen K, Gronbaek K, Klarlund M, Loft S, Tonnesen P, et al (1998) Randomized controlled smoking cessation study: transient increase in plasma high density lipoprotein but no change in lipoprotein oxidation resistance. Scand J Clin Lab Invest 58(1):11–18

230. Rabkin SW (1984) Effect of cigarette smoking cessation on risk factors for coronary athero-sclerosis. A control clinical trial. Atherosclerosis 53(2):173–184
231. Stubbe I, Eskilsson J, Nilsson-Ehle P (1982) High-density lipoprotein concentrations increase after stopping smoking. Br Med J (Clin Res Ed) 284(6328):1511–1513
232. Terres W, Becker P, Rosenberg A (1994) Changes in cardiovascular risk profile during the cessation of smoking. Am J Med 97(3):242–249
233. Hojnacki JL, Mulligan JJ, Cluette JE, Kew RR, Stack DJ, Huber GL (1981) Effect of cigarette smoke and dietary cholesterol on plasma lipoprotein composition. Artery 9(4):285–304
234. Tonstad S, Gorbitz C, Sivertsen M, Ose L (1999) Under-reporting of dietary intake by smok-ing and non-smoking subjects counselled for hypercholesterolaemia. J Intern Med 245(4):337–344
235. Assmann G, Schulte H, Schriewer H (1984) The effects of cigarette smoking on serum levels of HDL cholesterol and HDL apolipoprotein A-I. Findings of a prospective epidemiological study on employees of several companies in Westphalia, West Germany. J Clin Chem Clin Biochem 22(6):397–402
236. Hughes K, Choo M, Kuperan P, Ong CN, Aw TC (1998) Cardiovascular risk factors in relation to cigarette smoking: a population-based survey among Asians in Singapore. Atherosclerosis 137(2):253–258
237. Butowski P, Winder A (1998) The early cardiovascular toll of cigarette smoking in dyslipi-daemic patients in the United Kingdom. Eur J Med Res 3(4):189–193
238. Cuesta C, Sanchez-Muniz FJ, Garcia-La Cuesta A, Garrido R, Castro A, San Felix B, et al (1989) Effects of age and cigarette smoking on serum concentrations of lipids and apolipo-proteins in a male military population. Atherosclerosis 80(1):33–39
239. Glueck CJ, Heiss G, Morrison JA, Khoury P, Moore M (1981) Alcohol intake, cigarette smoking and plasma lipids and lipoproteins in 12–19-year-old children. The Collaborative Lipid Research Clinics Prevalence Study. Circulation 64(3 Pt 2):III-56
240. Jensen EX, Fusch C, Jaeger P, Peheim E, Horber FF (1995) Impact of chronic cigarette smok-ing on body composition and fuel metabolism. J Clin Endocrinol Metab 80(7):2181–2185
241. Razay G, Heaton KW (1995) Smoking habits and lipoproteins in British women. QJM 88(7):503–508
242. Shaten BJ, Kuller LH, Neaton JD (1991) Association between baseline risk factors, cigarette smoking, and CHD mortality after 10.5 years. MRFIT Research Group. Prev Med 20(5):655–659
243. Vincelj J, Sucic M, Bergovec M, Sokol I, Mirat J, Romic Z, et al (1997) Serum total, LDL, HDL cholesterol and triglycerides related to age, gender and cigarette smoking in patients with first acute myocardial infarction. Coll Antropol 21(2):517–524
244. Whitehead TP, Robinson D, Allaway SL (1996) The effects of cigarette smoking and alcohol consumption on blood lipids: a dose-related study on men. Ann Clin Biochem 33(Pt 2):99–106
245. Halfon ST, Green MS, Heiss G (1984) Smoking status and lipid levels in adults of different ethnic origins: the Jerusalem Lipid Research Clinic Program. Int J Epidemiol 13(2):177–183
246. Iscan A, Yigitoglu MR, Ece A, Ari Z, Akyildiz M (1997) The effect of cigarette smoking during pregnancy on cord blood lipid, lipoprotein and apolipoprotein levels. Jpn Heart J 38(4):497–502
247. Fuller CJ, May MA, Martin KJ (2000) The effect of vitamin E and vitamin C supplementation on LDL oxidizability and neutrophil respiratory burst in young smokers. J Am Coll Nutr 19(3):361–369
248. van Tits LJ, de Waart F, Hak-Lemmers HL, van Heijst P, de Graaf J, Demacker PN, et al (2001) Effects of alpha-tocopherol on superoxide production and plasma intercellular adhe-sion molecule-1 and antibodies to oxidized LDL in chronic smokers. Free Radic Biol Med 30:1122–1129

249. Allen SS, Hatsukami D, Gorsline J (1994) Cholesterol changes in smoking cessation using the transdermal nicotine system. Transdermal Nicotine Study Group. Prev Med 23(2):190–196

250. Haustein KO, Krause J, Haustein H (1999) Ergebnisse der Raucherentwöhnungsstudie mit Nicotin auf Parameter der Mikrozirkulation. In: Haustein KO (ed) Rauchen und Nikotin – Eine Kontroverse? 2. Dt. Nikotinkonferenz. Perfusion GmbH, Nürnberg, pp S.38–S.45

251. Ludviksdottir D, Blondal T, Franzon M, Gudmundsson TV, Sawe U (1999) Effects of nicotine nasal spray on atherogenic and thrombogenic factors during smoking cessation. J Intern Med 246:61–66

252. Lagrue G, Grimaldi B, Martin C, Demaria C, Jacotot B (1989) [Nicotine gum and lipid profile]. Pathol Biol (Paris) 37(8):937–939

253. Masarei JR, Puddey IB, Vandongen R, Beilin LJ, Lynch WJ (1991) Effect of smoking cessation-on serum apolipoprotein A-I and A-II concentrations. Pathology 23(2):98–102

254. Quensel M, Soderstrom A, Agardh CD, Nilsson-Ehle P (1989) High density lipoprotein concentrations after cessation of smoking: the importance of alterations in diet. Atherosclerosis 75(2–3):189–193

255. Colditz GA, Bonita R, Stampfer MJ, Willett WC, Rosner B, Speizer FE, et al (1988) Cigarette smoking and risk of stroke in middle-aged women. N Engl J Med 318(15):937–941

256. Fowkes FG, Housley E, Riemersma RA, Macintyre CC, Cawood EH, Prescott RJ, et al (1992) Smoking, lipids, glucose intolerance, and blood pressure as risk factors for peripheral atherosclerosis compared with ischemic heart disease in the Edinburgh Artery Study. Am J Epidemiol 135(4):331–340

257. Feskens EJ, Kromhout D (1989) Cardiovascular risk factors and the 25-year incidence of diabetes mellitus in middle-aged men. The Zutphen Study. Am J Epidemiol 130(6):1101–1108

258. Kawakami N, Takatsuka N, Shimizu H, Ishibashi H (1997) Effects of smoking on the incidence of non-insulin-dependent diabetes mellitus. Replication and extension in a Japanese cohort of male employees. Am J Epidemiol 145(2):103–109

259. Rimm EB, Manson JE, Stampfer MJ, Colditz GA, Willett WC, Rosner B, et al (1993) Cigarette-smoking and the risk of diabetes in women. Am J Public Health 83(2):211–214

260. Rimm EB, Chan J, Stampfer MJ, Colditz GA, Willett WC (1995) Prospective study of cigarette smoking, alcohol use, and the risk of diabetes in men. BMJ 310(6979):555–559

261. Uchimoto S, Tsumura K, Hayashi T, Suematsu C, Endo G, Fujii S, et al (1999) Impact of cigarette smoking on the incidence of Type 2 diabetes mellitus in middle-aged Japanese men: the Osaka Health Survey. Diabet Med 16(11):951–955

262. Perry IJ, Wannamethee SG, Walker MK, Thomson AG, Whincup PH, Shaper AG (1995) Prospective study of risk factors for development of non-insulin dependent diabetes in middle aged British men. BMJ 310(6979):560–564

263. Fushimi H, Inoue T, Yamada Y, Matsuyama Y, Kameyama M (1992) Profound vasoconstrictive effect of cigarette smoking in diabetics with autonomic neuropathy. Diabetes Res Clin Pract 16(3):191–195

264. Gay EC, Cai Y, Gale SM, Baron A, Cruickshanks KJ, Kostraba JN, et al (1992) Smokers with IDDM experience excess morbidity. The Colorado IDDM Registry. Diabetes Care 15(8):947–952

265. Celermajer DS, Sorensen KE, Georgakopoulos D, Bull C, Thomas O, Robinson J, et al (1993) Cigarette smoking is associated with dose-related and potentially reversible impairment of endothelium-dependent dilation in healthy young adults. Circulation 88(5 Pt 1):2149–2155

266. Cominacini L, Fratta PA, Garbin U, Davoli A, De Santis A, Campagnola M, et al (1995) Elevated levels of soluble E-selectin in patients with IDDM and NIDDM: relation to metabolic control. Diabetologia 38(9):1122–1124

267. Ridker PM, Hennekens CH, Roitman-Johnson B, Stampfer MJ, Allen J (1998) Plasma concentration of soluble intercellular adhesion molecule 1 and risks of future myocardial infarction in apparently healthy men. Lancet 351(9096):88–92

268. Zoppini G, Targher G, Cacciatori V, Guerriero A, Muggeo M (1999) Chronic cigarette smoking is associated with increased plasma circulating intercellular adhesion molecule 1 levels in young type 1 diabetic patients. Diabetes Care 22(11):1871–1874

269. Attvall S, Fowelin J, Lager I, Von Schenck H, Smith U (1993) Smoking induces insulin resistance – a potential link with the insulin resistance syndrome. J Intern Med 233(4):327–332

270. Frati AC, Iniestra F, Ariza CR (1996) Acute effect of cigarette smoking on glucose tolerance and other cardiovascular risk factors. Diabetes Care 19(2):112–118

271. Epifano L, Di Vincenzo A, Fanelli C, Porcellati F, Perriello G, De Feo P, et al (1992) Effect of cigarette smoking and of a transdermal nicotine delivery system on glucoregulation in type 2 diabetes mellitus. Eur J Clin Pharmacol 43(3):257–263

272. Eliasson B, Attvall S, Taskinen MR, Smith U (1994) The insulin resistance syndrome in smokers is related to smoking habits. Arterioscler Thromb 14(12):1946–1950

273. Facchini FS, Hollenbeck CB, Jeppesen J, Chen YD, Reaven GM (1992) Insulin resistance and cigarette smoking. Lancet 339(8802):1128–1130

274. Janzon L, Berntorp K, Hanson M, Lindell SE, Trell E (1983) Glucose tolerance and smoking: a population study of oral and intravenous glucose tolerance tests in middle-aged men. Diabetologia 25(2):86–88

275. Ronnemaa T, Ronnemaa EM, Puukka P, Pyorala K, Laakso M (1996) Smoking is independently associated with high plasma insulin levels in nondiabetic men. Diabetes Care 19(11): 1229–1232

276. Targher G, Alberiche M, Zenere MB, Bonadonna RC, Muggeo M, Bonora E (1997) Cigarette smoking and insulin resistance in patients with noninsulin-dependent diabetes mellitus. J Clin Endocrinol Metab 82(11):3619–3624

277. Anon (1996) The absence of a glycemic threshold for the development of long-term complications: the perspective of the Diabetes Control and Complications Trial. Diabetes 45(10): 1289–1298

278. Biesenbach G, Janko O, Zazgornik J (1994) Similar rate of progression in the predialysis phase in type I and type II diabetes mellitus. Nephrol Dial Transplant 9(8):1097–1102

279. Chase HP, Garg SK, Marshall G, Berg CL, Harris S, Jackson WE, et al (1991) Cigarette smoking increases the risk of albuminuria among subjects with type I diabetes. JAMA 265(5):614–617

280. Christiansen JS (1978) Cigarette smoking and prevalence of microangiopathy in juvenile-onset insulin-dependent diabetes mellitus. Diabetes Care 1(3):146–149

281. Couper JJ, Staples AJ, Cocciolone R, Nairn J, Badcock N, Henning P (1994) Relationship of smoking and albuminuria in children with insulin-dependent diabetes. Diabet Med 11(7): 666–669

282. Ekberg G, Grefberg N, Larsson LO, Vaara I (1990) Cigarette smoking and glomerular filtration rate in insulin-treated diabetics without manifest nephropathy. J Intern Med 228(3):211–217

283. Norden G, Nyberg G (1984) Smoking and diabetic nephropathy. Acta Med Scand 215(3): 257–261

284. Stegmayr B, Lithner F (1987) Tobacco and end stage diabetic nephropathy. Br Med J (Clin Res Ed) 295(6598):581–582

285. Biesenbach G, Zazgornik J (1996) Influence of smoking on the survival rate of diabetic patients requiring hemodialysis. Diabetes Care 19(6):625–628

286. Ishimura E, Shoji T, Emoto M, Motoyama K, Shinohara K, Matsumoto N, et al (2001) Renal insufficiency accelerates atherosclerosis in patients with type 2 diabetes mellitus. Am J Kidney Dis 38(4 Suppl 1):S186–S190

287. Ekberg G, Grefberg N, Larsson LO (1991) Cigarette smoking and urinary albumin excretion in insulin-treated diabetics without manifest nephropathy. J Intern Med 230(5):435–442

288. Ikeda Y, Suehiro T, Takamatsu K, Yamashita H, Tamura T, Hashimoto K (1997) Effect of smoking on the prevalence of albuminuria in Japanese men with non-insulin-dependent diabetes mellitus. Diabetes Res Clin Pract 36(1):57–61

289. Leonard MB, Lawton K, Watson ID, Patrick A, Walker A, MacFarlane I (1995) Cigarette smoking and free radical activity in young adults with insulin-dependent diabetes. Diabet Med 12(1):46–50

290. Biesenbach G, Grafinger P, Janko O, Zazgornik J (1997) Influence of cigarette-smoking on the progression of clinical diabetic nephropathy in type 2 diabetic patients. Clin Nephrol 48 (3):146–150

291. Sawicki PT, Didjurgeit U, Muhlhauser I, Bender R, Heinemann L, Berger M (1994) Smoking is associated with progression of diabetic nephropathy. Diabetes Care 17(2):126–131

292. Ravid M, Brosh D, Ravid-Safran D, Levy Z, Rachmani R (1998) Main risk factors for nephropathy in type 2 diabetes mellitus are plasma cholesterol levels, mean blood pressure, and hyperglycemia. Arch Intern Med 158(9):998–1004

293. Holl RW, Grabert M, Heinze E, Debatin KM (1998) Objective assessment of smoking habits by urinary cotinine measurement in adolescents and young adults with type 1 diabetes. Reliability of reported cigarette consumption and relationship to urinary albumin excretion. Diabetes Care 21(5):787–791

294. Hansen HP, Rossing K, Jacobsen P, Jensen BR, Parving HH (1996) The acute effect of smoking on systemic haemodynamics, kidney and endothelial functions in insulin-dependent diabetic patients with microalbuminuria. Scand J Clin Lab Invest 56(5):393–399

295. Hargrave DR, McMaster C, O'Hare MM, Carson DJ (1999) Tobacco smoke exposure in children and adolescents with diabetes mellitus. Diabet Med 16:31–34

296. Ford ES, Malarcher AM, Herman WH, Aubert RE (1994) Diabetes mellitus and cigarette smoking. Findings from the 1989 National Health Interview Survey. Diabetes Care 17(7): 688–692

297. Gaillard C, Borel GA, de Peyer R, Loizeau E (1984) [Peptic lesions of the upper digestive tract and drugs. Prospective study]. Schweiz Med Wochenschr 114(2):56–57

298. Hanson M, Almer LO, Ekman R, Janzon L, Trell E (1987) Motilin response to a glucose load aberrant in smokers. Scand J Gastroenterol 22(7):809–812

299. Boring CC, Squires TS, Tong T (1991) Cancer statistics, 1991. CA Cancer J Clin 41(1):19–36

300. Okumura T, Aruga H, Inohara H, Matsunaga T, Shiozaki H, Kobayashi K, et al (1993) Endoscopic examination of the upper gastrointestinal tract for the presence of second primary cancers in head and neck cancer patients. Acta Otolaryngol 501(Suppl):103–106

301. Zheng Z, Park JY, Guillemette C, Schantz SP, Lazarus P (2001) Tobacco carcinogen-detoxifying enzyme UGT1A7 and its association with orolaryngeal cancer risk. J Natl Cancer Inst 93:1411–1418

302. Mizobuchi S, Furihata M, Sonobe H, Ohtsuki Y, Ishikawa T, Murakami H, et al (2000) Association between p53 immunostaining and cigarette smoking in squamous cell carcinoma of the esophagus. Jpn J Clin Oncol 30(10):423–428

303. Newcomb PA, Carbone PP (1992) The health consequences of smoking. Cancer. Med Clin North Am 76(2):305–331

304. Brown LM, Silverman DT, Pottern LM, Schoenberg JB, Greenberg RS, Swanson GM, et al (1994) Adenocarcinoma of the esophagus and esophagogastric junction in white men in the United States: alcohol, tobacco, and socioeconomic factors. Cancer Causes Control 5(4): 333–340

305. Wu AH, Wan P, Bernstein L (2001) A multiethnic population-based study of smoking, alcohol and body size and risk of adenocarcinomas of the stomach and esophagus (United States). Cancer Causes Control 12(8):721–732

306. Castellsague X, Munoz N, De Stefani E, Victora CG, Castelletto R, Rolon PA, et al (1999) Independent and joint effects of tobacco smoking and alcohol drinking on the risk of esophageal cancer in men and women. Int J Cancer 82:657–664

307. Johnson N (2001) Tobacco use and oral cancer: a global perspective. J Dent Educ 65(4): 328–339

308. Kabat GC, Ng SK, Wynder EL (1993) Tobacco, alcohol intake, and diet in relation to adeno-carcinoma of the esophagus and gastric cardia. Cancer Causes Control 4(2):123–132
309. Kurata JH, Nogawa AN (1997) Meta-analysis of risk factors for peptic ulcer. Nonsteroidal antiinflammatory drugs, *Helicobacter pylori*, and smoking. J Clin Gastroenterol 24(1):2–17
310. Anda RF, Williamson DF, Escobedo LG, Remington PL (1990) Smoking and the risk of peptic ulcer disease among women in the United States. Arch Intern Med 150(7):1437–1441
311. Schabowski J (2001) Is there a territorial differentiation in the prevalence of peptic ulcer among rural population in Poland? Ann Agric Environ Med 8(1):57–62
312. Parasher G, Eastwood GL (2000) Smoking and peptic ulcer in the *Helicobacter pylori* era. Eur J Gastroenterol Hepatol 12(8):843–853
313. Bateson MC (1993) Cigarette smoing and *Helicobacter pylori* infection. Postgrad Med J 69 (807):41–44
314. Lynch DA, Mapstone NP, Lewis F, Pentith J, Axon AT, Dixon MF, et al (1996) Serum and gastric luminal epidermal growth factor in *Helicobacter pylori*-associated gastritis and peptic ulcer disease. Helicobacter 1(4):219–226
315. Ma L, Wang WP, Chow JY, Yuen ST, Cho CH (2000) Reduction of EGF is associated with the delay of ulcer healing by cigarette smoking. Am J Physiol Gastrointest Liver Physiol 278(1): G10–G17
316. Ma L, Chow JY, Cho CH (1999) Cigarette smoking delays ulcer healing: role of constitutive nitric oxide synthase in rat stomach. Am J Physiol 276(1 Pt 1):G238–G248
317. Martin-de-Argila C, Boixeda D, Canton R, Mir N, de Rafael L, Gisbert J, et al (1996) *Helicobacter pylori* infection in a healthy population in Spain. Eur J Gastroenterol Hepatol 8(12):1165–1168
318. Talley NJ, Evans JM, Fleming KC, Harmsen WS, Zinsmeister AR, Melton LJ III (1995) Nonsteroidal antiinflammatory drugs and dyspepsia in the elderly. Dig Dis Sci 40(6): 1345–1350
319. Chan FK, Sung JJ, Lee YT, Leung WK, Chan LY, Yung MY, et al (1997) Does smoking pre-dispose to peptic ulcer relapse after eradication of *Helicobacter pylori*? Am J Gastroenterol 92(3):442–445
320. Di Mario F, Battaglia G, Leandro G, Dotto P, Dal Bo N, Salandin S, et al (1994) Risk factors of duodenal ulcer bleeding: the role of smoking and nicotine. Ital J Gastroenterol 26(8):385–391
321. Ainsworth MA, Hogan DL, Koss MA, Isenberg JI (1993) Cigarette smoking inhibits acid-stimulated duodenal mucosal bicarbonate secretion. Ann Intern Med 119(9):882–886
322. Malesci A, Basilico M, Bersani M, Bonato C, Ballarin E, Ronchi G (1988) Serum pepsinogen I elevation in cigarette smokers. Scand J Gastroenterol 23(5):602–606
323. Eto K, Gomita Y, Furuno K, Yao K, Moriyama M, Araki Y (1991) Influences of cigarette smoke inhalation on pharmacokinetics of cimetidine in rats. Drug Metabol Drug Interact 9(2):103–114
324. Chen SP, Bei L, Wen SH (1993) [Study on omeprazole 20 mg twice weekly in prevention of duodenal ulcer relapse]. Zhonghua Nei Ke Za Zhi 32(8):538–541
325. Borsch G, Schmidt G, Wegener M, Sandmann M, Adamek R, Leverkus F, et al (1988) *Campylobacter pylori*: prospective analysis of clinical and histological factors associated with-colonization of the upper gastrointestinal tract. Eur J Clin Invest 18(2):133–138
326. Clodi PH (1988) [Nicotine and the gastrointestinal tract]. Wien Med Wochenschr 138(6–7): 132–134
327. Jedrychowski W, Boeing H, Wahrendorf J, Popiela T, Tobiasz-Adamczyk B, Kulig J (1992) Tobacco smoking and alcohol consumption as risk factors for stomach cancer in different locations and histologic types.. Przegl Epidemiol 46(4):357–367
328. Gammon MD, Schoenberg JB, Ahsan H, Risch HA, Vaughan TL, Chow WH, et al (1997) Tobacco, alcohol, and socioeconomic status and adenocarcinomas of the esophagus and gastric cardia. J Natl Cancer Inst 89(17):1277–1284

329. Ji BT, Chow WH, Yang G, McLaughlin JK, Gao RN, Zheng W, et al (1996) The influence of cigarette smoking, alcohol, and green tea consumption on the risk of carcinoma of the cardia and distal stomach in Shanghai, China. Cancer 77(12):2449–2457

330. Lagergren J, Bergstrom R, Lindgren A, Nyren O (2000) The role of tobacco, snuff and alcohol use in the aetiology of cancer of the oesophagus and gastric cardia. Int J Cancer 85(3): 340–346

331. Ye W, Ekstrom AM, Hansson LE, Bergstrom R, Nyren O (1999) Tobacco, alcohol and the risk of gastric cancer by sub-site and histologic type. Int J Cancer 83(2):223–229

332. Vaughan TL, Davis S, Kristal A, Thomas DB (1995) Obesity, alcohol, and tobacco as risk factors for cancers of the esophagus and gastric cardia: adenocarcinoma versus squamous cell carcinoma. Cancer Epidemiol Biomarkers Prev 4(2):85–92

333. Chen CC, Neugut AI, Rotterdam H (1994) Risk factors for adenocarcinomas and malignant carcinoids of the small intestine: preliminary findings. Cancer Epidemiol Biomarkers Prev 3(3):205–207

334. Zaridze D, Borisova E, Maximovitch D, Chkhikvadze V (2000) Alcohol consumption, smoking and risk of gastric cancer: case-control study from Moscow, Russia. Cancer Causes Control 11(4):363–371

335. Neugut AI, Jacobson JS, Suh S, Mukherjee R, Arber N (1998) The epidemiology of cancer of the small bowel. Cancer Epidemiol Biomarkers Prev 7(3):243–251

336. Gordis L, Gold EB (1984) Epidemiology of pancreatic cancer. World J Surg 8(6):808–821

337. Li D (2001) Molecular epidemiology of pancreatic cancer. Cancer J 7(4):259–265

338. Schwartz GG, Reis IM (2000) Is cadmium a cause of human pancreatic cancer? Cancer Epidemiol Biomarkers Prev 9(2):139–145

339. Talamini G, Bassi C, Falconi M, Sartori N, Salvia R, Rigo L, et al (1999) Alcohol and smoking as risk factors in chronic pancreatitis and pancreatic cancer. Dig Dis Sci 44(7):1303–1311

340. Band PR, Spinelli JJ, Threlfall WJ, Fang R, Le ND, Gallagher RP (1999) Identification of occupational cancer risks in British Columbia. Part I: Methodology, descriptive results, and analysis of cancer risks, by cigarette smoking categories of 15,463 incident cancer cases. J Occup Environ Med 41(4):224–232

341. Bray I, Brennan P, Boffetta P (2000) Projections of alcohol- and tobacco-related cancer mortality in Central Europe. Int J Cancer 87(1):122–128

342. Chiu BC, Lynch CF, Cerhan JR, Cantor KP (2001) Cigarette smoking and risk of bladder, pancreas, kidney, and colorectal cancers in Iowa. Ann Epidemiol 11(1):28–37

343. Fuchs CS, Colditz GA, Stampfer MJ, Giovannucci EL, Hunter DJ, Rimm EB, et al (1996) A prospective study of cigarette smoking and the risk of pancreatic cancer. Arch Intern Med 156(19):2255–2260

344. Harnack LJ, Anderson KE, Zheng W, Folsom AR, Sellers TA, Kushi LH (1997) Smoking, alcohol, coffee, and tea intake and incidence of cancer of the exocrine pancreas: the Iowa Women's Health Study. Cancer Epidemiol Biomarkers Prev 6(12):1081–1086

345. Shapiro JA, Jacobs EJ, Thun MJ (2000) Cigar smoking in men and risk of death from tobacco-related cancers. J Natl Cancer Inst 92(4):333–337

346. Bleyer AJ, Shemanski LR, Burke GL, Hansen KJ, Appel RG (2000) Tobacco, hypertension, and vascular disease: risk factors for renal functional decline in an older population. Kidney Int 57(5):2072–2079

347. Hesse E (1907) Der Einfluß des Rauchens auf den Kreislauf. Dtsch Arch Klin Med 89: 565–575

348. Black HR, Zeevi GR, Silten RM, Walker Smith GJ (1983) Effect of heavy cigarette smoking on renal and myocardial arterioles. Nephron 34(3):173–179

349. Stengel B, Watier L, Chouquet C, Cenee S, Philippon C, Hemon D (1999) Influence of renal biomarker variability on the design and interpretation of occupational or environmental studies. Toxicol Lett 106(1):69–77

350. Hansen HP, Rossing K, Jacobsen P, Jensen BR, Parving HH (1996) The acute effect of smoking on systemic haemodynamics, kidney and endothelial functions in insulin-dependent diabetic patients with microalbuminuria. Scand J Clin Lab Invest 56(5):393–399

351. Halimi JM, Philippon C, Mimran A (1998) Contrasting renal effects of nicotine in smokers and non-smokers. Nephrol Dial Transplant 13(4):940–944

352. Ritz E, Benck U, Franek E, Keller C, Seyfarth M, Clorius J (1998) Effects of smoking on renal hemodynamics in healthy volunteers and in patients with glomerular disease. J Am Soc Nephrol 9(10):1798–1804

353. Bump RC, McClish DM (1994) Cigarette smoking and pure genuine stress incontinence of urine: a comparison of risk factors and determinants between smokers and nonsmokers. Am J Obstet Gynecol 170(2):579–582

354. Cascorbi I, Roots I, Brockmoller J (2001) Association of NAT1 and NAT2 polymorphisms to urinary bladder cancer: significantly reduced risk in subjects with NAT1*10. Cancer Res 61 (13):5051–5056

355. Koskimaki J, Hakama M, Huhtala H, Tammela TL (1998) Association of smoking with lower urinary tract symptoms. J Urol 159(5):1580–1582

356. Nordlund LA, Carstensen JM, Pershagen G (1997) Cancer incidence in female smokers: a 26-year follow-up. Int J Cancer 73(5):625–628

357. Fels LM (1999) Risk assessment of nephrotoxicity of cadmium. Ren Fail 21(3–4):275–281

358. Benedetti JL, Samuel O, Dewailly E, Gingras S, Lefebvre MA (1999) Levels of cadmium in kidney and liver tissues among a Canadian population (province of Quebec). J Toxicol Environ Health A 56(3):145–163

359. Ellis KJ, Vartsky D, Zanzi I, Cohn SH, Yasumura S (1979) Cadmium: in vivo measurement in smokers and nonsmokers. Science 205(4403):323–325

360. Ala-Opas M, Tahvonen R (1995) Concentrations of cadmium and lead in renal cell cancer. J Trace Elem Med Biol 9(3):176–180

361. Friis L, Edling C (1998) [Reduced level of cadmium in the renal cortex. Due to less smoking or environmental improvement?]. Lakartidningen 95(37):3949–6

362. Friis L, Petersson L, Edling C (1998) Reduced cadmium levels in human kidney cortex in sweden. Environ Health Perspect 106(4):175–178

363. Ikeda M, Zhang ZW, Moon CS, Shimbo S, Watanabe T, Nakatsuka H, et al (2000) Possible effects of environmental cadmium exposure on kidney function in the Japanese general population. Int Arch Occup Environ Health 73(1):15–25

364. Stoner GD, Daniel FB, Schenck KM, Schut HA, Goldblatt PJ, Sandwisch DW (1982) Metabolism and DNA binding of benzoa.pyrene in cultured human bladder and bronchus. Carcinogenesis 3(2):195–201

365. Talaska G, al Juburi AZ, Kadlubar FF (1991) Smoking related carcinogen-DNA adducts in biopsy samples of human urinary bladder: identification of N-(deoxyguanosin-8-yl)-4-aminobiphenyl as a major adduct. Proc Natl Acad Sci U S A 88(12):5350–5354

366. Talaska G, Schamer M, Skipper P, Tannenbaum S, Caporaso N, Unruh L, et al (1991) Detection of carcinogen-DNA adducts in exfoliated urothelial cells of cigarette smokers: association with smoking, hemoglobin adducts, and urinary mutagenicity. Cancer Epidemiol Biomarkers Prev 1(1):61–66

367. Lodovici M, Dolara P, Caderni G, Carini M, Costantini A, Selli C, et al (1983) The effect of cigarette smoke on aryl-hydrocarbon hydroxylase (AHH) activity of the human kidney. Eur J Cancer Clin Oncol 19(11):1565–1568

368. Atawodi SE, Richter E (1996) Bacterial reduction of N-oxides of tobacco-specific nitrosamines (TSNA). Hum Exp Toxicol 15(4):329–334

369. Mothersill C, O'Malley K, Colucci S, Murphy D, Lynch T, Payne S, et al (1997) p53 protein expression and increased SSCP mobility shifts in the p53 gene in normal urothelium cultured from smokers. Carcinogenesis 18(6):1241–1245

370. Walker C (1998) Molecular genetics of renal carcinogenesis. Toxicol Pathol 26(1):113–120

371. Wilkens LR, Kadir MM, Kolonel LN, Nomura AM, Hankin JH (1996) Risk factors for lower urinary tract cancer: the role of total fluid consumption, nitrites and nitrosamines, and selected foods. Cancer Epidemiol Biomarkers Prev 5(3):161–166

372. Xu X, Stower MJ, Reid IN, Garner RC, Burns PA (1997) A hot spot for p53 mutation in transitional cell carcinoma of the bladder: clues to the etiology of bladder cancer. Cancer Epidemiol Biomarkers Prev 6(8):611–616

373. Bringuier PP, McCredie M, Sauter G, Bilous M, Stewart J, Mihatsch MJ, et al (1998) Carcinomas of the renal pelvis associated with smoking and phenacetin abuse: p53 mutations and polymorphism of carcinogen-metabolising enzymes. Int J Cancer 79(5):531–536

374. Bartsch H, Nair U, Risch A, Rojas M, Wikman H, Alexandrov K (2000) Genetic polymorphism of CYP genes, alone or in combination, as a risk modifier of tobacco-related cancers. Cancer Epidemiol Biomarkers Prev 9(1):3–28

375. Vineis P, Bartsch H, Caporaso N, Harrington AM, Kadlubar FF, Landi MT, et al (1994) Genetically based N-acetyltransferase metabolic polymorphism and low-level environmental exposure to carcinogens. Nature 369(6476):154–156

376. Badawi AF, Hirvonen A, Bell DA, Lang NP, Kadlubar FF (1995) Role of aromatic amine acetyltransferases, NAT1 and NAT2, in carcinogen-DNA adduct formation in the human urinary bladder. Cancer Res 55(22):5230–5237

377. Seree EM, Villard PH, Re JL, De Meo M, Lacarelle B, Attolini L, et al (1996) High inducibility of mouse renal CYP2E1 gene by tobacco smoke and its possible effect on DNA single strand breaks. Biochem Biophys Res Commun 219(2):429–434

378. Melikian AA, Wang X, Waggoner S, Hoffmann D, El Bayoumy K (1999) Comparative response of normal and of human papillomavirus-16 immortalized human epithelial cervical cells to benzoa.pyrene. Oncol Rep 6:1371–1376

379. Lehucher-Michel MP, Di Giorgio C, Amara YA, Laget M, Botta A (1995) The micronucleus assay in human exfoliated urothelial cells: effect of smoking. Mutagenesis 10(4):329–332

380. Helmert U, Bronder E, Klimpel A, Molzahn M, Pommer W (2000) Risk factors for urothelial carcinoma: drinking measures, smoking and other life style-related risk factors – results of the Berlin Urothelial Study (BUS). Rsikofaktoren fur das Urothelkarzinom: Trinkmenge, Rauchen und andere lebensstilbezogene Risikofaktoren – Ergebnisse der Berliner Urothelstudie (BUS). Gesundheitswesen 62(5):270–274

381. Lwaleed BA, Bass PS, Francis JL (1999) Urinary tissue factor: a potential marker of disease. J Pathol 188(1):3–8

382. Hultberg B, Isaksson A, Brattstrom L, Israelsson B (1992) Elevated urinary excretion of beta-hexosaminidase in smokers. Eur J Clin Chem Clin Biochem 30(3):131–133

383. Bray I, Brennan P, Boffetta P (2000) Projections of alcohol- and tobacco-related cancer mortality in Central Europe. Int J Cancer 87(1):122–128

384. Tavani A, Pregnolato A, Violante A, La Vecchia C, Negri E (1997) Attributable risks for kidney cancer in northern Italy. Eur J Cancer Prev 6(2):195–199

385. McCredie M, Stewart JH (1992) Risk factors for kidney cancer in New South Wales, Australia. II. Urologic disease, hypertension, obesity, and hormonal factors. Cancer Causes Control 3(4):323–331

386. Chiu BC, Lynch CF, Cerhan JR, Cantor KP (2001) Cigarette smoking and risk of bladder, pancreas, kidney, and colorectal cancers in Iowa. Ann Epidemiol 11(1):28–37

387. Moiche Bokobo P, Atxa de la Presa MA, Cuesta AJ (2001) [Transitional cell carcinoma in a young heavy marihuana smoker]. Carcinoma de celulas transicionales en un joven fumador severo de marihuana. Arch Esp Urol 54(2):165–167

388. Zhang ZF, Shu XM, Cordon-Cardo C, Orlow I, Lu ML, Millon TV, et al (1997) Cigarette smoking and chromosome 9 alterations in bladder cancer. Cancer Epidemiol Biomarkers Prev 6(5):321–326

389. D'Avanzo B, La Vecchia C, Negri E, Decarli A, Benichou J (1995) Attributable risks for bladder cancer in northern Italy. Ann Epidemiol 5(6):427–431

390. Chyou PH, Nomura AM, Stemmermann GN (1993) A prospective study of diet, smoking, and lower urinary tract cancer. Ann Epidemiol 3(3):211–216

391. Nomura A, Kolonel LN, Yoshizawa CN (1989) Smoking, alcohol, occupation, and hair dye use in cancer of the lower urinary tract. Am J Epidemiol 130(6):1159–1163

392. Sturgeon SR, Hartge P, Silverman DT, Kantor AF, Linehan WM, Lynch C, et al (1994) Associations between bladder cancer risk factors and tumor stage and grade at diagnosis. Epidemiology 5(2):218–225

393. Brinton LA, Fraumeni JF Jr (1986) Epidemiology of uterine cervical cancer. J Chronic Dis 39 (12):1051–1065

394. US Department of Health and Human Services. (1989) Reducing the health consequences of smoking: 25 years of progress: a report of the Surgeon General. Public Health Service, Certers of Disease Control, Center for Chronic Disease Prevention and Health Promotion, Office on Smoking and Health, Washington. DHHS Publ No (CDC) 89-8411

395. Vineis P, Frea B, Uberti E, Ghisetti V, Terracini B (1983) Bladder cancer and cigarette smoking in males: a case-control study. Tumori 69(1):17–22

396. Vineis P, Segnan N, Costa G, Terracini B (1981) Evidence of a multiplicative effect between cigarette smoking and occupational exposures in the aetiology of bladder cancer. Cancer Lett 14(3):285–290

397. Morrison AS, Buring JE, Verhoek WG, Aoki K, Leck I, Ohno Y, et al (1984) An international study of smoking and bladder cancer. J Urol 131(4):650–654

398. Thompson IM, Peek M, Rodriguez FR (1987) The impact of cigarette smoking on stage, grade and number of recurrences of transitional cell carcinoma of the bladder. J Urol 137(3): 401–403

399. Fleshner N, Garland J, Moadel A, Herr H, Ostroff J, Trambert R, et al (1999) Influence of smoking status on the disease-related outcomes of patients with tobacco-associated superficial transitional cell carcinoma of the bladder. Cancer 86(11):2337–2345

400. Pitard A, Brennan P, Clavel J, Greiser E, Lopez-Abente G, Chang-Claude J, et al (2001) Cigar, pipe, and cigarette smoking and bladder cancer risk in European men. Cancer Causes Control 12(6):551–556

401. Fortuny J, Kogevinas M, Chang-Claude J, Gonzalez CA, Hours M, Jockel KH, et al (1999) Tobacco, occupation and non-transitional-cell carcinoma of the bladder: an international case-control study. Int J Cancer 80:44–46

402. Coker AL, Rosenberg AJ, McCann MF, Hulka BS (1992) Active and passive cigarette smoke exposure and cervical intraepithelial neoplasia. Cancer Epidemiol Biomarkers Prev 1(5): 349–356

403. Daly SF, Doyle M, English J, Turner M, Clinch J, Prendiville W (1998) Can the number of cigarettes smoked predict high-grade cervical intraepithelial neoplasia among women-with mildly abnormal cervical smears? Am J Obstet Gynecol 179(2):399–402

404. Gram IT, Austin H, Stalsberg H (1992) Cigarette smoking and the incidence of cervical intraepithelial neoplasia, grade III, and cancer of the cervix uteri. Am J Epidemiol 135(4):341–346

405. Kanetsky PA, Gammon MD, Mandelblatt J, Zhang ZF, Ramsey E, Wright TC Jr, et al (1998) Cigarette smoking and cervical dysplasia among non-Hispanic black women. Cancer Detect Prev 22(2):109–119

406. Licciardone JC, Wilkins JR III, Brownson RC, Chang JC (1989) Cigarette smoking and alcohol consumption in the aetiology of uterine cervical cancer. Int J Epidemiol 18(3):533–537

407. Roteli-Martins CM, Panetta K, Alves VA, Siqueira SA, Syrjanen KJ, Derchain SF (1998) Cigarette smoking and high-risk HPV DNA as predisposing factors for high-grade cervical intraepithelial neoplasia (CIN) in young Brazilian women. Acta Obstet Gynecol Scand 77(6):678–682

408. Warwick AP, Redman CW, Jones PW, Fryer AA, Gilford J, Alldersea J, et al (1994) Progression of cervical intraepithelial neoplasia to cervical cancer: interactions of cytochrome P450 CYP2D6 EM and glutathione S-transferase GSTM1 null genotypes and cigarette smoking. Br J Cancer 70(4):704–708

409. Warwick A, Sarhanis P, Redman C, Pemble S, Taylor JB, Ketterer B, et al (1994) Theta class glutathione S-transferase GSTT1 genotypes and susceptibility to cervical neoplasia: interactions with GSTM1, CYP2D6 and smoking. Carcinogenesis 15(12):2841–2845

410. Lyon JL, Gardner JW, West DW, Stanish WM, Hebertson RM (1983) Smoking and carcinoma in situ of the uterine cervix. Am J Public Health 73(5):558–562

411. Trevathan E, Layde P, Webster LA, Adams JB, Benigno BB, Ory H (1983) Cigarette smoking and dysplasia and carcinoma in situ of the uterine cervix. JAMA 250(4):499–502

412. Slattery ML, Robison LM, Schuman KL, French TK, Abbott TM, Overall JC Jr, et al (1989) Cigarette smoking and exposure to passive smoke are risk factors for cervical cancer. JAMA 261(11):1593–1598

413. Sasson IM, Haley NJ, Hoffmann D, Wynder EL, Hellberg D, Nilsson S (1985) Cigarette smoking and neoplasia of the uterine cervix: smoke constituents in cervical mucus. N Engl J Med 312(5):315–316

414. Brinton LA, Schairer C, Haenszel W, Stolley P, Lehman HF, Levine R, et al (1986) Cigarette smoking and invasive cervical cancer. JAMA 255(23):3265–3269

415. McCann MF, Irwin DE, Walton LA, Hulka BS, Morton JL, Axelrad CM (1992) Nicotine and cotinine in the cervical mucus of smokers, passive smokers, and nonsmokers. Cancer Epidemiol Biomarkers Prev 1(2):125–129

416. Prokopczyk B, Cox JE, Hoffmann D, Waggoner SE (1997) Identification of tobacco-specific carcinogen in the cervical mucus of smokers and nonsmokers. J Natl Cancer Inst 89(12): 868–873

417. Szarewski A, Jarvis MJ, Sasieni P, Anderson M, Edwards R, Steele SJ, et al (1996) Effect of smoking cessation on cervical lesion size. Lancet 347(9006):941–943

418. Haidinger G, Temml C, Schatzl G, Brossner C, Roehlich M, Schmidbauer CP, et al (2000) Risk factors for lower urinary tract symptoms in elderly men. For the Prostate Study Group of the Austrian Society of Urology. Eur Urol 37(4):413–420

419. Platz EA, Rimm EB, Kawachi I, Colditz GA, Stampfer MJ, Willett WC, et al (1999) Alcohol consumption, cigarette smoking, and risk of benign prostatic hyperplasia. Am J Epidemiol 149(2):106–115

420. Hsing AW, McLaughlin JK, Schuman LM, Bjelke E, Gridley G, Wacholder S, et al (1990) Diet, tobacco use, and fatal prostate cancer: results from the Lutheran Brotherhood Cohort Study. Cancer Res 50(21):6836–6840

421. Hsing AW, McLaughlin JK, Hrubec Z, Blot WJ, Fraumeni JF Jr (1991) Tobacco use and prostate cancer: 26-year follow-up of US veterans. Am J Epidemiol 133(5):437–441

422. Mantel N (1992) Re: tobacco use and prostate cancer: 26-year follow-up of US veterans. Am J Epidemiol 135(3):327–328

423. Coughlin SS, Neaton JD, Sengupta A (1996) Cigarette smoking as a predictor of death from prostate cancer in 348,874 men screened for the Multiple Risk Factor Intervention Trial. Am J Epidemiol 143(10):1002–1006

424. Sharpe CR, Siemiatycki J (2001) Joint effects of smoking and body mass index on prostate cancer risk. Epidemiology 12(5):546–551

425. Stattin P, Soderberg S, Hallmans G, Bylund A, Kaaks R, Stenman UH, et al (2001) Leptin is associated with increased prostate cancer risk: a nested case-referent study. J Clin Endocrinol Metab 86(3):1341–1345

426. Lotufo PA, Lee IM, Ajani UA, Hennekens CH, Manson JE (2000) Cigarette smoking and risk of prostate cancer in the physicians' health study (United States). Int J Cancer 87:141–144

427. Vine MF (1996) Smoking and male reproduction: a review. Int J Androl 19(6):323–337

428. Vine MF, Tse CK, Hu P, Truong KY (1996) Cigarette smoking and semen quality. Fertil Steril 65(4):835–842

429. Dunphy BC, Barratt CL, von Tongelen BP, Cooke ID (1991) Male cigarette smoking and fecundity in couples attending an infertility clinic. Andrologia 23(3):223–225

430. Rubes J, Lowe X, Moore D, Perreault S, Slott V, Evenson D, et al (1998) Smoking cigarettes is associated with increased sperm disomy in teenage men. Fertil Steril 70(4):715–723

431. Joesoef MR, Beral V, Aral SO, Rolfs RT, Cramer DW (1993) Fertility and use of cigarettes, alcohol, marijuana, and cocaine. Ann Epidemiol 3(6):592–594

432. Sterzik K, Strehler E, De Santo M, Trumpp N, Abt M, Rosenbusch B, et al (1996) Influence of smoking on fertility in women attending an in vitro fertilization program. Fertil Steril 65 (4):810–814

433. Wong WY, Thomas CM, Merkus HM, Zielhuis GA, Doesburg WH, Steegers-Theunissen RP (2000) Cigarette smoking and the risk of male factor subfertility: minor association between cotinine in seminal plasma and semen morphology. Fertil Steril 74(5):930–935

434. Van Voorhis BJ, Dawson JD, Stovall DW, Sparks AE, Syrop CH (1996) The effects of smoking on ovarian function and fertility during assisted reproduction cycles. Obstet Gynecol 88 (5):785–791

435. Shiverick KT, Salafia C (1999) Cigarette smoking and pregnancy I: ovarian, uterine and placental effects. Placenta 20(4):265–272

436. Olsen J (1991) Cigarette smoking, tea and coffee drinking, and subfecundity. Am J Epidemiol 133(7):734–739

437. Florack EI, Zielhuis GA, Rolland R (1994) Cigarette smoking, alcohol consumption, and caffeine intake and fecundability. Prev Med 23(2):175–180

438. Gudmundsson JA, Ljunghall S, Bergquist C, Wide L, Nillius SJ (1987) Increased bone turnover during gonadotropin-releasing hormone superagonist-induced ovulation inhibition. J Clin Endocrinol Metab 65(1):159–163

439. Landin-Wilhelmsen K, Wilhelmsen L, Lappas G, Rosen T, Lindstedt G, Lundberg PA, et al (1995) Serum intact parathyroid hormone in a random population sample of men and women: relationship to anthropometry, life-style factors, blood pressure, and vitamin D. Calcif Tissue Int 56(2):104–108

440. Mellstrom D, Johansson C, Johnell O, Lindstedt G, Lundberg PA, Obrant K, et al (1993) Osteoporosis, metabolic aberrations, and increased risk for vertebral fractures after partial gastrectomy. Calcif Tissue Int 53(6):370–377

441. Ortego-Centeno N, Munoz-Torres M, Hernandez-Quero J, Jurado-Duce A, de la Higuera Torres-Puchol (1994) Bone mineral density, sex steroids, and mineral metabolism in premenopausal smokers. Calcif Tissue Int 55(6):403–407

442. Ortego-Centeno N, Munoz-Torres M, Jodar E, Hernandez-Quero J, Jurado-Duce A, de la Higuera Torres-Puchol (1997) Effect of tobacco consumption on bone mineral density in healthy young males. Calcif Tissue Int 60(6):496–500

443. Scragg R, Khaw KT, Murphy S (1995) Life-style factors associated with winter serum 25-hydroxyvitamin D levels in elderly adults. Age Ageing 24(4):271–275

444. Fisher CL, Mannino DM, Herman WH, Frumkin H (1997) Cigarette smoking and thyroid hormone levels in males. Int J Epidemiol 26(5):972–977

445. Kirschbaum C, Scherer G, Strasburger CJ (1994) Pituitary and adrenal hormone responses to pharmacological, physical, and psychological stimulation in habitual smokers and nonsmokers. Clin Investig 72(10):804–810

446. Salvini S, Stampfer MJ, Barbieri RL, Hennekens CH (1992) Effects of age, smoking and vitamins on plasma DHEAS levels: a cross-sectional study in men. J Clin Endocrinol Metab 74(1):139–143

447. Syversen U, Nordsletten L, Falch JA, Madsen JE, Nilsen OG, Waldum HL (1999) Effect of lifelong nicotine inhalation on bone mass and mechanical properties in female rat femurs. Calcif Tissue Int 65(3):246–249

448. Iwaniec UT, Fung YK, Akhter MP, Haven MC, Nespor S, Haynatzki GR, et al (2001) Effects of nicotine on bone mass, turnover, and strength in adult female rats. Calcif Tissue Int 68(6): 358–364

449. Chiba M, Masironi R (1992) Toxic and trace elements in tobacco and tobacco smoke. Bull World Health Organ 70(2):269–275

450. Orrenius S, McConkey DJ, Bellomo G, Nicotera P (1989) Role of Ca^{2+} in toxic cell killing. Trends Pharmacol Sci 10(7):281–285

451. Smith CJ, Livingston SD, Doolittle DJ (1997) An international literature survey of "IARC Group I carcinogens" reported in mainstream cigarette smoke. Food Chem Toxicol 35 (10–11):1107–1130

452. Hermann AP, Brot C, Gram J, Kolthoff N, Mosekilde L (2000) Premenopausal smoking and bone density in 2015 perimenopausal women. J Bone Miner Res 15(4):780–787

453. Brot C, Jorgensen NR, Sorensen OH (1999) The influence of smoking on vitamin D status and calcium metabolism. Eur J Clin Nutr 53(12):920–926

454. Spangler JG (1999) Smoking and hormone-related disorders. Prim Care 26(3):499–511

455. Kiel DP, Zhang Y, Hannan MT, Anderson JJ, Baron JA, Felson DT (1996) The effect of smoking at different life stages on bone mineral density in elderly men and women. Osteoporos Int 6(3):240–248

456. van Hoof HJ, van der Mooren MJ, Swinkels LM, Rolland R, Benraad TJ (1994) Hormone replacement therapy increases serum 1,25-dihydroxyvitamin D: a 2-year prospective study. Calcif Tissue Int 55(6):417–419

457. Michnovicz JJ, Hershcopf RJ, Naganuma H, Bradlow HL, Fishman J (1986) Increased 2-hydroxylation of estradiol as a possible mechanism for the anti-estrogenic effect of cigarette smoking. N Engl J Med 315(21):1305–1309

458. Geisler J, Omsjo IH, Helle SI, Ekse D, Silsand T, Lonning PE (1999) Plasma oestrogen fractions in postmenopausal women receiving hormone replacement therapy: influence of route of administration and cigarette smoking. J Endocrinol 162:265–270

459. Ewers U, Brockhaus A, Dolgner R, Freier I, Turfeld M, Engelke R, et al (1990) [Blood lead and blood cadmium concentrations in 55–66-year-old women fron different areas of Nordrhein-Westfalen – chronological trends during 1982–1988]. Zentralbl Hyg Umweltmed 189(5): 405–418

460. Kido T, Nogawa K, Yamada Y, Honda R, Tsuritani I, Ishizaki M, et al (1989) Osteopenia in inhabitants with renal dysfunction induced by exposure to environmental cadmium. Int Arch Occup Environ Health 61(4):271–276

461. Krall EA, Dawson-Hughes B (1991) Smoking and bone loss among postmenopausal women. J Bone Miner Res 6(4):331–338

462. Krall EA, Dawson-Hughes B (1999) Smoking increases bone loss and decreases intestinal calcium absorption. J Bone Miner Res 14(2):215–220

463. Fang MA, Frost PJ, Iida-Klein A, Hahn TJ (1991) Effects of nicotine on cellular function in UMR 106–01 osteoblast-like cells. Bone 12(4):283–286

464. Khaw KT, Sneyd MJ, Compston J (1992) Bone density parathyroid hormone and 25-hydroxyvitamin D concentrations in middle aged women. BMJ 305(6848):273–277

465. Martinez ME, del Campo MT, Sanchez-Cabezudo MJ, Garcia JA, Sanchez Calvin MT, Torrijos A, et al (1994) Relations between calcidiol serum levels and bone mineral density in postmenopausal women with low bone density. Calcif Tissue Int 55(4):253–256

466. Cooper C, Wickham C (1990) Cigarette smoking and the risk of age-related fractures. Oxford University Press, Oxford, pp 93–100

467. Law M (1990) Smoking and osteoporosis. Oxford University Press, Oxford, pp 83–92

468. Jensen GF (1986) Osteoporosis of the slender smoker revisited by epidemiologic approach. Eur J Clin Invest 16(3):239–242

469. Johnell O, Nilsson BE (1984) Life-style and bone mineral mass in perimenopausal women. Calcif Tissue Int 36(4):354–356

470. Sowers MR, Wallace RB, Lemke JH (1985) Correlates of mid-radius bone density among postmenopausal women: a community study. Am J Clin Nutr 41(5):1045–1053

471. Slemenda CW, Hui SL, Longcope C, Johnston CC Jr (1989) Cigarette smoking, obesity, and bone mass. J Bone Miner Res 4(5):737–741

472. Hollenbach KA, Barrett-Connor E, Edelstein SL, Holbrook T (1993) Cigarette smoking and bone mineral density in older men and women. Am J Public Health 83(9):1265–1270

473. Chapurlat RD, Ewing SK, Bauer DC, Cummings SR (2001) Influence of smoking on the antiosteoporotic efficacy of raloxifene. J Clin Endocrinol Metab 86(9):4178–4182

474. Komulainen M, Kroger H, Tuppurainen MT, Heikkinen AM, Honkanen R, Saarikoski S (2000) Identification of early postmenopausal women with no bone response to HRT: results of a five-year clinical trial. Osteoporos Int 11(3):211–218

475. Straub RH, Hense HW, Andus T, Scholmerich J, Riegger GA, Schunkert H (2000) Hormone replacement therapy and interrelation between serum interleukin-6 and body mass index in postmenopausal women: a population-based study. J Clin Endocrinol Metab 85(3):1340–1344

476. Egger P, Duggleby S, Hobbs R, Fall C, Cooper C (1996) Cigarette smoking and bone mineral density in the elderly. J Epidemiol Community Health 50(1):47–50

477. Slemenda CW (1994) Cigarettes and the skeleton. N Engl J Med 330(6):430–431

478. Cornuz J, Feskanich D, Willett WC, Colditz GA (1999) Smoking, smoking cessation, and risk of hip fracture in women. Am J Med 106(3):311–314

479. Jones G, Scott FS (1999) A cross-sectional study of smoking and bone mineral density in premenopausal parous women: effect of body mass index, breastfeeding, and sports participation. J Bone Miner Res 14(9):1628–1633

480. Bjarnason NH, Christiansen C (2000) The influence of thinness and smoking on bone loss and response to hormone replacement therapy in early postmenopausal women. J Clin Endocrinol Metab 85(2):590–596

481. Riggs BL, Melton LJ III (1992) The prevention and treatment of osteoporosis. N Engl J Med 327(9):620–627

482. Aloia JF, Cohn SH, Vaswani A, Yeh JK, Yuen K, Ellis K (1985) Risk factors for postmenopausal osteoporosis. Am J Med 78(1):95–100

483. Cummings SR, Nevitt MC, Browner WS, Stone K, Fox KM, Ensrud KE, et al (1995) Risk factors for hip fracture in white women. Study of Osteoporotic Fractures Research Group. N Engl J Med 332(12):767–773

484. Forsen L, Bjorndal A, Bjartveit K, Edna TH, Holmen J, Jessen V, et al (1994) Interaction between current smoking, leanness, and physical inactivity in the prediction of hip fracture. J Bone Miner Res 9(11):1671–1678

485. Kreiger N, Hilditch S (1986) Re: cigarette smoking and estrogen-dependent diseases. Am J Epidemiol 123(1):200

486. Paganini-Hill A, Chao A, Ross RK, Henderson BE (1991) Exercise and other factors in the prevention of hip fracture: the Leisure World study. Epidemiology 2(1):16–25

487. Seeman E, Melton LJ III, O'Fallon WM, Riggs BL (1983) Risk factors for spinal osteoporosis in men. Am J Med 75(6):977–983

488. Wickham CA, Walsh K, Cooper C, Barker DJ, Margetts BM, Morris J, et al (1989) Dietary calcium, physical activity, and risk of hip fracture: a prospective study. BMJ 299(6704):889–892

489. Felson DT, Kiel DP, Anderson JJ, Kannel WB (1988) Alcohol consumption and hip fractures: the Framingham Study. Am J Epidemiol 128(5):1102–1110

490. Holbrook TL, Barrett-Connor E, Wingard DL (1988) Dietary calcium and risk of hip fracture: 14-year prospective population study. Lancet 2(8619):1046–1049

491. Rockville M (1987) Smoking and health, a National Status Report: a report to Congress. Department of Health and Human Services, Rockville. DHHS publication No (CDC) 87-8396

492. Hoidrup S, Prescott E, Sorensen TI, Gottschau A, Lauritzen JB, Schroll M, et al (2000) Tobacco smoking and risk of hip fracture in men and women. Int J Epidemiol 29(2):253–259

493. Hoidrup S, Prescott EI, Sorensen TI, Gottschau A, Lauritzen JB, Schroll M, et al (2001) Tobacco smoking and risk of hip fracture in men and women. Results from the Hovedstadens Center for Prospective Population Studies. Tobaksrygning og risiko for hoftebrud hos maend og kvinder. Resultater fra Hovedstadens Center for Prospektive Befolkningsstudier. Ugeskr Laeger 163(40):5532–5536

494. Baron JA, Farahmand BY, Weiderpass E, Michaelsson K, Alberts A, Persson I, et al (2001) Cigarette smoking, alcohol consumption, and risk of hip fracture in women. Arch Intern Med 161(7):983–988

495. Michaelsson K, Weiderpass E, Farahmand BY, Baron JA, Persson PG, Ziden L, et al (1999) Differences in risk factor patterns between cervical and trochanteric hip fractures. Swedish Hip Fracture Study Group. Osteoporos Int 10:487–494

496. Willett W, Stampfer MJ, Bain C, Lipnick R, Speizer FE, Rosner B, et al (1983) Cigarette smoking, relative weight, and menopause. Am J Epidemiol 117(6):651–658

497. Fielding JE (1987) Smoking and women: tragedy of the majority. N Engl J Med 317(21): 1343–1345

498. Grando SA, Horton RM, Pereira EF, Diethelm-Okita BM, George PM, Albuquerque EX, et al (1995) A nicotinic acetylcholine receptor regulating cell adhesion and motility is expressed in human keratinocytes. J Invest Dermatol 105:774–781

499. Grando SA, Horton RM, Mauro TM, Kist DA, Lee TX, Dahl MV (1996) Activation of keratinocyte nicotinic cholinergic receptors stimulates calcium influx and enhances cell differentiation. J Invest Dermatol 107:412–418

500. Nguyen VT, Hall LL, Gallacher G, Ndoye A, Jolkovsky DL, Webber RJ, et al (2000) Choline acetyltransferase, acetylcholinesterase, and nicotinic acetylcholine receptors of human gingival and esophageal epithelia. J Dent Res 79(4):939–949

501. Macklin KD, Maus AD, Pereira EF, Albuquerque EX, Conti-Fine BM (1998) Human vascular endothelial cells express functional nicotinic acetylcholine receptors. J Pharmacol Exp Ther 287:435–439

502. Buchli R, Ndoye A, Rodriguez JG, Zia S, Webber RJ, Grando SA (1999) Human skin fibroblasts express m2, m4, and m5 subtypes of muscarinic acetylcholine receptors. J Cell Biochem 74:264–277

503. Kawashima K, Fujii T (2000) Extraneuronal cholinergic system in lymphocytes. Pharmacol Ther 86(1):29–48

504. Nguyen VT, Ndoye A, Hall LL, Zia S, Arredondo J, Chernyavsky AI, et al (2001) Programmed cell death of keratinocytes culminates in apoptotic secretion of a humectant upon secretagogue action of acetylcholine. J Cell Sci 114(Pt.6):1189–1204

505. Heeschen C, Jang JJ, Weis M, Pathak A, Kaji S, Hu RS, et al (2001) Nicotine stimulates angiogenesis and promotes tumor growth and atherosclerosis. Nat Med 7(7):833–839

506. Hagforsen E, Edvinsson M, Nordlind K, Michaelsson G (2002) Expression of nicotinic receptors in the skin of patients with palmoplantar pustulosis. Br J Dermatol 146(3):383–391

507. Eriksson MO, Hagforsen E, Lundin IP, Michaelsson G (1998) Palmoplantar pustulosis: a clinical and immunohistological study. Br J Dermatol 138(3):390–398

508. Scabbia A, Cho KS, Sigurdsson TJ, Kim CK, Trombelli L (2001) Cigarette smoking negatively affects healing response following flap debridement surgery. J Periodontol 72(1): 43–49

509. Goldminz D, Bennett RG (1991) Cigarette smoking and flap and full-thickness graft necrosis. Arch Dermatol 127(7):1012–1015

510. Partsch B, Jochmann W, Partsch H (1994) [Tobacco and the skin]. Wien Med Wochenschr 144(22–23):565–568

511. Wolf R, Lo Schiavo A, Ruocco V (1995) Smoking out the skin. J Appl Cosmetol 13:1–14

512. Solly S (1856) Clinical lectures on paralysis. Lancet (2):641–643

513. Martin J (1857) Effects of tobacco in Europeans in India. Lancet 1:226

514. Ippen M, Ippen H (1965) Approaches to a prophylaxis of skin aging. J Soc Cosmet Chem 16:305–308
515. Ernster VL, Grady D, Miike R, Black D, Selby J, Kerlikowske K (1995) Facial wrinkling in men and women, by smoking status. Am J Public Health 85(1):78–82
516. Model B (1985) Smokers' face: an underrated clinical sign? Br Med J 291:1760–1762
517. Wolf R, Tur E, Wolf D (1992) The effect of smoking on skin moisture and on surface lipids. Int J Cosmet 14:83–88
518. Allen HB, Johnson BL, Diamond SM (1973) Smoker's wrinkles? JAMA 225(9):1067–1069
519. Hind CR, Joyce H, Tennent GA, Pepys MB, Pride NB (1991) Plasma leucocyte elastase concentrations in smokers. J Clin Pathol 44(3):232–235
520. Weitz JI, Crowley KA, Landman SL, Lipman BI, Yu J (1987) Increased neutrophil elastase activity in cigarette smokers. Ann Intern Med 107(5):680–682
521. Pryor WA, Dooley MM, Church DF (1986) The inactivation of alpha-1-proteinase inhibitor by gas-phase cigarette smoke: protection by antioxidants and reducing species. Chem Biol Interact 57(3):271–283
522. Laurent P, Janoff A, Kagan HM (1983) Cigarette smoke blocks cross-linking of elastin in vitro. Am Rev Respir Dis 127(2):189–192
523. Janoff A (1985) Elastase in tissue injury. Annu Rev Med 36:207–216
524. Kramps JA, van Twisk C, Klasen EC, Dijkman JH (1988) Interactions among stimulated human polymorphonuclear leucocytes, released elastase and bronchial antileucoprotease. Clin Sci (Colch) 75(1):53–62
525. Peng YM, Peng YS, Lin Y, Moon T, Roe DJ, Ritenbaugh C (1995) Concentrations and plasma-tissue-diet relationships of carotenoids, retinoids, and tocopherols in humans. Nutr Cancer 23(3):233–246
526. Yin L, Morita A, Tsuji T (2000) Alterations of extracellular matrix induced by tobacco smoke extract. Arch Dermatol Res 292(4):188–194
527. Carnevali S, Nakamura Y, Mio T, Liu X, Takigawa K, Romberger DJ, et al (1998) Cigarette smoke extract inhibits fibroblast-mediated collagen gel contraction. Am J Physiol 274:L591–L598
528. Knuutinen A, Kokkonen N, Risteli J, Vahakangas K, Kallioinen M, Salo T, et al (2002) Smoking affects collagen synthesis and extracellular matrix turnover in human skin. Br J Dermatol 146(4):588–594
529. Mills CM, Peters TJ, Finlay AY (1993) Does smoking influence acne? Clin Exp Dermatol 18:100–101
530. Schafer T, Nienhaus A, Vieluf D, Berger J, Ring J (2001) Epidemiology of acne in the general population: the risk of smoking. Br J Dermatol 145(1):100–104
531. Mills CM, Srivastava ED, Harvey IM, Swift GL, Newcombe RG, Holt PJ, et al (1994) Cigarette smoking is not a risk factor in atopic dermatitis. Int J Dermatol 33:33–34
532. Lindegard B (1986) Diseases associated with psoriasis in a general population of 159,200 middle-aged, urban, native Swedes. Dermatologica 172(6):298–304
533. Olsen JH, Moller H, Frentz G (1992) Malignant tumors in patients with psoriasis. J Am Acad Dermatol 27(5 Pt 1):716–722
534. Stern RS, Lange R (1988) Cardiovascular disease, cancer, and cause of death in patients with psoriasis: 10 years prospective experience in a cohort of 1,380 patients. J Invest Dermatol 91(3):197–201
535. Kavli G, Forde OH, Arnesen E, Stenvold SE (1985) Psoriasis: familial predisposition and environmental factors. Br Med J (Clin Res Ed) 291(6501):999–1000
536. Mills CM, Srivastava ED, Harvey IM, Swift GL, Newcombe RG, Holt PJ, et al (1992) Smoking habits in psoriasis: a case control study. Br J Dermatol 127(1):18–21
537. Naldi L, Parazzini F, Brevi A, Peserico A, Veller FC, Grosso G, et al (1992) Family history, smoking habits, alcohol consumption and risk of psoriasis. Br J Dermatol 127(3):212–217

538. O'Doherty CJ, MacIntyre C (1985) Palmoplantar pustulosis and smoking. Br Med J (Clin Res Ed) 291(6499):861–864

539. Poikolainen K, Reunala T, Karvonen J (1994) Smoking, alcohol and life events related to psoriasis among women. Br J Dermatol 130(4):473–477

540. Poikolainen K (1990) Alcohol intake: a risk factor for psoriasis in young and middle-aged men? Br Med J 300:780–783

541. Naldi L, Peli L, Parazzini F (1999) Association of early-stage psoriasis with smoking and male alcohol consumption: evidence from an Italian case-control study. Arch Dermatol 135:1479–1484

542. Naldi L (1998) Cigarette smoking and psoriasis. Clin Dermatol 16(5):571–574

543. Gourlay SG, Forbes A, Marriner T, McNeil JJ (1999) Predictors and timing of adverse experiences during trandsdermal nicotine therapy. Drug Saf 20:545–555

544. Aubry F, MacGibbon B (1985) Risk factors of squamous cell carcinoma of the skin. A case-control study in the Montreal region. Cancer 55(4):907–911

545. Grodstein F, Speizer FE, Hunter DJ (1995) A prospective study of incident squamous cell carcinoma of the skin in the nurses' health study. J Natl Cancer Inst 87(14):1061–1066

546. Karagas MR, Stukel TA, Greenberg ER, Baron JA, Mott LA, Stern RS (1992) Risk of subsequent basal cell carcinoma and squamous cell carcinoma of the skin among patients with prior skin cancer. Skin Cancer Prevention Study Group. JAMA 267(24):3305–3310

547. Hunter DJ, Colditz GA, Stampfer MJ, Rosner B, Willett WC, Speizer FE (1990) Risk factors for basal cell carcinoma in a prospective cohort of women. Ann Epidemiol 1(1):13–23

548. Kune GA, Bannerman S, Field B, Watson LF, Cleland H, Merenstein D, et al (1992) Diet, alcohol, smoking, serum beta-carotene, and vitamin A in male nonmelanocytic skin cancer patients and controls. Nutr Cancer 18(3):237–244

549. Osterlind A, Tucker MA, Stone BJ, Jensen OM (1988) The Danish case-control study of cutaneous malignant melanoma. IV. No association with nutritional factors, alcohol, smoking or hair dyes. Int J Cancer 42(6):825–828

550. Osterlind A (1990) Malignant melanoma in Denmark. Occurrence and risk factors. Acta Oncol 29(7):833–854

551. Tuyp E, Burgoyne A, Aitchison T, MacKie R (1987) A case-control study of possible causative factors in mycosis fungoides. Arch Dermatol 123(2):196–200

552. Daling JR, Sherman KJ, Hislop TG, Maden C, Mandelson MT, Beckmann AM, et al (1992) Cigarette smoking and the risk of anogenital cancer. Am J Epidemiol 135(2):180–189

553. Hellberg D, Valentin J, Eklund T, Nilsson S (1987) Penile cancer: is there an epidemiological role for smoking and sexual behaviour? Br Med J (Clin Res Ed) 295(6609):1306–1308

554. Maden C, Sherman KJ, Beckmann AM, Hislop TG, Teh CZ, Ashley RL, et al (1993) History of circumcision, medical conditions, and sexual activity and risk of penile cancer. J Natl Cancer Inst 85(1):19–24

555. Daniel H (1985) Cause of anal cancer. J Amer Med Assoc 254:358–363

556. Mabuchi K, Bross DS, Kessler II (1985) Epidemiology of cancer of the vulva. A case-control study. Cancer 55(8):1843–1848

557. Newcomb PA, Weiss NS, Daling JR (1984) Incidence of vulvar carcinoma in relation to menstrual, reproductive, and medical factors. J Natl Cancer Inst 73(2):391–396

558. Smith JB, Fenske NA (1996) Cutaneous manifestations and consequences of smoking. J Am Acad Dermatol 34(5 Pt 1):717–732

559. Ashley FL, McConnell DV, Machida R, Sterling HE, Galloway D, Grazer F (1965) Carcinoma of the lip. A comparison of five year results after irradiation and surgical therapy. Am J Surg 110(4):549–551

560. Ratzkowski E, Hochman A, Buchner A, Michman J (1966) Cancer of the lip; review of 167 cases. Oncology 20(2):129–144

561. Spitzer WO, Hill GB, Chambers LW, Helliwell BE, Murphy HB (1975) The occupation of fishing as a risk factor in cancer of the lip. N Engl J Med 293(9):419–424
562. Koh HK, Sober AJ, Day CL Jr, Lew RA, Fitzpatrick TB (1984) Cigarette smoking and malignant melanoma. Prognostic implications. Cancer 53(11):2570–2573
563. Rohan TE, Miller AB (1999) A cohort study of cigarette smoking and risk of fibroadenoma. J Epidemiol Biostat 4:297–302
564. Braga C, Negri E, La Vecchia C, Filiberti R, Franceschi S (1996) Cigarette smoking and the risk of breast cancer. Eur J Cancer Prev 5:159–164
565. Chu SY, Stroup NE, Wingo PA, Lee NC, Peterson HB, Gwinn ML (1990) Cigarette smoking and the risk of breast cancer. Am J Epidemiol 131:244–253
566. Miller MD, Marty MA, Broadwin R, Johnson KC, Salmon AG, Winder B, Steinmaus C (2007) The association between exposure to environmental tobacco smoke and breast cancer: a review by the California Environmental Protection Agency. Prev Med 44(2):93–106
567. Austin H, Cole P (1986) Cigarette smoking and leukemia. J Chronic Dis 39(6):417–421
568. Brownson RC, Chang JC, Davis JR (1991) Cigarette smoking and risk of adult leukemia. Am J Epidemiol 134(9):938–941
569. Brownson RC, Novotny TE, Perry MC (1993) Cigarette smoking and adult leukemia. A meta-analysis. Arch Intern Med 153(4):469–475
570. Garfinkel L, Boffetta P (1990) Association between smoking and leukemia in two American Cancer Society prospective studies. Cancer 65(10):2356–2360
571. Kinlen LJ, Rogot E (1988) Leukaemia and smoking habits among United States veterans. BMJ 297(6649):657–659
572. Mills PK, Newell GR, Beeson WL, Fraser GE, Phillips RL (1990) History of cigarette smoking and risk of leukemia and myeloma: results from the Adventist health study. J Natl Cancer Inst 82(23):1832–1836
573. Severson RK, Davis S, Heuser L, Daling JR, Thomas DB (1990) Cigarette smoking and acute nonlymphocytic leukemia. Am J Epidemiol 132(3):418–422
574. Rollinson S, Roddam P, Willett E, Roman E, Cartwright R, Jack A, et al (2001) NAT2 acetylator genotypes confer no effect on the risk of developing adult acute leukemia: a case-control study. Cancer Epidemiol Biomarkers Prev 10(5):567–568
575. Roddam PL, Rollinson S, Kane E, Roman E, Moorman A, Cartwright R, et al (2000) Poor metabolizers at the cytochrome P450 2D6 and 2C19 loci are at increased risk of developing adult acute leukaemia. Pharmacogenetics 10(7):605–615
576. Cartwright RA, Darwin C, McKinney PA, Roberts B, Richards ID, Bird CC (1988) Acute myeloid leukemia in adults: a case-control study in Yorkshire. Leukemia 2(10):687–690
577. Schuz J, Kaatsch P, Kaletsch U, Meinert R, Michaelis J (1999) Association of childhood cancer with factors related to pregnancy and birth. Int J Epidemiol 28:631–639
578. Stagnaro E, Ramazzotti V, Crosignani P, Fontana A, Masala G, Miligi L, et al (2001) Smoking and hematolymphopoietic malignancies. Cancer Causes Control 12(4):325–334
579. Doll R, Peto R (1976) Mortality in relation to smoking: 20 years' observations on male British doctors. Br Med J 2(6051):1525–1536
580. Flodin U, Fredriksson M, Persson B, Axelson O (1988) Chronic lymphatic leukaemia and engine exhausts, fresh wood, and DDT: a case-referent study. Br J Ind Med 45(1):33–38
581. Kabat GC, Augustine A, Hebert JR (1988) Smoking and adult leukemia: a case-control study. J Clin Epidemiol 41(9):907–914
582. Spitz MR, Fueger JJ, Newell GR, Keating MJ (1990) Leukemia and cigarette smoking. Cancer Causes Control 1(2):195–196
583. Hirayama T (1990) Smoking and mortality. S.Karger, Basel, Switzerland, pp 28–59
584. Linet MS, McLaughlin JK, Hsing AW, Wacholder S, Co-Chien HT, Schuman LM, et al (1991) Cigarette smoking and leukemia: results from the Lutheran Brotherhood Cohort Study. Cancer Causes Control 2(6):413–417

585. Engeland A, Andersen A, Haldorsen T, Tretli S (1996) Smoking habits and risk of cancers other than lung cancer: 28 years' follow-up of 26,000 Norwegian men and women. Cancer Causes Control 7(5):497–506

586. Shu XO, Ross JA, Pendergrass TW, Reaman GH, Lampkin B, Robison LL (1996) Parental alcohol consumption, cigarette smoking, and risk of infant leukemia: a Childrens Cancer Group study. J Natl Cancer Inst 88(1):24–31

587. Deng J (1985) [The prevalence of the cigarette smoking habit among 110,000 adult residents-in the Shanghai urban area]. Zhonghua Yu Fang Yi Xue Za Zhi 19(5):271–274

588. Gong YL, Koplan JP, Feng W, Chen CH, Zheng P, Harris JR (1995) Cigarette smoking in China. Prevalence, characteristics, and attitudes in Minhang district. JAMA 274(15):1232–1234

589. Ji BT, Shu XO, Linet MS, Zheng W, Wacholder S, Gao YT, et al (1997) Paternal cigarette smoking and the risk of childhood cancer among offspring of nonsmoking mothers. J Natl Cancer Inst 89(3):238–244

590. Golding J, Paterson M, Kinlen LJ (1990) Factors associated with childhood cancer in a national cohort study. Br J Cancer 62(2):304–308

591. Li FP, Jamison DS, Meadows AT (1986) Questionnaire study of cancer etiology in 503 children. J Natl Cancer Inst 76(1):31–36

592. Anon (1986) Maternal smoking during pregnancy and the risk of childhood cancer. Lancet 2(8505):519–520

593. Pershagen G, Ericson A, Otterblad-Olausson P (1992) Maternal smoking in pregnancy: does it increase the risk of childhood cancer? Int J Epidemiol 21(1):1–5

594. Stjernfeldt M, Berglund K, Lindsten J, Ludvigsson J (1992) Maternal smoking and irradiation during pregnancy as risk factors for child leukemia. Cancer Detect Prev 16(2):129–135

595. Grufferman S, Delzell ES, Maile MC, Michalopoulos G (1983) Parents' cigarette smoking and childhood cancer. Med Hypotheses 12(1):17–20

596. John EM, Savitz DA, Sandler DP (1991) Prenatal exposure to parents' smoking and childhood cancer. Am J Epidemiol 133(2):123–132

597. Sorahan T, Lancashire R, Prior P, Peck I, Stewart A (1995) Childhood cancer and parental use of alcohol and tobacco. Ann Epidemiol 5(5):354–359

598. Sorahan T, Lancashire RJ, Hulten MA, Peck I, Stewart AM (1997) Childhood cancer and parental use of tobacco: deaths from 1953 to 1955. Br J Cancer 75(1):134–138

599. Stjernfeldt M, Berglund K, Lindsten J, Ludvigsson J (1986) Maternal smoking during pregnancy and risk of childhood cancer. Lancet 1(8494):1350–1352

600. Birch JM, Hartley AL, Teare MD, Blair V, McKinney PA, Mann JR, et al (1990) The interregional epidemiological study of childhood cancer (IRESCC): case-control study of children with central nervous system tumours. Br J Neurosurg 4(1):17–25

601. Buckley JD, Sather H, Ruccione K, Rogers PC, Haas JE, Henderson BE, et al (1989) A case-control study of risk factors for hepatoblastoma. A report from the Childrens Cancer Study Group. Cancer 64(5):1169–1176

602. Bunin GR, Meadows AT, Emanuel BS, Buckley JD, Woods WG, Hammond GD (1989) Pre- and postconception factors associated with sporadic heritable and nonheritable retinoblastoma. Cancer Res 49(20):5730–5735

603. Gold EB, Leviton A, Lopez R, Gilles FH, Hedley-Whyte ET, Kolonel LN, et al (1993) Parental-smoking and risk of childhood brain tumors. Am J Epidemiol 137(6):620–628

604. Howe GR, Burch JD, Chiarelli AM, Risch HA, Choi BC (1989) An exploratory case-control study of brain tumors in children. Cancer Res 49(15):4349–4352

605. Magnani C, Pastore G, Luzzatto L, Terracini B (1990) Parental occupation and other environmental factors in the etiology of leukemias and non-Hodgkin's lymphomas in childhood: a case-control study. Tumori 76(5):413–419

606. Severson RK, Buckley JD, Woods WG, Benjamin D, Robison LL (1993) Cigarette smoking and alcohol consumption by parents of children with acute myeloid leukemia: an analysis

within morphological subgroups – a report from the Childrens Cancer Group. Cancer Epidemiol Biomarkers Prev 2(5):433–439

607. Shu XO, Gao YT, Brinton LA, Linet MS, Tu JT, Zheng W, et al (1988) A population-based case-control study of childhood leukemia in Shanghai. Cancer 62(3):635–644

608. Tredaniel J, Boffetta P, Little J, Saracci R, Hirsch A (1994) Exposure to passive smoking during pregnancy and childhood, and cancer risk: the epidemiological evidence. Paediatr Perinat Epidemiol 8(3):233–255

609. Steensel-Moll HA, Valkenburg HA, Vandenbroucke JP, van Zanen GE (1985) Are maternal fertility problems related to childhood leukaemia? Int J Epidemiol 14(4):555–559

610. Michaelis J, Kaletsch U, Kaatsch P (2000) [Epidemiology of childhood brain tumors]. Epidemiologie von Hirntumoren im Kindesalter. Zentralbl Neurochir 61(2):80–87

611. Kane EV, Roman E, Cartwright R, Parker J, Morgan G (1999) Tobacco and the risk of acute leukaemia in adults. Br J Cancer 81:1228–1233

612. Fraga CG, Motchnik PA, Wyrobek AJ, Rempel DM, Ames BN (1996) Smoking and low antioxidant levels increase oxidative damage to sperm DNA. Mutat Res 351(2):199–203

613. Little J, Vainio H (1994) Mutagenic lifestyles? A review of evidence of associations between germ-cell mutations in humans and smoking, alcohol consumption and use of 'recreational' drugs. Mutat Res 313(2–3):131–151

614. Bottoms SF, Kuhnert BR, Kuhnert PM, Reese AL (1982) Maternal passive smoking and fetal serum thiocyanate levels. Am J Obstet Gynecol 144(7):787–791

615. Hauth JC, Hauth J, Drawbaugh RB, Gilstrap LC III, Pierson WP (1984) Passive smoking and thiocyanate concentrations in pregnant women and newborns. Obstet Gynecol 63(4):519–522

616. Van Vunakis H, Langone JJ, Milunsky A (1974) Nicotine and cotinine in the amniotic fluid of-smokers in the second trimester of pregnancy. Am J Obstet Gynecol 120(1):64–66

617. Brondum J, Shu XO, Steinbuch M, Severson RK, Potter JD, Robison LL (1999) Parental cigarette smoking and the risk of acute leukemia in children. Cancer 85(6):1380–1388

618. Korte JE, Hertz-Picciotto I, Schulz MR, Ball LM, Duell EJ (2000) The contribution of benzene to smoking-induced leukemia. Environ Health Perspect 108(4):333–339

619. Ong CN, Lee BL, Shi CY, Ong HY, Lee HP (1994) Elevated levels of benzene-related compounds in the urine of cigarette smokers. Int J Cancer 59(2):177–180

Smoking and Pregnancy

It is generally recognised that smoking during pregnancy is harmful to the foetus. When the risks associated with cigarette smoking are compared with other risks arising in the perinatal period, the harmful effects of smoking are clearly found to outweigh all other factors. The combustion products of tobacco are considered to be more harmful than nicotine, although uncertainty persists concerning the relative proportion of embryotoxic and faetotoxic effects that are attributable to nicotine or to the combustion products of tobacco. This problem is important because in 1994 more than 10% of women in Germany continued to smoke during pregnancy (Table 8.1)! The lowest prevalence rates for smoking among women were recorded in Saxony, Thuringia, Bavaria and Baden-Württemberg. More up-to-date statistics for Germany are not yet available but it is estimated that some 20% of all women continue to smoke during pregnancy [2]. Similarly high percentages are reported from the USA [3].

Salihu et al. perfomed a study in 2003 to (1) determine the risk of infant mortality associated with prenatal cigarette smoking, (2) assess whether the relationship, if existent, was dose-dependent, (3) explore the morbidity pathway that explains the effect of tobacco smoke on infant mortality and (4) compute excess infant deaths attributable to maternal smoking in the United States [4]. They performed a retrospective cohort study on 3,004,616 singleton live births that occurred in 1997 in the United States using the US national-linked birth/infant-death data. Excess infant deaths due to maternal smoking were computed using the population-attributable risk (PAR). The authors found that overall 13.2% of pregnant women who delivered live births in 1997 smoked during pregnancy. The rate of infant mortality was 40% higher in this group as compared to non-smoking gravidas ($p < 0.0001$). This risk increased with the amount of cigarettes consumed prenatally in a dose-dependent fashion (p for trend <0.0001). Small-for-gestational age rather than preterm birth is the main mechanism through which smoking causes excess infant mortality. We estimated that about 5% of infant deaths in the United States were attributable to maternal smoking while pregnant, with variations by race/ethnicity. The proportion of infant deaths attributable to maternal smoking was highest among American Indians at 13%, almost three times the national average. If pregnant smokers were to halt tobacco use, a total of 986 infant deaths would be averted annually. It can be concluded that smoking during pregnancy accounts for a sizeable number of infant deaths in the United States. This highlights the need for infusion of more resources into existing smoking cessation campaigns in order to achieve higher quit rates, and substantially diminish current levels of smoking-associated infant deaths [4].

K.-O. Haustein, D. Groneberg, *Tobacco or Health?* 221
DOI: 10.1007/978-3-540-87577-2_8, © Springer Verlag Berlin Heidelberg 2010

Table 8.1 Pregnancies in 1994 and associated risks based on perinatal surveys conducted as part of maternity care programmes [1]

German land	Smoke-free pregnancies		Pregnant women with evidence of risks		Smokers (>5 cigarettes/day)
	Absolute	Percent	Absolute	Percent	Percent
Schleswig-Holstein	–	–	8,234	33.6	15.7
Hamburg	5,827	32.7	5,632	31.4	15.9
Bremen	2,405	29.1	2,840	34.3	15.8
Lower Saxony	22,136	30.6	25,453	35.2	12.0
North Rhine/Westphalia	54,824	30.1	63,271	34.7	14.3
Hessen	20,136	35.0	17,454	30.3	8.4
Rheinland-Pfalz	12,464	33.2	11,174	29.8	12.8
Baden-Württemberg	–	–	29,020	27.3	7.7
Bavaria	40,943	37.4	29,297	26.8	7.0
Berlin	9,240	33.8	9,786	35.8	12.7
Saarland	2,739	29.0	3,336	35.3	16.6
Mecklenburg-Vorpommern	–	–	3,033	36.0	7.8
Brandenburg	3,458	30.1	4,923	42.9	9.1
Sachsen-Anhalt	4,260	30.4	5,855	41.8	8.6
Thuringia	3,610	29.9	3,834	31.8	6.2
Saxony	6,246	27.2	8,739	38.8	4.6
Germany (total)	188,288	26.1	231,881	32.1	10.8

A second study described the prevalence of spontaneous cessation of cigarette and alcohol use, alone and in combination and associated factors among low-income pregnant women [5]. Six hundred and one women were currently smoking or smoking when they became pregnant and participating in Special Supplemental Nutrition Program for Women, Infants, and Children (WIC) in the greater Boston, Massachusetts, area. Among the study group, spontaneous cessation of smoking and alcohol use was reported by 28 and 80% of the women, respectively; 25% spontaneously quit both, and 15% stopped neither. Multivariable analyses indicated that smoking cessation was less likely in women who had previous births, had a husband or partner who smoked, were born in the United States, were black (non-Hispanic, non-Portuguese), had less than a high-school education, were highly addicted, reported lower perceived risk to the foetus, and reported "too many other problems in life to stop". Hispanic ethnicity, younger age and more social support to quit smoking were related to spontaneous alcohol abstinence. It was concluded that targeted multiple strategies, including those aimed at increasing participation of partners, are needed for low-income pregnant smokers [5].

8.1
Effects of Smoking on the Placenta

Numerous effects of placenta-passing substances such carbon monoxide (CO) on the embryo and foetus are known. The blood of neonates born to active smoking mothers also contains significantly higher concentrations of polychlorinated biphenyls [6] (PCB) and hexachlorobenzene (HCB) than that of neonates born to passive-smoking mothers or to mothers who have had no contact whatsoever with tobacco smoke [7]. Diaplacentar transmission of toxic substances therefore plays a major role and the rate of adverse pregnancy outcomes in women who smoke may be as high as 33% [8–11]. Syncytial necrosis and thickening of the trophoblast membrane have been detected during the first weeks of pregnancy in the placenta of women who smoke [12]. During this period, stem cells for the formation of the syncytium or of cell groups fuse together and these become implanted in the uterus. According to experimental animal research, smoking interferes with these processes. Levels of the marker hormones, oestriol, oestradiol, human chorionic gonadotrophin (hCG) and placental lactogen, are reduced in smokers [13–15]. Similarly, the activity of placental aromatase is diminished by smoking [16]. Comparative investigations of placental tissue from smoking and non-smoking women (smoking status quantified objectively by the measurements of tissue cotinine levels) have revealed raised haematocrits and cadmium levels in the placental blood of smokers [17]. Furthermore, the relative surface areas of foetal capillaries as well as the relative and absolute volumes of foetal capillaries are reduced, primarily as a result of a decrease in mean capillary diameter rather than total capillary length [17]. Although haematocrits are increased, foetuses of smoking mothers suffer hypoxic stress; overall, it must be assumed that this is an all-or-none effect rather than one which is dose-dependent (i.e. on the number of cigarettes smoked) [17]. In the first trimester, the placental volume of smokers is already smaller than that of non-smokersbecause of resistance of high-perfusion. This state also persists in the second trimester, with the result that 3-dimensional ultrasound can be used to draw conclusions concerning smoking-related impairment of trophoblast invasion [18]. Women who smoke during pregnancy have a 2.6- to 4.4-fold higher risk of placenta praevia than non-smokers [19].

Several isoenzyms of the cytochrom oxygenase system occur not only in the liver, but also in several tissues such as the placenta. The activity of the monooxygenase system (CYP1A1) increases up to 100-fold and more if the pregnant mother is a smoker. This enzyme is induced by polyaromatic compounds, but not by phenobarbitone [20–25]. It could be demonstrated that the activity of the monooxygenase system is induced only by a smoking mother but not by a smoking father [26]. The extent of induction was dependent on the number of cigarettes smoked daily. Because of the lack of enzyme induction in the liver, the placenta seems to play a major role in protecting the foetus from the toxic-products of tobacco smoke (which are degraded before they reach the foetus) [27].

Cadmium levels are elevated in smokers [28, 29], hCG secretion is reduced and trophoblast proliferation is inhibited through interactions with calmodulin [30]. Nicotine, Cd^{2+} and polyaromatic hydrocarbons possibly also influence oestrogen synthesis and metabolism, as well as granulosa-luteal function [31]. Isolated stem villous arteries from the placentas of women who smoked heavily (≥ 15 cigarettes/day) responded in vitro to endothelin-1 by developing lower tension compared with vessels from non-smokers; however, the maximum vasoconstrictive response to endothelin-1 was more pronounced [32]. It is concluded from these experiments that the mechanical properties of stem villous arteries from heavy smokers are altered and these changes may ultimately compromise foetal placental blood flow and thereby contribute to lower birth weight [32].

Smoking is associated with increased Cd^{2+} levels, raised haematocrit and alterations in the fine-tissue structure of the placenta (smaller intervillous spaces, reduced foetal capillary volume), leading to hypoxic states characterised by diminished O_2 transfer [17]. Placental receptors for epidermal growth factor (EGF), a potent mitogen for trophoblasts, are reduced [31, 33–35]. Other investigators have attributed a pivotal harmful role to CO and lead, alongside numerous other harmful constituents of tobacco smoke [36]. Measurements of cadmium, zinc and copper levels in the placental tissue of women from Finland, Estonia and St. Petersburg [36] reveal that placental concentrations of Cd^{2+}, Cu^{2+} and Pb^{2+} are already markedly elevated in the first trimester [6], and a negative correlation was found between placental Cu^{2+} levels and neonatal birth weight [36]. The highest Cd^{2+} concentrations were detected in samples collected from women living in St. Petersburg [36].

The loss of EGF receptors because of benzo[*a*]pyrene is linked not only with reduced trophoblast proliferation and hCG secretion [37], but also with reduced c-myc expression (proto-oncogene) and increased transforming growth factor (TGF) β2 expression [38]. Tobacco smoke is therefore able to exert a deleterious effect on trophoblast gene expression via EGF receptors, c-myc (down-regulation) and TGFβ1 (up-regulation). Trophoblast growth is also affected because of smoking-induced hypoxia (see below) [31, 39].

Inhaled tobacco products such as cadmium and benzo[*a*]pyrene are toxic substances that act specifically on uterine villi, contributing to foetal hypoxemia and leading to miscarriage.

8.2
Complications of Pregnancy

It has been established for a number of years that women who smoke during pregnancy give birth to a high proportion of neonates with low birth weight (LBW) or growth retardation, sometimes with shortened pregnancies (preterm deliveries), and/or are more likely than non-smoking pregnant women to miscarry due to premature placental abruption (Table 8.2) [41]. Correlations have now been established in one study between reductions in birth weight of up to 500 g and CYP1A1 and GSTT1 enzyme activity (see Sect. 5.2.3.2 in Chap. 5) [42]. Genetic alterations in the two enzyme systems are linked with birth weight reductions, as shown by the data summarised in Table 8.3 [42], with the result that an association between the genetic changes, resultant metabolic capacity and cigarette smoking may be assumed. Despite the presence of adverse genotypes, reduced birth weights were not detected in neonates of non-smokers.

Table 8.2 Sequelae of tobacco consumption in the USA [40]

Sequelae	Risk (odds ratio)	Percent of all cases	Incidence/year
Tobacco-induced abortions	1.32	3–8	19,000–141,000
Infants with low birth weight (LBW)	1.99	11–21	32,000–61,000
Infant deaths due to adverse perinatal effects	1.23	3–8	1,900–4,800
Sudden infant death syndrome (SIDS)	2.98	22–41	1,200–2,200

Table 8.3 Influence of genetic variants of CYP1A1 and GSTT1 on the birth weight of infants born to 174 smoking and 567 non-smoking pregnant women [42]

Enzyme system	Genetic variant	n	Birth weight reduction (g)	OR (95% CI)
CYP1A1	(None)		-377 ± 89	2.1 (1.2–3.7)
CYP1A1	AA	75 (AA)	-252 ± 111	1.3 (0.6–2.6)
CYP1A1	AA/aa	43 (Aa), 6 (aa)	-520 ± 124	3.2 (1.6–6.4)
GSTT1	Present		-285 ± 99	1.7 (0.9–3.2
GSTT1	Absent		-642 ± 154	3.5 (1.5–8.3)
CYP1A1 – GSTT1	AA/aa + absent		$-1,285 \pm 234$	$p < 0.001$

Remarkably, the rate of pre-eclampsia has been reported to be lower in heavy smokers than in non-smokers (11.3 vs. 13.0%; OR = 0.85; CI: 0.73–0.99). However, smokers with pre-eclampsia had higher rates of infants with very low birth weight (OR = 1.85; CI: 1.55–2.20) and higher rates of placental abruption (OR = 3.49; CI: 1.65–7.28) [43].

More discriminating information on malformations is provided by a study from the USA in which 3,284 live births of women who smoked were compared with 4,500 live births of non-smokers. When all malformations were considered as a group, no increased risk was associated with maternal smoking. However, when specific malformations were considered separately, significant associations with maternal smoking were found for microcephalus, cleft defects and clubfoot, but not for Down syndrome (Table 8.5) [48]. Atrial septal defects are reported not to be attributable to smoking during pregnancy [52].

One survey of 12,914 pregnancies and 10,523 live births has shown that the risks of spontaneous abortion and congenital abnormality in smoking mothers are 1.7- and 2.3-fold higher, respectively, than in non-smokers [62]. Similar findings were reported in another study published in the same year showing that smokers (>20 cigarettes/day) had a 1.6-fold increased risk of giving birth to an infant with congenital malformations [63]. The infants' birth weight is reduced [64–67], and preterm deliveries are more common [68], because of the possibility of disturbances of placental maturation resulting from intrauterine O_2 deficiency. As demonstrated in a group of 770,744 babies born in Germany in 1999, 154,149 of them were born of smoking mothers [2]. A dose-dependent and age-dependent reduction of the mean birth weight was calculated (Fig. 8.1). It has also been suggested in this context that the infants affected have a lower IQ [69, 70], as substantiated by a prospective study in 19,117 children. Low IQ values were detected when no other neurological abnormalities were present. In a UK study conducted in children aged 9.4 years whose mothers had smoked during pregnancy, no adverse effects on IQ or cognitive development were detected compared with controls [71].

A study conducted in 227,791 live births in Westphalia clearly showed an association between LBW and cigarette consumption during pregnancy (>10 cigarettes/day) [72] (see Table 8.4). Similarly, smoking African American women from low-income groups were reported to be more likely to have LBW (<2,500 g) and preterm (<37 weeks' gestation) births. When lightsmokers were compared with non-smokers, the odds ratios were 1.89 (CI: 1.15–3.13) for LBW births and 1.74 (CI: 1.00–3.02) for preterm births. When heavy smokers were compared with non-smokers, the odds ratios were 3.03 (CI: 1.90–4.86) for LBW births and 2.60 (CI: 1.55–4.35) for preterm births [74]. According to a Swedish study in pregnant women who smoked, male foetuses were affected significantly more

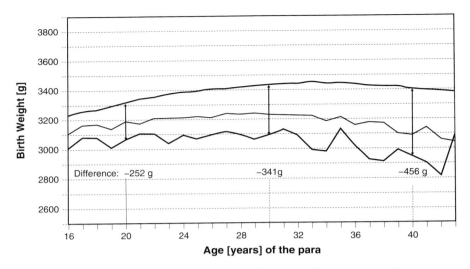

Fig. 8.1 Mean birth weight of children of non-smoking (*upper line*) and of smoking pregnant women (6–10 cigarettes/day; *middle line*; or 21–60 cigarettes/day; *lower line*). The data were calculated in dependence of the para's age [2]

Table 8.4 Risks to pregnancy associated with cigarette smoking

Risks	OR	References
Premature placental abruption (30,681 pregnancies)	In ca. 1%; OR 1.39	[42, 73]
Reduction in birth weight	−200–300 g	[2, 42, 64, 65, 74–78]
LBW (227,791 live births)	−239 g; −1.41 cm; BMI −0.6 kg/m²	[72]
LBW (1,011 pregnancies)	−205 g; −1.28 cm; −0.38 cm head circumference (>10 cigarettes/day)	[79]
Sudden infant death syndrome (SIDS)	Risk increased by 2.2- to 8.4-fold, depending on study, also depending on the number of cigarettes smoked	[80]
Spontaneous abortions (Sp) and malformations(MF) 12,914 pregnancies. +10,523 live births	1.7-fold (Sp) and 2.3-fold (MF) increase	[62]

frequently and severely than female foetuses in terms of growth retardation assessed in utero (biparietal diameter, subscapular fat accretion). In boys (but not girls) born to smokers, head circumference was also significantly smaller [81].

During a prospective cohort study of 30,681 pregnancies of at least 28 weeks' gestation, 307 women (ca. 1%) had placental abruptions. Each pack of cigarettes smoked per day increased the risk of placental abruption by 40% (OR = 1.39; CI: 1.09–1.79), with a concomitant increase in perinatal mortality. Placental abruption was also significantly associated with intrauterine growth retardation and foetal malformations [82].

The commonly detected presence of O_2 deficiency in the blood of women who smoke is attributable to the elevated CO levels [83], a phenomenon that is associated with the increased formation of CO–haemoglobin. The pathogenetic importance of CO is indicated by cases of CO poisoning during pregnancy culminating in the delivery of malformed infants (see Sect. 8.5).

According to other investigations, the *risk of spontaneous abortion* [84] and *perinatal mortality* are increased in pregnant women who smoke [85].

8.3
Malformations Possibly Caused by Smoking

Women who smoke during pregnancy must expect their neonates to display signs of embryotoxic and fetotoxic damage, even though the possibility of malformations, such as those known to occur with various medicinal products, was initially dismissed. Tables 8.4 and 8.5 summarise the risks of cigarette smoking during pregnancy, although the number of abortions may be subject to considerable variation [40]. In a study in more than 86,000 live births, negative associations were found between maternal smoking during pregnancy and increased risk for a number of malformations, including ventricular septal defects, hydroceles, clubfoot, pigmented naevi, haemangiomas and Down syndrome [44]. Similarly, following analysis of 288,067 live births during the period from 1980 to 1983 in Missouri, no association was detected between congenital malformations and maternal smoking during pregnancy (OR = 0.98) [45].

One problem frequently discussed in the literature is the possibility that maternal smoking during pregnancy may increase the occurrence of *Down syndrome*. Several studies [86–88] have failed to indicate any increased frequency among smokers compared with non-smokers (see Table 8.5). However, heavy smoking does increase co-morbidity in terms of additional malformations (tetralogy of Fallot, atrial septal defects without ventricular septal defects) [89]. These data have been confirmed by further studies in which maternal α-fetoprotein (AFP) and human chorionic gonadotrophin (hCG) were included as markers [90]. Slight changes in AFP, unconjugated oestriol (uE3) and hCG were reported in smokers in a population of 23,668 pregnant women: compared with non-smokers, AFP was raised by 3% while uE3 and hCG were reduced by 3 and 23%, respectively [91, 92]. Smoking has also been shown to affect the triple test (AFP, E3 and β-hCG) used to screen for trisomy 21, with β-hCG in particular being lowered by smoking [93–95]. However, the measured changes were inadequate to establish a prevalence for Down syndrome, and consequently it is not justifiable to use measurements of this type to predict a harmful effect [91]. Other investigators have reported opposite results with AFP determinations (21% increase) [96]. According to a Swedish study in 1,117,021 liveborn infants, an association was not found in multiparous women, but could not be ruled out totally in primiparous women [54]. The fact that somewhat fewer Down syndrome children are born to smoking mothers than to non-smoking mothers should therefore probably be interpreted as

Table 8.5 Malformations possibly caused by cigarette smoking

Malformations	Study population (*n*)	Risk or odds ratio (OR)	References
Malformations	86,000 and 288,067 live births	No association with smoking (OR 0.98)	[44, 45]
Cleft palate/cleft lip		3-and 11-fold increased risk	[46, 47]
Microcephalus, cleft defects, clubfoot	3,284 live births + 4,500 controls	Association confirmed	[48]
Cleft lip/palate		6.16-fold and 8.69-fold risk increase in smokers	[49]
Cleft lip/palate	1,002,742 live births	OR 1.16 (cleft lip), 1.29 (cleft palate)	[50]
Cleft lip/palate	Meta-analysis 1966–1996	OR 1.29 (cleft lip + palate) and 1.32 (cleft palate)	[51]
Atrial septal defects		No association with smoking	[52]
Down syndrome	1,117,021 live births	No association in multiparous women, but cannot be ruled out in primiparous women	[53]
Limb defects and limb reduction defects	1,575,904 and 1,109,299 live births (610 infants)	OR 1.26–1.70	[54–56]
Urinary tract malformations and polycystic kidneys	118 live births + 369 controls, and 1,117,021 live births	OR 2.3 and 1.22 respectively	[57, 58]
Aortopulmonary septal defects		OR 1.9	[56]
Craniosynostosis		Increased risk with higher antenatal maternal altitude	[59, 60]
Gastroschisis	Children born to mothers below 25 years of age	OR 2.0	[61]

a chance event [86]. The development of neural tube defects is a controversial topic [97, 98] but the association with maternal smoking during pregnancy is less likely.

The risk of *oral clefts (cleft lip and palate)* has been considered repeatedly in the context of maternal smoking (Table 8.5) [97, 99]. Studies rejecting such an association have occasionally appeared: for example, one recently published study has reported higher odds ratios (1.09–1.85) for oral clefts with increasing cigarette consumption, but no associations were identified between clefting type and smoking habits [100].

The association between maternal smoking during pregnancy and the development of cleft lip and palate in infants has been demonstrated elsewhere [97, 99]. One case -control study conducted in Maryland between 1992 and 1996 revealed no statistically significant association between maternal smoking and oral cleft development, although there was a slight increase in the C2 allele on the TGFα genotype among cases of oral cleft [46]. In contrast, another US study showed increased risks for isolated cleft lip (OR = 2.1) and for isolated cleft palate (OR = 2.2) when the mothers smoked 20 or more cigarettes/day. This corresponds to a 3- to 11-fold risk increase compared with non-smokers [101]. In a study conducted in almost 3.9 million live births in the USA, 2,207 live births with cleft lip/palate were identified [102]. A significant association was found between any amount of maternal cigarette use during pregnancy and having a child with a cleft lip/palate (OR = 1.55). Additional factors such as maternal education level, age, race and maternal medical conditions (e.g. diabetes or pregnancy-associated hypertension) were potential confounders. After adjusting for these confounders, a dose-response association with smoking was shown, by comparison with the non-smoking reference group: the odds ratios were 1.50 (1–10 cigarettes/day), 1.55 (11–20 cigarettes/day) and 1.78 (>20 cigarettes/day) [102]. Infants carrying the rarer C2 allele at the TaqI site in the TGFα locus who were exposed to maternal smoking were more likely to develop cleft palate (6.16-fold risk increase at 10 or fewer cigarettes/day, 8.69-fold risk increase at more than 10 cigarettes/day) [49, 103].

TGFα, TGFβ3, RARA (retinolic acid receptor) and the proto-oncogene BCL-3 have been found to be useful markers, although allocation of the various clefting types to the described genes, TGFα, TGFβ3 and MSX1, is possibly premature [104], as is conjecture whether multivitamin juice consumption during pregnancy interferes with the TGFα gene [105]. An association between smoking and the occurrence of this anomaly has not been demonstrated.

Further malformations were identified in a study conducted in four Polish districts: these occurred in between 1.1 and 1.9% of neonates and manifested themselves principally as *limb reduction defects* and *functional disturbances of striated muscle* [106–108]. An association with smoking was less likely than with harmful environmental factors. It is also debatable whether *neural tube defects* are more likely to develop during pregnancy when the mother smokes [109]. Serious defects that have also been linked with smoking include changes consistent with *holoprosencephaly*, a condition characterised by abnormal forebrain and midfacial development and by failure of cleavage into left and right hemispheres. Compared with controls, maternal periconceptional exposures associated with increased risks for holoprosencephaly included cigarette smoking (OR = 4.1), and combined alcohol and smoking (OR = 5.4), and these increased risk levels were only surpassed by women with insulin-dependent diabetes (OR = 10.2) [110].

Mothers who smoke during pregnancy are more likely to have offspring with congenital urinary tract anomalies (OR = 2.3). This risk was higher (OR = 3.7) among light smokers (1–1,000 cigarettes during the pregnancy) than among heavy smokers (OR = 1.4) [57]. Polycystic renal changes have been reported most commonly [58].

Child behaviour has also been studied in terms of maternal smoking during pregnancy: where the mothers were smokers, externalising behaviour problems (aggressive, oppositional, overactive) were more prominent in the children than internalising behaviour problems (depressed, anxious, withdrawn), and the effect of maternal smoking was almost identical for boys and girls [111]. According to analyses of lead levels in the blood, the first behavioural problems in children of smokers coincide with raised lead levels [6]. Smoking 10 or more cigarettes/day during pregnancy doubles the risk (OR = 2.0) of infants being non-babblers at the examination at 8 months [112]. The child's cognitive development is not affected by maternal smoking behaviour; in this context, social background and lifestyle are more important determinants (see also Sect. 7.1.4 in Chap. 7, [113]). According to other estimates, prenatal exposure of the foetus to nicotine may lead to behavioural disturbances and can indicate higher risk for psychiatric problems, including substance abuse [114]. One French study suggests that being born small for gestational age at full term is associated with poorer school performance at 12 and 18 years and later entry into secondary school than children born appropriate for gestational age (OR = 2.3) [115].

8.4
Smoking and Sudden Infant Death Syndrome (SIDS)

An association between smoking and sudden infant death syndrome (SIDS) has been reported in several publications (Table 8.4). It has been suggested that hypoxia and raised CO levels in foetal blood during pregnancy play a crucial role in the context of SIDS. These two factors exert a noxious effect on the respiratory control mechanisms in the foetal brain which then remains susceptible to further insults in the early post-natal period from infection and hyperthermia, resulting in death from central respiratory dysfunction [116]. Infants born to smoking mothers have a reduced drive to breathe and a blunted ventilatory response to hypoxia, possibly contributing to SIDS [117].

According to investigations carried out in piglets, infusions of nicotine (5 μg/kg), IL-1β (10-pmole/kg) and nicotine plus IL-1β cause prolonged periods of apnoea without a subsequent hyperventilatory response, with the result that the O_2 pressure falls and CO_2 pressure rises. IL-1β has a powerful depressant effect on respiration; in the case of nicotine, it has not been clarified whether the plasma levels achieved correspond to those in the foetus or infant [118].

Protein kinase C and nitric oxide synthase activities in the dorsocaudal brainstem of rats exposed to cigarette smoke from day 2 to 22 of pregnancy are also clearly reduced [119]; these findings possibly explain the decreased respiratory drive and enhanced hypoxic vulnerability seen in infants born to smoking mothers. According to more recent studies, prenatal nicotine exposure reduces vigilance (altered sleep–wake rhythm) by increasing the expression of nAChRs in the brain regions responsible for regulating these processes, possibly predisposing to SIDS [120].

In a case-control study from Sweden [80] comparing 244 SIDS cases with 869 controls, maternal smoking was reported to be associated with a 4-fold increased risk for SIDS. It is now known that over a period of 25 years since the early 1970s there has been a rise in the incidence of SIDS in Sweden for which no conclusive explanation can be found [121]. It has been reported that 29% of mothers whose infants die of SIDS are smokers [122]. Histological examination has revealed increases in the inner and epithelial wall areas of the airways in infants whose mothers were smokers, a finding that may also be associated with SIDS [123]. Research conducted in Shanghai in 2,227 children [124] to investigate the synergistic effect of passive smoking and artificial feeding detected a dose-dependent increased risk of hospitalisation for respiratory illnesses during the first 18 months of life: this was shown separately for boys and girls, low and normal birth weight, and for breastfed and artificially-fed infants (Fig. 8.2). Similarly, in a US case-control study, a dose-dependent increased risk for SIDS was reported as a function of the number of smokers living in the household and the number of cigarettes smoked daily (Fig. 8.2) [125].

Increased risk has been confirmed in another study [126] and a secondary role has been assigned to *alcohol consumption* [127]. Where mothers reduced or ceased cigarette

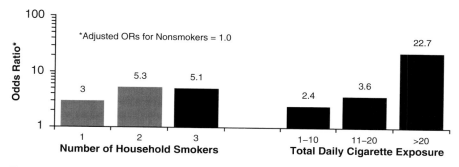

Fig. 8.2   Results of a SIDS case-control study from the USA. Smokers in the household included the children's parents and other live in adults [125]

consumption during pregnancy, the risk of SIDS was reduced. Causal differences have been reported, depending on age at death (before or after 120 days) [128]. Late SIDS occurred predominantly in winter, and a variety of risk conditions (low parental social and educational level, smoking status, and the prone sleeping position) were important in both early and late SIDS. The risk of SIDS was increased 8.4-fold in preterm babies, 3.4-fold in low-birth-weight babies (<2,500 g) and 2.2-fold when the mothers smoked during pregnancy [129, 130]. These factors underline a multiple-cause hypothesis for SIDS [126]. The SIDS rate was reduced when infants were changed to sleeping on their backs [131]. Apart from smoking, numerous other sociocultural factors (young maternal age, low educational level of mother and father, frequent pregnancies etc.) increase the risk for SIDS, as demonstrated by a study recently conducted in Norway [132]. In further studies, the infants' risk level for SIDS was reported to be increased 6.2-fold [133] and 5.01-fold [127]. According to the Westphalia study, the SIDS risk increased dose-dependently from 2.4-fold in moderate smokers (>10 cigarettes/day) to 7.2-fold in heavy smokers(>20 cigarettes/day) [70]. Only preterm babies had an even higher risk (16-fold increase). Very similar risk assessments have also been published by researchers in the USA [134] and Scotland [135]. A plasma cotinine level >30 ng/ml has been recorded in about 25% of SIDS children [124], evidence that tobacco smoke and hence the inhaled nicotine is transferred to the foetus.

LBW is an important risk factor, given the proven ethnic differences in the subsequent occurrence of SIDS. An association between infant LBW and SIDS has been reported among whites and American Indians, and to a lesser extent among blacks, but not among Asians or Hispanics [136].

Investigations have recently been conducted into the fine tissue changes in the brainstem of SIDS victims [137]. It was found that in SIDS victims there was 41% probability that the more the mothers smoked during pregnancy, the more gliosis in the nucleus olivaris inferior was found in their infants ($p < 0.01$). Similarly, associations were found between gliosis in the nucleus olivaris inferior and hypoxic-ischaemic events during pregnancy, birth and the perinatal period [137].

Children of women suffering from *schizophrenia* are at increased risk for SIDS (RR = 2.76; CI: 1.67–4.56) and for congenital malformations among their children (RR = 1.70; CI:

1.04–2.77). These findings should be interpreted not merely in the light of increased drug consumption, including smoking, but also in socio-economic terms [138].

Overall, 30–40% of all cases of SIDS would be preventable if women were to completely cease smoking during and after pregnancy [139].

8.5
Foetotoxic Effects of CO

Animal experiments in pregnant rats confirm that inhalation of high concentrations of smoke leads to changes in the foetus that are reflected among other things in LBW, depending on the duration and extent of exposure [140]. Findings following CO inhalation in mice and rabbits confirm the LBWs of the animals and slight changes in the skeletal system [141], but do not support a teratogenic effect of CO. Studies in pregnant, CO-exposed guinea-pigs (200 ppm for 10 h) confirm reduced tyrosine hydroxylase-immunoreactivity in the medulla oblongata and increased choline acetyltransferase-immunoreactivity [142]. Consequently, more extensive changes may be assumed to occur in the cholinergic and adrenergic system in the medulla, with particular implications for the cardiorespiratory centres, regions thought to be compromised in SIDS [142]. In experiments of similar design, changes were detected following exposure to a combination of sulphur dioxide (SO_2) and CO, but not to SO_2 alone [143]. In mice, CO levels of 180 ppm in air markedly reduced oxyhaemoglobin levels while carboxyhaemoglobin levels were increased. This resulted in increases in the incidence of resorbed embryos and of cleft lip/palate [144]. In a different experimental design, pregnant CD-1 mice underwent exposure to increasing concentrations of CO (0–500 ppm CO) and were fed diets with differing protein contents (4, 8 and 16%). Foetal weights were reduced in the CO-exposed groups receiving protein-deficient diets. There was also an increased incidence of brachygnathia, microstomia, microcephalus, open mouth, open eyes, skull and jaw malformations, scoliosis and limb unossifications [145]. The protein-deficient diet had a synergistic effect with chronic CO intoxication on the animals' development.

According to recently published research, maternal smoking during pregnancy reduces foetal heart rate and the regulation of heart rate range. This change may be attributed to chronic hypoxaemia [146]. End-tidal CO measurements in neonates reveal differing values, following correction for inhaled air: 10.0 ± 7.7 ppm in neonates born to smokers, 2.51 ± 1.4 ppm in neonates of passively exposed mothers and 1.74 ± 0.98 ppm in neonates of non-smoking mothers ($p < 0.0001$) [147]. Thus, neonatal CO exposure can be demonstrated as a result of maternal smoking immediately before delivery.

Important evidence for the teratogenic effect of CO can be deduced from reports of CO intoxication in pregnant women: for example, women who experienced CO intoxication during pregnancy have given birth to children with telencephalic dysgenesis [148].

Case report: Owing to defective household appliances, a pregnant woman was exposed on several occasions to raised ambient CO concentrations up to 100 ppm. In week 41 of pregnancy she gave birth to an underdeveloped infant with bilateral cleft formation, ear dysplasia, micropenis and general muscle weakness. The child died on day 12 in cardiogenic

Table 8.6 Maternal CO poisoning and implications for the foetus or child; summary of 42 out of 60 cases of CO exposure from the literature for which adequate information was available [150]

Outcome for the foetus	Severity of maternal CO exposure		
	Minimal	Moderate	Severe (death)
No sequelae	4	2	–
Survived with malformations and/or functional impairment	–	10	–
Death	–	15	11

shock and post-mortem examination revealed multiple brain malformations [149]. The mother's CO–Hb level was 14%, and she also smoked about 15 cigarettes/day.

Sixty cases of CO poisoning in pregnant women were collected in a retrospective survey: adequate information concerning the severity of CO exposure was available for 42 of these cases (Table 8.6). Overall, ten cases of CO poisoning subsequently led to malformations in the children (absent or malformed extremities, brachycephaly, craniosynostosis, multiple contractures of the extremities, hypoplastic lungs, hydrocephalus, ear anomalies etc.) [148, 150–152] and a high proportion of the mothers ($n = 26$) gave birth to stillborn infants [150].

Maternal CO–Hb levels are particularly important in this context. One prospective study conducted between 1985 and 1989 examined foetal outcomes in 32 women following accidental CO poisoning due to a variety of causes. The sources of CO were malfunctioning furnaces, hot-water heaters, car exhaust fumes and methylene chloride inhalation. Pregnancy outcome was adversely affected in 3 out of 5 pregnancies with severe toxicity: two stillbirths and one cerebral palsy because of ischaemic damage. The women received hyperbaric oxygen therapy immediately after poisoning, with the result that 31 neonates showed normal physical development despite mild or moderate CO poisoning in utero. Severe maternal CO toxicity was associated with significantly more adverse foetal effects [153]. In a further six women with CO poisoning, there were two abortions and one preterm delivery with numerous morphological anomalies [151]. Several studies indicate that hyperbaric oxygen ventilation is the treatment of choice for reversing the effects of CO toxicity [153, 154].

In women with pregnancy-induced hypertension and pre-eclampsia, endogenous CO formation is somewhat lower than in normotensive pregnant controls (1.17 ± 0.35 vs. 1.70 ± 0.54 ppm) [153], with CO being accorded a contributory role in the paradox of the seemingly protective effect of smoking to decrease the risk of pre-eclampsia [155].

8.6
Effects of Nicotine on the Foetus

Little has been published concerning the teratogenic or embryotoxic and fetotoxic effects of nicotine. Instead of pure nicotine, a few animal experiments have used aqueous extracts of chewing tobacco, involving pre- and postconceptional intragastric administration of doses of 4, 12 and 20 mg/kg body weight three times daily to CD-1 mice. The plasma nicotine levels measured 30 min after administration ranged from 99 to 623 ng/ml. This overdosing led to the death of 18 and 31% of the dams in the two highest dosage groups. Following administration of the highest dose, the foetal weights of the mice were reduced by 7.4%, and external malformations were few and only minor in extent. Otherwise, precocious ossification was observed (in the top dosage group) [156]. Only minimal changes were noted in a second study in mice following administration of 12 mg nicotine/kg, and fatalities and malformations were not detected [157]. In another study, pregnant rats were exposed to cigarette smoke or injected with nicotine for 20 days. Markedly reduced weight gain during pregnancy was detected only in the smoke-exposed rats [158]. Short-term administration of high doses of nicotine in animal experiments adversely affects the maternal and foetal cardiovascular system whereas the nicotine doses used in pregnant humans to achieve smoking cessation (nicotine replacement therapy; see Chap. 11) do not affect the cardiovascular system [36]. In particular, CO and Pb^{2+} from tobacco smoke have been cited as reproductive toxins [36]. Breast-feeding over the first 4–5 months of life is also useful for reducing the risk of childhood asthma [159].

Following treatment of pregnant rhesus monkeys with 1.5 mg nicotine/kg/day from day 26 to day 160 of gestation, the absolute birth weights of neonatal monkeys was not changed, although there was a 10% reduction in birth weights with nicotine exposure when they were normalised to maternal weight. Plasma leptin levels measured on postnatal day 1 were reduced by 50% in the nicotine treatment group, reflecting a decrease in NPY-mRNA expression in the neonatal monkeys [160]. It has been suggested that nicotine exposure during pregnancy may increase energy expenditure in hypothalamic structures, resulting in lower birth weights and body fat levels [160].

Rat pups were exposed to nicotine (6 mg/kg/day) under controlled conditions from postnatal days 4 to 9, using a procedure that ensured that observed effects are not due to nutritional deficits. Examination of the animals on postnatal day 18–19 revealed that nicotine-exposed animals were overactive compared with those with controls [161]. Transposed to the situation in humans, this could mean that maternal smoking during pregnancy is associated with an increased prevalence of children with hyperactivity disorder [162].

No differences in 3H-nicotine binding were detected in 14 different brainstem regions in SIDS victims compared with healthy controls. In contrast, in controls whose mothers smoked during pregnancy, up-regulation of the 3H-nicotine binding sites was detected in three different regions responsible for cardiorespiratory functions. This up-regulation was absent in the corresponding brainstem regions of SIDS victims [163]; however, this finding does not yet permit any conclusions regarding the pathophysiology or pathogenesis of SIDS.

8.7
Smoking and Breast-feeding

A study was conducted in Norway between 1970 and 1991 to investigate smoking behaviour during pregnancy in 24,438 mothers. During that period, the number of smoking mothers fell from 38 to 26%. The proportion of breast-feeding non-smokers was twice that of breastfeeding smokers. Where only the father smoked, mothers stopped breast-feeding earlier than where the father was a non-smoker [164]. These data are probably also representative for other countries.

Because of its lipophilic character, nicotine passes very rapidly into breast milk where it attains threefold higher concentrations than in blood [165, 166]. On the basis of the volume of breast milk consumed, this means that the infant receives 6 µg nicotine/kg body weight daily [165]. Cotinine levels are an indicator of smoking habits and correlate with the number of cigarettes smoked [167]. The infant's urinary cotinine comes from the cotinine in the mother's breast milk. It is difficult to assess what proportion derives from inhalation because of passive exposure by being in the same room as smokers [168]. The elimination half-life for nicotine in breast milk is somewhat higher than that in the mother's blood (97 ± 20 vs. 81 ± 9 min; $p > 0.05$), whereas cotinine concentrations remain fairly consistent during a 4-h interval without smoking [166]. Newborn infants breast-fed by smokers and unexposed to passive smoking show low plasma levels of nicotine (0.2–1.6 ng/ml) and cotinine (5–30 ng/ml). Newborn infants breast-fed by non-smokers did not have measurable amounts of the two substances in plasma [169]. As shown by the data presented in Table 8.7, breast-feeding mothers clearly contribute to raised plasma nicotine levels.

Nicotine and cotinine concentrations in breast milk increase with the number of cigarettes smoked daily, with concentrations up to 1.6 ng nicotine/ml and 20 ng cotinine/ml having been measured [170]. Concentrations arising as a result of passive smoking are markedly lower. Nicotine and cotinine levels were measured by gas chromatography in 34 human milk samples: nicotine was not found in the 6 samples of milk from non-smokers but was detected in the 28 samples from smokers (average: 91 ppb; ranging from 20 to 512 ppb) [171]. The varying nicotine levels did not cause any adverse effects in the breast-fed children [171]. Urinary cotinine levels in breast-fed infants of smoking mothers were ten times higher than those in bottle-fed infants of smoking mothers [172]. Cotinine levels were also increased when infants of non-smoking mothers lived in households with other smokers. In this group the differences compared with infants of smoking mothers were very minimal [172], suggesting that passive smoking must be recognised as a pivotal cause of the accumulation of products of combustion. In addition, Cd^{2+} levels in breast milk are raised in smokers [27].

Overall, breast-feeding is useful because the risk of childhood wheezing is reduced, even where mothers smoke [173]. It is still better – but far from ideal – to smoke and breastfeed than to smoke and not breastfeed [174, 175], although it is known that smokers breastfeed for a clearly shorter period than non-smokers [176], owing possibly to a reduction in prolactin levels [177]. Initial investigations also suggest that breast-feeding for 5–6 months benefits the child's cognitive development to a greater extent than breast-feeding for 3 months [178].

Table 8.7 Urinary excretion of nicotine and cotinine in breast-fed infants [169]

Infant exposure pattern	Nicotine/creatinine ratio (ng nicotine/mg creatinine)	Cotinine/creatinine ratio (ng cotinine/mg creatinine)
Newborn infants breast-fed by smoking mothers and unexposed to passive smoking	14 (5.0–110.0)	110 (10–550)
Non-breast-fed infants exposed only to passive smoking	35 (4.7–218.0)	327 (117–780)
Infants exposed to passive smoking and to smoke via breast milk	12 (3.0–42.0)	550 (225–870)

Median nicotine/creatinine and cotinine/creatinine ratios (and ranges)

8.8
Medical Care Costs Attributable to Smoking During Pregnancy

In recent years, several calculations have been made in an attempt to estimate the financial burden on the health insurance schemes, and hence on society, arising from smoking during pregnancy [179–182]. In 1993, in the USA medical care expenditures attributable to smoking were estimated to be US$50 billion [179]. The pregnant smoker runs considerable risks for herself, her pregnancy and her child, and this behaviour by pregnant women places a major economic burden on society, estimated at US$135–167 million in the USA in 1993 [183] although others have suggested a figure as high as US$1.4 billion [184]. Some studies have exclusively considered costs as they relate to the newborn child or infant [185]. One recent study of birth and first-year costs for mothers and infants demonstrated incremental costs of US$23,697 for placental abruption and US$21,944 for respiratory distress syndrome [186]. In contrast, costs have been reported as US$914 for LBW and US$428 for lower respiratory tract infection. The sum of the additional costs attributable to maternal smoking during pregnancy for all conditions yielded a total ranging from US$1,142–1,358 per smoking pregnant woman [186]. Similar results have been reported in a German study from 1999 in 770,744 live births and with a 20.3% smoking prevalence among pregnant women: from this population of pregnant women, preterm deliveries in a hospital setting incurred additional expenditure of 36 million [187].

In view of these facts it is an urgent priority that effective programmes be initiated among women to encourage smoking cessation at the very start of pregnancy.

8.9
Concluding Remarks

- Current knowledge indicates that cigarette smoking during pregnancy and the breast-feeding period has considerable harmful effects on foetal health and on the infant's initial growth phase.
- Smoking mothers run a major risk for their child, not only in terms of higher rates of abortion, premature placental abruption and LBW, but also of malformations (cleft lip/palate, limb defects etc.), while differing views persist concerning the risk of Down syndrome.
- These harmful effects are evidently caused by hypoxic reactions during smoking, with subsequent increased levels of carboxyhaemoglobin, as has also been observed in cases of CO poisoning which have resulted in the birth of malformed infants. To this must be added the now proven placenta-toxic properties of cadmium, a substance which pregnant women absorb in increased amounts during smoking.
- During the first months of life, large numbers of infants die from SIDS, a condition that is also triggered by maternal and passive smoking, as shown by the detected presence of cotinine in victims' urine and hair.
- No unified view currently exists concerning the involvement of nicotine in these harmful effects, particularly since only animal experiments have been conducted in this area, and

it is questionable whether the findings obtained can be transposed to human pregnancy. On the basis of at least the experimental animal studies to date, no malformations have come to light. The regulation of dopaminergic receptors is altered, and while it has been postulated that cardiopulmonary regulation is disturbed, this has by no means been proved.

- Overall, almost all complications in the unborn child occurring during pregnancy can be attributed to the combustion products of tobacco, including the formation of CO. This body of evidence might also justify reconsideration of the use of smoking cessation therapy with nicotine products in pregnant women.
- Alongside the harmful effects to the child, the additional economic burden imposed on the state and society should be sufficient reason for implementing effective smoking cessation programmes.

References

1. Anonym (1994) Dokumentation über Mutterschaftsvorsorge und Entbindungen, Tabelle 3. Kassenärztliche Bundesvereinigung, Köln
2. Voigt M, Hesse V, Wermke K, Friese K (2001) Rauchen in der Schwangerschaft. Risiko für das Wachstum des Feten. Kinderärztl Praxis 72:26–29
3. Andres RL, Day MC (2000) Perinatal complications associated with maternal tobacco use. Semin Neonatol 5(3):231–241
4. Salihu HM, Aliyu MH, Pierre-Louis BJ, Alexander GR (2003) Levels of excess infant deaths attributable to maternal smoking during pregnancy in the United States. Matern Child Health J 7(4):219–227
5. Ockene J, Ma Y, Zapka J, Pbert L, Valentine GK, Stoddard A (2002) Spontaneous cessation of smoking and alcohol use among low-income pregnant women. Am J Prev Med 23(3):150–159
6. Wasserman GA, Liu X, Pine DS, Graziano JH (2001) Contribution of maternal smoking during pregnancy and lead exposure to early child behavior problems. Neurotoxicol Teratol 23(1):13–21
7. Lackmann GM, Angerer J, Tollner U (2000) Parental smoking and neonatal serum levels of polychlorinated biphenyls and hexachlorobenzene. Pediatr Res 47(5):598–601
8. Ahluwalia IB, Grummer-Strawn L, Scanlon KS (1997) Exposure to environmental tobacco smoke and birth outcome: increased effects on pregnant women aged 30 years or older. Am J Epidemiol 146(1):42–47
9. Ananth CV, Savitz DA, Luther ER (1996) Maternal cigarette smoking as a risk factor for placental abruption, placenta previa, and uterine bleeding in pregnancy. Am J Epidemiol 144(9):881–889
10. Cnattingius S, Axelsson O, Eklund G, Lindmark G (1985) Smoking, maternal age, and fetal growth. Obstet Gynecol 66(4):449–452
11. Wang X, Tager IB, Van Vunakis H, Speizer FE, Hanrahan JP (1997) Maternal smoking during pregnancy, urine cotinine concentrations, and birth outcomes. A prospective cohort study. Int J Epidemiol 26(5):978–988
12. Poppe WA, Drijkoningen M, Ide PS, Lauweryns JM, Van Assche FA (1996) Langerhans' cells and L1 antigen expression in normal and abnormal squamous epithelium of the cervical transformation zone. Gynecol Obstet Invest 41(3):207–213
13. Bernstein L, Pike MC, Lobo RA, Depue RH, Ross RK, Henderson BE (1989) Cigarette smoking in pregnancy results in marked decrease in maternal hCG and oestradiol levels. Br J Obstet Gynaecol 96(1):92–96
14. Boyce A, Schwartz D, Hubert C, Cedard L, Dreyfus J (1975) Smoking, human placental lactogen and birth weight. Br J Obstet Gynaecol 82(12):964–967

15. Mochizuki M, Maruo T, Masuko K, Ohtsu T (1984) Effects of smoking on fetoplacental-maternal system during pregnancy. Am J Obstet Gynecol 149(4):413–420
16. Barbieri RL, Gochberg J, Ryan KJ (1986) Nicotine, cotinine, and anabasine inhibit aromatase in human trophoblast in vitro. J Clin Invest 77(6):1727–1733
17. Bush PG, Mayhew TM, Abramovich DR, Aggett PJ, Burke MD, Page KR (2000) A quantitative study on the effects of maternal smoking on placental morphology and cadmium concentration. Placenta 21(2–3):247–256
18. Hafner E, Metzenbauer M, Dillinger-Paller B, Hoefinger D, Schuchter K, Sommer-Wagner H, et al (2001) Correlation of first trimester placental volume and second trimester uterine artery Doppler flow. Placenta 22(8–9):729–734
19. Chelmow D, Andrew DE, Baker ER (1996) Maternal cigarette smoking and placenta previa. Obstet Gynecol 87:703–706
20. Gurtoo HL, Williams CJ, Gottlieb K, Mulhern AI, Caballes L, Vaught JB, et al (1983) Population distribution of placental benzo(a)pyrene metabolism in smokers. Int J Cancer 31:29–37
21. Juchau MR (1971) Human placental hydroxylation of 3,4-benzpyrene during early gestation and at term. Toxicol Appl Pharmacol 18:665–675
22. Kapitulnik J, Levin W, Poppers PJ, Tomaszewski JE, Jerina DM, Conney AH (1976) Comparison of the hydroxylation of zoxazolamine and benzo[a]pyrene in human placenta: effect of cigarette smoking. Clin Pharmacol Ther 20:557–564
23. Pelkonen O, Jouppila P, Karki NT (1972) Effect of maternal cigarette smoking on 3,4-benzpyrene and N-methylaniline metabolism in human fetal liver and placenta. Toxicol Appl Pharmacol 23:399–407
24. Welch RM, Harrison YE, Gommi BW, Poppers PJ, Finster M, Conney AH (1969) Stimulatory effect of cigarette smoking on the hydroxylation of 3,4-benzpyrene and the N-demethylation of 3-methyl-4-monomethylaminoazobenzene by enzymes in human placenta. Clin Pharmacol Ther 10:100–109
25. Wong TK, Everson RB, Hsu ST (1985) Potent induction of human placental mono-oxygenase activity by previous dietary exposure to polychlorinated biphenyls and their thermal degradation products. Lancet 1:721–724
26. Manchester DK, Jacoby EH (1981) Sensitivity of human placental monooxygenase activity to maternal smoking. Clin Pharmacol Ther 30:687–692
27. Remmer H (1987) Passively inhaled tobacco smoke: a challenge to toxicology and preventive medicine. Arch Toxicol 61:89–104
28. Kuhnert PM, Kuhnert BR, Bottoms SF, Erhard P (1982) Cadmium levels in maternal blood, fetal cord blood, and placental tissues of pregnant women who smoke. Am J Obstet Gynecol 142(8):1021–1025
29. Radisch B, Luck W, Nau H (1987) Cadmium concentrations in milk and blood of smoking mothers. Toxicol Lett 36(2):147–152
30. Powlin SS, Keng PC, Miller RK (1997) Toxicity of cadmium in human trophoblast cells (JAr choriocarcinoma): role of calmodulin and the calmodulin inhibitor, zaldaride maleate. Toxicol Appl Pharmacol 144(2):225–234
31. Shiverick KT, Salafia C (1999) Cigarette smoking and pregnancy I: ovarian, uterine and placental effects. Placenta 20:265–272
32. Clausen HV, Jorgensen JC, Ottesen B (1999) Stem villous arteries from the placentas of heavy smokers: functional and mechanical properties. Am J Obstet Gynecol 180:476–482
33. Gabriel R, Alsat E, Evain-Brion D (1994) Alteration of epidermal growth factor receptor in placental membranes of smokers: relationship with intrauterine growth retardation. Am J Obstet Gynecol 170(5 Pt 1):1238–1243
34. Lucier GW, Nelson KG, Everson RB, Wong TK, Philpot RM, Tiernan T, et al (1987) Placental markers of human exposure to polychlorinated biphenyls and polychlorinated dibenzofurans. Environ Health Perspect 76:79–87

35. Wang SL, Lucier GW, Everson RB, Sunahara GI, Shiverick KT (1988) Smoking-related alterations in epidermal growth factor and insulin receptors in human placenta. Mol Pharmacol 34 (3):265–271

36. Dempsey DA, Benowitz NL (2001) Risks and benefits of nicotine to aid smoking cessation in pregnancy. Drug Saf 24(4):277–322

37. Zhang L, Connor EE, Chegini N, Shiverick KT (1995) Modulation by benzo[a]pyrene of epidermal growth factor receptors, cell proliferation, and secretion of human chorionic gonadotropin in human placental cell lines. Biochem Pharmacol 50(8):1171–1180

38. Zhang L, Shiverick KT (1997) Benzo(a)pyrene, but not 2,3,7,8-tetrachlorodibenzo-p-dioxin, alters cell proliferation and c-myc and growth factor expression in human placental choriocarcinoma JEG-3 cells. Biochem Biophys Res Commun 231(1):117–120

39. Genbacev O, Bass KE, Joslin RJ, Fisher SJ (1995) Maternal smoking inhibits early human cytotrophoblast differentiation. Reprod Toxicol 9(3):245–255

40. DiFranza JR, Lew RA (1995) Effect of maternal cigarette smoking on pregnancy complications and sudden infant death syndrome. J Fam Pract 40(4):385–394

41. Cnattingius S, Nordstrom ML (1996) Maternal smoking and feto-infant mortality: biological pathways and public health significance. Acta Paediatr 85(12):1400–1402

42. Wang X, Zuckerman B, Pearson C, Kaufman G, Chen C, Wang G, et al (2002) Maternal cigarette smoking, metabolic gene polymorphism, and infant birth weight. JAMA 287(2):195–202

43. Newman MG, Lindsay MK, Graves W (2001) Cigarette smoking and pre-eclampsia: their association and effects on clinical outcomes. J Matern Fetal Med 10(3):166–170

44. Shiono PH, Klebanoff MA, Berendes HW (1986) Congenital malformations and maternal smoking during pregnancy. Teratology 34(1):65–71

45. Malloy MH, Kleinman JC, Bakewell JM, Schramm WF, Land GH (1989) Maternal smoking during pregnancy: no association with congenital malformations in Missouri 1980–83. Am J Public Health 79(9):1243–1246

46. Beaty TH, Maestri NE, Hetmanski JB, Wyszynski DF, Vanderkolk CA, Simpson JC, et al (1997) Testing for interaction between maternal smoking and TGFA genotype among oral-cleft cases born in Maryland 1992–1996. Cleft Palate Craniofac J 34(5):447–454

47. Ericson A, Kallen B, Lofkvist E (1988) Environmental factors in the etiology of neural tube defects: a negative study. Environ Res 45(1):38–47

48. Van den Eeden SK, Karagas MR, Daling JR, Vaughan TL (1990) A case-control study of maternal smoking and congenital malformations. Paediatr Perinat Epidemiol 4(2):147–155

49. Hwang SJ, Beaty TH, Panny SR, Street NA, Joseph JM, Gordon S, et al (1995) Association study of transforming growth factor alpha (TGF alpha) TaqI polymorphism and oral clefts: indication of gene-environment interaction in a population-based sample of infants with birth defects. Am J Epidemiol 141(7):629–636

50. Kallen K (1997) Maternal smoking and orofacial clefts. Cleft Palate Craniofac J 34(1):11–16

51. Wyszynski DF, Duffy DL, Beaty TH (1997) Maternal cigarette smoking and oral clefts: a meta-analysis. Cleft Palate Craniofac J 34(3):206–210

52. Tikkanen J, Heinonen OP (1992) Risk factors for conal malformations of the heart. Eur J Epidemiol 8(1):48–57

53. Kallen K (1997) Down's syndrome and maternal smoking in early pregnancy. Genet Epidemiol 14(1):77–84

54. Kallen K (1997) Maternal smoking during pregnancy and limb reduction malformations in Sweden. Am J Public Health 87(1):29–32

55. Czeizel AE, Kodaj I, Lenz W (1994) Smoking during pregnancy and congenital limb deficiency. BMJ 308(6942):1473–1476

56. Wasserman CR, Shaw GM, O'Malley CD, Tolarova MM, Lammer EJ (1996) Parental cigarette smoking and risk for congenital anomalies of the heart, neural tube, or limb. Teratology 53(4):261–267

57. Li DK, Mueller BA, Hickok DE, Daling JR, Fantel AG, Checkoway H, et al (1996) Maternal smoking during pregnancy and the risk of congenital urinary tract anomalies. Am J Public Health 86(2):249–253
58. Kallen K (1997) Maternal smoking and urinary organ malformations. Int J Epidemiol 26(3): 571–574
59. Alderman BW, Bradley CM, Greene C, Fernbach SK, Baron AE (1994) Increased risk of craniosynostosis with maternal cigarette smoking during pregnancy. Teratology 50(1):13–18
60. Alderman BW, Zamudio S, Baron AE, Joshua SC, Fernbach SK, Greene C, et al (1995) Increased risk of craniosynostosis with higher antenatal maternal altitude. Int J Epidemiol 24(2):420–426
61. Goldbaum G, Daling J, Milham S (1990) Risk factors for gastroschisis. Teratology 42(4): 397–403
62. Himmelberger DU, Brown BW Jr, Cohen EN (1978) Cigarette smoking during pregnancy and the occurrence of spontaneous abortion and congenital abnormality. Am J Epidemiol 108(6): 470–479
63. Kelsey JL, Dwyer T, Holford TR, Bracken MB (1978) Maternal smoking and congenital malformations: an epidemiological study. J Epidemiol Community Health 32(2):102–107
64. Cooke RW (1998) Smoking, intra-uterine growth retardation and sudden infant death syndrome. Int J Epidemiol 27(2):238–241
65. Cornelius MD, Taylor PM, Geva D, Day NL (1995) Prenatal tobacco and marijuana use among adolescents: effects on offspring gestational age, growth, and morphology. Pediatrics 95(5):738–743
66. Martin TR, Bracken MB (1986) Association of low birth weight with passive smoke exposure in pregnancy. Am J Epidemiol 124(4):633–642
67. Martinez-Frias ML, Prieto VL, Bermejo SE, Gaya MF (1990) [Birth weight of infants born without congenital defects. II. Effect of tobacco and parity of the mother on the weight of the newborn infant]. An Esp Pediatr 33(1):16–20
68. Shah NR, Bracken MB (2000) A systematic review and meta-analysis of prospective studies on the association between maternal cigarette smoking and preterm delivery. Am J Obstet Gynecol 182(2):465–472
69. Naeye RL, Peters EC (1984) Mental development of children whose mothers smoked during pregnancy. Obstet Gynecol 64(5):601–607
70. Naeye RL, Peters EC (1987) Antenatal hypoxia and low IQ values. Am J Dis Child 141(1): 50–54
71. MacArthur C, Knox EG, Lancashire RJ (2001) Effects at age nine of maternal smoking in pregnancy: experimental and observational findings. BJOG 108(1):67–73
72. Schellscheidt J, Jorch G, Menke J (1998) Effects of heavy maternal smoking on intrauterine growth patterns in sudden infant death victims and surviving infants. Eur J Pediatr 157(3): 246–251
73. Naeye RL (1980) Abruptio placentae and placenta previa: frequency, perinatal mortality, and cigarette smoking. Obstet Gynecol 55(6):701–704
74. Moore ML, Zaccaro DJ (2000) Cigarette smoking, low birth weight, and preterm births in low-income African American women. J Perinatol 20(3):176–180
75. Hruba D, Kachlik P (2000) Influence of maternal active and passive smoking during pregnancy on birthweight in newborns. Cent Eur J Public Health 8(4):249–252
76. Kukla L, Hruba D, Tyrlik M (2001) Smoking and damages of reproduction: evidence of ELSPAC. Cent Eur J Public Health 9(2):59–63
77. Naeye RL (1981) Influence of maternal cigarette smoking during pregnancy on fetal and childhood growth. Obstet Gynecol 57(1):18–21
78. Schwartz-Bickenbach D, Schulte-Hobein B, Abt S, Plum C, Nau H (1987) Smoking and passive smoking during pregnancy and early infancy: effects on birth weight, lactation period, and cotinine concentrations in mother's milk and infant's urine. Toxicol Lett 35(1):73–81

79. Vlajinac H, Petrovic R, Marinkovic J, Kocev N, Sipetic S (1997) [The effect of cigarette smoking during pregnancy on fetal growth]. Srp Arh Celok Lek 125(9–10):267–271
80. Alm B, Milerad J, Wennergren G, Skjaerven R, Oyen N, Norvenius G, et al (1998) A case-control study of smoking and sudden infant death syndrome in the Scandinavian countries, 1992 to 1995. The Nordic Epidemiological SIDS Study. Arch Dis Child 78(4):329–334
81. Zaren B, Lindmark G, Bakketeig L (2000) Maternal smoking affects fetal growth more in the male fetus. Paediatr Perinat Epidemiol 14(2):118–126
82. Raymond EG, Mills JL (1993) Placental abruption. Maternal risk factors and associated fetal conditions. Acta Obstet Gynecol Scand 72(8):633–639
83. Haustein KO (1999) [Smoking, cardiovascular diseases and possibilities for treating nicotine dependence]. Wien Med Wochenschr 149(1):19–24
84. Kline J, Stein ZA, Susser M, Warburton D (1977) Smoking: a risk factor for spontaneous abortion. N Engl J Med 297(15):793–796
85. Longo LD (1982) Some health consequences of maternal smoking: issues without answers. Birth Defects Orig Artic Ser 18(3 Pt A):13–31
86. Cuckle HS, Alberman E, Wald NJ, Royston P, Knight G (1990) Maternal smoking habits and Down's syndrome. Prenat Diagn 10(9):561–567
87. Hook EB, Cross PK (1985) Cigarette smoking and Down syndrome. Am J Hum Genet 37(6): 1216–1224
88. Perona M, Mancini G, Dall'Amico D, Guaraldo V, Carbonara A (1998) Influence of smoking habits on Down's syndrome risk evaluation at mid-trimester through biochemical screening. Int J Clin Lab Res 28(3):179–182
89. Torfs CP, Christianson RE (1999) Maternal risk factors and major associated defects in infants with Down syndrome. Epidemiology 10(3):264–270
90. Spencer K (1998) The influence of smoking on maternal serum AFP and free beta hCG levels-and the impact on screening for Down syndrome. Prenat Diagn 18(3):225–234
91. Palomaki GE, Knight GJ, Haddow JE, Canick JA, Wald NJ, Kennard A (1993) Cigarette smoking and levels of maternal serum alpha-fetoprotein, unconjugated estriol, and hCG: impact on Down syndrome screening. Obstet Gynecol 81(5 Pt 1):675–678
92. Palomaki GE, Knight GJ, Haddow JE (1994) Human chorionic gonadotropin and unconjugated oestriol measurements in insulin-dependent diabetic pregnant women being screened for fetal Down syndrome. Prenat Diagn 14(1):65–68
93. de Graaf IM, Cuckle HS, Pajkrt E, Leschot NJ, Bleker OP, van Lith JM (2000) Co-variables in first trimester maternal serum screening. Prenat Diagn 20(3):186–189
94. Hafner E, Stangl G, Rosen A, Schuchter K, Plattner M, Philipp K (1999) Influence of cigarette-smoking on the result of the triple test. Gynecol Obstet Invest 47(3):188–190
95. Tislaric D, Brajenovic-Milic B, Ristic S, Latin V, Zuvic-Butorac M, Bacic J, et al (2002) The influence of smoking and parity on serum markers for Down's syndrome screening. Fetal Diagn Ther 17(1):17–21
96. Bartels I, Hoppe-Sievert B, Bockel B, Herold S, Caesar J (1993) Adjustment formulae for maternal serum alpha-fetoprotein, human chorionic gonadotropin, and unconjugated oestriol to maternal weight and smoking. Prenat Diagn 13(2):123–130
97. Ericson A, Kallen B, Westerholm P (1979) Cigarette smoking as an etiologic factor in cleft lip and palate. Am J Obstet Gynecol 135(3):348–351
98. Evans DR, Newcombe RG, Campbell H (1979) Maternal smoking habits and congenital malformations: a population study. Br Med J 2(6183):171–173
99. Khoury MJ, Adams MM, Rhodes P, Erickson JD (1987) Monitoring for multiple malformations in the detection of epidemics of birth defects. Teratology 36(3):345–353
100. Lieff S, Olshan AF, Werler M, Strauss RP, Smith J, Mitchell A (1999) Maternal cigarette smoking during pregnancy and risk of oral clefts in newborns. Am J Epidemiol 150(7): 683–694

101. Shaw GM, Wasserman CR, Lammer EJ, O'Malley CD, Murray JC, Basart AM, et al (1996) Orofacial clefts, parental cigarette smoking, and transforming growth factor-alpha gene variants. Am J Hum Genet 58(3):551–561

102. Chung KC, Kowalski CP, Kim HM, Buchman SR (2000) Maternal cigarette smoking during pregnancy and the risk of having a child with cleft lip/palate. Plast Reconstr Surg 105(2):485–491

103. Christensen K, Olsen J, Norgaard-Pedersen B, Basso O, Stovring H, Milhollin-Johnson L, et al (1999) Oral clefts, transforming growth factor alpha gene variants, and maternal smoking: a population-based case-control study in Denmark, 1991–1994. Am J Epidemiol 149(3):248–255

104. Romitti PA, Lidral AC, Munger RG, Daack-Hirsch S, Burns TL, Murray JC (1999) Candidate genes for nonsyndromic cleft lip and palate and maternal cigarette smoking and alcohol consumption: evaluation of genotype-environment interactions from a population-based case-control study of orofacial clefts. Teratology 59(1):39–50

105. Shaw GM, Wasserman CR, Murray JC, Lammer EJ (1998) Infant TGF-alpha genotype, orofacial clefts, and maternal periconceptional multivitamin use. Cleft Palate Craniofac J 35(4):366–370

106. Christianson RE (1980) The relationship between maternal smoking and the incidence of congenital anomalies. Am J Epidemiol 112(5):684–695

107. Kallen B (1989) A prospective study of some aetiological factors in limb reduction defects in Sweden. J Epidemiol Community Health 43(1):86–91

108. Sitarek K, Berlinska B (1997) [Comparative evaluation of the frequency of congenital defects in newborns from the provinces of Walbrzych, Piotrkow Trybunalski and Suwalki]. Przegl Epidemiol 51(3):349–358

109. Shaw GM, Velie EM, Morland KB (1996) Parental recreational drug use and risk for neural tube defects. Am J Epidemiol 144(12):1155–1160

110. Croen LA, Shaw GM, Lammer EJ (2000) Risk factors for cytogenetically normal holoprosencephaly in California: a population-based case-control study. Am J Med Genet 90(4):320–325

111. Orlebeke JF, Knol DL, Verhulst FC (1997) Increase in child behavior problems resulting from maternal smoking during pregnancy. Arch Environ Health 52(4):317–321

112. Obel C, Henriksen TB, Hedegaard M, Secher NJ, Ostergaard J (1998) Smoking during pregnancy and babbling abilities of the 8-month-old infant. Paediatr Perinat Epidemiol 12(1):37–48

113. Niemela A, Jarvenpaa AL (1996) Is breastfeeding beneficial and maternal smoking harmful to the cognitive development of children? Acta Paediatr 85(10):1202–1206

114. Ernst M, Moolchan ET, Robinson ML (2001) Behavioral and neural consequences of prenatal exposure to nicotine. J Am Acad Child Adolesc Psychiatry 40(6):630–641

115. Larroque B, Bertrais S, Czernichow P, Leger J (2001) School difficulties in 20-year-olds who were born small for gestational age at term in a regional cohort study. Pediatrics 108(1):111–115

116. Hutter CD, Blair ME (1996) Carbon monoxide – does fetal exposure cause sudden infant death syndrome? Med Hypotheses 46(1):1–4

117. Ueda Y, Stick SM, Hall G, Sly PD (1999) Control of breathing in infants born to smoking mothers. J Pediatr 135:226–232

118. Froen JF, Akre H, Stray-Pedersen B, Saugstad OD (2000) Adverse effects of nicotine and interleukin-1beta on autoresuscitation after apnea in piglets: implications for sudden infant death syndrome. Pediatrics 105(4):E52

119. Hasan SU, Simakajornboon N, MacKinnon Y, Gozal D (2001) Prenatal cigarette smoke exposure selectively alters protein kinase C and nitric oxide synthase expression within the neonatal rat brainstem. Neurosci Lett 301(2):135–138

120. Frank MG, Srere H, Ledezma C, O'Hara B, Heller HC (2001) Prenatal nicotine alters vigilance states and AchR gene expression in the neonatal rat: implications for SIDS. Am J Physiol Regul Integr Comp Physiol 280(4):R1134–R1140

121. Alm B, Norvenius SG, Wennergren G, Skjaerven R, Oyen N, Milerad J, et al (2001) Changes in the epidemiology of sudden infant death syndrome in Sweden 1973–1996. Arch Dis Child 84(1):24–30

122. Alm B, Norvenius SG, Wennergren G, Lagercrantz H, Helweg-Larsen K, Irgens LM (2000) Living conditions in early infancy in Denmark, Norway and Sweden 1992–95: results from the Nordic Epidemiological SIDS study. Acta Paediatr 89(2):208–214

123. Elliot J, Vullermin P, Robinson P (1998) Maternal cigarette smoking is associated with increased inner airway wall thickness in children who die from sudden infant death syndrome. Am J Respir Crit Care Med 158(3):802–806

124. Chen Y (1989) Synergistic effect of passive smoking and artificial feeding on hospitalization for respiratory illness in early childhood. Chest 95:1004–1007

125. Klonoff-Cohen HS, Edelstein SL, Lefkowitz ES, Srinivasan IP, Kaegi D, Chang JC, et al (1995) The effect of passive smoking and tobacco exposure through breast milk on sudden infant death syndrome. JAMA 273(10):795–798

126. Rajs J, Rasten-Almqvist P, Falck G, Eksborg S, Andersson BS (1997) Sudden infant death syndrome: postmortem findings of nicotine and cotinine in pericardial fluid of infants in relation to morphological changes and position at death. Pediatr Pathol Lab Med 17(1):83–97

127. Mitchell EA, Ford RP, Stewart AW, Taylor BJ, Becroft DM, Thompson JM, et al (1993) Smoking and the sudden infant death syndrome. Pediatrics 91(5):893–896

128. Kohlendorfer U, Kiechl S, Sperl W (1998) Sudden infant death syndrome: risk factor profiles for distinct subgroups. Am J Epidemiol 147(10):960–968

129. Anderson HR, Cook DG (1997) Passive smoking and sudden infant death syndrome: review of the epidemiological evidence. Thorax 52(11):1003–1009

130. Schlaud M, Kleemann WJ, Poets CF, Sens B (1996) Smoking during pregnancy and poor antenatal care: two major preventable risk factors for sudden infant death syndrome. Int J Epidemiol 25(5):959–965

131. Hollebecque V, Briand E, Bouvier-Colle MH (1998) [Information campaign on child care practices: measure of the effects on sleep position and sudden infant death syndrome]. Rev Epidemiol Sante Publique 46(2):115–123

132. Daltveit AK, Irgens LM, Oyen N, Skjaerven R, Markestad T, Alm B, et al (1998) Sociodemographic risk factors for sudden infant death syndrome: associations with other risk factors. The Nordic Epidemiological SIDS Study. Acta Paediatr 87(3):284–290

133. Nilsen ST, Laerdal A (1991) [Crib death and smoking during pregnancy]. Tidsskr Nor Laegeforen 111(29):3493–3495

134. MacDorman MF, Cnattingius S, Hoffman HJ, Kramer MS, Haglund B (1997) Sudden infant death syndrome and smoking in the United States and Sweden. Am J Epidemiol 146(3):249–257

135. Brooke H, Gibson A, Tappin D, Brown H (1997) Case-control study of sudden infant death syndrome in Scotland, 1992–5. BMJ 314(7093):1516–1520

136. Li DK, Daling JR (1991) Maternal smoking, low birth weight, and ethnicity in relation to sudden infant death syndrome. Am J Epidemiol 134(9):958–964

137. Storm H, Nylander G, Saugstad OD (1999) The amount of brainstem gliosis in sudden infant death syndrome (SIDS) victims correlates with maternal cigarette smoking during pregnancy. Acta Paediatr 88(1):13–18

138. Bennedsen BE, Mortensen PB, Olesen AV, Henriksen TB (2001) Congenital malformations, stillbirths, and infant deaths among children of women with schizophrenia. Arch Gen Psychiatry 58(7):674–679

139. Wisborg K, Kesmodel U, Henriksen TB, Olsen SF, Secher NJ (2000) A prospective study of smoking during pregnancy and SIDS. Arch Dis Child 83(3):203–206

140. Reznik G, Marquard G (1980) Effect of cigarette smoke inhalation during pregnancy in Sprague-Dawley rats. J Environ Pathol Toxicol 4(5–6):141–152

141. Schwetz BA, Ioset HD, Leong BK, Staples RE (1979) Teratogenic potential of dichlorvos given by inhalation and gavage to mice and rabbits. Teratology 20(3):383–387

142. Tolcos M, McGregor H, Walker D, Rees S (2000) Chronic prenatal exposure to carbon monoxide results in a reduction in tyrosine hydroxylase-immunoreactivity and an-increase in

choline acetyltransferase-immunoreactivity in the fetal medulla: implications for sudden infant death syndrome. J Neuropathol Exp Neurol 59(3):218–228

143. Murray FJ, Schwetz BA, Crawford AA, Henck JW, Quast JF, Staples RE (1979) Embryotoxicity of inhaled sulfur dioxide and carbon monoxide in mice and rabbits. J Environ Sci Health C 13(3):233–250

144. Bailey LJ, Johnston MC, Billet J (1995) Effects of carbon monoxide and hypoxia on cleft lip in A/J mice. Cleft Palate Craniofac J 32(1):14–19

145. Singh J, Aggison L Jr, Moore-Cheatum L (1993) Teratogenicity and developmental toxicity of carbon monoxide in protein-deficient mice. Teratology 48(2):149–159

146. Coppens M, Vindla S, James DK, Sahota DS (2001) Computerized analysis of acute and chronic changes in fetal heart rate variation and fetal activity in association with maternal smoking. Am J Obstet Gynecol 185(2):421–426

147. Seidman DS, Paz I, Merlet-Aharoni I, Vreman H, Stevenson DK, Gale R (1999) Noninvasive validation of tobacco smoke exposure in late pregnancy using end-tidal carbon monoxide measurements. J Perinatol 19:358–361

148. Woody RC, Brewster MA (1990) Telencephalic dysgenesis associated with presumptive maternal carbon monoxide intoxication in the first trimester of pregnancy. J Toxicol Clin Toxicol 28(4):467–475

149. Courtens W, Hennequin Y, Blum D, Vamos E (1996) CHARGE association in a neonate exposed in utero to carbon monoxide. Birth Defects Orig Artic Ser 30(1):407–412

150. Norman CA, Halton DM (1990) Is carbon monoxide a workplace teratogen? A review and evaluation of the literature. Ann Occup Hyg 34(4):335–347

151. Caravati EM, Adams CJ, Joyce SM, Schafer NC (1988) Fetal toxicity associated with maternal carbon monoxide poisoning. Ann Emerg Med 17(7):714–717

152. Zourbas J (1947) Congenital encephalopathy with the effects of the neuromuscular tone apparently following carbon monoxide poisoning. Archs franc Pédiat 4:513–515

153. Koren G, Sharav T, Pastuszak A, Garrettson LK, Hill K, Samson I, et al (1991) A multicenter, prospective study of fetal outcome following accidental carbon monoxide poisoning in pregnancy. Reprod Toxicol 5(5):397–403

154. Van Hoesen KB, Camporesi EM, Moon RE, Hage ML, Piantadosi CA (1989) Should hyperbaric oxygen be used to treat the pregnant patient for acute carbon monoxide poisoning? A case report and literature review. JAMA 261(7):1039–1043

155. Baum M, Schiff E, Kreiser D, Dennery PA, Stevenson DK, Rosenthal T, et al (2000) End-tidal carbon monoxide measurements in women with pregnancy-induced hypertension and preeclampsia. Am J Obstet Gynecol 183(4):900–903

156. Paulson R, Shanfeld J, Sachs L, Price T, Paulson J (1989) Effect of smokeless tobacco on the development of the CD-1 mouse fetus. Teratology 40(5):483–494

157. Paulson RB, Shanfeld J, Prause L, Iranpour S, Paulson JO (1991) Pre- and post-conceptional tobacco effects on the CD-1 mouse fetus. J Craniofac Genet Dev Biol 11(1):48–58

158. Bertolini A, Bernardi M, Genedani S (1982) Effects of prenatal exposure to cigarette smoke and nicotine on pregnancy, offspring development and avoidance behavior in rats. Neurobehav Toxicol Teratol 4(5):545–548

159. Oddy WH (2000) Breastfeeding and asthma in children: findings from a West Australian study. Breastfeed Rev 8(1):5–11

160. Grove KL, Sekhon HS, Brogan RS, Keller JA, Smith MS, Spindel ER (2001) Chronic maternal nicotine exposure alters neuronal systems in the arcuate nucleus that regulate feeding behavior in the newborn rhesus macaque. J Clin Endocrinol Metab 86(11): 5420–5426

161. Thomas JD, Garrison ME, Slawecki CJ, Ehlers CL, Riley EP (2000) Nicotine exposure during the neonatal brain growth spurt produces hyperactivity in preweanling rats. Neurotoxicol Teratol 22(5):695–701

162. Milberger S, Biederman J, Faraone SV, Jones J (1998) Further evidence of an association between maternal smoking during pregnancy and attention deficit hyperactivity disorder: findings from a high-risk sample of siblings. J Clin Child Psychol 27:352–358

163. Nachmanoff DB, Panigrahy A, Filiano JJ, Mandell F, Sleeper LA, Valdes-Dapena M, et al (1998) Brainstem 3H-nicotine receptor binding in the sudden infant death syndrome. J Neuropathol Exp Neurol 57(11):1018–1025

164. Haug K, Irgens LM, Baste V, Markestad T, Skjaerven R, Schreuder P (1998) Secular trends in breastfeeding and parental smoking. Acta Paediatr 87(10):1023–1027

165. Dahlstrom A, Lundell B, Curvall M, Thapper L (1990) Nicotine and cotinine concentrations in the nursing mother and her infant. Acta Paediatr Scand 79(2):142–147

166. Luck W, Nau H (1984) Nicotine and cotinine concentrations in serum and milk of nursing smokers. Br J Clin Pharmacol 18(1):9–15

167. Labrecque M, Marcoux S, Weber JP, Fabia J, Ferron L (1989) Feeding and urine cotinine values in babies whose mothers smoke. Pediatrics 83(1):93–97

168. Woodward A, Grgurinovich N, Ryan P (1986) Breast feeding and smoking hygiene: major influences on cotinine in urine of smokers' infants. J Epidemiol Community Health 40(4):309–315

169. Luck W, Nau H (1985) Nicotine and cotinine concentrations in serum and urine of infants exposed via passive smoking or milk from smoking mothers. J Pediatr 107(5):816–820

170. Luck W, Nau H (1987) Nicotine and cotinine concentrations in the milk of smoking mothers: influence of cigarette consumption and diurnal variation. Eur J Pediatr 146(1):21–26

171. Ferguson BB, Wilson DJ, Schaffner W (1976) Determination of nicotine concentrations in human milk. Am J Dis Child 130(8):837–839

172. Mascola MA, Van Vunakis H, Tager IB, Speizer FE, Hanrahan JP (1998) Exposure of young infants to environmental tobacco smoke: breast-feeding among smoking mothers. Am J Public Health 88(6):893–896

173. McConnochie KM, Roghmann KJ (1986) Breast feeding and maternal smoking as predictors-of wheezing in children age 6 to 10 years. Pediatr Pulmonol 2(5):260–268

174. Lagerlov P (1991) [Breast feeding and smoking - a study at a health center]. Tidsskr Nor Laegeforen 111(29):3496–3498

175. Minchin MK (1991) Smoking and breastfeeding: an overview. J Hum Lact 7(4):183–188

176. Cabello G, Hrepic N, Astudillo I, Benitez R, Ortega L, Poblete S, et al (1991) [Cigarette smoking and its relation to pregnancy and lactation in Africa (Chile)]. Rev Chil Pediatr 62(6):386–389

177. Andersen AN, Lund-Andersen C, Larsen JF, Christensen NJ, Legros JJ, Louis F, et al (1982) Suppressed prolactin but normal neurophysin levels in cigarette smoking breast-feeding women. Clin Endocrinol (Oxf) 17(4):363–368

178. Angelsen NK, Vik T, Jacobsen G, Bakketeig LS (2001) Breast feeding and cognitive development at age 1 and 5 years. Arch Dis Child 85(3):183–188

179. Center for Disease Control (1994) Medical-care expenditures attributable to cigarette smoking - United States, 1993. MMWR Morb Mortal Wkly Rep 43:469–472

180. Hauswald M (1989) The cost of smoking: an emergency department analysis. Am J Emerg Med 7:187–190

181. Miller VP, Ernst C, Collin F (1999) Smoking-attributable medical care costs in the USA. Soc Sci Med 48:375–391

182. Shultz JM, Novotny TE, Rice DP (1991) Quantifying the disease impact of cigarette smoking with SAMMEC II software. Public Health Rep 106:326–333

183. Adams EK, Melvin CL (1998) Costs of maternal conditions attributable to smoking during pregnancy. Am J Prev Med 15:212–219

184. Center for Disease Control (1997) Medical-care expenditures attributable to cigarette smoking during pregnancy - United States, 1995. MMWR Morb Mortal Wkly Rep 46:1048–1050

185. Aligne CA, Stoddard JJ (1997) Tobacco and children. An economic evaluation of the medical effects of parental smoking. Arch Pediatr Adolesc Med 151(7):648–653

186. Miller DP, Villa KF, Hogue SL, Sivapathasundaram D (2001) Birth and first-year costs for mothers and infants attributable to maternal smoking. Nicotine Tob Res 3(1):25–35
187. Voigt M, Hesse V, Honke B, Wermke K, Olbertz D, Friese K (2001) Kosten des Rauchens der Mütter in der Schwangerschaft für die Perinatalmedizin. In: K.-O Haustein (ed) Rauchen und kindliche Entwicklung - Raucherschäden und Primärprävention. Perfusion GmbH, Nürnberg, pp 29–34

Passive Smoking

9

Controversy has raged for decades concerning the importance of environmental tobacco smoke (ETS), with some claiming that it is "almost irrelevant" while others have labelled it a "substantial risk to health" [1, 2]. Main arguments against causal relation between ETS and lung cancer are based on quantitative differences in the main constituents of active and passive tobacco smoking [3–6]. On the basis of earlier calculations, a non-smoker inhales 1/10 to 1/5 of a cigarette. In terms of occupational exposure to carcinogens in the European Union (see Table 9.1), the CAREX (carcinogen exposure) database indicates that ETS is the second most common exposure after solar radiation [7]. Regrettably, the controversy surrounding ETS has been heightened because research results from the cigarette industry's own laboratories have blurred the overall assessment [8, 9]. For example, it has been claimed that, in terms of cigarettes smoked, the passive smoker's exposure might be equivalent to 1 cigarette/day at most [10]. Side-stream smoke is known to be more toxic than exhaled mainstream smoke [6, 11], and the cardiovascular system response to exhaled smoke is more sensitive in passive smokers than in active smokers.

The likelihood of exposure to ETS has been shown to vary across sociodemographic characteristics, health behaviours, and the type of smoking restrictions at work [12]. Therefore, Stamatakis et al. assessed differences in the likelihood of exposure to ETS at home and at work among an ethnically diverse sample of women of age 40 and older in the United States. They used data from the U.S. Women's Determinants Study and restricted the sample to include only non-smoking women ($n = 2,326$). Unadjusted and adjusted odds ratios (aOR) for exposure to ETS by sociodemographic characteristics, health risk behaviours and the type of workplace smoking policy were calculated using logistic regression. They found out that exposure to ETS at home was associated with being American Indian/Alaska Native (aOR 1.5, 95%; CI 1.0, 2.6), age 40–44 (aOR 1.6, 95%; CI 1.0, 2.6) and 45–54 (aOR 1.8, 95%; CI 1.2, 2.6), having eighth grade (aOR 2.1, 95%; CI 1.3, 3.6) or high school education (aOR 2.2, 95%; CI 1.4, 3.3), inadequate fruit and vegetable consumption (aOR 1.5, 95%; CI 1.0, 2.1), and not getting screened for breast cancer (aOR 1.5, 95%; CI 1.1, 2.0) [12]. Women who did not have regular breast (aOR 1.3, 95%; CI 1.9, 1.9) and cervical (aOR 2.0, 95%; CI 1.5, 5.3) cancer screening were more likely to be exposed to ETS at work. Exposure to ETS at work was higher among women with some high school education (aOR 2.8, 95%; CI 1.5, 5.3) and high school graduates (aOR 3.1, 95%; CI 1.9, 5.1) and substantially higher for women who worked where smoking was allowed in some (aOR 15.1, 95%; CI 10.2, 22.4) or all (aOR 44.8, 95%; CI 19.6, 102.4) work areas.

K.-O. Haustein, D. Groneberg, *Tobacco or Health?*
DOI: 10.1007/978-3-540-87577-2_9, © Springer Verlag Berlin Heidelberg 2010

Table 9.1 Carcinogen
exposure of industrial
workers in the European
Union, based on the
CAREX database maintained
by the International Agency
of Research on Cancer
(IARC) [7]

Carcinogen type	Workers exposed (million)
Group 1 carcinogens	22
Solar radiation	9.1 (75% of working time)
ETS	7.5 (75% of working time)
Crystalline silica	3.2
Diesel exhaust	3.0
Radon	2.7
Wood dust	2.6

Table 9.2 Comparison of the amounts of toxic, cocancerogenic and cancerogenic main constituents of tobacco smoke determined in the room air of restaurants and bureaus, which passive smokers and active smokers, consuming ten cigarettes, inhale during 8 h [6]

	Passive smokers (P)	Active smokers (A)	Ratio A/P
Smoke particles	0.4–2.4 mg	100 mg	100
Nicotine	0.04–0.2 mg	10–20 mg	100
CO	4–24 mg	200 mg	10–50
Benzo(a)pyrene	4–80 ng	100–500 ng	10–50
Acroleine	0.1–0.5 mg	1.5 mg	3–10
NO_x	0.4–20 mg	2–5 mg	2–6
Formaldehyde	0.5–1.0 µg	0.1–0.4 µg	2–5
Dimethylnitrosamine	40–400 ng	100–500 ng	1–2

Larger effect sizes were also observed for the relationship between selected risk factors and ETS exposure at work than for ETS exposure at home. Among individual risk factors, lower education level was most strongly related to ETS exposure at work [12].

The amounts of inhaled toxic products are lower in passive than active smokers (cf. Table 9.2) [6]. As shown with cultured cells, the toxic action of undiluted side-stream smoke are far more pronounced than those of mainstream smoke [13, 14].

Exposure to tobacco smoke is extensive among the general population [15]. Children, especially in the first months and years of life, are at extreme risk. On the basis of published research from large population samples or on meta-analyses, chiefly from the USA, a number of extensive studies have presented data on the extent of the additional risk to health from several sources, including diet, environmental toxins and alcohol [16].

Three groups may be distinguished in terms of smoke exposure:

1. *Smokers* (who may also be passive smokers at the same time).
2. *Passive smokers* (non-smokers themselves but are exposed to ETS at home or in the workplace).
3. *Non-smokers* (not exposed to ETS either at home or in the workplace).

Non-smokers are at risk in their own homes, in the workplace, at social gatherings and in public buildings. The NHANES III Study [17], published in 1996, presents data on the extent of ETS exposure among the US population and on the contribution of the home and workplace to ETS exposure. The plasma cotinine data illustrated in Fig. 9.1 show that while levels for non-smokers and passive smokers are clearly lower than those for smokers, cotinine can be detected in small amounts in non-smokers and in individuals exposed to ETS (passive smokers).

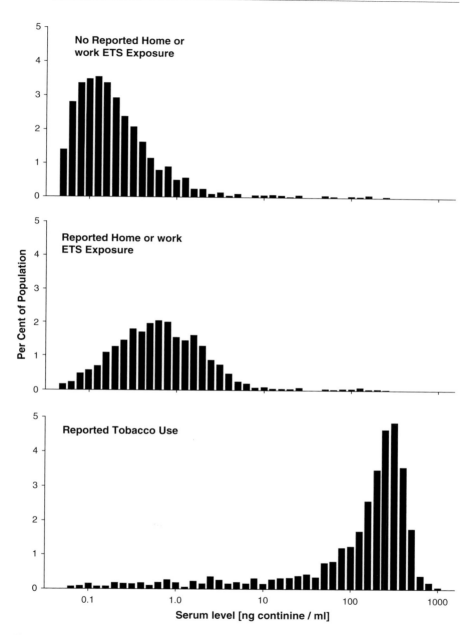

Fig. 9.1   Distribution of serum cotinine levels in a US population (minimum age: 4 years) in non-smokers (*upper panel*), passive smokers (*middle panel*) and smokers (*lower panel*) [17]

9.1
ETS in the Workplace and at Home

If the medical consequences of ETS are to be understood, air monitoring for toxic substances must be performed in cities, rural areas, and in buildings designed for a variety of purposes (offices, public buildings, homes etc.); in addition, on the basis of epidemiological studies ETS exposure must be investigated in comparisons with smokers and non-exposed individuals. For this purpose, depending on circumstances, samples of blood, urine, saliva etc. may be used, as well as determinations of toxic substances (nicotine, cotinine, benzopyrenes, ethenyl pyridine, DNA adducts etc.) in the body [18]. Since 80% of the nicotine absorbed by the body is converted into cotinine, this metabolite can be regarded as a reliable marker [19].

ETS markers also include respirable suspended particulate matter (RSPM), ultraviolet-absorbing particulate matter (UVPM) and fluorescing particulate matter (FPM). Solanesol (SolPM), a terpenoid alcohol from tobacco leaves, as well as nicotine and 3-ethenyl pyridine may also be used. On the basis of human respiratory capacity, the values measured per cubic metre may then be converted to cumulative exposures (expressed, for example, in μg/24 h). Methodological details have now been published concerning the use of ETS constituents as markers of exposure [20, 21].

The problem of incorrect classification of non-smokers, passive smokers and smokers is inherent in all population-based studies because the self-reported smoking status of the subjects recruited is likely to be unreliable. Misinterpretation of the data collected can be avoided to some extent thanks to optimised analytical techniques with improved detection limits [22, 23]. ETS studies have now been published for numerous European and US cities: these will not be discussed further in the present context. With any study, however, it is important to note the sponsor and to check that publication has been preceded by objective and unbiased scientific review [24, 25].

One study conducted in several hundred passive smokers in 12 major US cities indicates that ETS exposure is heavier away from the workplace (Fig. 9.2). Moreover, the differences measured between passive smokers and people not exposed to ETS are clearly evident. According to a study from Basel, workplaces where smoking is permitted make a 34–46% contribution to passive smoking [27]. Heavily ETS-exposed housewives potentially smoke 18 cigarette equivalents/year, while workers who are heavily exposed to ETS in the workplace and at home potentially smoke 61 cigarette equivalents/year [27]. According to a study conducted concurrently in ten countries, an increase in cotinine levels of 5 ng/mg in non-smoking ETS-exposed women was predicted by exposure to 7.2-cigarettes/8 h/40 m^3 from the husband and 17.9 cigarettes/8 h/40 m^3 in the workplace [28].

Restaurant and bar workers constitute one group of passive smokers with particularly high ETS exposure because in many countries it is not possible to ban smoking in restaurants/bars or to separate smokers and non-smokers. Extremely high levels of these toxic products were measured in these locations [29, 30]. A study of barkeepers and other bar staff for ETS exposure compared the bar area with other areas and found that bar staff were clearly more exposed than other staff (Fig. 9.3) [31]. The bar area (and barkeepers) were more heavily exposed to UVPM, FPM, SolPM and the gaseous constituents of ETS than other areas (and other staff). The exception to this general pattern was the concentration of

Fig. 9.2 (**a**, **b**) Comparison of ETS exposure of individuals in and away from the workplace [26]. Mean values in µg/m³ in 24 h. RPr-RAR ($n = 119$): passive smokers both privately and in workplace; RPr-NRAR ($n = 109$): passive smokers privately but not in workplace; NRPr-RAR ($n = 163$): passive smokers in workplace but not privately; NRPr-NRAR ($n = 497$): no ETS exposure either privately or in workplace. *3-EP* 3-ethenyl pyridine; *Nic* nicotine; *RSP* respirable suspended particles; *FPM* fluorescing particulate matter; *Solan* solanesol particulate matter

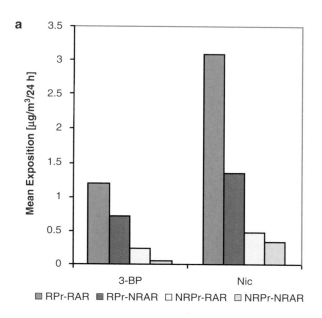

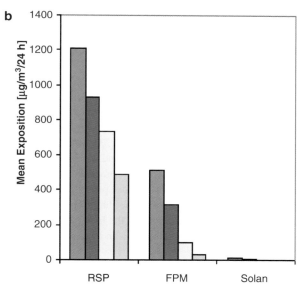

RSPM: in this case, exposure was found to be heavier to other staff than to other areas [31]. Hair nicotine levels were also higher in ETS-exposed staff. Nicotine levels were only lower where there was an absolute ban on smoking [32]. A high proportion of ETS-exposed bar and restaurant staff (77%) reported respiratory tract irritation and 75% of interviewees would have liked some smoking restriction in bars [33].

Despite a high air exchange rate in intercontinental aircraft, considerable differences in cabin air quality have been reported between smoking allowed flights (respirable particles:

Fig. 9.3 Particle concentrations in bar area and other areas, and exposure of barkeepers and other staff. Mean concentrations of ETS components in g/m³ [31]. *RSP* respirable suspended particles; *UVPM* ultraviolet-absorbing particulate matter; *Sol-PM* solanesol particulate matter; *Nic* nicotine

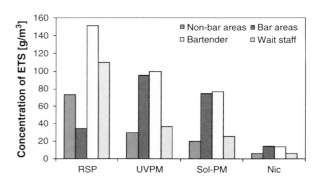

66 ± 56 µg/m³) and smoking-not-allowed flights (3 ± 0.8 µg/m³). ETS exposure on smoking allowed flights is associated with ocular symptoms, decreased tear-film stability, headache and fatigue among cabin attendants and passengers [34]. Despite the spatial separation between smokers and non-smokers on intercontinental flights, non-smoking cabin attendants had higher ETS exposure in the rear cabin section than in the front cabin section [35]. Median urinary cotinine levels in cabin attendants increased from 3.71 (2.08–8.67) µg/g creatinine before take-off to 6.37 (3.98–19) µg/g creatinine after landing; however, attendants working in the front cabin section had no appreciable increase in urinary cotinine levels during the flight [35].

A study performed in Norway tested the hypothesis that nurses' aides who were exposed to ETS at home during childhood have an increased risk of long-term sick leave [36]. The study sample comprised 5,563 Norwegian nurses' aides, who were not on sick leave when they completed a mailed questionnaire in 1999. Of these, 4,744 (85.3%) completed a second questionnaire 15 months later. The outcome measure was the incidence proportion of long-term sick leave during the 12 months prior to the follow-up. It was found that respondents who reported at baseline that they had been exposed to ETS at home during childhood had increased risk of sick leave exceeding 14 days attributed to neck pain (odds ratio (OR), 1.34; 95% confidence interval (CI), 1.04–1.73), high back pain (OR, 1.49; CI, 1.07–2.06), low back pain (OR, 1.21; CI, 0.97–1.50), and any illness (OR, 1.23; CI, 1.07–1.42), after adjustments for demographic and familial characteristics, former smoking, current smoking, physical leisure-time activities, work factors, prior neck injury, and affective symptoms. They also had increased risk of sick leave exceeding 8 weeks (OR, 1.29; CI, 1.08–1.55). The authors concluded that the study supported the hypothesis that nurses' aides who were exposed to ETS at home during childhood have an increased risk of long-term sickness absence [36].

9.2
Changes at the Molecular and Cellular Level

Smokers display increased activity of coagulation variables, including elevations of plasma fibrinogen and platelet reactivity. The rise in fibrinogen levels also causes an increase in viscosity, leading to a deterioration in the flow properties of the blood [37, 38]. In addition, endothelial cells become damaged in response to an increase in total cholesterol (TC) and a reduction in HDL cholesterol (for review, see [37]).

9.2.1
Fibrinogen

Plasma fibrinogen levels in 1,140 Japanese women aged between 45 and 74 years and exposed passively to smoking were compared with those in 524 non-smokers, controlling for age, cholesterol, body mass index, ethanol intake and menopausal status [39]. Plasma fibrinogen concentrations were 8.6 (1.6–15.6) mg/dl higher in women exposed to ETS outside the home, and 11.2 (3.0–19.3) mg/dl higher in women exposed to ETS both in and outside the home. Compared with non-smokers, plasma fibrinogen levels in a subgroup aged 45–59 years were increased by 15.3 mg/dl in women who were exposed to ETS in both locations. Women exposed to ETS only in their own homes showed hardly any elevation of fibrinogen, a finding that is attributable to sociocultural practices in Japan (men tend to spend the evenings with friends away from the home). Compared with cigarette smoke-derived SO_2, NO_2 or ozone, smoke particlulate matter with a diameter <10 μm (PM_{10}) correlate more closely with the increase in fibrinogen [40]. These particles have been assigned causal significance in the development of harmful cardiovascular effects.

9.2.2
Cholesterol

Raised *cholesterol* levels, represented by the total cholesterol/HDL cholesterol (TC/HDL-C) ratio, are regarded as a marker for atherogenic potential and hence for the development of coronary heart disease [41–43]. Cholesterol levels may already be altered in childhood and adolescence [44, 45]. After controlling for dietary factors, the TC/HDL-C ratio was investigated in 444 adolescent schoolchildren (age 14.8 ± 1.6 years), together with cotinine determinations as a marker of passive smoking [46]. Smokers and subjects with very elevated plasma cotinine levels (>25 ng/ml) were excluded from the study. The TC/HDL-C ratio was found to be greater where plasma cotinine levels were ≥2.5 ng/ml (Fig. 9.4). The raised ratios were attributable in particular to lowered HDL cholesterol values, with ETS exposure being associated with an 8.9% greater TC/HDL-C ratio ($p = 0.003$) and a 6.8% lower HDL-C ($p = 0.03$). The disadvantage of the study was that insufficient account was taken of the socioeconomic status of the schoolchildren and their parents, including their dietary habits. Nevertheless, the raised TC/HDL-C ratio measured in passive smokers must be viewed as a risk factor for the development of CHD [47]. Reduced HDL-C levels had already been reported in an earlier study in ETS-exposed children [48].

9.2.3
Endothelium and Platelets

Passive smoking may be expected to cause *endothelial* damage and activation of *platelet* function – additional risk factors for the development of arteriosclerosis [49, 50]. Debris from endothelial cells is encountered increasingly in the bloodstream in response to passive smoking [51–53]. Similarly, increased platelet aggregate formation has been detected both in active [54] and in passive smokers [55].

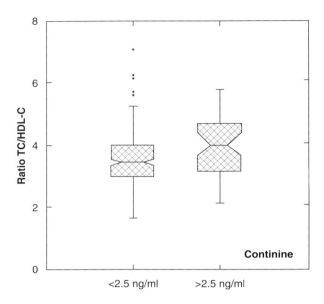

Fig. 9.4 Cholesterol ratio in passive smokers and non-exposed non-smokers. Ratio TC/HDL-C. *Asterisk* indicates outliers [46]

When ten healthy male non-smokers sat for 20 min in an open hospital corridor beside two cigarette smokers already smoking there on their own initiative, the non-smokers' plasma nicotine concentrations rose from 0 to 2.8 ng/ml. Concurrently, their platelet aggregate ratio fell from 0.87 to 0.78, and their endothelial cell count increased from 2.8 to 3.7 per counting chamber. As a result of ETS exposure, carboxyhaemoglobin levels increased from 0.9 to 1.3% (+44%). Although these investigations were conducted in a small study population, the findings have been confirmed by other workers [15, 54–56].

Platelet sensitivity to the anti-aggregatory properties of prostacyclin is lowered by ETS [57]. Platelet aggregation (increase in 2,3-dinor-thromboxane B and in 2,3-dinor-6-keto-prostaglandin F) and oxidative stress (measured by 8-hydroxy-2''-deoxyguanosine) are increased in passive smokers [58].

9.2.4
Markers of Inflammation

Cigarette smoking is known to produce chronic inflammatory responses in the bronchial system, because of increased numbers of neutrophils and macrophages in the blood and lungs [59, 60], leading in turn to oxidative membrane damage [61–64]. Neutrophil functions were studied in eight passive smokers exposed to six active smokers (consuming a maximum of 14 cigarettes) in a poorly ventilated room for 3 h. Passive smoking was associated with significant increases in leucocyte counts (33%), neutrophil chemotaxis (57%) and reactive-oxidant release (71%) [65]. The CO concentration in the room where the experiment was conducted was between 17 and 22 ppm. Although the experimental conditions were not consistent with the home situation, they are comparable to some extent with conditions in nightclubs and discotheques.

Table 9.3 Recurrent respiratory tract infections: a comparison of selected inflammatory variables in children (aged 9–11 years) of smoking and non-smoking parents [66]

Group	n	Infections/ year	TLC (c/mm^3)	EC (c/mm^3)	IL-4 (pg/ml)	IgE (IU/ml)
Children with frequent infections	41	4.5 ± 1.1^a	$7,889 \pm 989^a$	651 ± 121^a	1.8 ± 0.5	605 ± 365
Children with infrequent infections	29	2.0 ± 0.6	$6,771 \pm 1131$	364 ± 85	1.31 ± 0.45	557 ± 354
All children of smoking parents	70	3.4 ± 0.8^b	$7,426 \pm 899^b$	482 ± 96^b	1.6 ± 0.46^b	587 ± 359^b
Children of non-smoking parents	50	1.2 ± 0.6	$6,040 \pm 530$	239 ± 51	0.8 ± 0.5	189 ± 21

TLC total leucocyte count; *EC* eosinophil count; *IL-4* interleukin-4; *IgE* immunoglobulin E
[a] $p < 0.05$, between children of smoking parents
[b] $p < 0.05$: group vs. control

In 79 children exposed to ETS, concentrations of IgE and interleukin-4 (IL-4) and eosinophil counts were higher in cases where the children experienced more frequent respiratory illness (average 3.4 illnesses/year). In contrast, the children of non-smoking parents only experienced 1.2 episodes of respiratory illness/year and their IgE, IL-4 and eosinophil values were unchanged (Table 9.3).

Many studies have shown that cigarette smoking is associated with elevated concentrations of total serum IgE. Few studies, however, have examined total IgE in relation to passive smoking exposure, especially in adults. In a cross-sectional study, Miyake et al. investigated the association of active and passive smoking exposure with levels of total serum IgE in Japan [67]. They examined 981 pregnant women in Osaka and found out that current smoking of at least 15 cigarettes a day and 8.0 or more pack-years of smoking were independently related to an increased prevalence of elevated total serum IgE (aORs 3.40 and 2.51, 95% CIs 2.12–5.47 and 1.55–4.06, respectively), and both cigarette smoking status and pack-years of smoking were significantly positively associated with total serum IgE levels, especially in subjects with a positive familial allergic history. There was no measurable association of exposure to ETS at home or at work with total serum IgE concentrations among those who had never smoked. It was concluded that there is a positive relationship between active smoking and total serum IgE levels; however, this study failed to substantiate a positive association of ETS exposure with total IgE. Investigations with more precise and detailed exposure measurements are warranted [67].

Another study assessed the correlation of ETS exposure with the expression of pro-inflammatory mediators in airway secretions, including IFN-γ and IL-12, as well as IL-5 and IL-13, in allergic asthmatic schoolchildren and healthy control subjects [68]. By using the nasopharyngeal aspiration technique, airway secretions were collected from 24 atopic children with asthma (age, 6–16 years) and 26 healthy control subjects, and the concentration of cytokines was measured with immunoenzymatic methods. It was shown that IL-13 levels were highly increased in patients with asthma ($p < 0.005$), and parental tobacco smoke resulted in a significant increase in airway IL-13 secretion in these children compared with that seen in non-exposed children and healthy control subjects (median, 860 vs. 242 and 125 pg/ml, respectively). Furthermore, a positive correlation between IL-13 levels and serum IgE concentrations (r(s) = 0.55) was found in children with allergic asthma. The study indicated that ETS augments the expression and secretion of IL-13 in allergic asthma and that nasopharyngeal aspiration is a suitable method to assess cytokine measurements in the airways of children. Measurements of IL-13 in secretions might be taken into account as a non-invasive marker of airway inflammation and to assess the detrimental effects of ETS [68].

9.2.5
ETS and Drug Metabolism

The influence of passive smoking in children and adults on the metabolism of medicinal drugs and toxic substances cannot yet be gauged. Where the parents had a minimum 1-pack/day habit, ETS-exposed children displayed intensified metabolism of medicines such as theophylline. Compared with children without ETS exposure, total body clearance of theophylline was significantly elevated (1.36 ± 0.09 vs. 0.90 ± 0.04 ml/min/kg; $p < 0.0001$) and serum concentrations were significantly lower (55.3 ± 2.8 vs. 73.2 ± 3.3 µg/ml; $p < 0.00001$). Hospital stay times were also longer in the group exposed to passive smoking (4.4 ± 2.6 vs. 2.9 ± 1.3 days; $p < 0.05$) [69]. These findings suggest that the metabolism of other medicinal drugs may also be accelerated in children exposed to ETS.

9.3
Passive Smoking During and After Pregnancy

ETS-exposed children born to mothers who smoke during pregnancy are 2–4-times more likely than children without ETS exposure to be born small for gestational age (see Chap. 8) [70]. A 50–100% increase in acute respiratory disorders has been reported in children as a result of passive smoking [71]. Children born to mothers exposed to ETS during pregnancy have increased number of nucleated red blood cells [72], indicating reduced O_2 supplies during pregnancy [73]. The same finding has been made in children born to women who were active smokers during pregnancy [69]. Infants have a 2.5-fold increased risk of dying from sudden infant death syndrome (SIDS) where their mothers continue to smoke after giving birth [1, 74]. The presence of nicotine and cotinine in children's hair after birth is an important marker of foetal exposure to tobacco smoke (Table 9.4) [56]. The detected presence of cotinine (10-50 to >50 ng/nl pericardiac fluid) in four infants is indicative of absorption due to passive smoking [20]. However, it is highly improbable that raised nicotine and cotinine levels in the pericardiac region are contributory factors in SIDS [20].

While there are sufficient data regarding the negative effect of exposure to the constituents of tobacco smoke on newborn infants' birth weights, it is still unclear whether this effect may originate in early pregnancy. Therefore, Hanke et al. evaluated the impact of exposure to tobacco smoke components in early pregnancy (20–24 weeks) on foetal biometry [75].

Table 9.4 Hair concentrations (mean ± SEM) of nicotine and cotinine in women and their newborn infants [56]

	Nicotine (ng/ml)		Cotinine (ng/ml)	
Active smoking women ($n = 36$)	19.2	(4.9)	6.3	(4.0)
Newborns of active smoking women	2.4	(0.9)	2.8	(0.8)
Passive smoking women[a] ($n = 23$)	3.2	(0,8)	0.9	(0.3)[b]
Newborns of passive smoking women	0.28	(0.05)	0.6	(0.15)
Non-smoking women ($n = 35$)	1.2	(0.4)	0.3	(0.06)
Newborns of non-smoking women	0.4	(0.09)	0.26	(0.04)

[a]Defined as regular and steady gestational exposure to other person's cigarette smoke, either at home or in the workplace

[b]$p < 0.01$ when compared to newborns of active smoking women and newborns of non-smokers

The study population comprised 183 women consecutively enrolled at 20–24 weeks of pregnancy at the two antenatal care units and ultrasound biometric measurements of foetal bi-parietal diameter (BPD), abdominal circumference (AC) and femur length (FL) were performed. Also, serum cotinine concentration was determined at 20–24 weeks of gestation by gas chromatography with mass spectrometry detector (GC/MS) to assess ETS exposure during the previous evening and the morning of the same day (blood collection at 1,200–1,300 h). ETS exposure (passive smoking) was assumed to occur when the level of serum cotinine ranged from 2 to 10 ng/ml. The authors demonstrated that a statistically significant negative association was present between the BPD and serum cotinine concentration. A similar association was identified for subjects with serum cotinine concentrations below 10 ng/ml (corresponding to passive smoking) ($p = 0.06$). After controlling for pregnancy duration, maternal pre-pregnancy weight and infant's gender, we found that serum cotinine levels at 20–24 weeks of gestation was inversely associated with infant birth weight ($p = 0.004$). For the subjects with serum cotinine levels below 10 ng/ml, a borderline association ($p = 0.09$) with infant birth weight was found. It was concluded that maternal exposure to tobacco smoke in early pregnancy, as measured by serum cotinine concentrations at 20–24 weeks of gestation, adversely affects foetal BPD [75].

In children with low birth weight following ETS exposure, the vasodilator response following forearm cuff occlusion and release was still reduced at age 9–11 years compared with that in normal birth weight children born to non-smoking mothers. The physiological vasodilator response is triggered by NO release from endothelial cells [76]. Among other things, this harmful effect has its origins in the prenatal period and is related to the smoking behaviour of the mother-to-be during pregnancy; it manifests itself as early as the first decade of life as a prelude to later atherogenic changes. Evidently, in the developmental phases characterised by rapid growth (such as the foetal period), the endothelial cells also undergo adverse changes which limit physiological function [77].

Urinary cotinine levels were determined in 199 ETS-exposed children between the ages of 4 months and 4 years with obstructive bronchitis. Compared with healthy children of the same age, urinary cotinine levels were found to be 5.7 µg/l, instead of 4.4 µg/l. The risk of developing bronchitis was increased in line with the extent of passive smoking and the rise in urinary cotinine. This risk was increased threefold at a urinary cotinine concentration of 20 µg/l [78]. Similar results have been reported in 69 children [79]. The incidence of

spastic bronchitis increased by 14% where maternal tobacco consumption was 4 ciga-
rettes/day, and by 49% at >14 cigarettes/day [80].

ETS-induced hypoxia causes chronic pulmonary hypoventilation in children at the risk
of SIDS [81]. In response to hypoxia, a decline in mitochondrial cytochrome oxidase has
been observed in conjunction with reduced succinate oxidase and palmitoyl carnitine
capacity during circulatory collapse. The brown mitochondria of adipose tissue were activated in response to increased blood flow, causing the tissue apparently to take on a brown
discolouration [82]. The hypoxia hypothesis is thus a more likely starting point for foetal
and postpartum harmful effects, ahead of nicotine and its metabolites.

Although so far demonstrated only in animal experiments (rats), exposure of pregnant
animals to smoke causes the development of hypoplastic lungs with fewer or larger sacculi
and a reduced lung surface area for gas exchange. Transposed to the situation in humans,
this would mean that the pulmonary changes have their origin in utero and are thus consistent with reduced respiratory capacity at birth [52].

Overall, ETS exposure is harmful for paediatric development, starting with the smoking behaviour of the mother (and to a lesser extent, of the father) before birth, but of both
parents after birth. Exposure of children to ETS in rooms where smokers are actively
smoking should be viewed as similarly harmful.

Maternal smoking during and after pregnancy exerts substantial harmful effects on the
health of the neonate or infant [83]: smoking cessation should therefore be encouraged in
the mother either before she becomes pregnant or during the early weeks of pregnancy.

9.4
Cardiovascular Disease

9.4.1
Coronary Heart Disease

CHD is the leading cause of death in various industrialised countries. In 1995, a total of
481,287 people in the USA alone died from the consequences of CHD [76], and active
smoking is one of the key risk factors for its development. Studies have also been published
to indicate that ETS is implicated in CHD [84], and plasma or serum levels of cotinine are a
useful index of smoke exposure [85, 86]. One comprehensive meta-analysis of ten prospective cohort studies and eight case-control studies involving between 513 [87] and 479,680
subjects [88] used myocardial infarction or death from CHD as endpoints. The follow-up
observation period ranged from 6 to 20 years. Even though the assessment criteria for inclusion in the meta-analysis were varied, ETS exposure was associated with a 25% increase
in the risk of acquiring CHD with all its sequelae (Table 9.5). Another meta-analysis has
shown that the risk of CHD in non-smokers was higher when their spouses continued to
smoke (RR, 1.16; CI, 1.06–1.28) than when their spouses were former smokers (RR, 0.98;
CI, 0.89–1.08) [89]. When the number of passively smoked cigarettes and the duration of exposure (years) were taken into account, there was a slight increase in CHD risk compared with
non-smokers (Fig. 9.5) [84]. The relative risk for the development of CHD in ETS-exposed
non-smokers has been estimated at 1.30 (California Environmental Protection Agency,

Table 9.5   Relative risk of coronary heart disease associated with passive smoking among non-smokers [84]

Studies included in the meta-analysis	Number	Relative risk (95% CI)	p-value
All studies	18	1.25 (1.17–1.32)	<0.001
Peer-reviewed studies	15	1.25 (1.17–1.33)	<0.001
Studies using death from AMI or CHD as an outcome measure	14	1.24 (1.17–1.32)	0.001
Studies controlling for important risk factors for CHD	10	1.26 (1.16–1.38)	0.001

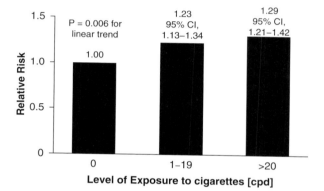

Fig. 9.5   Relative risk of coronary heart disease associated with passive smoking among non-smokers [84]. Number of cigarettes smoked *(above)* and duration of exposure *(below)*. *95% CI* 95% confidence interval

CAEPA) and 1.23 (Scientific Committee on Tobacco and Health, SCOTH) [90]. Platelet aggregation induced by tobacco smoke products has been proposed as the mechanism responsible for this non-linear dose–response anomaly [90].

The purpose of studies by Pitsavos et al. performed in Greece was to investigate the association between passive smoking and the risk of acute coronary syndromes (ACS) among non-smokers [91]. In total, 848 patients with the first event of ACS and 1,078 cardiovascular disease-free matched controls completed a detailed questionnaire regarding their exposure to environmental smoke. Two hundred and ninety-seven (35%) of the patients and 259 (24%) of the controls were defined as non-smokers and passive smokers, respectively. After controlling for several potential confounders, the results showed that non-smokers exposed to cigarette smoke increased the risk of ACS by 51% (OR, 1.51; 95% CI, 1.21–2.99) compared with non-smokers not exposed to smoke. It was estimated that 34 coronary events per 134 subjects would occur as a result of passive smoking during their lifetime. Consequently, this study supported the hypothesis that passive smoking increases the risk of developing ACS [91].

A British study examined the associations between a biomarker of overall passive exposure to tobacco smoke (serum cotinine concentration), and risk of CHD and stroke by the use of a prospective population-based study design (the British regional heart study) [92]. In total, 4,729 men in 18 towns, who provided baseline blood samples (for cotinine assay) and a detailed smoking history in 1978–1980, it was shown that 2,105 men who said they did not smoke and who had cotinine concentrations <14.1 ng/ml were divided into four equal-sized groups on the basis of cotinine concentrations. Relative hazards (95% CIs) for CHD in the second (0.8–1.4 ng/ml), third (1.5–2.7 ng/ml), and fourth (2.8–14.0 ng/ml) quarters of cotinine concentration compared with the first (≥0.7 ng/ml) were 1.45 (1.01–2.08), 1.49 (1.03–2.14), and 1.57 (1.08–2.28), respectively, after adjustment for established risk factors for CHD. Hazard ratios (for cotinine 0.8–14.0 nu ≥0.7 ng/ml) were particularly increased during the first (3.73, 1.32–10.58) and second 5-year follow-up periods (1.95, 1.09–3.48) compared with later periods. There was no consistent association between cotinine concentration and risk of stroke. In conclusion, this study indicated that the studies based on reports of smoking in a partner alone seem to underestimate the risks of exposure to passive smoking. Further prospective studies relating biomarkers of passive smoking to the risk of CHD are needed [92].

However, all ETS-studies clearly show that ETS represents a smaller risk than active smoking in terms of the development of CHD. The findings from a cancer prevention study indicate that the risk of CHD for smokers is 1.7 times higher than for non-smokers, and for women the factor is 1.6 [93]. Related lifestyle variables in passive smokers must be taken into account in a consistent manner if the conclusions reached are to be usable [94, 95]. Various studies suggest that passive smokers differ from non-smokers in terms of diet (less fruit and vegetables, more fat and meat) [96–99]. ETS causes increases in CO and CO-Hb, whereas heart rate and blood pressure rise only minimally [37].

9.4.2
Arteriosclerosis

Cigarette smoking is beyond doubt a major factor in the development of cardiovascular disease [100]. A direct association has been established between carotid artery calcification and smoking [71, 101]. However, crossover studies indicate that ETS exposure also correlates with atherosclerotic changes [71, 102]. The Atherosclerosis Risk in Communities (ARIC) Study investigated the impact of active smoking and of ETS exposure on atherosclerosis progression in 10,914 subjects between 1987 and 1989. Carotid intima-media thickness (IMT) was measured by ultrasound at baseline and again after 3 years, and correlations

Fig. 9.6 Atherosclerosis progression, assessed in terms of the increase in intima-media thickness of the carotid artery within 3 years, in non-smokers (N), past smokers (P) and current smokers (C) and taking ETS exposure (+E) into account. Mean values and 95% CIs [103]

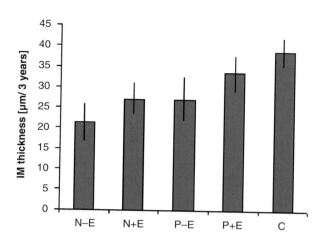

were investigated with other risk factors and lifestyle variables. After adjustment for these factors, it was compared with a carotid IMT in never-smokers of 28.7 μm; current cigarette smokers had a 50% increase (43.0 μm) and passive smokers had a 20% increase (35.2 μm) (Fig. 9.6) [103]. The most pronounced impact was detected in subjects with hypertension and diabetes and in smokers of more than one pack/day. In these subjects, the changes were found to be irreversible even after smoking cessation [103]. Atherosclerosis progression has therefore been demonstrated in response to ETS and the process is irreversible in heavy smokers [104]. The extent of atherosclerosis progression due to ETS is reported to be 34% (5.9 μm) compared with 17.1 μm in smokers [103]. The ARIC Study was the first to demonstrate in a large patient population that, in contrast with non-smoking, ETS causes an 11% progression in atherosclerosis.

Differences in the profile of cardiovascular risk factors may potentially be due to differences in atherosclerosis progression between active smokers and passive smokers [72, 105]. All cardiovascular and lifestyle variables are less implicated than smoking in the progression of atherosclerosis. After a prolonged smoking career, smoking cessation possibly has no influence on progression [106], although other observations suggest that 3–5 years after smoking cessation the risk of cardiovascular events approximates to that in non-smokers [107].

In terms of IMT, diabetic patients show marked atherosclerosis progression because their underlying diabetes is already associated with vascular damage [108]. The relative risk of death from cardiac arrest is 2.5 times higher for smoking than for non-smoking diabetic patients [109]. Other studies also indicate that the smoking diabetic patient is at extreme risk in terms of morbidity and mortality (see Sect. 7.4.2.2 in Chap. 7) [110–112].

To date, however, no correlation has been shown between ETS exposure (number of hours) and atherosclerosis progression [113]. Pack-years of smoking are not crucial for ex-smokers, especially since no differences in atherosclerosis progression have been found in this group between ETS-exposed and non-ETS-exposed individuals. By comparison with non-smokers, the effect of ETS exposure has been demonstrated. IMT is an excellent marker of atherosclerosis progression [114].

9.4.3
Stroke and Subarachnoid Haemorrhage

The risk of acute stroke was investigated in a population-based case-control study from New Zealand in which 521 patients were compared with 1,851 controls [115]. Exposure to ETS among non-smokers and long-term ex-smokers was associated with an increased risk of stroke (OR, 1.82; CI, 1.34–2.49), and the risk increase was greater in men (OR, 2.10; CI, 1.33–3.32) than in women (OR, 1.66; CI, 1.07–2.57) (Fig. 9.7). Active smokers had a four-fold higher risk of stroke compared with people who reported that they had never smoked cigarettes (OR, 4.14; CI, 3.04–5.63), and the risk was increased even further when active smokers were compared with people who had never smoked or had quit smoking more than 10 years earlier and who were not exposed to ETS (OR, 6.33; CI, 4.50–8.91). A further study assessed the independent effect of exposure to ETS on the risk of stroke using a cohort study design among 27,698 lifelong non-smokers with no prior history of stroke (62% women, aged 30–85 years at enrolment; 1979–1985) [116]. Self-reported ETS exposure at home and outside home (in h/week) and stroke risk factors were collected in San Francisco and Oakland and data on follow-up for hospitalization and death was available through the end of 2000 (median = 16 years). It was found in multivariate analysis adjusting for age, race/ethnicity, educational attainment, marital status, hypertension, diabetes and serum TC, ETS exposure at home for 20 h or more/week (in relation to <1 h/week) was associated with a 1.29-fold (95% CI, 0.75–2.20) and a 1.50-fold (95% CI, 1.07–2.09) increased risk of first ischemic stroke among men and women, respectively. No significant associations were found between ETS exposure outside home and ischemic stroke, or between exposure to ETS at home or out of home and the risk of transient ischemic attack. It can be concluded from this study that although potentially important confounders (such as dietary habits) were not included in the analysis, high-level ETS exposure at home was independently associated with increased risk of first ischemic stroke among never-smoking women [116].

It can be stated that:

- Male and female smokers have a clearly increased risk of stroke [117–129].
- ETS also contributes to an increased stroke risk in men and women, although an objective statement concerning the extent of ETS exposure – for example, by measuring cotinine levels – cannot be done so far.

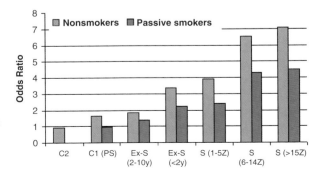

Fig. 9.7 Increased risk of acute stroke: a comparison of non-smokers (group 2), passive smokers (PS, group 1), ex-smokers (<2 years and 2–10 years) and smokers (1–5, 6–14 and >15 cigarettes/day) [115]

For subarachnoid haemorrhage (SAH), one study has examined 432 incident cases of SAH frequency matched to 473 community SAH-free controls to determine dose-dependent associations of active and passive smoking (at home) and smoking cessation with SAH [130]. Compared with never-smokers not exposed to passive smoking, the aOR for SAH among current smokers was 5.0 (95% CI, 3.1–8.1); for past smokers, 1.2 (95% CI, 0.8–2.0); and for passive smokers, 0.9 (95% CI, 0.6–1.5). Current and lifetime exposures showed a clear dose-dependent effect, and risks appeared more prominent in women and for aneurysmal SAH. Approximately 1 in 3 cases of SAH could be attributed to current smoking, but risks decline quickly after smoking cessation, even among heavy smokers. From this study, it was concluded that there is a strong positive association present between cigarette smoking and SAH, especially for aneurysmal SAH and women, which is virtually eliminated within a few years of smoking cessation. Large opportunities exist for preventing SAH through smoking avoidance and cessation programs [130].

9.5
Respiratory Tract

ETS clearly impairs lung function variables. Forced expiratory volume in the first second (FEV_1) and forced vital capacity (FVC) were studied in ETS-exposed workers (Scottish MONICA Survey): FEV_1 fell by 254 (84–420) ml and FVC by 273 (60–480) ml compared with values in workers not exposed to ETS. An inverse correlation between cotinine levels and FVC was found only in those workers who had had blood collected in the morning [131].

When male and female non-smokers were exposed for 7.33 h/day to fresh diluted sidestream smoke with a respirable suspended particle concentration of 179 $\mu g/m^3$, significant reductions in FVC and FEV_1 (1.6%, $p < 0.05$) and in PEF (1.3%, $p < 0.03$) were detected within 5 days [132]. The observed decline in pulmonary function was accompanied by a noradrenaline-induced alteration in blood flow, leading to transient bronchoconstriction [132].

9.5.1
Respiratory Tract in Children and Teenagers

Studies and meta-analyses have focused in particular on the effects of ETS exposure on the respiratory tract in children [78, 133–137]. ETS exposure, airway symptoms and respiratory history were assessed in an urban population of 8,008 randomly selected inhabitants [137]. In never-smokers with childhood ETS exposure, the prevalence of physician-diagnosed asthma was 7.6% compared with 5.9% in non-exposed subjects ($p = 0.036$), and ETS was reported to be the most common lower airway irritant ahead of exercise in cold air, dust, perfume, pollen and pets [137].

A study by Manning et al. examined the prevalence of bronchitis (cough with phlegm) symptoms in teenagers who either smoked cigarettes on a regular basis (active smokers) or were non-smokers but who are exposed to passive smoking (passive smokers) in the home

[138]. The study was undertaken in 1995 and repeated in 1998. The 1995 study was a cross-sectional questionnaire survey of smoking habits in secondary school children aged 13–14 years and was undertaken as part of the ISAAC questionnaire survey. Thirty representative and randomly selected schools from throughout the Republic of Ireland took part in the study. In the 1995 study, 3,066 students completed a questionnaire on their current smoking habits and symptoms of cough and phlegm. The authors found that 634 (20.7%) of these young teenagers actively smoked cigarettes with significantly more females smoking than males with 23.3% of girls compared to 17.6% boys ($p = 0.0001$). Percentage of non-smoking children exposed to smoking in the home (passive smokers) with parental smoking accounting for most of the passive smoking is 46.3%. Bronchitis symptoms were more commonly reported in active smokers compared to non-smokers with an OR of 3.02 (95% CI, 2.34–3.88) ($p < 0.0001$) or in passive smokers compared to those not exposed to smoking with OR of 1.82 (95% CI, 1.32–2.52) ($p < 0.0001$). The 1998 study showed similar results for smoking habits, passive smoking and prevalence of bronchitis symptoms as with the 1995 study. In conclusion, the results of this study documented that increased bronchitis symptoms occur in teenagers exposed to active or passive smoking [138].

A study by Kabesch et al. was performed to determine whether the consequences of parental smoking could be traced in adulthood [139]. Information from interviewer-led questionnaires was available for 18,922 subjects aged 20–44 years from random population samples in 37 areas participating in the European Community Respiratory Health Survey. Lung function data were available for 15,901 subjects. It was found that in men, father's smoking in childhood was associated with more respiratory symptoms (ORwheeze 1.13 (95% CI, 1.00–1.28); never-smokers: ORwheeze 1.21 (95% CI, 0.96–1.50)) and there was a dose-dependent association between number of parents smoking and wheeze (one: OR 1.08 (95% CI, 0.94–1.24); both: OR 1.24 (95% CI, 1.05–1.47); ptrend = 0.010). A reduced ratio of forced expiratory volume in FEV_1 to FVC was related to father's smoking (−0.3% (95% CI, −0.6 to 0)) and number of parents smoking (ptrend <0.001) among men. In women, mother's smoking was associated with more respiratory symptoms and poorer lung function (ORwheeze 1.15 (95% CI, 1.01–1.31), never-smokers: ORwheeze 1.21 (95% CI, 0.98–1.51); FEV1 −24 ml (95% CI, −45 to −3); FEV1/FVC ratio −0.6% (95% CI, −0.9 to −0.3)). These effects were possibly accounted for by maternal smoking in pregnancy (ORwheeze 1.39 (95% CI, 1.17–1.65); FEV1 −23 ml (95% CI, −52 to 7); FEV1/FVC ratio −0.9% (95% CI, −1.3 to −0.4)) as there was no association with paternal smoking among women (interaction by sex, $p < 0.05$). These results were homogeneous across centres. The authors concluded that both intrauterine and environmental exposure to parental tobacco smoking was related to more respiratory symptoms and poorer lung function in adulthood in this multicultural study. The age window of particular vulnerability appeared to differ by sex, postnatal exposure being important only in men and a role for prenatal exposure being more evident in women [139]. Only one study focussed on the effects of domestic passive smoking by narghile (water pipe) and/or cigarettes on the development of respiratory ailments among children aged 10–15 years [140]. In this study, students were recruited from five private schools in Beirut, and information on demographic, in-home smoking, and students' respiratory tract illnesses (cough, wheezing, runny nose, or nasal congestion) were collected from each participant (results: of 625 students surveyed, 438 (70.1%) had at least one individual smoking at home). Compared with the non-exposed group, the OR of having respiratory illness for children exposed to narghile or cigarette smoke were 2.3 (95% CI, 1.1–5.1) and 3.2 (95% CI, 1.9–5.4), respectively. It can be concluded that domestic passive smoking of the misconceived "innocuous" habitual smoking device, narghile, is associated with significant respiratory health ailments [140]. Only one study has reported a reduced risk of respiratory illness in children exposed to ETS. In children exposed to the smoke of >15 cigarettes/day, ETS was associated with cellular infiltrates in the nasal mucosa containing increased numbers of IgE+ cells and eosinophils but not of IgE+ mast cells. It is concluded that exposure to ETS produces reactions resembling those seen in the nasal mucosa of allergic children [141].

Parental atopy is an important marker of response in ETS-exposed children [132]. Parental atopy alone has been shown to increase the risk of bronchial obstruction (OR, 1.62; CI, 1.10–2.40) and asthma (OR, 1.66; CI, 1.08–2.54). In children without parental atopy, the effect of ETS exposure on risk for both symptoms was clearly less pronounced (bronchial obstruction: OR, 1.29; CI, 0.88–1.89; and asthma: OR, 0.84; CI, 0.53–1.34). The presence of parental atopy and ETS exposure increased the risks substantially (bronchial obstruction: OR, 2.88; CI, 1.91–4.32; and asthma: OR, 2.68; CI, 1.70–4.22), indicating that ETS exposure and genetic constitution should in future be considered jointly as trigger factors for these respiratory problems [142].

Urinary cotinine levels, measured using the cotinine/creatinine ratio (CCR), were significantly lower in asthmatic children living in homes with a total smoking ban (7.6 nmole/mmole) [143]. Children's CCR levels from homes in which smoking was allowed in rooms the children rarely frequented (14.1 nmole/mmole) were lower than those in children from homes where unrestricted smoking was allowed (26.0 nmole/mmole) [143].

The risk of respiratory illness with possible hospitalisation was increased in ETS-exposed children (up to 3 years of age) by 57% where both parents smoke and by 72% where only the mother smoked. Smoking by other household members in families where the mother does not smoke was associated with a 29% risk increase. Evidence for a dose-dependent increase in lower respiratory tract illness has also been demonstrated in most studies in which this has been investigated [144]. The increased risk of ETS-induced lung disease in children resulting primarily from the harmful effects of maternal smoking has been confirmed in numerous studies (Table 9.6) [145]. In any event, this is a causal phenomenon.

Table 9.6   Parental smoking and respiratory tract infections in infancy and early childhood: ORs and 95% CIs [144]

	Both parents	Mother	Father
All studies	1.57 (1.42–1.74)	1.72 (1.55–1.91)	1.29 (1.16–1.44)
Community-based studies on lower respiratory tract infections, bronchitis and/or pneumonia	1.54 (1.31–1.80)	1.57 (1.33–1.86)	a
Community-based studies on childhood wheeze	1.55 (1.16–2.08)	2.08 (1.59–2.71)	a
Hospital admission for lower respiratory illness, bronchitis, bronchiolitis or pneumonia	1.71 (1.21–2.40)	1.53 (1.25–1.86)	1.32 (0.87–2.00)

aNo conclusion possible because of insufficient number of studies

One survey of 43,732 adults in the USA assessed the number of days on which respiratory symptoms had occurred during the 2 weeks prior to the survey. Only 20.2% of never-smokers and 23.1% of former smokers reported ETS-induced symptoms at home or in the workplace, compared with 87.2% of current smokers [146]. Among never-smokers, people who were exposed to ETS were more likely to report one or more days of restricted activity (RR, 1.27; CI, 1.10–1.46), one or more days of bed confinement (RR, 1.43; CI, 1.19–1.73) and one or more days of work absence (RR, 1.33; CI, 1.05–1.73). These correlations were less strong for former smokers and current smokers. Overall, never-smokers (RR, 1.47; CI, 1.34–1.62), former smokers (RR, 1.22; CI, 1.07–1.39) and current smokers (RR, 1.31; CI, 1.10–1.56) exposed to ETS were more likely to report a less than very good health status than were people without such exposure. Overall, during the 2 weeks covered by the survey, exacerbations of chronic respiratory illness were reported in 1.8% of never-smokers, 2.6% of former smokers and 2.7% of current smokers. It may be concluded that never-smokers exposed to ETS report greater health impairment than smokers. Additional ETS exposure also increased respiratory symptoms in former and current smokers [146].

A study conducted in 4,281 children aged 0–4 years concluded that 45% of very young children live in households with at least one current smoker; the current smoker was the child's own mother in 28.5% of cases and the father in 31.8% [147]. In non-smoking households, bronchial asthma was reported in 9.3% and asthma wheeze in 19.8% of children. In smoking households, asthma wheeze was detected in 38% of children where mothers smoked less than 15 cigarettes/day (47% of the mothers), and in 70% of children where maternal cigarette consumption was >15 cigarettes/day. The corresponding figures for bronchial asthma were 33 and 76% [147], and quantitative associations were found between cigarette consumption and asthma symptoms in the children (<15 vs. >15 cigarettes/day; OR, 1.33; CI, 0.98–1.81 vs. OR, 1.76; CI, 1.36–2.12; $p < 0.001$). On the basis of this study, it was calculated that 13% of bronchial asthma or asthma wheeze in 0- to 4-year-old Australian children in 1989–1990 was due to maternal smoking, and this conclusion is confirmed by other studies [133, 148–150]. The effects of ETS on childhood wheeze are particularly pronounced among children exposed to two smokers, especially where the mother has smoked during pregnancy and the diagnosis of bronchial asthma was made during the first year of life [151]. In these cases, ETS operates as a co-factor with intercurrent infections as a trigger for wheezing attacks.

It is assumed furthermore that parents who model smoking also encourage smoking in their children at a later date [133, 150, 152]. Compared with non-asthmatic children of smokers, children with bronchial asthma from smoker households have plasma nicotine levels that are twofold higher for the same exposure, a finding also confirmed by cotinine determinations in urine and hair (see also Table 9.4) [153]. It may thus be assumed that the renal excretion of nicotine and its metabolite is delayed in these children [153].

Another meta-analysis of respiratory tract changes induced by passive smoking and covering 21 publications from the period 1966 to 1995 reached the following conclusions:

- As a result of ETS exposure, infants and young children (<2 years of age) have a twofold higher risk (OR, 1.93; CI, 1.66–2.25) of developing lower respiratory tract infections with subsequent hospitalisation.
- In older children (3–6 years old), the OR is lower (1.25; CI, 0.88–1.78) [154].

In some cases, the risk was more than doubled where the children had a low birth weight (<2.5 kg) or were still very young [78, 155].

Infants and young children possibly show increased susceptibility to respiratory tract infections because:

- Their immune system is less well developed [156].
- Mucociliary clearance is still developing, possibly in conjunction with the additional harmful effects of the toxic substances present in mainstream and side-stream cigarette smoke [157].
- Their epithelium (due to the action of NO_2) displays increased sensitivity to pathogenic bacteria [158].

9.5.2
Bronchial Carcinoma

The association between cigarette smoking and the development of small cell lung cancer in men and of adenocarcinoma, mainly in women, is incontrovertible. Less certain is the question as to whether cancers of this type may also develop following exposure to ETS [159–161]. However, studies in preschool children of smoking and non-smoking mothers have revealed the presence of polycyclic aromatic hydrocarbon–albumin (PAH-albumin) adducts – components of ETS with carcinogenic potential (Table 9.7) [162].

The literature contains contradictory findings concerning the carcinogenicity of ETS. One study of ETS exposure and lung cancer risk has reported lower ORs for ETS from all sources combined (OR, 1.39; CI, 0.96–2.01) than for ETS in the workplace (OR, 1.93; CI, 1.04–3.58) and ETS in vehicles (OR, 2.64; CI, 1.30–5.36) [163]. The workplace and other public indoor settings are thus identified as important risk factors for the passive smoker in terms of lung cancer development. One meta-analysis cites similar ORs for various ETS-exposed groups [16].

In particular, several genetic components – polymorphisms of N-acetyltransferase (NAT2) and glutathione S-transferase (GSTM1) – have been considered in the development

Table 9.7 Cotinine and PAH-albumin levels in mothers and their preschool children (mean ± SE) [162]

	Cotinine (ng/ml)		PAH-albumin level (fmole/μg)	
Active smoking women ($n = 31$)	170	(21.2)	0.80	(0.15)
Preschool children of active smoking women	4.14	(0.54)	0.35	(0.07)
Passive smoking women[a] ($n = 32$)	1.64	(0.97)	0.49	(0.08)
Preschool children of passive smoking women	0.87	(0.20)[b]	0.18	(0.04)[c]
Non-smoking women ($n = 24$)	0.96	(0.79)	0.31	(0.08)
Preschool children of non-smoking women	0.25	(0.12)	0.15	(0.02)

[a]Exposure to ETS at home from other household members and visitors
[b]Levels in preschool children in households with ETS exposure were significantly higher ($p < 0.01$) than those in children in non-smoking households
[c]Levels in preschool children in households with ETS exposure were not significantly higher than those in children in non-smoking

of lung cancer [164–170]. No differences in GST polymorphism have been discovered between active smokers and passive smokers [171]. NAT2 slow acetylators evidently display reduced metabolism of carcinogenic arylamines. In addition, a significant association has been demonstrated between GST M1 (allele 0: GSTM1-0) and lung cancer (OR, 1.41; CI, 1.23–1.61) [172]. Smokers with the GSTM1(null) genotype have considerably higher PAH–DNA adduct levels than smokers with the GSTM1(+) genotype [170]. Combination of GSTM1-0 together with two allelic variants of cytochrome P4501A1 (m2/m2 and Val/Val) further increases the risk of lung cancer (see Table 5.3 in Chap. 5). Combination of GSTM1-0 and NAT2 slow acetylation is associated with a 7.8-fold increase (CI: 1.4–78.7) in the risk of bronchial carcinoma [172]. The non-smoker is at greater risk as a slow acetylator, whereas the smoker is at a greater risk as a rapid acetylator, as a function of pack-years of smoking [168, 173]. Other authors have disputed this association. NAT1 polymorphism is reported to be important for the development of lung cancer [174]. p53 mutations are clearly increased in smokers compared with ex-smokers and non-smokers (OR, 9.08; CI, 2.06–39.98), whereas K-ras mutations displayed no differences between the various groups defined in terms of smoker status [175].

Early studies on ETS exposure in women focused on countries in Asia and the Far East: increased cancer risks were reported for ETS-exposed women who also inhaled carcinogens from cooking oils at high temperatures [176–178]. As an additional factor, these ETS-exposed women may also themselves have been smokers in the past. Epidemiological studies from the USA and other industrialised countries have shown a slight but detectable risk increase for bronchial carcinoma in passive smokers: in New Zealand, for example, relative risks of 1.3 (CI: 1.1–1.5) have been reported for both men and women exposed to passive smoking at home, and of 2.2 (CI: 1.4–3.0) for both men and women exposed to passive smoking in the workplace [179, 180]. In a further study, the risk of lung cancer more than doubled for women who reported 40 or more smoke-years of household exposure during adulthood (OR, 2.4; CI, 1.1–5.3), or 22 or more-smoke-years of exposure during childhood or adolescence (OR, 2.4; CI, 1.1–5.4) [181]. Recent research has confirmed that never-smoking women exposed to ETS from spouses are at increased risk of lung cancer compared with unexposed never-smoking women (OR, 1.29; CI, 1.17–1.43) [161].

The possible association between ETS exposure during childhood and the development of bronchial carcinoma in later years has been investigated in a multicentre case-control study (Fig. 9.8). While the association was rejected on the basis of the results [182], weak evidence emerged for a positive correlation emerged between the risk of lung cancer and exposure to workplace and spousal ETS [182].

Other studies have reported lower lung cancer risk levels for passive smokers (OR, 1.3; CI, 0.8–1.8) [183–185]. The risk of lung cancer was increased where ETS exposure occurred at a young age: the risk was highest for children exposed below the age of 7 years (OR, 3.46; CI, 1.80–6.65), but was also significant for children aged between 7 and 14 years (OR, 3.08; CI, 1.62–5.57) and for adolescents aged between 15 and 22 years (OR, 3.10; CI, 1.52–6.31) [186]. Similarly, high risk rates have been recorded in women whose husbands smoked particularly strong Russian cigarettes known as "papirosy" (OR, 2.12; CI, 1.32–3.40) [187]. The data recorded in ETS-exposed children were not confirmed in another study [182] or the lung cancer risk was increased only for women exposed

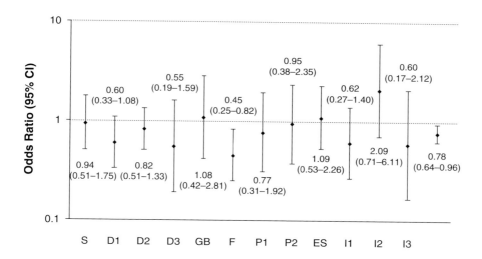

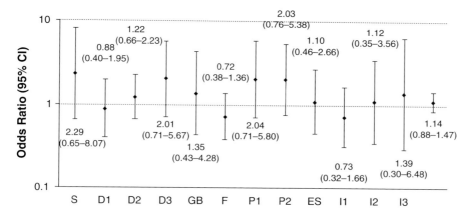

Fig. 9.8 Risk of bronchial carcinoma (odds ratio (OR)) associated with passive smoking, based on studies in various countries [170]. *Upper panel*: ETS exposure during childhood; heterogeneity test between centres: $\chi^2 = 10.45$, df = 11, $p = 0.49$. *Lower panel*: Exposure to workplace or spousal ETS; heterogeneity: $\chi^2 = 6.76$, df = 11, $p = 0.82$. *Ov* overall

to ETS in the workplace (OR, 1.5; CI, 0.8–3.0) [188]. In a comparison of 3,138 ETS-exposed non-smoking women with 1,747 smoking women, death from bronchial carcinoma was recorded in 0.2% of non-exposed non-smoking women, 0.9% of the ETS-exposed non-smoking women and 8.0% of the women who smoked, indicating that ETS-exposed women had a 4.5-fold higher risk of lung cancer than non-exposed non-smokers [189].

Not all studies ever conducted to assess the risk of lung cancer with ETS exposure can be accepted [190]. While an evaluation of numerous studies indicates that the excess risk of lung cancer is 24% [190], it is recommended that all the data should be re-analysed with caution. Similar risk increases have been reported for ETS-exposed women (24%) and men (34%) [191]. According to another meta-analysis of ETS exposure and lung cancer based on 14 published studies, the increase in lung cancer risk is 39% for non-smoking women whose husbands smoke 25 cigarettes/day, and 91% where ETS exposure occurs predominantly in the workplace [192].

In ETS-exposed non-smokers, additional radon exposure is reported to be particularly dangerous in terms of the development of lung cancer (maximal OR increase from 1.08 [0.8–1.5] to 1.44 [1.0–2.1]) [193].

9.6
Complications of Anaesthesia

In younger children, in particular, ETS exposure is associated with delayed growth of the lungs, with reduced FEV_1 and diminished respiratory capacity [194–196]. ETS exposure causes an increase in children's plasma cotinine levels [197–202]. Since cotinine has an elimination half-life of 19–40 h, the plasma cotinine level reflects smoke exposure over the preceding 3–4 days [199]. N_2O/O_2-halothane anaesthesia was implemented as indicated in 575 children aged between 1 month and 12 years who were free from respiratory tract and cardiovascular disease. The children's urine was collected for the determination of cotinine levels. At the end of anaesthesia, the recovery room nurse documented any airway complications that may have occurred. Urinary cotinine levels (>40 ng cotinine/ml urine) correlated with the number of unwanted complications of anaesthesia (OR, 2.3; CI, 1.2–4.5; Fig. 9.9). Children whose parents smoked >30 cigarettes/day had a 44% airway complication rate, compared with only 25.5% in children whose parents were non-smokers [203]. The urinary cotinine levels measured in the children were too low for them to have been active smokers themselves. Ultimately, the incidence of airway complications following anaesthesia is doubled when the parents are smokers [203]!

A study by Reisli et al. evaluated the effects of ETS on onset and recovery time after single dose of rocuronium in children. Forty children between 4 and 10 years were enrolled

Fig. 9.9 Unwanted respiratory complications in 88 out of 365 children with a urinary cotinine level <10 ng/ml, in 30 out of 91 children with an intermediate urinary cotinine level, and in 18 out of 43 children (42%) with a urinary cotinine level >40 ng/ml (significant differences between the groups; $p = 0.01$) [203]

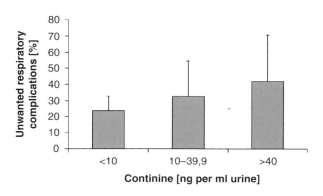

into the study [204]. Children who have no familial smoking history were included in the first group whereas passive smokers included in the second group. Sevoflurane in 50% O_2 and 50% N_2O was used for induction of anaesthesia. Evoked adductor pollicis electromyography was used to monitor neuromuscular block. The T95 and T25 values were recorded. It was shown that the T95 values ($\pm SD$) for rocuronium were 110.1 ± 39.3 s and 79.3 ± 35.6 s for group 1 and group 2, respectively ($p < 0.05$). The T25 value of group 2 was 40.1 ± 10.6 min; compared with group 1 values (30.85 ± 7.02 min), it was significantly longer ($p < 0.01$). Therefore, it can be concluded that passive smoking children consume less rocuronium than non-smokers during similar anaesthesia. A history of passive smoking must also be taken into consideration during preoperative evaluation of paediatric patients [204].

Overall, it should be noted that:

- Girls are more susceptible than boys to such complications [205, 206] because of the more favourable ratio of respiratory tract to lung size in boys [206, 207].
- Girls respond more sensitively than boys to cholinergic stimuli [208].
- Low maternal socioeconomic status is associated with persistent lower respiratory tract infections and influences the complication rate [209].
- According to one retrospective study, laryngospasm is ten times more common in children exposed to ETS compared with non-exposed children [210].
- Oxygen desaturation following anaesthesia was observed more frequently in the recovery room in ETS-exposed children than in non-exposed children [211].
- By using a pre-anaesthesia questionnaire or by determining urinary cotinine-levels, the paediatric anaesthetist should take steps to prevent those complications of anaesthesia that are more likely to occur in ETS-exposed children.

9.7
Otitis Media

Otitis media affects up to 46% of young children up to the age of 3 years and is the condition most commonly prompting medical consultations in this age group (Table 9.8) [213–217].

Table 9.8 Influence of maternal smoking on the risk of otitis media in young children. Calculations based on a multivariate logistic regression model [212]

Variable	Odds ratio (95% CI)	p
Number of cigarettes smoked (<10 vs. ≥10)	1.89 (1.22–2.91)	0.004
Child's place of residence during the first year of life (household vs. day care vs. private creche)	2.94 (1.55–5.54)	0.001
Maternal educational level (<12 vs. ≥13 years)	1.55 (1.05–2.30)	0.03
Doctor visits (number during the past 12 months)		
≤3	1.00	
4–10	2.50 (1.70–3.67)	<0.001
≥11	2.01 (0.96–4.18)	0.06

Fig. 9.10 Correlation between hair cotinine concentration and number of smokers in household, according to parental self-report. Medians including 25th and 75th percentiles. Data outside the confidence range. Significant differences between the groups ($p = 0.03$) [212]

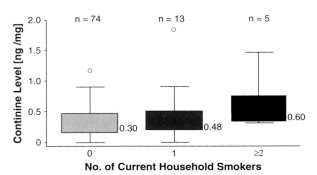

Moreover, otitis media frequently marks the starting point for surgical intervention [74, 213]. Since 38–60% of young children are exposed to ETS in their parents' homes, passive smoking is an important factor in the development of this condition [218–221]. The frequency of otitis media, surgery and antimicrobial therapy during the preceding 12 months was assessed (hair cotinine measurements, physician medical records, home visits) in a study in 227 cases and 398 healthy controls who satisfied the inclusion criteria for the study (Fig. 9.10) [212]. Otitis media developed in 23.9% of the children and 9.8% had to undergo myringotomy. Children exposed to ETS had a 2–3 times higher risk of otitis media than non-exposed children (Table 9.8). These results are consistent with those reported in other studies [222–225] (OR, 1.80; CI, 1.1–3.0 [222]).

To estimate the relative risk for otitis media (OM) in children from ETS, maternal smoking during pregnancy (gestational exposure), or both, a national cross-sectional health survey was analysed by the use of questionnaire information and serum cotinine measurements [226]. Children younger than 12 years ($N = 11,728$) were examined who participated in the Third National Health and Nutrition Examination Survey (NHANES III), conducted from 1988 to 1994. The outcome of the study was the occurrence and recurrence of ear infections. It was found that the cumulative incidence of ear infections was 69%. Of all participants, 38% were exposed to passive smoke, 23% were exposed to gestational smoke, and 19% were exposed to combined passive and gestational smoke. The occurrence of any ear infection was not increased by passive smoke exposure (adjusted risk ratio [RR], 1.01; 95% CI, 0.95–1.06), but was slightly increased by gestational (adjusted RR, 1.08; 95% CI, 1.01–1.14) and combined (adjusted RR, 1.07; 95% CI, 1.00–1.14) smoke exposures. The risk of recurrent ear infections (≥6 lifetime episodes) was significantly increased with combined smoke exposure (adjusted RR, 1.44; 95% CI, 1.11–1.81). Other risk factors for ear infection identified in multivariable analysis were race/ethnicity, poverty–income ratio of 2.00 or more, attendance in day care, history of asthma and presence of allergic symptoms. From this study, it can be concluded that passive smoke exposure was not associated with an increased risk of ever developing an ear infection. The increased risk found with gestational and combined smoke exposures has marginal clinical significance. For recurrent ear infections, however, combined smoke exposure had a clinically and statistically significant effect [226].

9.8
Meningococcal Infections

Sepsis and meningitis caused by *Neisseria meningitidis* frequently have a fatal outcome, and tobacco smoke should be regarded as a vehicle for the nasopharyngeal transport of the bacteria [227–229]. In particular, NO_2 from tobacco smoke increases the incidence of viral respiratory tract infections [230]; by impairing defence mechanisms, the gas encourages viral spread on the mucosa. Cigarette smoke inhibits mucociliary clearance, increases bacterial adhesion and ruptures respiratory tract epithelium [231–233]. In vitro experiments indicate that tobacco smoke harms neutrophil migration, and inhibits the phagocytic activity of macrophages and the production of immunoglobulins [231, 232, 234].

Passive smokers are more likely than individuals not exposed to ETS to be infected by pathogenic meningococci. Alongside numerous other causes [235], ETS is an important factor in promoting meningococcal infection in young children [236–238]. In a comparison of 129 cases with 274 controls matched for age, sex, ethnic group etc., having a mother who smoked was the strongest independent risk factor for invasive meningococcal disease in children <18 years of age, compared with non-smoking mothers (OR, 3.8; CI, 1.6–8.9; $p < 0.01$). This risk was additionally increased where the children were in school classes of >30 pupils (OR, 5.7; CI, 1.3–24.2; $p = 0.02$). Similarly, the risk of meningococcal infection showed a dose–response relationship with increasing number of maternal pack-years of smoking. Ultimately, according to this study the incidence of meningococcal infection in ETS-exposed children was 37% higher than in non-exposed children. Younger children (<5 years old) were at greater risk than older children (5–17 years old) [235].

In view of the risk of meningococcal infection, frequently a fatal condition, it is therefore recommended that mothers with young children should give up smoking.

9.9
Breast Cancer

Although a causal association between passive smoking and an increased risk of breast cancer is not immediately evident [239] (see Sect. 7.8.4 in Chap. 7), initial findings indicate that an association does exist. Evidently, in genetically "sensitive" individuals [240–242] the inhaled ETS produces hormonal changes consistent with an anti-oestrogen effect and oestrogen-induced mitogenesis [243, 244]. According to a study conducted in 334 women with breast cancer, ever-active smokers had an OR of 2.0 (CI: 1.1–3.6) when compared with never-active, never-passive smokers. Risk levels were higher in women who smoked only before their first pregnancy (OR, 5.6; CI, 1.5–21) and in women who quit smoking 5–15 years before their index year (OR, 3.9; CI, 1.4–10). Passive-only smokers had an OR of 2.0 (CI: 1.1–3.7). Among those women who were exposed to ETS before the age of 12 years, the ORs were 4.5 (CI: 1.2–16) for passive-only smokers, and 7.5 (CI: 1.6–36) for ever-active smokers [245]. It is possible that ETS exposure needs to occur at a very early stage, shortly before the development of breast tissue, in order to induce mitogenic changes consistent with carcinogenesis [246]. More extensive studies are certainly required in this area before a definitive verdict can be given.

Johnson and Glantz compared the strength of evidence from epidemiologic studies of second hand smoke of the US Surgeon General's 1986 conclusion that secondhand smoke caused lung cancer with the California Environmental Protection Agency's (CalEPA) similar 2005 conclusion on breast cancer in younger, primarily premenopausal women [247]. They reviewed each report for criteria used to assess causality: number of studies, statistically significant increases in risk, and pooled summary risk estimates. The authors showed that both the Surgeon General and CalEPA used updated Bradford Hill criteria for assessing causality and found that the evidence met those criteria. Six of 13 lung cancer studies (46%) had statistically significant increases (one of three cohort studies). Pooled risk estimates for lung cancer for spousal exposure were 1.53 for ten combined case-control studies and 1.88 for seven studies with dose–response results. The CalEPA reported 10 of 14 studies (71%) had statistically significant increases in breast cancer risk (two of four cohort studies). Pooled relative risk estimates for younger, primarily premenopausal women were 1.68 (95% CI: 1.33, 2.12) for all exposed women and 2.19 (95% CI: 1.68, 2.84) for five studies with better exposure assessment. It was concluded that the evidence from epidemiologic studies of passive smoke in 2005 for breast cancer in younger, primarily premenopausal women was stronger than for lung cancer in 1986.

9.10
Psychosocial Changes

Children exposed to ETS display behavioural changes that can be linked with ETS. Within a family setting, lifestyle habits evolve (e.g. smoking, fat consumption, sedentary lifestyle increased alcohol consumption) which in turn may be regarded as risk factors for the children because they adopt these lifestyle habits [248, 249]. Body measurements were performed in a study of 804 children aged 10–12 years; additionally, smoking behaviour and dietary characteristics were identified. Among the children from these families, 19% of boys and 10% of girls were already smokers. Among the children who smoked, 57% (boys) and 68% (girls) came from families in which at least one parent smoked (OR, 2.1; CI, 1.2–3.8). In the longer term, however, girls were less likely to adopt the smoking habits of their parents (OR, 0.4; CI, 0.2–0.6). Parental smoking behaviour was an additive predictor in children of lower physical activity and more television watching, regardless of which parent smoked. Children's fat intake was significantly greater if either parent smoked, whereas children's body mass index and waist-to-hip ratio were significantly greater if mothers smoked [250].

Overall, children who grow up in "smoker households" take health risks upon themselves regardless of the risks already present as a result of smoking during pregnancy [251]. Parental smoking is formative in encouraging an unhealthy lifestyle in children, expressed as a preference for sitting around [96], earlier alcohol consumption [252], increased fat intake [252, 253] or an accumulation of these unhealthy behaviours [254]. The smoking habits of the children also correlate with those of their parents, as has been demonstrated in several studies [255–257]. Readers are referred to Chap. 12 for further discussion of this aspect.

9.11
Concluding Remarks

The data presented in the literature permit a range of conclusions, several of which are of major importance in terms of public health policy:

- Adult non–smokers exposed to ETS become ill more frequently than non-smokers without ETS exposure, prompting the conclusion that smoking should be banned in the workplace and in public buildings.
- Non-smokers and smokers should be educated about the dangers of ETS, the objective being to reduce or prevent ETS in their own homes.
- Any study of the medical consequences of smoking and any comparison with the situation in non-smokers must always consider the role played by ETS because this factor already leads to health-related changes.
- Despite contradictory data, it has now been proved that extensive ETS exposure (a minimum of 20–30 pack-years) increases the risk of bronchial carcinoma by at least 30%, and in extreme cases this risk may be increased two- to threefold. Ethnic differences appear to exist, with Asian populations being at even greater risk than those in Western Europe or North America.
- Female smokers planning to become pregnant or unexpectedly becoming pregnant should make every effort to stop smoking either before pregnancy or during the first weeks of pregnancy. They should also refrain from smoking during the first years after their child has been born. The same applies for fathers living in the same household.
- The mother is the key figure in determining a healthy lifestyle for the family, and this should be the starting point increasingly for health education programmes in future.
- Before infants and young children undergo a general anaesthetic, parental smoking status should always be ascertained. Where parents are smokers, the risk of anaesthetic complications during the recovery phase is doubled. Urinary cotinine measurements can be helpful in this context.
- If the health of the majority is not to be further endangered by ETS, there is an urgent need to introduce strict legislation for the protection of non-smokers (Fig. 9.11).
- The general population should also be kept aware of the latest findings on ETS: the danger to health must be clearly communicated so that children and adolescents in particular are protected effectively.

Fig. 9.11   Poster from the German Museum for Public Health (Deutsches Hygiene-Museum) encouraging smokers to show consideration for the non-smoking majority (source: DHM 1995-641)

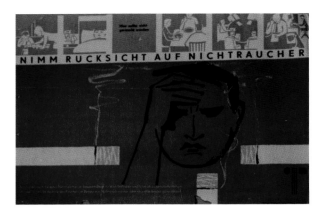

References

1. Hammond SK, Sorensen G, Youngstrom R, Ockene JK (1995) Occupational exposure to environmental tobacco smoke. JAMA 274:956–960
2. Manuel J (1999) Double exposure. Environmental tobacco smoke. Environ Health Perspect 107:A196–A201
3. Lee PN (1986) Passive smoking. Br J Cancer 54:1019–1021
4. Lee PN, Chamberlain J, Alderson MR (1986) Relationship of passive smoking to risk of lung cancer and other smoking-associated diseases. Br J Cancer 54:97–105
5. Vutuc C (1984) Quantitative aspects of passive smoking and lung cancer. Prev Med 13:698–704
6. Remmer H (1987) Passively inhaled tobacco smoke: a challenge to toxicology and preventive medicine. Arch Toxicol 61:89–104
7. Kauppinen T, Toikkanen J, Pedersen D, Young R, Ahrens W, Boffetta P, et al (2000) Occupational exposure to carcinogens in the European Union. Occup Environ Med 57(1):10–18
8. Drope J, Chapman S (2001) Tobacco industry efforts at discrediting scientific knowledge of environmental tobacco smoke: a review of internal industry documents. J Epidemiol Community Health 55(8):588–594
9. Nellen MA, De Blij BA (1999) The "success" of Philip Morris' campaign on environmental tobacco smoke in The Netherlands. Tob Control 8:221–222
10. Anonym (1995) Second hand smoke: is it a hazard? Consume Rep 20:27–33
11. Glantz SA, Parmley WW (1995) Passive smoking and heart disease. Mechanisms and risk. JAMA 273:1047–1053
12. Stamatakis KA, Brownson RC, Luke DA (2002) Risk factors for exposure to environmental tobacco smoke among ethnically diverse women in the United States. J Womens Health Gend Based Med 11(1):45–51
13. Leuchtenberger C, Leuchtenberger R, Zbinden I (1974) Gas vapour phase constituents and-SH reactivity of cigarette smoke influence lung cultures. Nature 247:565–567
14. Sonnenfeld G, Griffith RB, Hudgens RW (1985) The effect of smoke generation and manipulation variables on the cytotoxicity of mainstream and sidestream cigarette smoke to monolayer cultures of L-929 cells. Arch Toxicol 58:120–122
15. Davis RM (1997) Passive smoking: history repeats itself. BMJ 315:961–962
16. Zhong L, Goldberg MS, Parent ME, Hanley JA (2000) Exposure to environmental tobacco-smoke and the risk of lung cancer: a meta-analysis. Lung Cancer 27(1):3–18

17. Pirkle JL, Flegal KM, Bernert JT, Brody DJ, Etzel RA, Maurer KR (1996) Exposure of the US population to environmental tobacco smoke: the Third National Health and Nutrition Examination Survey, 1988 to 1991. JAMA 275:1233–1240

18. Vainiotalo S, Vaaranrinta R, Tornaeus J, Aremo N, Hase T, Peltonen K (2001) Passive monitoring method for 3-ethenylpyridine: a marker for environmental tobacco smoke. Environ Sci Technol 35(9):1818–1822

19. Benowitz NL (1996) Cotinine as a biomarker of environmental tobacco smoke exposure. Epidemiol Rev 18:188–204

20. LaKind JS, Ginevan ME, Naiman DQ, James AC, Jenkins RA, Dourson ML, et al (1999) Distribution of exposure concentrations and doses for constituents of environmental tobacco smoke. Risk Anal 19:375–390

21. LaKind JS, Jenkins RA, Naiman DQ, Ginevan ME, Graves CG, Tardiff RG (1999) Use of environmental tobacco smoke constituents as markers for exposure. Risk Anal 19:359–373

22. Phillips K, Bentley MC, Howard DA, Alvan G (1998) Assessment of environmental tobacco smoke and respirable suspended particle exposures for nonsmokers in Prague using personal monitoring. Int Arch Occup Environ Health 71:379–390

23. Wells AJ, English PB, Posner SF, Wagenknecht LE, Perez-Stable EJ (1998) Misclassification rates for current smokers misclassified as nonsmokers. Am J Public Health 88:1503–1509

24. Barnes DE, Bero LA (1996) Industry-funded research and conflict of interest: an analysis of research sponsored by the tobacco industry through the Center for Indoor Air Research. J Health Polit Policy Law 21:515–542

25. Bero LA, Glantz SA (1993) Tobacco industry response to a risk assessment of environmental tobacco smoke. Tobacco Control 2:103–113

26. Jenkins RA, Palausky MA, Counts RW, Guerin MR, Dindal AB, Bayne CK (1996) Determination of personal exposure of non-smokers to environmental tobacco smoke in the United States. Lung Cancer 14(Suppl 1):S195–S213

27. Phillips K, Howard DA, Bentley MC, Alván G (1999) Assessment of environmental tobacco smoke and respirable suspended particle exposures for nonsmokers on Basel by personal monitoring. Atmos Environ 33:1889–1904

28. Riboli E, Preston-Martin S, Saracci R, Haley NJ, Trichopoulos D, Becher H, et al (1990) Exposure of nonsmoking women to environmental tobacco smoke: a 10-country collaborative study. Cancer Causes Control 1:243–252

29. Hiller FC, McCusker KT, Mazumder MK, Wilson JD, Bone RC (1982) Deposition of sidestream cigarette smoke in the human respiratory tract. Am Rev Respir Dis 125:406–408

30. Mitchell RI (1962) Controlled measurement of smoke-particle retention in the respiratory tract. Am Rev Respir Dis 85:526–533

31. Maskarinec MP, Jenkins RA, Counts RW, Dindal AB (2000) Determination of exposure to environmental tobacco smoke in restaurant and tavern workers in one US city. J Expo Anal Environ Epidemiol 10(1):36–49

32. Al Delaimy W, Fraser T, Woodward A (2001) Nicotine in hair of bar and restaurant workers. N Z Med J 114(1127):80–83

33. Jones S, Love C, Thomson G, Green R, Howden-Chapman P (2001) Second-hand smoke at work: the exposure, perceptions and attitudes of bar and restaurant workers to environmental tobacco smoke. Aust N Z J Public Health 25(1):90–93

34. Wieslander G, Lindgren T, Norback D, Venge P (2000) Changes in the ocular and nasal signs and symptoms of aircrews in relation to the ban on smoking on intercontinental flights. Scand J Work Environ Health 26(6):514–522

35. Lindgren T, Willers S, Skarping G, Norback D (1999) Urinary cotinine concentration in flight attendants, in relation to exposure to environmental tobacco smoke during intercontinental flights. Int Arch Occup Environ Health 72:475–479

36. Eriksen W (2004) Do people who were passive smokers during childhood have increased risk of long-term work disability? A 15-month prospective study of nurses' aides. Eur J Public Health 14(3):296–300
37. Haustein KO (1999) Smoking tobacco, microcirculatory changes and the role of nicotine. Int J Clin Pharmacol Ther 37:76–85
38. Wilhelmsen L, Svardsudd K, Korsan-Bengtsen K, Larsson B, Welin L, Tibblin G (1984) Fibrinogen as a risk factor for stroke and myocardial infarction. N Engl J Med 311:501–505
39. Iso H, Shimamoto T, Sato S, Koike K, Iida M, Komachi Y (1996) Passive smoking and plasma fibrinogen concentrations. Am J Epidemiol 144:1151–1154
40. Schwartz J (2001) Air pollution and blood markers of cardiovascular risk. Environ Health Perspect 109(Suppl 3):405–409
41. Brischetto CS, Connor WE, Connor SL, Matarazzo JD (1983) Plasma lipid and lipoprotein profiles of cigarette smokers from randomly selected families: enhancement of hyperlipidemia and depression of high-density lipoprotein. Am J Cardiol 52:675–680
42. Criqui MH, Wallace RB, Heiss G, Mishkel M, Schonfeld G, Jones GT (1980) Cigarette smoking and plasma high-density lipoprotein cholesterol. The Lipid Research Clinics Program Prevalence Study. Circulation 62:IV70–IV76
43. Freedman DS, Srinivasan SR, Shear CL, Hunter SM, Croft JB, Webber LS, et al (1986) Cigarette smoking initiation and longitudinal changes in serum lipids and lipoproteins in early adulthood: the Bogalusa Heart Study. Am J Epidemiol 124:207–219
44. Gordon T, Castelli WP, Hjortland MC, Kannel WB, Dawber TR (1977) High density lipoprotein as a protective factor against coronary heart disease. The Framingham Study. Am J Med 62: 707–714
45. Wallace RB, Anderson RA (1987) Blood lipids, lipid-related measures, and the risk of atherosclerotic cardiovascular disease. Epidemiol Rev 9:95–119
46. Feldman J, Shenker IR, Etzel RA, Spierto FW, Lilienfield DE, Nussbaum M, et al (1991) Passive smoking alters lipid profiles in adolescents. Pediatrics 88:259–264
47. Helsing KJ, Sandler DP, Comstock GW, Chee E (1988) Heart disease mortality in nonsmokers living with smokers. Am J Epidemiol 127:915–922
48. Moskowitz WB, Mosteller M, Schieken RM, Bossano R, Hewitt JK, Bodurtha JN, et al (1990) Lipoprotein and oxygen transport alterations in passive smoking preadolescent children. The MCV Twin Study. Circulation 81:586–592
49. Fuster V, Chesebro JH (1981) Antithrombotic therapy: role of platelet-inhibitor drugs. I. Current concepts of thrombogenesis: role of platelets (first of three parts). Mayo Clin Proc 56:102–112
50. Ross R (1986) The pathogenesis of atherosclerosis – an update. N Engl J Med 314:488–500
51. Prerovsky I, Hladovec J (1979) Suppression of the desquamating effect of smoking on the human endothelium by hydroxyethylrutosides. Blood Vessels 16:239–240
52. Collins MH, Moessinger AC, Kleinerman J, Bassi J, Rosso P, Collins AM, et al (1985) Fetal lung hypoplasia associated with maternal smoking: a morphometric analysis. Pediatr Res 19(4): 408–412
53. Renaud S, Blache D, Dumont E, Thevenon C, Wissendanger T (1984) Platelet function after cigarette smoking in relation to nicotine and carbon monoxide. Clin Pharmacol Ther 36:389–395
54. Davis JW, Hartman CR, Lewis HD Jr, Shelton L, Eigenberg DA, Hassanein KM, et al (1985) Cigarette smoking – induced enhancement of platelet function: lack of prevention by aspirin in men with coronary artery disease. J Lab Clin Med 105:479–483
55. Davis JW, Shelton L, Watanabe IS, Arnold J (1989) Passive smoking affects endothelium and platelets. Arch Intern Med 149:386–389
56. Eliopoulos C, Klein J, Phan MK, Knie B, Greenwald M, Chitayat D, et al (1994) Hair concentrations of nicotine and cotinine in women and their newborn infants. JAMA 271:621–623
57. Burghuber OC, Punzengruber C, Sinzinger H, Haber P, Silberbauer K (1986) Platelet sensitivity to prostacyclin in smokers and non-smokers. Chest 90:34–38

58. Smith CJ, Fischer TH, Heavner DL, Rumple MA, Bowman DL, Brown BG, et al (2001) Urinary thromboxane, prostacyclin, cortisol, and 8-hydroxy-2'-deoxyguanosine in nonsmokers exposed and not exposed to environmental tobacco smoke. Toxicol Sci 59(2):316–323

59. Corre F, Lellouch J, Schwartz D (1971) Smoking and leucocyte-counts. Results of an epidemiological survey. Lancet 2:632–634

60. Ludwig PW, Schwartz BA, Hoidal JR, Niewoehner DE (1985) Cigarette smoking causes accumulation of polymorphonuclear leukocytes in alveolar septum. Am Rev Respir Dis 131: 828–830

61. Anderson R, Theron AJ, Ras GJ (1987) Regulation by the antioxidants ascorbate, cysteine, and dapsone of the increased extracellular and intracellular generation of reactive oxidants by activated phagocytes from cigarette smokers. Am Rev Respir Dis 135:1027–1032

62. Hoidal JR, Fox RB, LeMarbe PA, Perri R, Repine JE (1981) Altered oxidative metabolic responses in vitro of alveolar macrophages from asymptomatic cigarette smokers. Am Rev Respir Dis 123:85–89

63. Hoidal JR, Niewoehner DE (1982) Lung phagocyte recruitment and metabolic alterations induced by cigarette smoke in humans and in hamsters. Am Rev Respir Dis 126:548–552

64. Ludwig PW, Hoidal JR (1982) Alterations in leukocyte oxidative metabolism in cigarette smokers. Am Rev Respir Dis 126:977–980

65. Anderson R, Theron AJ, Richards GA, Myer MS, van Rensburg AJ (1991) Passive smoking by humans sensitizes circulating neutrophils. Am Rev Respir Dis 144:570–574

66. el Nawawy A, Soliman AT, el Azzouni O, Amer e, Demian S, el Sayed M (1996) Effect of passive smoking on frequency of respiratory illnesses and serum immunoglobulin-E (IgE) and interleukin-4 (IL-4) concentrations in exposed children. J Trop Pediatr 42:166–169

67. Miyake Y, Miyamoto S, Ohya Y, Sasaki S, Matsunaga I, Yoshida T, Hirota Y, Oda H (2004) Relationship between active and passive smoking and total serum IgE levels in Japanese women: baseline data from the Osaka Maternal and Child Health Study. Int Arch Allergy Immunol 135(3):221–228

68. Feleszko W, Zawadzka-Krajewska A, Matysiak K, Lewandowska D, Peradzyńska J, Dinh QT, Hamelmann E, Groneberg DA, Kulus M (2006) Parental tobacco smoking is associated with augmented IL-13 secretion in children with allergic asthma. J Allergy Clin Immunol 117(1): 97–102

69. Mayo PR (2001) Effect of passive smoking on theophylline clearance in children. Ther Drug Monit 23(5):503–505

70. Misra DP, Nguyen RH (1999) Environmental tobacco smoke and low birth weight: a hazard in the workplace? Environ Health Perspect 107(Suppl 6):897–904

71. Howard G, Burke GL, Szklo M, Tell GS, Eckfeldt J, Evans G, et al (1994) Active and passive smoking are associated with increased carotid wall thickness. The Atherosclerosis Risk in Communities Study. Arch Intern Med 154:1277–1282

72. Willard JC, Schoenborn CA (1995) Relationship between cigarette smoking and other unhealthy behaviors among our nation's youth: United States, 1992. Adv Data 24(263):1–11

73. Yeruchimovich M, Dollberg S, Green DW, Mimouni FB (1999) Nucleated red blood cells in infants of smoking mothers. Obstet Gynecol 93:403–406

74. Black N (1984) Surgery for glue ear – a modern epidemic. Lancet 1:835–837

75. Hanke W, Sobala W, Kalinka J (2004) Environmental tobacco smoke exposure among pregnant women: impact on fetal biometry at 20–24 weeks of gestation and newborn child's birth weight. Int Arch Occup Environ Health 77(1):47–52

76. Leeson CP, Whincup PH, Cook DG, Donald AE, Papacosta O, Lucas A, et al (1997) Flow-mediated dilation in 9- to 11-year-old children: the influence of intrauterine and childhood factors. Circulation 96:2233–2238

77. Widdowson EM, McCance RA (1975) A review: new thoughts on growth. Pediatr Res 9:154–156

78. Rylander E, Pershagen G, Eriksson M, Nordvall L (1993) Parental smoking and other risk factors for wheezing bronchitis in children. Eur J Epidemiol 9:517–526
79. Schulte-Hobein B, Schwartz-Bickenbach D, Abt S, Plum C, Nau H (1992) Cigarette smoke exposure and development of infants throughout the first year of life: influence of passive smoking and nursing on cotinine levels in breast milk and infant's urine. Acta Paediatr 81(6–7): 550–557
80. Neuspiel DR, Rush D, Butler NR, Golding J, Bijur PE, Kurzon M (1989) Parental smoking and post-infancy wheezing in children: a prospective cohort study. Am J Public Health 79(2):168–171
81. Naeye RL (1980) Abruptio placentae and placenta previa: frequency, perinatal mortality, and cigarette smoking. Obstet Gynecol 55(6):701–704
82. Reid GM, Tervit H (1991) Sudden infant death syndrome (SIDS) and disordered blood flow. Med Hypotheses 36(3):295–299
83. Taylor B, Wadsworth J (1987) Maternal smoking during pregnancy and lower respiratory tract illness in early life. Arch Dis Child 62:786–791
84. He J, Vupputuri S, Allen K, Prerost MR, Hughes J, Whelton PK (1999) Passive smoking and the risk of coronary heart disease – a meta-analysis of epidemiologic studies. N Engl J Med 340: 920–926
85. Tunstall-Pedoe H, Brown CA, Woodward M, Tavendale R (1995) Passive smoking by self report and serum cotinine and the prevalence of respiratory and coronary heart disease in the Scottish heart health study. J Epidemiol Community Health 49:139–143
86. Wagenknecht LE, Manolio TA, Sidney S, Burke GL, Haley NJ (1993) Environmental tobacco smoke exposure as determined by cotinine in black and white young adults: the CARDIA Study. Environ Res 63:39–46
87. Humble C, Croft J, Gerber A, Casper M, Hames CG, Tyroler HA (1990) Passive smoking and 20-year cardiovascular disease mortality among nonsmoking wives, Evans County, Georgia. Am J Public Health 80:599–601
88. Steenland K, Thun M, Lally C, Heath C Jr (1996) Environmental tobacco smoke and coronary heart disease in the American Cancer Society CPS-II cohort. Circulation 94:622–628
89. Thun M, Henley J, Apicella L (1999) Epidemiologic studies of fatal and nonfatal cardiovascular disease and ETS exposure from spousal smoking. Environ Health Perspect 107(Suppl 6): 841–846
90. Smith CJ, Fischer TH, Sears SB (2000) Environmental tobacco smoke, cardiovascular disease, and the nonlinear dose–response hypothesis. Toxicol Sci 54(2):462–472
91. Pitsavos C, Panagiotakos DB, Chrysohoou C, Tzioumis K, Papaioannou I, Stefanadis C, Toutouzas P (2002) Association between passive cigarette smoking and the risk of developing acute coronary syndromes: the CARDIO2000 study. Heart Vessels 16(4):127–130
92. Whincup PH, Gilg JA, Emberson JR, Jarvis MJ, Feyerabend C, Bryant A, Walker M,Cook DG (2004) Passive smoking and risk of coronary heart disease and stroke: prospective study with cotinine measurement. BMJ 329(7459):200–205
93. Labarthe DR (1998) Smoking and other tobacco use. In: Epidemiology and prevention of cardiovascular diseases: a global challenge. Aspen, Gaithersburg, MD, pp 323–346
94. Aronow WS (1978) Effect of passive smoking on angina pectoris. N Engl J Med 299:21–24
95. Denson KWE (1996) Smoke in the face, diet, and harm to the heart. Lancet 348(1663):1664
96. Matanoski G, Kanchanaraksa S, Lantry D, Chang Y (1995) Characteristics of nonsmoking women in NHANES I and NHANES I epidemiologic follow-up study with exposure to spouses who smoke. Am J Epidemiol 142:149–157
97. Osler M (1998) The food intake of smokers and nonsmokers: the role of partner's smoking behavior. Prev Med 27:438–443
98. Thornton A, Lee P, Fry J (1994) Differences between smokers, ex-smokers, passive smokers and non-smokers. J Clin Epidemiol 47:1143–1162
99. Sidney S, Caan BJ, Friedman GD (1989) Dietary intake of carotene in nonsmokers with and without passive smoking at home. Am J Epidemiol 129:1305–1309

100. Law MR, Morris JK, Wald NJ (1997) Environmental tobacco smoke exposure and ischaemic heart disease: an evaluation of the evidence. BMJ 315:973–980

101. Tell GS, Polak JF, Ward BJ, Kittner SJ, Savage PJ, Robbins J (1994) Relation of smoking with carotid artery wall thickness and stenosis in older adults. The Cardiovascular Health Study. The Cardiovascular Health Study (CHS) Collaborative Research Group. Circulation 90: 2905–2908

102. Diez-Roux AV, Nieto FJ, Comstock GW, Howard G, Szklo M (1995) The relationship of active and passive smoking to carotid atherosclerosis 12–14 years later. Prev Med 24:48–55

103. Howard G, Wagenknecht LE, Burke GL, Diez-Roux A, Evans GW, McGovern P, et al (1998) Cigarette smoking and progression of atherosclerosis: The Atherosclerosis Risk in Communities (ARIC) Study. JAMA 279:119–124

104. Li R, Duncan BB, Metcalf PA, Crouse JR III, Sharrett AR, Tyroler HA, et al (1994) B-mode-detected carotid artery plaque in a general population. Atherosclerosis Risk in Communities (ARIC) Study Investigators. Stroke 25:2377–2383

105. Kannel WB, Wolf PA, Castelli WP, D'Agostino RB (1987) Fibrinogen and risk of cardiovascular disease. The Framingham Study. JAMA 258:1183–1186

106. Tell GS, Howard G, McKinney WM, Toole JF (1989) Cigarette smoking cessation and extracranial carotid atherosclerosis. JAMA 261:1178–1180

107. Rich-Edwards JW, Manson JE, Hennekens CH, Buring JE (1995) The primary prevention of coronary heart disease in women. N Engl J Med 332:1758–1766

108. Deckert T, Feldt-Rasmussen B, Borch-Johnsen K, Jensen T, Kofoed-Enevoldsen A (1989) Albuminuria reflects widespread vascular damage. The Steno hypothesis. Diabetologia 32: 219–226

109. Ford ES, Merritt RK, Heath GW, Powell KE, Washburn RA, Kriska A, et al (1991) Physical activity behaviors in lower and higher socioeconomic status populations. Am J Epidemiol 133: 1246–1256

110. Gay EC, Cai Y, Gale SM, Baron A, Cruickshanks KJ, Kostraba JN, et al (1992) Smokers with IDDM experience excess morbidity. The Colorado IDDM Registry. Diabetes Care 15:947–952

111. Stamler J, Vaccaro O, Neaton JD, Wentworth D (1993) Diabetes, other risk factors, and 12-yr cardiovascular mortality for men screened in the Multiple Risk Factor Intervention Trial. Diabetes Care 16:434–444

112. Suarez L, Barrett-Connor E (1984) Interaction between cigarette smoking and diabetes mellitus in the prediction of death attributed to cardiovascular disease. Am J Epidemiol 120: 670–675

113. Wagenknecht LE, Burke GL, Perkins LL, Haley NJ, Friedman GD (1992) Misclassification of smoking status in the CARDIA study: a comparison of self-report with serum cotinine levels. Am J Public Health 82:33–36

114. Chambless LE, Heiss G, Folsom AR, Rosamond W, Szklo M, Sharrett AR, et al (1997) Association of coronary heart disease incidence with carotid arterial wall thickness and major risk factors: the Atherosclerosis Risk in Communities (ARIC) Study, 1987–1993. Am J Epidemiol 146:483–494

115. Bonita R, Duncan J, Truelsen T, Jackson RT, Beaglehole R (1999) Passive smoking as well as active smoking increases the risk of acute stroke. Tob Control 8:156–160

116. Iribarren C, Darbinian J, Klatsky AL, Friedman GD (2004) Cohort study of exposure to environmental tobacco smoke and risk of first ischemic stroke and transient ischemic attack. Neuroepidemiology 23(1–2):38–44

117. Bonita R, Scragg R, Stewart A, Jackson R, Beaglehole R (1986) Cigarette smoking and risk of premature stroke in men and women. Br Med J (Clin Res Ed) 293:6–8

118. Gill JS, Shipley MJ, Tsementzis SA, Hornby R, Gill SK, Hitchcock ER, et al (1989) Cigarette smoking. A risk factor for hemorrhagic and nonhemorrhagic stroke. Arch Intern Med 149:2053–2057

119. Haheim LL, Holme I, Hjermann I, Leren P (1996) Smoking habits and risk of fatal stroke: 18 years follow up of the Oslo Study. J Epidemiol Community Health 50:621–624

120. Kawachi I, Colditz GA, Stampfer MJ, Willett WC, Manson JE, Rosner B, et al (1993) Smoking cessation and decreased risk of stroke in women. JAMA 269:232–236

121. Lindenstrom E, Boysen G, Nyboe J (1993) Lifestyle factors and risk of cerebrovascular disease in women. The Copenhagen City Heart Study. Stroke 24:1468–1472

122. Meade TW, Mellows S, Brozovic M, Miller GJ, Chakrabarti RR, North WR, et al (1986) Haemostatic function and ischaemic heart disease: principal results of the Northwick Park Heart Study. Lancet 2:533–537

123. Wannamethee SG, Shaper AG, Whincup PH, Walker M (1995) Smoking cessation and the risk of stroke in middle-aged men. JAMA 274:155–160

124. Wolf PA, D'Agostino RB, Kannel WB, Bonita R, Belanger AJ (1988) Cigarette smoking as a risk factor for stroke. The Framingham Study. JAMA 259:1025–1029

125. Shinton R, Beevers G (1989) Meta-analysis of relation between cigarette smoking and stroke. BMJ 298:789–794

126. Berger K, Schulte H, Stogbauer F, Assmann G (1998) Incidence and risk factors for stroke in an occupational cohort: the PROCAM Study. Prospective Cardiovascular Muenster Study. Stroke 29:1562–1566

127. Bonita R, Broad JB, Beaglehole R (1997) Ethnic differences in stroke incidence and case fatality in Auckland, New Zealand. Stroke 28:758–761

128. Donnan GA, McNeil JJ, Adena MA, Doyle AE, O'Malley HM, Neill GC (1989) Smoking as a risk factor for cerebral ischaemia. Lancet 2:643–647

129. Zhang X, Shu XO, Yang G, Li HL, Xiang YB, Gao YT, Li Q, Zheng W (2005) Association of passive smoking by husbands with prevalence of stroke among Chinese women nonsmokers. Am J Epidemiol 161(3):213–218

130. Anderson CS, Feigin V, Bennett D, Lin RB, Hankey G, Jamrozik K (2004) Active and passive smoking and the risk of subarachnoid hemorrhage: an international population-based case-control study. Stroke 35(3):633–637

131. Chen R, Tunstall-Pedoe H, Tavendale R (2001) Environmental tobacco smoke and lung function in employees who never smoked: the Scottish MONICA study. Occup Environ Med 58(9): 563–568

132. Smith CJ, Bombick DW, Ryan BA, Morton MJ, Doolittle DJ (2001) Pulmonary function in nonsmokers following exposure to sidestream cigarette smoke. Toxicol Pathol 29(2): 260–264

133. Charlton A (1994) Children and passive smoking: a review. J Fam Pract 38:267–277

134. Colley JR, Holland WW, Corkhill RT (1974) Influence of passive smoking and parental phlegm on pneumonia and bronchitis in early childhood. Lancet 2:1031–1034

135. Leeder SR, Corkhill RT, Irwig LM, Holland WW (1976) Influence of family factors on asthma-and wheezing during the first five years of life. Br J Prev Soc Med 30:213–218

136. Tager IB, Hanrahan JP, Tosteson TD, Castile RG, Brown RW, Weiss ST, et al (1993) Lung function, pre- and post-natal smoke exposure, and wheezing in the first year of life. Am Rev Respir Dis 147:811–817

137. Larsson ML, Frisk M, Hallstrom J, Kiviloog J, Lundback B (2001) Environmental tobacco smoke exposure during childhood is associated with increased prevalence of asthma in adults. Chest 120(3):711–717

138. Manning P, Goodman P, Kinsella T, Lawlor M, Kirby B, Clancy L (2002) Bronchitis symptoms in young teenagers who actively or passively smoke cigarettes. Ir Med J 95(7):202–204

139. Svanes C, Omenaas E, Jarvis D, Chinn S, Gulsvik A, Burney P (2004) Parental smoking in childhood and adult obstructive lung disease: results from the European Community Respiratory Health Survey. Thorax 59(4):295–302

140. Tamim H, Musharrafieh U, El Roueiheb Z, Yunis K, Almawi WY (2003) Exposure of children to environmental tobacco smoke (ETS) and its association with respiratory ailments. J Asthma 40(5):571–576

141. Vinke JG, KleinJan A, Severijnen LW, Fokkens WJ (1999) Passive smoking causes an 'allergic' cell infiltrate in the nasal mucosa of non-atopic children. Int J Pediatr Otorhinolaryngol 51: 73–81

142. Jaakkola JJ, Nafstad P, Magnus P (2001) Environmental tobacco smoke, parental atopy, and childhood asthma. Environ Health Perspect 109(6):579–582

143. Wakefield M, Banham D, Martin J, Ruffin R, McCaul K, Badcock N (2000) Restrictions on smoking at home and urinary cotinine levels among children with asthma. Am J Prev Med 19(3): 188–192

144. Strachan DP, Cook DG (1997) Health effects of passive smoking. 1. Parental smoking and lower respiratory illness in infancy and early childhood. Thorax 52:905–914

145. DiFranza JR, Lew RA (1996) Morbidity and mortality in children associated with the use of tobacco products by other people. Pediatrics 97:560–568

146. Mannino DM, Siegel M, Rose D, Nkuchia J, Etzel R (1997) Environmental tobacco smoke exposure in the home and worksite and health effects in adults: results from the 1991 National Health Interview Survey. Tob Control 6:296–305

147. Lister SM, Jorm LR (1998) Parental smoking and respiratory illnesses in Australian children aged 0–4 years: ABS 1989–90 National Health Survey results. Aust N Z J Public Health 22: 781–786

148. Infante-Rivard C (1993) Childhood asthma and indoor environmental risk factors. Am J Epidemiol 137:834–844

149. Stoddard JJ, Miller T (1995) Impact of parental smoking on the prevalence of wheezing respiratory illness in children. Am J Epidemiol 141:96–102

150. Haby MM, Peat JK, Woolcock AJ (1994) Effect of passive smoking, asthma, and respiratory infection on lung function in Australian children. Pediatr Pulmonol 18:323–329

151. Gilliland FD, Li YF, Peters JM (2001) Effects of maternal smoking during pregnancy and environmental tobacco smoke on asthma and wheezing in children. Am J Respir Crit Care Med 163(2):429–436

152. Peat JK (1997) Environmental tobacco smoke. In: Barnes P, et al (ed) Asthma. Lippincott-Raven, Philadelphia, pp 12–33

153. Knight JM, Eliopoulos C, Klein J, Greenwald M, Koren G (1998) Pharmacokinetic predisposition to nicotine from environmental tobacco smoke: a risk factor for pediatric asthma. J Asthma 35:113–117

154. Li JS, Peat JK, Xuan W, Berry G (1999) Meta-analysis on the association between environmental tobacco smoke (ETS) exposure and the prevalence of lower respiratory tract infection in early childhood. Pediatr Pulmonol 27:5–13

155. Chen Y (1994) Environmental tobacco smoke, low birth weight, and hospitalization for respiratory disease. Am J Respir Crit Care Med 150:54–58

156. Abel EL (1980) Smoking during pregnancy: a review of effects on growth and development of offspring. Hum Biol 52:593–625

157. Spektor DM, Yen BM, Lippmann M (1989) Effect of concentration and cumulative exposure of inhaled sulfuric acid on tracheobronchial particle clearance in healthy humans. Environ Health Perspect 79:167–172

158. Koenig JQ (1987) Pulmonary reaction to environmental pollutants. J Allergy Clin Immunol 79:833–843

159. Boffetta P, Tredaniel J, Greco A (2000) Risk of childhood cancer and adult lung cancer after childhood exposure to passive smoke: a meta-analysis. Environ Health Perspect 108(1):73–82

160. Sugita M, Izuno T, Kanamri M, Otahara Y, Kasuga H (1998) Per capita gross national product and summarized odds ratio for epidemiologic studies on the relationship between passive smoking and lung cancer. Tokai J Exp Clin Med 23:235–240

161. Taylor R, Cumming R, Woodward A, Black M (2001) Passive smoking and lung cancer: a cumulative meta-analysis. Aust N Z J Public Health 25(3):203–211

162. Crawford FG, Mayer J, Santella RM, Cooper TB, Ottman R, Tsai WY, et al (1994) Biomarkers of environmental tobacco smoke in preschool children and their mothers. J Natl Cancer Inst 86:1398–1402
163. Kreuzer M, Krauss M, Kreienbrock L, Jockel KH, Wichmann HE (2000) Environmental tobacco smoke and lung cancer: a case-control study in Germany. Am J Epidemiol 151(1): 241–250
164. Henning S, Cascorbi I, Munchow B, Jahnke V, Roots I (1999) Association of arylamine N-acetyltransferases NAT1 and NAT2 genotypes to laryngeal cancer risk. Pharmacogenetics 9:103–111
165. Hirvonen A (1999) Chapter 20. Polymorphic NATs and cancer predisposition. IARC Sci Publ (148)251–270
166. Hirvonen A (1995) Genetic factors in individual responses to environmental exposures. J Occup Environ Med 37:37–43
167. Martinez C, Agundez JA, Olivera M, Martin R, Ladero JM, Benitez J (1995) Lung cancer and-mutations at the polymorphic NAT2 gene locus. Pharmacogenetics 5:207–214
168. Nyberg F, Hou SM, Hemminki K, Lambert B, Pershagen G (1998) Glutathione S-transferase mu1 and N-acetyltransferase 2 genetic polymorphisms and exposure to tobacco smoke in nonsmoking and smoking lung cancer patients and population controls. Cancer Epidemiol Biomarkers Prev 7:875–883
169. Seow A, Zhao B, Poh WT, Teh M, Eng P, Wang YT, et al (1999) NAT2 slow acetylator genotype is associated with increased risk of lung cancer among non-smoking Chinese women in Singapore. Carcinogenesis 20:1877–1881
170. Butkiewicz D, Grzybowska E, Phillips DH, Hemminki K, Chorazy M (2000) Polymorphisms of the GSTP1 and GSTM1 genes and PAH-DNA adducts in human mononuclear white blood cells. Environ Mol Mutagen 35(2):99–105
171. Malats N, Camus-Radon AM, Nyberg F, Ahrens W, Constantinescu V, Mukeria A, et al (2000) Lung cancer risk in nonsmokers and GSTM1 and GSTT1 genetic polymorphism. Cancer Epidemiol Biomarkers Prev 9(8):827–833
172. Hengstler JG, Arand M, Herrero ME, Oesch F (1998) Polymorphisms of N-acetyltransferases, glutathione S-transferases, microsomal epoxide hydrolase and sulfotransferases: influence on cancer susceptibility. Recent Results Cancer Res 154:47–85
173. Cascorbi I, Brockmoller J, Mrozikiewicz PM, Bauer S, Loddenkemper R, Roots I (1996) Homozygous rapid arylamine N-acetyltransferase (NAT2) genotype as a susceptibility factor for lung cancer. Cancer Res 56:3961–3966
174. Bouchardy C, Mitrunen K, Wikman H, Husgafvel-Pursiainen K, Dayer P, Benhamou S, et al (1998) N-acetyltransferase NAT1 and NAT2 genotypes and lung cancer risk. Pharmacogenetics 8:291–298
175. Vahakangas KH, Bennett WP, Castren K, Welsh JA, Khan MA, Blomeke B, et al (2001) p53 and K-ras mutations in lung cancers from former and never-smoking women. Cancer Res 61(11): 4350–4356
176. Ko YC, Lee CH, Chen MJ, Huang CC, Chang WY, Lin HJ, et al (1997) Risk factors for primary-lung cancer among non-smoking women in Taiwan. Int J Epidemiol 26:24–31
177. Wang TJ, Zhou BS, Shi JP (1996) Lung cancer in nonsmoking Chinese women: a case-control study. Lung Cancer 14(Suppl 1):S93–S98
178. Shen XB, Wang GX, Zhou BS (1998) Relation of exposure to environmental tobacco smoke and pulmonary adenocarcinoma in non-smoking women: a case control study in Nanjing. Oncol Rep 5:1221–1223
179. Jockel KH, Pohlabeln H, Ahrens W, Krauss M (1998) Environmental tobacco smoke and lung cancer. Epidemiology 9:672–675
180. Kawachi I, Pearce NE, Jackson RT (1989) Deaths from lung cancer and ischaemic heart disease due to passive smoking in New Zealand. N Z Med J 102:337–340

181. Stockwell HG, Goldman AL, Lyman GH, Noss CI, Armstrong AW, Pinkham PA, et al (1992) Environmental tobacco smoke and lung cancer risk in nonsmoking women. J Natl Cancer Inst 84:1417–1422

182. Boffetta P, Agudo A, Ahrens W, Benhamou E, Benhamou S, Darby SC, et al (1998) Multicenter case-control study of exposure to environmental tobacco smoke and lung cancer in Europe. J Natl Cancer Inst 90:1440–1450

183. Brownson RC, Alavanja MC, Hock ET, Loy TS (1992) Passive smoking and lung cancer in nonsmoking women. Am J Public Health 82:1525–1530

184. Fontham ET, Correa P, Reynolds P, Wu-Williams A, Buffler PA, Greenberg RS, et al (1994) Environmental tobacco smoke and lung cancer in nonsmoking women. A multicenter study. JAMA 271:1752–1759

185. Hackshaw AK, Law MR, Wald NJ (1997) The accumulated evidence on lung cancer and environmental tobacco smoke. BMJ 315:980–988

186. Wang FL, Love EJ, Liu N, Dai XD (1994) Childhood and adolescent passive smoking and the risk of female lung cancer. Int J Epidemiol 23:223–230

187. Zaridze D, Maximovitch D, Zemlyanaya G, Aitakov ZN, Boffetta P (1998) Exposure to environmental tobacco smoke and risk of lung cancer in non-smoking women from Moscow, Russia. Int J Cancer 75:335–338

188. Boffetta P, Ahrens W, Nyberg F, Mukeria A, Bruske-Hohlfeld I, Fortes C, et al (1999) Exposure to environmental tobacco smoke and risk of adenocarcinoma of the lung. Int J Cancer 83: 635–639

189. Miller GH, Golish JA, Cox CE, Chacko DC (1994) Women and lung cancer: a comparison of active and passive smokers with nonexposed nonsmokers. Cancer Detect Prev 18:421–430

190. Copas JB, Shi JQ (2000) Reanalysis of epidemiological evidence on lung cancer and passive smoking. BMJ 320(7232):417–418

191. Lubin JH (1999) Estimating lung cancer risk with exposure to environmental tobacco smoke. Environ Health Perspect 107(Suppl 6):879–883

192. Brown KG (1999) Lung cancer and environmental tobacco smoke: occupational risk to non-smokers. Environ Health Perspect 107(Suppl 6):885–890

193. Lagarde F, Axelsson G, Damber L, Mellander H, Nyberg F, Pershagen G (2001) Residential radon and lung cancer among never-smokers in Sweden. Epidemiology 12(1):396–404

194. Berkey CS, Ware JH, Dockery DW, Ferris BG Jr, Speizer FE (1986) Indoor air pollution and pulmonary function growth in preadolescent children. Am J Epidemiol 123:250–260

195. Tager IB, Weiss ST, Munoz A, Rosner B, Speizer FE (1983) Longitudinal study of the effects of-maternal smoking on pulmonary function in children. N Engl J Med 309:699–703

196. Wang X, Wypij D, Gold DR, Speizer FE, Ware JH, Ferris BG Jr, et al (1994) A longitudinal study of the effects of parental smoking on pulmonary function in children 6–18 years. Am J Respir Crit Care Med 149:1420–1425

197. Boyle P (1993) The hazards of passive- and active-smoking. N Engl J Med 328:1708–1709

198. Chilmonczyk BA, Salmun LM, Megathlin KN, Neveux LM, Palomaki GE, Knight GJ, et al (1993) Association between exposure to environmental tobacco smoke and exacerbations of asthma in children. N Engl J Med 328:1665–1669

199. Greenberg RA, Haley NJ, Etzel RA, et al (1984) Measuring the exposure of infants to tobacco smoke. Nicotine and cotinine in urine and saliva. N Engl J Med 310:1075–1078

200. Henderson FW, Reid HF, Morris R, Wang OL, Hu PC, Helms RW, et al (1989) Home air nicotine levels and urinary cotinine excretion in preschool children. Am Rev Respir Dis 140:197–201

201. Wright AL, Holberg C, Martinez FD, Taussig LM (1991) Relationship of parental smoking to wheezing and nonwheezing lower respiratory tract illnesses in infancy. Group Health Medical Associates. J Pediatr 118:207–214

202. Axelrad CM, Sepkovic DW, Colosimo SG, Haley NJ (1987) Biochemical validation of cigarette smoke exposure and tobacco use. In: Sandhu SS, DeMarini DM, Mass MJ, Moore MM,

Mumford JL (eds) Short-term bioassays in the analysis of complex environmental mixtures V. Plenum, New York, pp 115–126

203. Skolnick ET, Vomvolakis MA, Buck KA, Mannino SF, Sun LS (1998) Exposure to environmental tobacco smoke and the risk of adverse respiratory events in children receiving general anesthesia. Anesthesiology 88:1144–1153

204. Reisli R, Apilliogullari S, Reisli I, Tuncer S, Erol A, Okesli S (2004) The effect of environmental tobacco smoke on the dose requirements of rocuronium in children. Paediatr Anaesth 14(3):247–250

205. Forastiere F, Agabiti N, Corbo GM, Pistelli R, Dell'Orco V, Ciappi G, et al (1994) Passive smoking as a determinant of bronchial responsiveness in children. Am J Respir Crit Care Med 149:365–370

206. Paoletti P, Carrozzi L, Viegi G, Modena P, Ballerin L, Di Pede F, et al (1995) Distribution of bronchial responsiveness in a general population: effect of sex, age, smoking, and level of pulmonary function. Am J Respir Crit Care Med 151:1770–1777

207. Schwartz J, Katz SA, Fegley RW, Tockman MS (1988) Sex and race differences in the development of lung function. Am Rev Respir Dis 138:1415–1421

208. Zamel N (1984) Threshold of airway response to inhaled methacholine in healthy men and women. J Appl Physiol 56:129–132

209. Margolis PA, Greenberg RA, Keyes LL, LaVange LM, Chapman RS, Denny FW, et al (1992) Lower respiratory illness in infants and low socioeconomic status. Am J Public Health 82:1119–1126

210. Lakshmipathy N, Bokesch PM, Cowen DE, Lisman SR, et al (1996) Environmental tobacco smoke: a risk factor for pediatric laryngospasm. Anesth Analg 82:724–727

211. Lyons B, Frizelle H, Kirby F, Casey W (1996) The effect of passive smoking on the incidence of airway complications in children undergoing general anaesthesia. Anaesthesia 51:324–326

212. Adair-Bischoff CE, Sauve RS (1998) Environmental tobacco smoke and middle ear disease in preschool-age children. Arch Pediatr Adolesc Med 152:127–133

213. Bluestone CD (1982) Otitis media in children: to treat or not to treat? N Engl J Med 306:1399–1404

214. Hakansson A (1989) Health complaints and drug consumption during the first 18 months of life. Fam Pract 6:210–216

215. Klein JO (1994) Lessons from recent studies on the epidemiology of otitis media. Pediatr Infect Dis J 13:1031–1034

216. Teele DW, Klein JO, Rosner B (1989) Epidemiology of otitis media during the first seven years of life in children in greater Boston: a prospective, cohort study. J Infect Dis 160: 83–94

217. Schappert SM (1992) Office visits for otitis media: United States, 1975–90. Adv Data 18(253):1–19

218. Overpeck MD, Moss AJ (1991) Children's exposure to environmental cigarette smoke before and after birth. Health of our nation's children, United States, 1998. Adv Data (202):1–11

219. Cook DG, Whincup PH, Jarvis MJ, Strachan DP, Papacosta O, Bryant A (1994) Passive exposure to tobacco smoke in children aged 5–7 years: individual, family, and community factors. BMJ 308:384–389

220. Teele DW (1994) Long term sequelae of otitis media: fact or fantasy? Pediatr Infect Dis J 13:1069–1073

221. Ilicali OC, Keles N, De er K, Sa un OF, Guldiken Y (2001) Evaluation of the effect of passive smoking on otitis media in children by an objective method: urinary cotinine analysis. Laryngoscope 111(1):163–167

222. Collet JP, Larson CP, Boivin JF, Suissa S, Pless IB (1995) Parental smoking and risk of otitis media in pre-school children. Can J Public Health 86:269–273

223. Ey JL, Holberg CJ, Aldous MB, Wright AL, Martinez FD, Taussig LM (1995) Passive smoke exposure and otitis media in the first year of life. Group Health Medical Associates. Pediatrics 95:670–677

224. Kitchens GG (1995) Relationship of environmental tobacco smoke to otitis media in young children. Laryngoscope 105:1–13

225. Gryczynska D, Kobos J, Zakrzewska A (1999) Relationship between passive smoking, recurrent respiratory tract infections and otitis media in children. Int J Pediatr Otorhinolaryngol 49(Suppl 1):S275–S278

226. Lieu JE, Feinstein AR (2002) Effect of gestational and passive smoke exposure on ear infections in children. Arch Pediatr Adolesc Med 156(2):147–154

227. Blackwell CC, Tzanakaki G, Kremastinou J, Weir DM, Vakalis N, Elton RA, et al (1992) Factors affecting carriage of *Neisseria meningitidis* among Greek military recruits. Epidemiol Infect 108:441–448

228. Caugant DA, Hoiby EA, Magnus P, Scheel O, Hoel T, Bjune G, et al (1994) Asymptomatic carriage of *Neisseria meningitidis* in a randomly sampled population. J Clin Microbiol 32:323–330

229. Stuart JM, Cartwright KA, Robinson PM, Noah ND (1989) Effect of smoking on meningococcal carriage. Lancet 2:723–725

230. Becker S, Soukup JM (1999) Effect of nitrogen dioxide on respiratory viral infection in airway epithelial cells. Environ Res 81:159–166

231. Dye JA, Adler KB (1994) Effects of cigarette smoke on epithelial cells of the respiratory tract. Thorax 49:825–834

232. Green GM, Carolin D (1967) The depressant effect of cigarette smoke on the in vitro antibacterial activity of alveolar macrophages. N Engl J Med 276:421–427

233. Raman AS, Swinburne AJ, Fedullo AJ (1983) Pneumococcal adherence to the buccal epithelial cells of cigarette smokers. Chest 83:23–27

234. Merrill WW, Goodenberger D, Strober W, Matthay RA, et al (1980) Free secretory component and other proteins in human lung lavage. Am Rev Respir Dis 122:156–161

235. Fischer M, Hedberg K, Cardosi P, Plikaytis BD, Hoesly FC, et al (1997) Tobacco smoke as a risk factor for meningococcal disease. Pediatr Infect Dis J 16:979–983

236. Haneberg B, Tonjum T, Rodahl K, Gedde-Dahl TW (1983) Factors preceding the onset of meningococcal disease, with special emphasis on passive smoking, symptoms of ill health. NIPH Ann 6:169–173

237. Stuart JM, Cartwright KA, Dawson JA, Rickard J (1988) Risk factors for meningococcal disease: a case control study in south west England. Community Med 10:139–146

238. Stanwell-Smith RE, Stuart JM, Hughes AO, Robinson P, Griffin MB, Cartwright K (1994) Smoking, the environment and meningococcal disease: a case control study. Epidemiol Infect 112:315–328

239. Madigan MP, Ziegler RG, Benichou J, Byrne C, Hoover RN (1995) Proportion of breast cancer cases in the United States explained by well-established risk factors. J Natl Cancer Inst 87:1681–1685

240. Ambrosone CB, Freudenheim JL, Graham S, Marshall JR, Vena JE, Brasure JR, et al (1996) Cigarette smoking, *N*-acetyltransferase 2 genetic polymorphisms, and breast cancer risk. JAMA 276:1494–1501

241. Ambrosone CB, Shields PG (1997) Molecular epidemiology of breast cancer. Prog Clin Biol Res 396:83–99

242. Shields PG, Ambrosone CB, Graham S, Bowman ED, Harrington AM, Gillenwater KA, et al (1996) A cytochrome P4502E1 genetic polymorphism and tobacco smoking in breast cancer. Mol Carcinog 17:144–150

243. Baron JA, La Vecchia C, Levi F (1990) The antiestrogenic effect of cigarette smoking in women. Am J Obstet Gynecol 162:502–514

244. MacMahon B, Trichopoulos D, Cole P, Brown J (1982) Cigarette smoking and urinary estrogens. N Engl J Med 307:1062–1065

245. Lash TL, Aschengrau A (1999) Active and passive cigarette smoking and the occurrence of breast cancer. Am J Epidemiol 149:5–12

246. Wartenberg D, Calle EE, Thun MJ, Heath CW Jr, Lally C, Woodruff T (2000) Passive smoking exposure and female breast cancer mortality. J Natl Cancer Inst 92(20):1666–1673

247. Johnson KC, Glantz SA (2008) Evidence secondhand smoke causes breast cancer in 2005 stronger than for lung cancer in 1986. Prev Med 46(6):492–496

248. Cunnane SC (1993) Childhood origins of lifestyle-related risk factors for coronary heart disease in adulthood. Nutr Health 9:107–115

249. Wild RA, Taylor EL, Knehans A, Cleaver V (1994) Matriarchal model for cardiovascular prevention. Obstet Gynecol Surv 49:147–152

250. Burke V, Gracey MP, Milligan RA, Thompson C, Taggart AC, Beilin LJ (1998) Parental smoking and risk factors for cardiovascular disease in 10- to 12-year-old children. J Pediatr 133: 206–213

251. Haustein KO (1999) Cigarette smoking, nicotine and pregnancy. Int J Clin Pharmacol Ther 37:417–427

252. Raitakari OT, Porkka KV, Taimela S, Telama R, Rasanen L, Viikari JS (1994) Effects of persistent physical activity and inactivity on coronary risk factors in children and young adults. The Cardiovascular Risk in Young Finns Study. Am J Epidemiol 140:195–205

253. McPhillips JB, Eaton CB, Gans KM, Derby CA, Lasater TM, McKenney JL, et al (1994) Dietary differences in smokers and nonsmokers from two southeastern New England communities. J Am Diet Assoc 94:287–292

254. Prattala R, Karisto A, Berg MA (1994) Consistency and variation in unhealthy behaviour among Finnish men, 1982–1990. Soc Sci Med 39:115–122

255. Green G, Macintyre S, West P, Ecob R (1991) Like parent like child? Associations between drinking and smoking behaviour of parents and their children. Br J Addict 86:745–758

256. Greenlund KJ, Liu K, Kiefe CI, Yunis C, Dyer AR, Burke GL (1995) Impact of father's education and parental smoking status on smoking behavior in young adults. The CARDIA study. Coronary Artery Risk Development in Young Adults. Am J Epidemiol 142:1029–1033

257. Hill DJ, White VM, Williams RM, Gardner GJ (1993) Tobacco and alcohol use among Australian secondary school students in 1990. Med J Aust 158:228–234

Non-Drug Treatments to Promote Smoking Cessation

10

Smoking cessation should be the prime objective of medical treatment for people who smoke, particularly since most smokers who require treatment are dependent on tobacco. Statistics on readiness to quit smoking show wide variations. For some 20–30% of smokers, an external event marks the starting point for giving up. Further undecided smokers – the figures vary between 25 and 40% – may possibly be persuaded to quit by extensive education campaigns directed at the smoking public [1, 2].

Besides techniques employed worldwide in which patient education is combined chiefly with the pharmacological approach (see Chap. 11), a wide range of counselling methods have found application, ranging from physician advice through to psychological withdrawal programmes, such as those used in other forms of dependence. Scientific assessment of these techniques is only possible if they also adhere to defined standards. The technique used must, therefore, also be scientifically justified or justifiable and the success of treatment must be quantifiable by measuring biochemical markers (e.g. CO in expired air or, preferably, cotinine levels in plasma, urine or saliva). In addition, the consensus definition of cessation is that the smoker remains abstinent for at least 6 (or preferably 12) months after the start of treatment, i.e. the ex-smoker should no longer smoke any cigarettes. A reduction in cigarette smoking (e.g. by 20 cigarettes/day) may be termed a partial success, but does not qualify as smoking cessation in the sense defined above. Given the millions of smokers who are potentially willing to quit, the techniques employed must be practicable and economically viable, and this explains the dominant position of nicotine replacement therapy (NRT) worldwide [3].

Smokers often set themselves the goal of giving up smoking and the factors prompting this decision may be a planned pregnancy [4], a sense of responsibility towards their own children or even financial considerations [5]. A prerequisite for any intervention intended to promote smoking cessation is the development of a strong determination to quit smoking. It may take several weeks before these contemplative processes can be transposed into a practicable reality. This is connected with a behavioural change vis-à-vis smoking [6].

A study by Carlson et al., community-based cognitive-behavioural intervention, evaluated the predictive value of aspects of the Transtheoretical model (TTM) of behaviour change as applied to smoking cessation in a large group [7]. A cognitive-behavioural intervention was followed by a 3-month assessment of the smoking status in a regional outpatient cancer centre with a total of 2,069 participants in smoking

K.-O. Haustein, D. Groneberg, *Tobacco or Health?*
DOI: 10.1007/978-3-540-87577-2_10, © Springer Verlag Berlin Heidelberg 2010

cessation clinics. Eight 90-min sessions over 4 months utilizing education, self-monitoring, a group quit date and behaviour modification techniques were performed, and as main outcome measures, the cessation rates at 3 months post-quit date were used. Also, differences were monitored between successful and unsuccessful participants on the baseline TTM variables of stages of change, processes of change, decisional balance and situational temptations, as well as of precessation demographic, smoking history and smoking behaviour variables. It was shown that non-smokers at 3 months endorsed using more of only one of the processes of change (reinforcement management) more than smokers prior to starting the programme. They also endorsed more Cons of Smoking and had a more negative Decisional Balance score. When the variables of tobacco tolerance on the Fagerstrom Test for Nicotine Dependence (FTND), marital status, association with the Cancer Centre and amount of vigorous exercise were first entered in a logistic regression model, Reinforcement Management and Cons of Smoking continued to be predictive of smoking cessation success, but again none of the other TTM variables added explanatory power. The authors concluded that TTM variables measured prior to programme attendance added little predictive value for cessation outcome beyond that explained by demographic and smoking history variables. Future studies may benefit from reassessing the TTM variables at the quit date and the 3-month assessment of smoking status to evaluate how the programme impacted these variables [7].

A further study examined the association between stage of change and smoking cessation outcomes among youth receiving two interventions of varying intensity: a 10-min brief self-help smoking cessation intervention (BI) or the American Lung Association's 10-week Not-on-Tobacco (N-O-T) smoking cessation programme [8]. At baseline, the participants were classified into three stages (e.g. pre-contemplation, contemplation and preparation) based on their intention to change their smoking behaviour. Smoking behaviour, stage of change, self-efficacy and beliefs about smoking were assessed at baseline and 3 months post-baseline. It was found that the relationship between stage of change and cessation outcomes varied by treatment intensity. Logistic regression analyses revealed that BI participants in the preparation stage were 25 times more likely to quit smoking at post-baseline than participants in the contemplation or pre-contemplation stages. In contrast, N-O-T was effective for youth regardless of baseline stage. Additionally, N-O-T participants demonstrated greater forward stage movement from baseline to post-baseline than did BI participants [8].

Smokers who think about stopping smoking ("contemplation"; Stage II) have already moved beyond contented unawareness of the problem ("pre-contemplation"; Stage I). They next have to consider how they might handle quitting (preparation phase; "deciding to try to quit"; Stage III). Once they stop smoking ("action"; Stage IV), they have taken a decisive step, but initially they are short-term ex-smokers ("maintenance"; Stage V) and are constantly at risk of slipping back into old ways ("relapse"; Stage VI). Smokers may find themselves repeating the cycle from Stage II or III to Stage VII several times, depending on how they cope with relapses (Fig. 10.1). In many cases (Chap. 11), this short-term abstinence may become "sustained abstinence" (Stage VII). It is important for ex-smokers to extend their smoking cessation at

Fig. 10.1 Smoking cessation
as a potentially protracted
process (see text) [6]

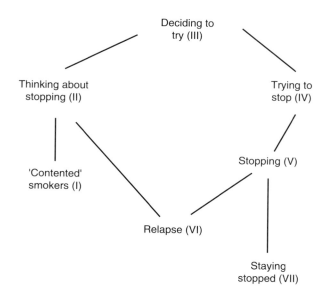

least over a period of months or even 1 year or longer; they will then have a sense that cessation is "tough to handle," something which preferably they would not wish to go through a second time.

10.1
Indications and Diagnostic Considerations

In principle, given the many and well-known harmful effects of smoking, any intervention to achieve smoking cessation is to be recommended. There are the following four important indications for smoking cessation:

1. To prevent a wide range of diseases.
2. To allow treatment for smoking-related diseases, e.g. chronic obstructive pulmonary disease (COPD), peptic ulcer, hypertension, coronary heart disease, peripheral arterial occlusive disease (PAOD), hyper cholesterolaemia, diabetes, psychiatric illnesses, etc.
3. As a component of rehabilitation during recovery from smoking-related diseases (e.g. myocardial infarction, stroke, limb amputation).
4. To protect non-smokers.

Before treatment starts, smokers should be questioned concerning the strength of their resolve to quit smoking absolutely. Their degree of dependence should be assessed (using the Fagerström test, Chap 4, Sect. 4.5.1) and, as a minimum requirement, measurements should be taken of CO in expired air (see Table 10.1 and Chap. 11, Sect. 11.4).

An overview of the studies on the non-pharmacological treatment of nicotine dependence is provided in Haustein [9] and Table 10.2.

Table 10.1 Diagnostic considerations in smoker counselling [113]

Daily cigarette consumption (regular or irregular consumption)
Cigarette brand (subsequently classified as light – medium – strong)
CO levels in expired air (specifying time of measurement)
Fagerström test for nicotine dependence
Interview to establish whether the smoker is dissonant (loathes smoking, cannot quit without medical assistance: nicotine pre-abstinence syndrome) or consonant (unwilling to quit)
Tar exposure level (TEL): correlates with the risk of bronchial carcinoma; depends on the number of years of smoking, daily cigarette consumption and the tar yield of the cigarette brand (<15 mg, 15–24 mg or >24 mg)
Carbohydrate dependence (may be present additionally in dependent smokers)
Height and body weight (calculate body mass index: subsequent weight gain!)
Smoker's past experience of attempted smoking cessation (number of successes/ failures)
Occurrence of nocturnal sleep disturbances and smoking while sleep is interrupted (nocturnal sleep-disturbing nicotine craving: NSDNC)
Presence of additional cardiovascular or pulmonary disease (previous angina attacks, myocardial infarction, hypertension, chronic obstructive pulmonary disease, bronchial carcinoma, etc.), concurrent psychoses or depressive illness (may complicate smoking cessation)
Concomitant medication (neuroleptics, clozapine, antidepressants, antihypertensive agents, lipid-lowering drugs, etc)

10.2
Objective of Treatment

Treatment of the smoker should aim at complete cessation, and stopping smoking abruptly is indicated. Only <1–2% of heavily dependent smokers achieve this goal without any medical intervention and through willpower alone, and the number of cigarettes smoked/ day need not be a decisive factor. This (abrupt) method of smoking cessation can be achieved with psychological support, but the outcome is more promising with pharmacological support.

It has subsequently become known that many smokers, because of their heavy dependence and/or considerable habituation, are unable to give up smoking completely, with the result that "harm reduction" or partial cessation is then a necessary option. The goal here is for smokers (simultaneously patients at risk) to cut their consumption to <10 cigarettes/ day with pharmacological support. After a longer period of reduced cigarette consumption, some smokers may possibly themselves recognise the sense of stopping completely, though this does not automatically imply any change in dependence. According to the AHQR (Agency for Healthcare Quality and Research) guidelines, the following five "A"s should be used: Ask – Advice – Assess – Assist – Arrange (fragen, raten, beurteilen, helfen, arrangieren) [10].

Reducing tobacco use is a leading goal of the nation's Healthy People 2010. To improve the health of all Americans during the first decade of the twenty-first century, tobacco control practices must also be a top priority in older adults [11]. Older adult smokers are often less educated, have a low socio-economic status, are more likely to be female and have reduced self-efficacy with the cessation process. Older adults suffer disproportionately

Table 10.2 Assessment of non-drug treatment modalities to promote smoking cessation, compiled from the Cochrane Database

	Odds ratio	Assessment	Reference
Reduced smoking	–	⇩⇩	–
Self-help interventions	1.23 (1.01–1.49)	⇔	[25]
Self-help intervention with telephone counselling	1.62 (1.33–1.97)	⇑	[25]
Training by health care professionals	1.48 (1.20–1.83)	⇔	[56]
Nurse-managed counselling	1.43 (1.24–1.66)	⇑	[65]
Physician counselling	1.69 (1.45–1.98)	⇑	[59]
Individual counselling (short counselling session, booklet, etc.)	1.55 (1.27–1.90)	⇔	[114]
Group therapy (behavioural therapy)	2.10 (1.64–2.70)	⇑⇑⇑	[70, 114]
Hypnotherapy	+	⇔	[115]
Aversion therapy (aversive stimulation)	2.08 (1.39–3.12)	⇑	[77]
Aversion therapy (general)	1.19 (0.77–1.83)	⇔	[77]
Acupuncture	1.22 (0.99–1.49)	⇩⇩	[106]

⇑⇑⇑ Claim (e.g. on efficacy) supported by several suitable, valid clinical studies (e.g. randomised clinical trials) or by one or more valid meta-analyses or systematic reviews. Positive claim clearly confirmed

⇑ Claim (e.g. on efficacy) supported by at least one suitable, valid clinical study (e.g. randomised clinical trial). Positive claim confirmed

⇩⇩ Negative claim (e.g. on efficacy) supported by one or more suitable, valid clinical studies (e.g. randomised clinical trials) or by one or more valid meta-analyses or systematic reviews. Negative claim clearly confirmed

⇔ No reliable study results available to confirm a positive or negative effect. This may be due to the absence of suitable studies, but also to the availability of several studies with contradictory results

+ No usable studies

from smoking-related diseases, yet experience physical, social and psychological rewards from cessation. Clinicians managing the care of smokers can be effective in promoting smoking cessation, regardless of the smoker's age or duration of smoking history. The AHRQ guideline recommends clinicians to ask, advice, assess, assist and arrange follow-up for all smokers. Pharmacological and behavioural therapies are recommended to assist with the cessation process. Gerontological nurses can play a key role in optimizing health and successful aging by reducing tobacco use in older adults [11].

10.3
Self-Help Interventions by the Smoker

Undoubtedly, the ideal situation is for the smoker to decide one day, more or less spontaneously, to give up smoking and from that time onwards never to smoke. This type of decision is commonly taken on special days of the year (e.g. as a New Year's resolution) and, more rarely, is also acted upon. Greater seriousness is attached to decisions that are prompted by personal illness or by the illness or death of a family member or close friend. From our own experience of counselling smokers, we know that even heavy smokers (40–60 cigarettes/day) can carry through such decisions without major effort. The 6 studies published to date in which self-help interventions led to successful smoking cessation for 6–9 months (OR = 1.08; CI: 0.81–1.44) or 12 months (OR = 1.0; CI: 0.75–1.34) are of limited value because biochemical variables were measured in only isolated cases [12]. The support of a partner was described as an increasing successful aspect for quitting in only 2 of the 6 studies [12]. Smokers whose partners are non-smokers or ex-smokers are more likely to be successful at quitting [13, 14]. Currently married smokers have a higher chance of success than divorced, widowed or never married smokers [15]. The support of the spouse may be beneficial for success [16, 17]. If smokers are constantly nagged, face complaints about their behaviour or are repeatedly criticised for failed attempts to quit smoking, then their position becomes entrenched [18]. Studies indicating the positive influence of the spouse/partner in this context are countered by others which are critical of their role [19, 20]. Two systematic studies report the supportive effect of a partner in achieving smoking cessation [21, 22], in one case including the recommendations of the AHQR [21].

However, numerous organisations also provide self-help manuals designed to assist smokers who wish to quit [23, 24]. Consulting a therapist, in addition, may enhance the effectiveness of the method [23]. Standard instructions have been found to be less effective than personalised instructions tailored for a group of smokers (OR = 1.41; CI: 1.14–1.75) [25]. Overall, instructions on smoking cessation are assessed as useful and more effective than attempting smoking cessation without instructions.

Sporting activities are a key aspect of self-help to achieve smoking cessation [26]. Physical exercise has a beneficial effect on cravings [27], depressed mood [28], sleep disturbances [29], feelings of tension [30], stress situations [31] and on weight gain following smoking cessation, an aspect that is especially important for women [32–34]. Sport also has a positive effect on relapses [35], coping with the smoking problem [36] and self-esteem [37]. Overall, of course, physical activity confers health benefits on the ex-smoker [38]; heavy smokers often already notice this just 2 or 3 weeks after stopping smoking and they volunteer this information spontaneously during counselling sessions. Out of a total of 8 studies of this aspect published to date, 6 could not be assessed because patient numbers were too small. In the final analysis, therefore, only 1 study provided positive evidence of the effect of vigorous exercise in terms of smoking cessation (OR = 2.36; CI: 0.97–5.70) [39], with a definite increase in continuous abstinence compared with controls (11.9% vs. 5.4%; $p = 0.05$) [39].

To determine whether exercise-based interventions alone or combined with a smoking cessation programme are more effective than a smoking cessation intervention alone, Ussher searched the Cochrane Tobacco Addiction Group specialized register for studies including the terms "exercise" or "physical activity" and MEDLINE, EMBASE, PsycINFO, CINAHL, Dissertation Abstracts and SPORTDiscus. Randomized trials which compared an exercise programme alone or an exercise programme as an adjunct to a cessation programme with a cessation programme recruiting smokers or recent quitters, and with a follow-up of 6 months or more were included in the [40]. Eleven trials were identified, six of which had fewer than 25 people in each treatment arm. They varied in the timing and intensity of the smoking cessation and exercise programmes. Three studies showed significantly higher abstinence rates in a physically active group vs. a control group at the end of treatment. One of these studies also showed a benefit for exercise vs. control on abstinence at both the 3 month and 12 month follow-up points. One study showed significantly higher abstinence rates for the exercise group vs. a control group at the 3 month follow–up, but not at the end of treatment or at 12 month follow-up. The other studies showed no significant effect for exercise on abstinence. The study concluded that only one of the 11 trials offered evidence for exercise aiding smoking cessation. All but one of the other trials were too small to conclude that the intervention was ineffective, or included an exercise intervention which was insufficiently intense to achieve the desired level of exercise. Trials are needed with larger sample sizes, sufficiently intense exercise interventions, equal contact control conditions and measures of exercise adherence [40].

The effectiveness of *telephone counselling* has been investigated in 23 studies, the results of which are extremely heterogeneous. In 4 studies, telephone counselling was followed by face-to-face counselling. However, telephone counselling can help to prevent further relapses or stabilise smoking cessation [41]. Since telephone counselling is usually performed on an individual basis, it is preferable to group counselling, a modality that is often rejected by smokers [42]. Counselling then becomes a hotline to request a wide range of information. Counselling services have been set up specifically for smokers (e.g. Quitline/Australia, Quit/England, Heidelberger Telefon/Germany) or they may operate within the broader framework of an integrated smoking cessation support service [43]. Similarly, the Erfurt Smoker Counselling Centre provides free information and advice, but also offers individual treatment free-of-charge over a period of weeks or months with the goal of achieving smoking cessation (see Appendix).

10.4
Physician Advice for Smoking Cessation

Seventeen different studies used 5-min standard interviews to point out the dangers of smoking and issued smokers with an information booklet without offering any further consultation. Three of these 17 studies were conducted in a hospital setting. The studies revealed no clear differences in terms of success, not even when biochemical markers were measured (plasma nicotine levels or CO).

Where the studies were conducted with additional physician input (spirometry, CO measurement, oral or written medical counselling, post-cessation support or a combination of interventions), different success outcomes were achieved ($p < 0.001$), a fact that was also attributable, among other things, to non-standardised methods and individually tailored physician input in the individual studies.

Group sessions with a medical expert to discuss the health consequences of smoking also showed no significant success. In *pregnant women* attending three sessions, success was reported in 9 independent studies in which biochemical markers were measured.

Effectiveness was greater than in non-pregnant women undergoing the same procedure. Higher success rates were recorded in 7 studies in pregnant women with self-help instructions (9%; $p = 0.01$) than in 11 similar studies in non-pregnant women (Table 10.2).

Hospital-based interventions for smoking cessation are not necessarily more successful than interventions outside a hospital setting, even though a 30% increase in smoking cessation has been achieved (OR = 1.09; CI: 0.91–1.31) [44]. However, where these interventions are combined with after-care, a marked rise in effectiveness is reported (OR = 1.82; CI: 1.49–2.22) [44].

Clinicians achieved a 35% success rate in group sessions with high-risk *patients with coronary heart disease* who had survived a myocardial infarction [45]. Even higher success rates were recorded in one uncontrolled study [46]. In 4 further studies where counselling was made available to high-risk smokers with no history of infarction [47–49], differing success rates for smoking cessation were achieved (range: 7–31.3%). Where smokers were simply counselled to stop smoking, success was no worse in comparison with the other 3 studies with additional interventions such as repeated reminders of the risk of infarction, support for successful smoking cessation, etc. [47–49] (21% success rate; $p < 0.001$). A change in smoking habits (cigar, pipe) was reported in 1 study [50].

Individual counselling [51–55] is more effective than no counselling at all (OR = 1.55; CI: 1.27–1.90) and the extent of counselling does not appear to be decisive because brief information (OR = 1.17; CI: 0.59–2.34) as well as group-counselling sessions (OR = 1.33; CI: 0.83–2.13) have proved useful [56]. Follow-up telephone contact with patients has been shown to be beneficial [54].

A study by Picardi et al. assessed the effectiveness of a behavioural group intervention for smoking cessation, which included the recommendation to participate with a relative or close friend as its most original feature [57]. In this study, a total of 1,060 subjects took part in the programme, which consisted of nine group sessions over a period of 5 weeks. The intervention consisted of a modified version of the Five-Day Plan, the main differences being the use of behavioural therapy techniques and small group work, and the addition of 4 weekly booster sessions. About two-thirds of the participants came with a relative or close friend. Long-term abstinence from smoking was assessed with follow-up telephone interviews. It was also found that very few subjects were lost to follow-ups (9.2% at 6 months, 9.7% at 1 year, 10.8% at 2 years). The observed quit rates were 42.6% at 6 months, 35.5% at 1 year and 32% at 2 years. When considering as smokers all subjects who were lost to follow-ups, quit rates were also satisfactory (38.7% at 6 months, 32.1% at 1 year and 28.6% at 2 years). The main predictors of a good outcome were being male, smoking <20 cigarettes/day, having started smoking after 18 years of age, having made previous quitting attempts, not having a history of unsuccessful participation to smoking cessation interventions and attending the sessions with a relative or close friend. From this study, it was concluded that although some limitations inherent in the design of the study suggested caution in interpreting the results and in making comparisons, the long-term effectiveness of the intervention was satisfactory. The inclusion of a relative or close friend appeared useful. This simple and inexpensive strategy may deserve recommendation, though in the future it should be tested in controlled trials [57].

10.5
Nursing Involvement

Since nurses constitute a very much larger professional body than doctors worldwide, training efforts are warranted to qualify nursing staff for involvement in smoking cessation programmes, given the enormity of the task. The effectiveness of physician counselling for smoking cessation is well-established [58, 59]. By contrast, counselling by nursing professionals is reported to be less effective [60]. The different [61, 62] studies should be regarded as successful (OR = 1.50; CI: 1.29–1.73), though some investigators used NRT to promote smoking cessation (see Chap. 11, Sect. 11.1). Nevertheless, counselling delivered by nurses and respiratory care therapists etc. is viewed as useful [63]. Following the example of the USA, this activity should be incorporated into nurse education programmes worldwide [64]. One recent analysis [65] summarising 17 studies indicates that the odds of quitting are increased by nursing intervention (OR = 1.43; 95% CI: 1.24–1.66) and this improved effectiveness was found for both intensive (OR = 1.39; CI: 1.19–1.64) and less intensive interventions (OR = 1.67; CI: 1.14–2.65). Where post-infarction patients took part in nurse-managed programmes in a cardiology clinic, effectiveness was very much higher (OR = 2.14; CI: 1.39–3.31) [33, 60, 66]. In 1 study, the effectiveness of nurse-managed counselling in non-hospitalised patients with cardiovascular health problems was very low (OR = 0.19; CI: 0.08–0.46) [61]. However, this study should be viewed critically in as much as the control group included more coronary artery bypass graft patients who also quit smoking without counselling. In a further 8 studies, an 80% increase in effectiveness was reported in non-hospitalised patients (OR = 1.81; CI: 1.39–2.36) [67, 68]. Additional telephone contact increased the effectiveness of smoking cessation interventions in some studies (OR = 1.40; CI: 1.00–1.96) [59].

Overall, counselling by trained nursing professionals may be regarded as useful, with statistically significant though moderate effects having been achieved to date [65]. In selected hospitals and outpatient departments, nurses should, therefore, be included in the system of patient education to promote smoking cessation [59].

10.6
Group Behaviour Therapy Programmes

Dependence experts and psychiatrists, in particular, consider that behaviour therapy programmes are also very effective to promote smoking cessation (OR = 2.10; CI: 1.64–2.70) [62, 69]. The hypothesis that smoking is a learned and consolidated behaviour based on many years of conditioning has prompted the development of treatment strategies using the same practices to "unlearn" the resultant dependence.

Behaviours learned as a result of smoking (situations in which the smoker reaches for a cigarette; the act of lighting up and smoking; automatisation and ritualisation of smoking) have to be unlearned in the course of treatment. Self-monitoring of smoking behaviour (for example, by keeping a smoker's journal) is a commonly used method in which habits have to be broken down in stages (by recording them). Key aspects of the treatment strategy are the initial boosting of motivation (non-smoking is better!), increased self-observation (documenting cigarette consumption to make smoking habits transparent) and developing individual techniques for coping with cravings. Smokers must gradually realise that abstinence is attractive and they must be prepared for the possibility of relapses. The system also enables smokers to learn a relaxation technique that should always be used when cravings arise. Since the possibility of weight gain can undo the benefit of cessation, quitting smokers should be prepared for this eventuality (Chap. 11, Sect. 11.5.3). It is important to develop new behaviours and to set rewards for goals achieved. However, since the physical dependence also has to be treated, adjunctive NRT also alleviates the symptoms of withdrawal (see Chap. 11, Sect. 11.1.1).

The treatment uses elements of behavioural therapy (sanctions or "punishments" [formerly also learning aversive responses such as nausea and vomiting], identifying alternative actions, support measures for quitting smoking) and may be conducted individually, in a group or with a self-help manual. In 13 studies comparing a group programme with a self-help programme, there was an increase in smoking cessation with a group programme (OR = 2.10; CI: 1.64–2.70). Group programmes were more effective than no intervention or minimal-contact interventions (OR = 1.91; CI: 1.20–3.04). There was no evidence that manipulating the social interactions between participants in a group programme had an effect on outcome [70]. In every case, however, biochemical markers should be included when assessing success. Overall, interpretation of results is rendered difficult because the study objectives were very differently defined. Behavioural therapy can be implemented in weekly group sessions (10–15 smokers), particularly since individual treatment is far too personnel-intensive and will, therefore, fail. For the most part, a 5–10-week course of treatment is required [71, 72]. Shorter treatments often leave the ex-smoker to cope alone with the late symptoms of withdrawal.

10.7
Aversion Therapy

Aversion therapy is based on pairing the "pleasurable" event with an unpleasant physical stimulus. It may be regarded as a form of behavioural therapy designed to correct certain behaviours such as dependence (e.g. on cigarettes) or excessive eating [73]. In this context, the best-known technique is that of rapid and increased cigarette consumption [74], the target being one puff every 6–10 s. After 3 min, generally, the smoker reaches the point at which nausea develops. Some smokers need three cigarettes in this period. This "mild" nicotine overdose (dizziness, nausea, vomiting) is intended to develop aversion. These methods are hardly used at all today and they may even be dangerous for patients who are at risk (coronary heart disease, etc.) [75], though the contrary view also exists [9, 26, 76]. As soon as the symptoms of overdose have resolved, the procedure may be repeated, with 3–10 such sessions being reported in different studies. As far as possible, smokers should not smoke between sessions. One summary review of 35,000 smokers who have been treated with this technique did not detect any major negative effects [30]. In 10 studies of rapid smoking, compared with control, the overall odds ratio for abstinence was 2.08 (CI: 1.39–3.12) [77]. However, this finding should be interpreted cautiously because the funnel plot of included studies was asymmetrical due to the relative absence of small studies with negative results (Table 10.2) [77]. The single trial using biochemical validation of all self-reported cessation did not show a significant result.

Other aversion methods (e.g. application of electric shocks, intensive puffing, holding the smoke in the mouth for longer periods while continuing to breathe through the nose, cough stimulus provocation, taking bitter pills before smoking a cigarette, silver acetate chewing gum) are reported to be only marginally effective (OR = 1.19; CI: 0.77–1.83) [77].

10.8
Mass Media Communication Strategies

Over the past 10–15 years, several attempts have been made via the mass media to influence smoking behaviour among the wider population. The following media formats have been utilised for this purpose: television, cinema, radio broadcasts, print media of all types, posters, personal discussions, smoker helplines and even personal direct mailings. These campaigns communicated factual information or they took the form of appeals; they also employed a counter-advertising strategy, tantamount to a condemnation of the tobacco industry's marketing strategies. When assessing the usefulness of such methods, of course, the decisive point is the achievement of smoking cessation (or at least a definite reduction in smoking) over a period of several months (≥6 months).

In citing a number of such campaigns from the past, attention here will focus primarily on Australia and the UK [78]:

- *"Every cigarette is doing you damage"* (Australia). This campaign gained international recognition because it used hard-hitting TV adverts, in conjunction with radio broadcasts, billboards and full-page magazine adverts, to depict the adverse consequences of tobacco consumption [79]. The initially positive results were seen most clearly among adolescents (14–17-years old), even though this group was not part of the intended target audience; nevertheless, 67% of them were motivated to quit smoking. The mean national smoker prevalence was lowered by 1.7% (from 23.5 to 21.8%). The campaign was run again in Singapore with slight modifications [80].
- The *John Cleese Campaign* featured this celebrity comic actor to stimulate the interest of smokers between the ages of 25 and 44 years; it sought to promote smoking cessation by presenting serious messages (e.g. *"Smoking can kill,"* *"Smoking harms your children,"* *"Smoking is not the only way to enjoy yourself"*) in a humorous way. The campaign was supported by a telephone helpline. Following the campaign, smoking prevalence fell by 1.2% (from 28.0 to 26.8%) over a 3-year period (1992–1995) [78, 81, 82].
- The target group for the *"Break Free Campaign"* was smokers who were already seriously considering quitting smoking. The *"You can be free"* slogan was shown on TV

and posters. This 2-year campaign had minimal success, reflected in the fact that a high proportion of the key target audience no longer recalled the adverts and only 49% believed they could be motivated to quit smoking by these campaigns [78, 82].

- The "*Quit for Life*" campaign used TV and radio adverts to deliver messages designed to encourage smoking cessation, primarily with practical tips on quitting. Despite positive pre-testing, the TV adverts were not sufficiently powerful to stimulate smokers into taking action, whereas the radio adverts were received more favourably [78, 82].
- Running from 1997–1999, the "*Testimonials*" campaign used older smokers to tell younger smokers about their tobacco-related illnesses in the hope that for younger smokers the future consequences of smoking would be brought into a more immediate time frame. Special TV adverts also drew the attention of female smokers to these problems. Surveys revealed that 72% of women agreed that the adverts were aimed at people like them and 67% stated that the adverts made them realise the possible health risks of smoking. The adverts were ineffective among younger (16–24-year old) female smokers [78, 82].

As shown by data from the various campaigns (Table 10.3), the "*John Cleese Campaign*" produced the most sustained effect (92% recognition). One year after the campaign ended, 90% of those surveyed could still remember it.

Smoking cessation programmes using a range of mass media were initiated almost simultaneously in Holland *("Quit smoking together")* and in the USA (Bellingham, Washington: "*Broadcast cessation clinics*") [83, 84]; these showed initial successes in terms of smoking cessation, with the combination of TV and radio proving to be beneficial and having a lasting effect [84].

Population surveys indicate that the combined use of various mass media components (TV, radio, billboards, print media), as in the *California Tobacco Control Program*, is

Table 10.3   Results reported from four UK anti-smoking campaigns and their associated media cost [79–82]

Question	Campaign			
	"Cleese" 1992–1995	"Break" 1995–1996	"Quit" 1996–1997	"Testimonial" 1997–1999
Prompted awareness of the campaign	92	54	63	66
"Fed up with seeing the adverts"	20–22*	16	–	–
"Encouraged me to think about giving up"	–	50	44	57–60*
"More confidence to give up"	35	42	49	41
"Made me feel guilty about smoking"	42–43*	38	38	49–55*
"Unfair to smokers"	20–24*	19	23	20–21*
Cost (in £ millions)	3,183	2,326	2,484	4,886

– Question not asked; *Statistics from various surveys

Table 10.4 Assumed effectiveness of various mass media messages [95]: survey of 1,500 adolescents and adults in California, Michigan and Massachusetts

Message content	Adolescents	Adults
Tobacco industry manipulation	++	++
Passive smoking	++	++
Nicotine as a powerful addictive substance	+	+
Reasons for and information on quitting smoking	±	+
Easy youth access to cigarettes	−−	−
Short-term negative effects	−	−−
Long-term health effects	−−	−
Romantic rejection	−−	−−

++ Very effective; + effective; ± uncertain; − minimally effective; −− not effective

advantageous: 6.7% of those surveyed quit smoking as a result of media-led motivation. Among ex-smokers, 69.1% confirmed awareness of the campaign and 34.3% subsequently cited this campaign as justifying their decision to quit smoking [85].

As shown by the survey results summarised in Table 10.4, only a very limited number of messages communicated in the mass media have a positive effect, and this needs to be borne in mind for future campaigns. Quit smoking TV campaigns ("television clinics") in the USA have been more successful and in Texas, an abstinence rate of 22% has even been reported with one such campaign over a 6-week period [84]. Even though numerous professional groups work together in campaigns of this kind, the role of the physician in personal counselling assumes high importance [86].

Experience indicates that younger smokers are unreachable or very hard to reach with such campaigns, whereas middle-aged smokers already have health issues related to cigarette smoking and also express a desire to quit smoking for the most varied reasons. Elderly smokers are frequently heavily dependent: they are aware of this and know in some cases that they already have major health problems. Left to their own devices, however, they are not capable of achieving smoking cessation. This is where medical intervention comes into its own, with extensive counselling being a necessary prerequisite for longer-term success. For ex-smokers and non-smokers, mass media campaigns also strengthen their resolve not to smoke in future.

Fewer than 10% of the numerous studies (6 out of 63) satisfy the criteria of evidence-based medicine [84, 87]. These 6 studies also used a controlled trial design. Two of the studies underline the effectiveness of mass media campaigns also in terms of influencing adolescents. On the one hand, these campaigns reach several tens or even hundreds of thousands of people. On the other hand, given the considerable levels of media spend (see Table 10.3), their effectiveness in terms of achieving smoking cessation is low to moderate, as also shown by numerous studies in other countries. Mass media campaigns have been conducted in Holland [83, 88], California [83, 89], Switzerland [90], the UK [91], and in California with a centralised telephone counselling service [92], in Chicago with a media-based workplace smoking cessation programme [93] and in Australia with a directly mailed smoking cessation intervention [94]. The results of the studies were generally not very encouraging, a finding revealed by the analysis performed by the Cochrane Group [87, 95].

Thought also needs to be given to the messages communicated during these campaigns because these determine success to a considerable extent in terms of motivating people to quit smoking or to think about doing so. Several campaigns frequently failed to reach >2% of the target audience, while others reached up to 10% [96]. In this context, the determining factors were found to be the type of programme and the programme sponsor, as well as the type of communication channel used (including TV, radio) and the segmentation of the message by stage of change. In one campaign, the telephone was identified as being a particularly important recruitment channel: the number of smokers recruited was clearly higher with the telephone than with passive recruitment strategies (42.5% vs. 10%) [96].

10.9
Hypnosis

Hypnosis is a suggestive technique that aims to overcome short-term withdrawal symptoms and to cancel out the cues for smoking. Hypnotherapy lacks any capacity to prevent relapse and is of no consequence in coping with cravings.

Hypnotherapy was investigated in 10 studies, but none of them measured biochemical markers (nicotine, cotinine, CO, etc.), with the result that success rates self-reported by ex-smokers (in many cases the information was elicited only over the telephone) should be categorised as uncertain [27].

In addition, the studies differ quite considerably in terms of design [97–99]. Older uncontrolled studies have also repeatedly reported abstinence success rates as high as 50% over 6–12 months, but here too no biochemical markers were included.

Over a follow-up observation period of 6 months, hypnotherapy to promote smoking cessation did not prove more effective than programmes without interventions. Studies reporting higher success rates for hypnotherapy, compared with no intervention groups, displayed methodological defects, particularly since the effects of hypnotherapy may be quite non-specific: overall, the assessment of such studies is complicated by the heterogeneity of the results (Table 10.2) [77]. The highly significant effects reported for hypnotherapy in an earlier study are due to the absence of a control group [100].

10.10
Acupuncture

In a review of 18 studies of the efficacy of acupuncture, only one showed a significant effect after 12 months (OR = 2.44; CI: 1.15–5.20) [101]. In a comparison of 18 studies using hard criteria, acupuncture was not superior to sham acupuncture in terms of achieving smoking cessation (OR = 1.22; CI: 0.99–1.49 after a few days; OR = 1.38; CI: 0.90–2.11 after 6 months; and OR = 1.02; CI: 0.72–1.43 after 12 months) [102–105]. Also, in a comparison with other smoking cessation methods, the odds ratios were similar (OR = 0.80–1.05) for the best and worst results. Comparison of acupuncture with other interventions for promoting smoking cessation did not reveal differences in outcome at any time point. Acupuncture appeared to be superior to no intervention in terms of early results (OR = 5.88; CI: 2.66–13.01), but this effect could not be confirmed after 6-months (OR = 0.99; CI: 0.30–3.24) (Table 10.2) [106]. Differences in acupuncture technique (auricular vs. other body location) also had no effect on success rates. It remains to be seen whether acupuncture is useful during the acute withdrawal phase [104].

10.11
Reduced Smoking

Gradual reduction of the nicotine dose administered in cigarettes has been tested as a method of promoting smoking cessation. These studies were designed to investigate the following:

1. Different filter sizes to reduce the absorbed nicotine dose
2. Cigarettes with differing nicotine yields
3. Gradual daily reduction in cigarette consumption [100, 107–109]

The statistically non-significant success rate associated with this technique was 5% (2–11%) on average. Methods based on smokers' intentions to quit smoking by a gradual reduction in consumption or other related techniques (e.g. using filter tips of differing lengths) are unusable and should be discarded.

10.12
Pregnancy

As is evident from the data reviewed in Chap. 9, pregnant women who smoke run a considerable risk for their children – and this risk increases as a function of the number of cigarettes smoked daily. Since women ideally should not receive any medication during pregnancy, numerous smoking cessation programmes have been designed, based solely on the provision of counselling to women. Data obtained in 37 trials including 16,916 women offer grounds for optimism: a significant reduction in smoking (smoking cessation) was achieved by medical counselling in 34 studies (OR = 0.53; CI: 0.47–0.60) and the percentage of women continuing to smoke was lowered by 6.4% [105]. In 8 studies with validated smoking cessation, high-intensity counselling and very stringent assessment criteria, the percentage of women continuing to smoke fell by 8.1% (OR = 0.53; CI: 0.44–0.63) [105]. The subset of trials with information on fetal outcome revealed reductions in low birth weight (OR = 0.80; CI: 0.67–0.95) and preterm births (OR = 0.83; CI: 0.69–0.99) and an increase in mean birth weight of 28 g (9–49 g). Ultimately, therefore, these techniques may be regarded as useful for reducing perinatal mortality [110].

Counselling guidelines for use in gynaecological practice have been published in Germany, providing advice to pregnant women and indicating where additional information can be purchased [23].

10.13
E-Learning, Email and Internet for Smoking Cessation

In the past few years, internet or email-driven programmes for smoking cessation were established [111]. A study by Riley et al. sought to test the feasibility of two self-help behavioural interventions to reduce and maintain a 50% reduction in smoking among those unable or unwilling to quit, and to evaluate the impact of smoking reduction on subsequent quit attempts [112]. Ninety-three smokers who desired to reduce rather than quit smoking were entered in the study and randomly assigned to either computerized scheduled gradual reduction (CSGR) or a manual-based selective elimination reduction (SER). Both groups produced significant reductions in smoking (approximately 10 cigarettes/day, during the 7-week treatment phase), which were maintained over 1 year. The CSGR group reported greater mean percent reductions in smoking from pre- to post-treatment (37% for CSGR, 20% for SER) and a greater percentage of subjects meeting the 50% reduction goal (30% for CSGR, 16% for SER) compared with the SER group. The groups were comparable, however, on all other outcome measures at post-treatment and at 6- and 12-month follow-up. Although subjects with a current desire for smoking cessation were excluded from this study, one-third of the subjects reported a 24-h quit attempt in the year following study initiation, and 8.6% of the subjects met 7-day point-prevalence criteria for abstinence (CO validated) at the 12-month follow-up. The results of this study lend support to the feasibility of self-help behavioural interventions to produce sustained reductions in smoking rates without apparent negative impact on subsequent quit attempts [112].

10.14
Concluding Remarks

- The counselling of smokers by a physician or other trained health care professionals is an essential component of smoking cessation.
- Behavioural therapy programmes have proved effective in terms of non-pharmacological counselling and treatment, and these should also be used in pregnant women.
- Mass media campaigns reach larger segments of the population, but differ widely in terms of their effectiveness, and the financial cost of the media spend can be considerable. Projects of this kind should, therefore, be discussed on a case-to-case basis before the decision is taken to implement them.
- Like many other interventions, hypnotherapy and acupuncture may be effective in individual smokers. Overall, however, the results of treatment in the published literature do not satisfy the efficacy criteria of evidence-based medicine.

References

1. Velicer WF, Fava JL, Prochaska JO, Abrams DB, Emmons KM, Pierce JP (1995) Distribution of smokers by stage in three representative samples. Prev Med 24(4):401–411
2. Kommission der Europäischen Gemeinschaften (ed) (1988) Die Europäer und die Krebsverhütung: Eine Studie über Einstellung und Verhalten der Bevölkerung
3. Hajek P (1994) Treatments for smokers. Addiction 89(11):1543–1549
4. Bock BC, Marcus BH, King TK, Borrelli B, Roberts MR (1999) Exercise effects on withdrawal and mood among women attempting smoking cessation. Addict Behav 24(3):399–410
5. Tölle R, Buchkremer G (1989) Zigarettenrauchen - Epidemiologie, Psychologie, Pharmakologie und Therapie, 2 edn.Springer, Heidelberg
6. Prochaska JO, DiClemente CC (1983) Stages and processes of self-change of smoking: toward an integrative model of change. J Consult Clin Psychol 51:390–395
7. Carlson LE, Taenzer P, Koopmans J, Casebeer A (2003) Predictive value of aspects of the Transtheoretical Model on smoking cessation in a community-based, large-group cognitive behavioral program. Addict Behav 28(4):725–740
8. Dino G, Kamal K, Horn K, Kalsekar I, Fernandes A (2004) Stage of change and smoking cessation outcomes among adolescents. Addict Behav 29(5):935–940
9. Haustein KO (2000) Pharmacotherapy of nicotine dependence. Int J Clin Pharmacol Ther 38(6):273–290
10. US Department of Health and Human Services. Clinical practice guideline: Treating tobacco use and dependence. 2000. Report No.: Publication No. 00–0032
11. Andrews JO, Heath J, Graham-Garcia J (2004) Management of tobacco dependence in older adults: using evidence-based strategies. J Gerontol Nurs 30(12):13–24
12. Park EW, Schultz JK, Tudiver F, Campbel T, Becker L (2002) Enhancing partner support to improve smoking cessation (Cockraine Review). Issue 1. Oxford, Update Software. The Cochrane Library
13. McBride CM, Curry SJ, Grothaus LC, Nelson JC, Lando H, Pirie PL (1998) Partner smoking status and pregnant smoker's perceptions of support for and likelihood of smoking cessation. Health Psychol 17:63–69
14. Hanson BS, Isacsson SO, Janzon L, Lindell SE (1990) Social support and quitting smoking for good. Is there an association? Results from the population study, "Men born in 1914," Malmo, Sweden. Addict Behav 15:221–233
15. Waldron I, Lye D (1989) Family roles and smoking. Am J Prev Med 5:136–141
16. Coppotelli HC, Orleans CT (1985) Partner support and other determinants of smoking cessation maintenance among women. J Consult Clin Psychol 53:455–460
17. Gulliver SB, Hughes JR, Solomon LJ, Dey AN (1995) An investigation of self-efficacy, partner support and daily stresses as predictors of relapse to smoking in self-quitters. Addiction 90:767–772
18. Roski J, Schmid LA, Lando HA (1996) Long-term associations of helpful and harmful spousal behaviors with smoking cessation. Addict Behav 21:173–185
19. McIntyre-Kingsolver K, Lichtenstein E, Mermelstein RJ (1986) Spouse training in a multicomponent smoking-cessation program. Behav Ther 17:67–74
20. Ginsberg D, Hall SM, Rosinski M (1992) Partner support, psychological treatment, and nicotine gum in smoking treatment: an incremental study. Int J Addict 27:503–514
21. Fiore MC (2000) Treating tobacco use and dependence: an introduction to the US Public Health Service Clinical Practice Guideline. Respir Care 45(10):1196–1199
22. May S, West R (2000) Do social support interventions ("buddy systems") aid smoking cessation? A review. Tob Control 9(4):415–422

23. Brecklinghaus I, Lang P, Greiser E (1999) Rauchfrei in der Schwangerschaft. Beratungsleitfaden für die gynäkologische Fachpraxis. Loseblatt-Sammlung, Köln

24. Glynn TJ, Boyd GM, Gruman JC (1990) Essential elements of self-help/minimal intervention strategies for smoking cessation. Health Educ Q 17(3):329–345

25. Lancaster T, Stead LF (2000) Self-help interventions for smoking cessation. Cochrane Database Syst Rev (2):CD001118

26. Hill JS (2001) Health behaviour: the role of exercise in smoking cessation. CAPHER J 28:15–18

27. Ashenden R, Silagy CA, Lodge M, Fowler G (1997) A meta-analysis of the effectiveness of acupuncture in smoking cessation. Drugs Alcohol Rev (16):33–40

28. Brown SL, Owen N (1992) Self-help smoking cessation materials. Aust J Public Health 16(2):188–191

29. O'Connor PJ, Youngstedt SD (1995) Influence of exercise on human sleep. Exerc Sport Sci Rev 23:105–134

30. Danaher BG (1977) Rapid smoking and self-control in the modification of smoking behaviour. J Consult Clin Psychol 45:1068–1075

31. King AC, Taylor CB, Haskell WL (1993) Effects of differing intensities and formats of 12 months of exercise training on psychological outcomes in older adults. Health Psychol 12(4):292–300

32. Sorensen G, Goldberg R, Ockene J, Klar J, Tannenbaum T Lemeshow S (1992) Heavy smoking among a sample of employed women. Am J Prev Med 8(4):207–214

33. Miller NH, Smith PM, DeBusk RF, Sobel DS, Taylor CB (1997) Smoking cessation in hospitalized patients. Results of a randomized trial. Arch Intern Med 157(4):409–415

34. Kawachi I, Troisi RJ, Rotnitzky AG, Coakley EH, Colditz GA (1996) Can physical activity minimize weight gain in women after smoking cessation? Am J Public Health 86(7):999–1004

35. Gritz ER, Klesges RC, Meyers AW (1989) The smoking and the body weight relationship: implications for interventions and postcessation weight control. Ann Behav Med 11:144–153

36. Steptoe A, Bolton J (1988) The short-term influence of high and low intensity physical exercise on mood. Psychol Health 2:91–106

37. McAuley E, Mihalko SL, Bane SM (1997) Exercise and self-esteem in middle-aged adults: multidimensional relationships and physical fitness and self-efficacy influences. J Behav Med 20(1):67–83

38. Pate RR, Pratt M, Blair SN, Haskell WL, Macera CA, Bouchard C, et al (1995) Physical activity and public health. A recommendation from the Centers for Disease Control and Prevention and the American College of Sports Medicine. JAMA 273(5):402–407

39. Marcus BH, Albrecht AE, King TK, Parisi AF, Pinto BM, Roberts M, et al (1999) The efficacy of exercise as an aid for smoking cessation in women: a randomized controlled trial. Arch Intern Med 159(11):1229–1234

40. Ussher M (2005) Exercise interventions for smoking cessation. Cochrane Database Syst Rev (1):CD002295

41. Brandon TH, Collins BN, Juliano LM, Lazev AB (2000) Preventing relapse among former smokers: a comparison of minimal interventions through telephone and mail. J Consult Clin Psychol 68(1):103–113

42. Lichtenstein E, Glasgow RE, Lando HA, Ossip-Klein DJ, Boles SM (1996) Telephone counseling for smoking cessation: rationales and meta-analytic review of evidence. Health Educ Res 11:243–257

43. Glasgow RE, Hollis JF, McRae SG, Lando HA, LaChance P (1991) Providing an integrated program of low intensity tobacco cessation services in a health maintenance organization. Health Educ Res 6:87–99

44. Rigotti NA, Munafo MR, Murphy MFG, Stead LF (2002) Interventions for smoking cessation in hospitalised patients. Issue 1. Oxford, Update Software. The Cochrane Library

45. Brenner H, Mielck A (1993) The role of childbirth in smoking cessation. Prev Med 22(2):225–236
46. Manley MW, Epps RP, Glynn TJ (1992) The clinician's role in promoting smoking cessation among clinic patients. Med Clin North Am 76(2):477–494
47. Hjermann I, Velve BK, Holme I, Leren P (1981) Effect of diet and smoking intervention on the incidence of coronary heart disease. Report from the Oslo Study Group of a randomised trial in healthy men. Lancet 2(8259):1303–1310
48. Multiple Risk Factor Intervention Trial Research Group (1982) Multiple risk factor intervention trial. Risk factor changes and mortality results. JAMA 248(12):1465–1477
49. World Health Organization European Collaborative Group (1982) Multifactorial trial in the prevention of coronary heart disease, II: risk factor changes at two and four years. Eur Heart J 3:184–190
50. Miller NS, Gold MS (1998) Comorbid cigarette and alcohol addiction: epidemiology and treatment. J Addict Dis 17(1):55–66
51. Rigotti NA, Arnsten JH, McKool KM, Wood-Reid KM, Pasternak RC, Singer DE (1997) Efficacy of a smoking cessation program for hospital patients. Arch Intern Med 157(22):2653–2660
52. Simon JA, Solkowitz SN, Carmody TP, Browner WS (1997) Smoking cessation after surgery. A randomized trial. Arch Intern Med 157(12):1371–1376
53. Stevens VJ, Glasgow RE, Hollis JF, Lichtenstein E, Vogt TM (1993) A smoking-cessation intervention for hospital patients. Med Care 31(1):65–72
54. Weissfeld JL, Holloway JL (1991) Treatment for cigarette smoking in a Department of Veterans Affairs outpatient clinic. Arch Intern Med 151(5):973–977
55. Windsor RA, Lowe JB, Bartlett EE (1988) The effectiveness of a worksite self-help smoking cessation program: a randomized trial. J Behav Med 11(4):407–421
56. Lancaster T, Silagy C, Fowler G, Soiers I (2000) Training health professionals in smoking cessation (Cochrane Review). Cochrane Database Syst Rev (2):CD000214
57. Picardi A, Bertoldi S, Morosini P (2002) Association between the engagement of relatives in a behavioural group intervention for smoking cessation and higher quit rates at 6-, 12- and 24-month follow-ups. Eur Addict Res 8(3):109–117
58. Kottke TE, Battista RN, DeFriese GH, Brekke ML (1988) Attributes of successful smoking cessation interventions in medical practice. A meta-analysis of 39 controlled trials. JAMA 259(19):2883–2889
59. Silagy C (2000) Physician advice for smoking cessation (Cochrane Review). Cochrane Database Syst Rev (4):CD000165
60. Taylor CB, Houston-Miller N, Killen JD, DeBusk RF (1990) Smoking cessation after acute myocardial infarction: effects of a nurse-managed intervention. Ann Intern Med 113:118–123
61. Rice VH, Fox DH, Lepczyk M, Sieggreen M, Mullin M, Jarosz P, et al (1994) A comparison of nursing interventions for smoking cessation in adults with cardiovascular health problems. Heart Lung 23(6):473–486
62. AHCPR (1996) The agency for Health Care Polity and Research. Smoking cessation: Clinical Practice Guidline. J Amer Med Assoc 275:1270–1280
63. Law M, Tang L (1995) An analysis of the effectiveness of interventions intended to help people stop smoking. Arch Intern Med 155:1933–1941
64. Nurses Assosiation Position Statement (1995) Cessation of tobacco use. The Association, Indianapolis
65. Rice VH, Stead LF (2000) Nursing interventions for smoking cessation. Cochrane Database Syst Rev (2):CD001188
66. Taylor CB, Miller NH, Herman S, Smith PM, Sobel D, Fisher L, et al (1996) A nurse-managed smoking cessation program for hospitalized smokers. Am J Public Health 86(11):1557–1560
67. Janz NK, Becker MH, Kirscht JP, Eraker SA, Billi JE, Woolliscroft JO (1987) Evaluation of a minimal-contact smoking cessation intervention in an outpatient setting. Am J Public Health 77:805–809

68. Vetter NJ, Ford D (1990) Smoking prevention among people aged 60 and over: a randomized controlled trial. Age Ageing 19:164–168
69. Stead LF, Lancaster T (2002) Group behaviour therapy programmes for smoking cessation (Cochrane Review). Issue 1. Oxford, Copyright Update Software Ltd. The Cochrane Library
70. Stead LF, Lancaster T (2000) Group behaviour therapy programmes for smoking cessation. Cochrane Database Syst Rev (2):CD001007
71. Hajek P (1989) Withdrawal-oriented therapy for smokers. Br J Addict 84(6):591–598
72. Hajek P, Belcher M, Stapleton J (1985) Enhancing the impact of groups: an evaluation of two group formats for smokers. Br J Clin Psychol 24(Pt 4):289–294
73. Davison G, Naele J (1994) Abnormal psychology. Wiley, New York
74. Lublin I, Joslyn L (1968) Aversive conditioning of cigarette addiction. Paper presented at the meeting of the Western Psychological Association, Los Angeles, CA
75. Burt A, Thornley P, Illingworth D, White P, Shaw TR, Turner R (1974) Stopping smoking after myocardial infarction. Lancet 1(7852):304–306
76. Hall RG, Sachs DP, Hall SM, Benowitz NL (1984) Two-year efficacy and safety of rapid smoking therapy in patients with cardiac and pulmonary disease. J Consult Clin Psychol 52(4):574–581
77. Hajek P, Stead LF (2000) Aversive smoking for smoking cessation. Cochrane Database Syst Rev (2):CD000546
78. Health and Developing Agency (ed) (2000) A breath of fresh air tackling smoking through the media. London
79. Commonwealth Department of Health and Aged Care (2000) Evaluation Report. Australia's National Tobacco Campaign (ed), vol 1 and 2. Canberra, NTC
80. Yeong CC, Yap E, Heng V, Law F, Cheong K (2000) Singapore's experience in adapting Australia's National Tobacco Campaign. 11th World Conference on Tobacco or Health, Chicago, 6 August2000
81. McVey D, Stapleton J (2000) Can anti-smoking television advertising affect smoking behaviour? controlled trial of the Health Education Authority for England's anti-smoking TV campaign. Tob Control 9:273–282
82. . John Cleese Campaign (2002) www.public.health.wa.gov.au/smoking/quit95.pdf
83. Mudde AN, De Vries H (1999) The reach and effectiveness of a national mass media-led smoking cessation campaign in The Netherlands. Am J Public Health 89:346–350
84. Sparks RE, Green LW (1998) Mass Media in support of smoking cessation. In: Institute of Health Promotion Research (ed) Smoking cessation: a synthesis of the literature on program effectiveness. University of British Columbia, Victoria
85. Popham WJ, Potter LD, Hetrick MA, Muthen LK, Duerr JM, Johnson MD (1994) Effectiveness of the California 1990–1991 tobacco education media campaign. Am J Prev Med 10:319–326
86. Fiore MC, Bailey WC, Cohen SJ, Dorfman SF, Goldstein MG, Gritz ER, et al (2000) Treating tobacco use and dependence. US Department of Health and Human Services, Public Health Service. AHCPR Supported Guidelines
87. Sowden AJ, Arblaster L (2001) Mass media interventions for preventing smoking in young people (Cochrane Review). [Issue 4]. Oxford, The Cochrane Library
88. Mudde AN, De Vries H, Dolders MG (1995) Evaluation of a Dutch community-based smoking cessation intervention. Prev Med 24:61–70
89. Pierce JP, Gilpin EA, Emery SL, White MM, Rosbrook B, Berry CC, et al (1998) Has the California tobacco control program reduced smoking? JAMA 280:893–899
90. Etter JF, Ronchi A, Perneger T (1999) Short-term impact of a university based smoke free campaign. J Epidemiol Community Health 53:710–715
91. Owen L (2000) Impact of a telephone helpline for smokers who called during a mass media campaign. Tob Control9(2):148–154

92. Zhu SH, Anderson CM, Johnson CE, Tedeschi G, Roeseler A (2000) A centralised telephone service for tobacco cessation: the California experience. Tob Control 9(Suppl 2):II48–II55

93. Salina D, Jason LA, Hedeker D, Kaufman J, Lesondak L, McMahon SD, et al (1994) A follow-up of a media-based, worksite smoking cessation program. Am J Community Psychol 22:257–271

94. Schofield PE, Hill DJ, Johnston CI, Streeton JA (1999) The effectiveness of a directly mailed smoking cessation intervention to Australian discharged hospital patients. Prev Med 29:527–534

95. Goldman LK, Glantz SA (1998) Evaluation of antismoking advertising campaigns. JAMA 279:772–777

96. McDonald PW (1999) Population-based recruitment for quit-smoking programs: an analytic review of communication variables. Prev Med 28:545–557

97. Hyman GJ, Stanley RO, Burrows GD, Horne DJ (1986) Treatment effectiveness of hypnosis and behaviour therapy in smoking cessation: a methodological refinement. Addict Behav 11(4):355–365

98. Lambe R, Osier C, Franks P (1986) A randomized controlled trial of hypnotherapy for smoking cessation. J Fam Pract 22(1):61–65

99. Rabkin SW, Boyko E, Shane F, Kaufert J (1984) A randomized trial comparing smoking cessation programs utilizing behaviour modification, health education or hypnosis. Addict Behav 9(2):157–173

100. von Dedenroth TE (1968) The use of hypnosis in 1000 cases of "tobaccomaniacs". Am J Clin Hypn 10(3):194–197

101. White AR, Rampes H, Ernst E (2000) Acupuncture for smoking cessation (Cochrane Review). Issue 3. Oxford, Update Software. The Cochrane Library

102. He D, Berg JE, Hostmark AT (1997) Effects of acupuncture on smoking cessation or reduction for motivated smokers. Prev Med 26(2):208–214

103. Lacroix JC, Besancon F (1977) [Tobacco withdrawal. Efficacy of acupuncture in a comparative trial]. Ann Med Interne (Paris) 128(4):405–408

104. Waite NR, Clough JB (1998) A single-blind, placebo-controlled trial of a simple acupuncture treatment in the cessation of smoking. Br J Gen Pract 48(433):1487–1490

105. White AR, Resch KL, Ernst E (1998) Randomized trial of acupuncture for nicotine withdrawal symptoms. Arch Intern Med 158(20):2251–2255

106. White AR, Rampes H, Ernst E (2000) Acupuncture for smoking cessation. Cochrane Database Syst Rev (2):CD000009

107. Kendler KS, Neale MC, MacLean CJ, Heath AC, Eaves LJ, Kessler RC (1993) Smoking and major depression. A causal analysis. Arch Gen Psychiatry 50(1):36–43

108. Marks MJ, Burch JB, Collins AC (1983) Effects of chronic nicotine infusion on tolerance development and nicotinic receptors. J Pharmacol Exp Ther 226(3):817–825

109. Nicklas BJ, Tomoyasu N, Muir J, Goldberg AP (1999) Effects of cigarette smoking and its cessation on body weight and plasma leptin levels. Metabolism 48(6):804–808

110. Lumley J, Oliver S, Waters E (2004) Interventions for promoting smoking cessation during pregnancy (Cochrane Review). Cochrane Database Syst Rev (4):CD001055

111. Lenert L, Munoz RF, Perez JE, Bansod A (2004) Automated e-mail messaging as a tool for improving quit rates in an internet smoking cessation intervention. J Am Med Inform Assoc 11(4):235–240

112. Riley W, Jerome A, Behar A, Weil J (2002) Computer and manual self-help behavioral strategies for smoking reduction: initial feasibility and one-year follow-up. Nicotine Tob Res 4(Suppl 2):S183–S188

113. Schoberberger R, Kunze M (1999) Nikotinabhängigkeit: Diagnostik und Therapie. Springer, Berlin

114. Lancaster T, Stead LF (2000) Individual behavioural counselling for smoking cessation. Cochrane Database Syst Rev (2):CD001292

115. Abbot NC, Stead LF, White AR, Barnes J, Ernst E (2000) Hypnotherapy for smoking cessation. Cochrane Database Syst Rev (2):CD001008

Pharmacotherapy of Nicotine Dependence   **11**

Pharmacotherapy to promote smoking cessation has been studied in recent decades using a variety of medicinal products: currently, the most commonly employed method (and the one that is recommended by the World Health Organization) involves the use of nicotine products (for review, see [1]). All other pharmacological agents have either not fully proved their usefulness or else, like bupropion, whose efficacy has been demonstrated, require further investigation because of a smaller risk-benefit ratio. Consensus papers on the treatment of tobacco use and nicotine dependence have now appeared in the USA [2, 3] and, like the publications of the Cochrane Group [4], these have formed the basis for treatment recommendations in other countries and have provided a major stimulus to the formulation of our own recommendations (Table 11.1).

In addition to general *history-taking*, specific information should be elicited from patients concerning any concurrent illnesses of importance that may have resulted from years or decades of tobacco consumption (see Chap. 10). The diagnostic considerations summarised in Table 10.1 in Chap. 10 should be addressed in detail [18].

In principle, against the background of the many known harmful effects of smoking any measures designed to help patients achieve smoking cessation are to be recommended. Chapter 10 contains further details on the indications for and the objectives of treatment. Reduced smoking can only be achieved in conjunction with pharmacotherapy (e.g. with nicotine products).

11.1
Nicotine

In the past decades, nicotine replacement therapy (NRT) has been employed in some 40 million smokers: NRT has also been assessed scientifically in over 40,000 smokers in more than 180 studies and these have been reviewed in several meta-analyses [19–21].

A Cochrane database review study by Stead and colleagues aimed to determine the effect of NRT compared to placebo in aiding smoking cessation, and to consider whether there is a difference in effect for the different forms of NRT (chewing gum, transdermal patches, nasal spray, inhalers and tablets/lozenges) in achieving abstinence from cigarettes [22]. They also analysed whether the effect is influenced by the dosage, form and timing of use

K.-O. Haustein, D. Groneberg, *Tobacco or Health?*
DOI: 10.1007/978-3-540-87577-2_11, © Springer Verlag Berlin Heidelberg 2010

Table 11.1 Assessment of treatment methods to achieve smoking cessation (also based on the treatment recommendations on smoking cessation issued by the Pharmaceutical Commission of the German Medical Profession) [5]

Pharmacological methods	Odds ratio	Assessment	References
Nicotine replacement (total)[a]	1.73 (1.60–1.82)	⇈⇑	[5]
Chewing gum	1.63 (1.49–1.79)	⇈⇑	[5]
2 vs. 4 mg chewing gum	2.67 (1.69–4.22)	⇈⇑	[6]
Patch	1.73 (1.56–1.93)	⇈⇑	[7]
Nasal spray	2.27 (1.61–3.20)	⇈⇑	[8]
Inhaler	2.08 (1.43–3.04)	⇈⇑	[9]
Sublingual tablet	1.73 (1.07–2.80)	⇈⇑	[10]
Lozenge 2 mg	2.10 (1.59–2.79)	⇑[b]	[11]
Lozenge 4 mg	3.69 (2.74–4.96)	⇑[b]	[11]
Bupropion	2.73 (1.90–3.94)	⇈⇑	[12]
Combined with nicotine	2.65 (1.58–4.40)	⇑	[13]
Lobeline	–	⇊	[14]
Clonidine	1.89 (1.30–2.74)	⇑[c]	[15]
Buspirone	–	⇔	[16]
Anxiolytics and antidepressants	–	⇊	[16]
Nortriptyline[d]	2.83 (1.59–5.03)	⇈⇑	[16]
Aversion therapy with silver acetate	1.05 (0.63–1.73)	⇊	[17]

⇈⇑ Claim (e.g. on efficacy) supported by several suitable, valid clinical studies (e.g. randomised clinical trials) or by one or more valid meta-analyses or systematic reviews. Positive claim clearly confirmed
⇑ Claim (e.g. on efficacy) supported by at least one suitable, valid clinical study (e.g. randomised clinical trial). Positive claim confirmed
⇊ Negative claim (e.g. on efficacy) supported by one or more suitable, valid clinical studies (e.g. randomised clinical trials) or by one or more valid meta-analyses or systematic reviews. Negative claim clearly confirmed
⇔ No reliable study results available to confirm a positive or negative effect. This may be due to the absence of suitable studies but also to the availability of several studies with contradictory results
–No usable studies
[a]Additional counselling may increase efficacy
[b]Twenty-eight-day abstinence at 6 weeks [11]
[c]Efficacy after 1-year follow-up is even poorer (OR = 1.02; CI: 0.72–1.43)
[d]Not used because of AEs

of NRT; the intensity of additional advice and support offered to the smoker, or the clinical setting in which the smoker is recruited and treated. Finally, it was determined whether combinations of NRT are more likely to lead to successful quitting than one type alone and whether NRT is more, or less, likely to lead to successful quitting compared to other pharmacotherapies. As a result, a total of 132 trials were identified; 111 with over 40,000 participants contributed to the primary comparison between any type of NRT and a placebo or non-NRT control group [22]. The analysis found out that the RR of abstinence for any form of NRT relative to control was 1.58 (95% confidence interval [CI]: 1.50–1.66). The pooled RR for each type were: 1.43 (95% CI: 1.33–1.53, 53 trials) for nicotine gum; 1.66 (95% CI: 1.53–1.81, 41 trials) for nicotine patch; 1.90 (95% CI: 1.36–2.67, 4 trials) for nicotine inhaler; 2.00 (95% CI: 1.63–2.45, 6 trials) for oral tablets/lozenges and 2.02 (95% CI: 1.49–3.73, 4 trials) for nicotine nasal spray. The effects were largely independent of the duration of therapy, the intensity of additional support provided or the setting in which the NRT was offered. The effect was similar in a small group of studies that aimed to assess the use of NRT obtained without a prescription [22]. In highly dependent smokers, there was a significant benefit of 4 mg gum compared with 2 mg gum, but weaker evidence of a benefit from higher doses of patch. There was evidence that combining a nicotine patch with a rapid delivery form of NRT was more effective than a single type of NRT. Only one study directly compared NRT to another pharmacotherapy. In this study, quit rates with nicotine patch were lower than with the antidepressant bupropion. It was concluded that all of the commercially available forms of NRT (gum, transdermal patch, nasal spray, inhaler and sublingual tablets/lozenges) are efficient for smokers who make a quit attempt to increase their chances of successfully stopping smoking. The different forms of NRT increase the rate of quitting by 50–70%, regardless of setting. It was also concluded that the effectiveness of NRT appears to be largely independent of the intensity of additional support provided to the individual [22].

Treatment of the dependent smoker with nicotine replacement (in the form of patches, chewing gum, nasal sprays, sublingual tablets, inhalers) can be implemented without any major concerns over safety (for list of studies, see Table 11.1 and Fig. 11.1).

Smokers with severe "physical" dependence derive the greatest benefit from NRT. However, a heavy smoker (e.g. 20–30 cigarettes/day) is not automatically a dependent smoker. The following criteria should be applied when initiating treatment with nicotine products:

1. Daily cigarette consumption.
2. Deep and frequent inhalation on the cigarette.
3. Increased CO levels measured in expired air.
4. Difficulty in not smoking in response to "external compulsions".
5. A score of ≥3 points in the Fagerström test for nicotine dependence (FTND) (see Table 4.5 in Chap. 4).

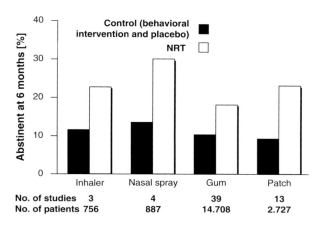

Fig. 11.1 Efficacy of nicotine products as aids to smoking cessation, based on 6-month abstinence from cigarettes. Efficacy is at least twice as great as that of behavioural therapy alone. Data summarised from [8, 9, 19, 20, 23]

11.1.1
Evaluation of Nicotine Products

Nicotine products are licensed as aids to smoking cessation for the relief of withdrawal from tobacco dependence. Cigarette smoking with its bolus-like input to the brain is regarded as the most reinforcing and dependence-producing form of nicotine administration [24]. The rationale for NRT is that the various nicotine products alleviate withdrawal symptoms by providing an alternative source of nicotine. Initially, smokers continue at a reduced dose and speed of nicotine delivery while coping with the loss of the behavioural side of their dependence (cf. Figs. 11.2 and 11.3). Several weeks later, smokers then break the nicotine dependence by stopping their use of the various nicotine formulations.

In its analysis of the now numerous publications on the subject, the Cochrane Group includes only trials which are placebo-controlled or comparator-controlled (pharmacotherapy or non-drug therapy) and which assess smoking cessation by stating the number of "failures" over a follow-up period of 6 months or longer [5]. Out of 108 studies selected on the basis of the defined criteria, 94 were performed with a control group (no nicotine product), 51 with chewing gum, 33 with patches, 4 with nasal sprays, 4 with inhalers, 2 with sublingual tablets and 4 with two products administered in combination [5]. These studies employed objective criteria (measurements of plasma nicotine concentrations, CO etc.) (see Table 11.1).

All nicotine products are suitable for use in promoting smoking cessation. The 4 mg nicotine chewing gum reportedly yields higher success rates (odds ratio [OR] = 2.67; CI: 1.69–4.22) than the 2 mg strength, but only in heavily dependent smokers (Table 11.1) [26–29], and for this reason it is better to replace the 2 mg chewing gum with the 4 mg

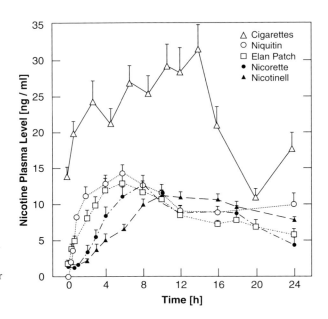

Fig. 11.2 Differing plasma nicotine concentrations after smoking (1 cigarette/h) and following application of four different transdermal nicotine patches [25]

Fig. 11.3 Plasma nicotine concentrations measured after different nicotine formulations [21]. The curves illustrate that none of the nicotine products attains the plasma concentrations or the rapid delivery achieved by cigarette smoking

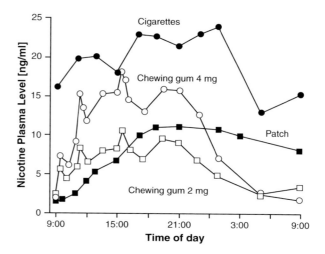

strength. To date, the prescribing information invariably recommends that the nicotine replacement product should be administered singly. However, some studies [30] indicate that combined administration, for example, of a nicotine patch + chewing gum or a patch + nasal spray in the more severe forms of dependence is more likely to achieve success than administration of a single formulation (OR = 1.55; CI: 1.17–2.05) [24].

Additional individual counselling of patients helps to increase the success rate. One study has shown that an 8-week course of treatment with nicotine patches was just as effective as longer courses of treatment [31]. Stopping smoking abruptly was just as effective as gradual smoking reduction. Furthermore, success rates do not differ depending on whether the patch remains on the skin for 16 or 24 h a day [23, 32, 33].

11.1.2
Nicotine Chewing Gum

Chewing gum was the first type of NRT to become widely available. Nicotine is absorbed directly through the buccal mucosa, resulting in plasma concentrations which are approximately half those produced by smoking a cigarette [34] (cf. Figs. 4.5 in Chap. 4, Fig. 11.3). Both 2- and 4-mg preparations are available in many countries and these are sold over-the-counter (OTC) (2 mg more than 4 mg). Several factors, including oral and gastric side effects, and dental prostheses etc., limit the usefulness of nicotine gum in some smokers [35]. It has been reported that some smokers may be at risk of switching their former cigarette addiction across to the nicotine gum [36]; however, we have observed this addiction transfer extremely rarely. According to the Cochrane Group, 51 trials have been carried out with nicotine gum (cf. Table 11.1), and two trials have compared the gum with combination of patch plus gum [37, 38]. Apart from eight of the individual trials [5], the use of nicotine chewing gum (4 mg more than 2 mg) has been reported to be more effective than placebo in promoting smoking cessation. The advantage of nicotine chewing gum over the patch is that its dosage can be adjusted individually over the course of a day in response to any cravings that may be experienced.

11.1.3
Nicotine Patch

Nicotine patches were developed as transdermal delivery systems to ensure constant release of the active ingredient over a period of 16–24 h. These systems should be applied to a dry area of hairless skin, and the application site should be varied daily. Nicorette® patches are available in strengths of 15, 10 and 5 mg. The 15-mg patch contains 25 mg nicotine. The Nicorette patch is intended to be worn for only 16 h, i.e. not during the night (Figs. 11.2 and 11.3).

By contrast, NiQuitin® and Nicotinell® aim to administer nicotine over a 24 h period. The three patch strengths of NiQuitin® and Nicotinell® deliver 7, 14 and 21 mg nicotine to the body every 24 h. Thanks to the special pharmaceutical formulation of NiQuitin® (incorporating a membrane type that releases nicotine for transcutaneous delivery), they contain 36, 78 and 114 mg nicotine on patch areas of 7, 15 and 22 cm^2 respectively. Nicotinell® contains 52.5 mg nicotine on an area of 30 cm^2. During the first 2 h after patch application, differences have been detected in terms of body area selected (chest > leg > back > gluteal region). One other study comparing absorbtion from hip and arm did not find any difference. The observed differences between application sites are without clinical relevance.

Nicotine attains maximum concentrations between 4 and 10 h following single application, and levels then plateau over 16–24 h. Significant differences exist between the area under the curve (AUC) values and the mean plasma concentration curve between single dose and steady state for the 24-h patches. The 16-h patch has similar plasma concentrations during steady state as after a single dose, as the plasma level decline over night. Separate investigations have established that nicotine is not inactivated (metabolised) during transdermal passage, whereas minimal metabolism to the analogous N-oxide or N-methyl compounds has been demonstrated under in vitro conditions following 6 day incubation [39, 40]. Overall, the metabolism of nicotine to cotinine during transdermal passage is estimated to be minimal.

Nicotine release from patches has also been studied in terms of differences due to gender, age and obesity. While gender and age differences have been excluded, a correlation with body weight has been confirmed, with AUC declining as body weight increases [41]. However, it was immaterial whether the patches were applied to the upper arm or upper body. These investigations did not reveal any consequences for therapy.

Plasma nicotine concentrations rise if cigarettes are smoked in addition to patch application (see Fig. 11.4). Naturally, nicotine absorption from cigarettes is subject to numerous influences already discussed, even where the smoker is required to smoke one cigarette at 30 min intervals over a 15 h experimental period [42, 43]. Mean nicotine concentrations at all time points are almost doubled. Mean concentrations of approximately 40 ng/ml (day 3) and 50 ng/ml (day 7) are achieved with the patch + smoking combination, whereas very much lower concentrations (<30 ng/ml) are found with an ad libitum smoking option. In practice, however, the differences in measured plasma nicotine concentrations are of minor

Fig. 11.4 Mean plasma nicotine concentrations following 2-day therapy with a 21-mg nicotine patch without (*open circle*) and with additional cigarette consumption at 30-min intervals (*open triangle*) ($n = 14$) under experimental conditions. Vertical bars represent the standard deviations of the mean (see [42])

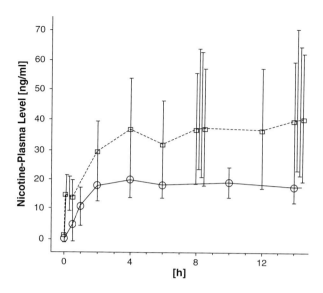

importance because external factors determine the smoker's daily cigarette consumption. Furthermore, experience shows that cigarette consumption is reduced when nicotine products are administered concurrently because the accustomed nicotine concentrations are achieved by smoking fewer cigarettes.

11.1.4
Nicotine Sublingual Tablet

Two studies (one of which has been published [10]) have been conducted to date with nicotine sublingual tablets, a formulation that is intended particularly for smokers who want to give up smoking but who do not like chewing gum [10]. Approximately 50% of absorption from the 2-mg tablet occurs through the buccal mucosa, but the tablet should be left under the tongue. The plasma nicotine profiles were similar following repeated administration of the 2-mg tablet and a 2-mg gum although absorption of nicotine from the 2-mg tablet at higher doses (2 or 3 tablets) was non-linear [44].

11.1.5
Nicotine Nasal Spray

Nicotine nasal spray is the formulation that allows the most rapid absorption of active ingredient (through the nasal mucosa), thus enabling cravings to be relieved more effectively than with chewing gum. The nasal spray is a formulation that is commonly associated with adverse effects (see Sect. 11.1.9). Four published studies with nicotine nasal spray alone [8, 45–47] and one study describing the combined application of nicotine nasal spray + patch [30] confirm its high level of efficacy (Table 11.1).

11.1.6
Nicotine Inhaler

The inhaler consists of a plastic housing with mouthpiece designed to hold a disposable porous cartridge impregnated with 10 mg nicotine. When the patient draws air into the mouth through the inhaler, nicotine from the cartridge is vaporised. At room temperature, 13 µg nicotine is released by one draw on the 10-mg inhaler [48]. In total, approximately 4 mg is absorbed from a 10-mg inhaler; a maximum of 50% is available to the systemic circulation and the inhalation technique (buccal or pulmonary) is of marginal importance in terms of the dose and steady-state plasma concentrations achieved (see Fig. 11.5). Following the use of the inhaler for 20 min, bioavailability is not higher with pulmonary inhalation (deep drawing) than with buccal inhalation (shallow puffing). Thus, the blood nicotine levels produced with the inhaler are approximately 30% of those seen in chronic cigarette smokers (see Fig. 11.5) [49, 50]. Details of the effectiveness of the inhaler in smoking cessation are presented in Table 11.2.

11.1.7
Nicotine Lozenge

Two new oral forms of nicotine formulations have recently been introduced: the 1-mg lozenge (UK and Sweden) without published pharmacokinetic or efficacy data, and a

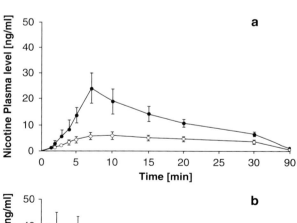

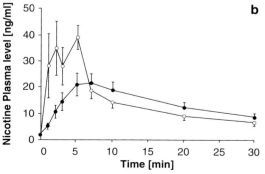

Fig. 11.5 (**a**) Mean arterial (*open circle*) and jugular venous (*closed circle*) plasma nicotine level after using one inhaler for 5 min (*n* = 7). (**b**) Mean arterial (*open circle*) and jugular venous (*closed circle*) plasma nicotine level after smoking one cigarette over 5 min (*n* = 7). Note that the AV difference is reversed for the inhaler relative to the cigarette [49]

Table 11.2 Study results of smoking cessation with the nicotine inhaler

Inhaler	n	Parameter	Effectiveness (active treatment vs. placebo)	References
3 months ad libitum	222	CO, cotinine	21 vs. 6% (6 months)	[48]
6 months	286	CO	15 vs. 5% (1 year)	[51]
6 months	223	CO, cotinine	13 vs. 8% (1 year)	[9]
6 months ad libitum	247	CO, cotinine	35 vs. 22% (1 year)	[52]
4 months	400	CO	9.5 vs. 3% (2 years)	[53]
12 weeks (combined with nicotine patch)	30	Cotinine	30% (12 weeks)[a]	[25]

[a]No placebo group

2- and 4-mg lozenge. Compared with the analogous gum formulations, the lozenges deliver small amounts more nicotine than the gum formulations if the area under curves were measured [54]. The efficacy of the 2- and 4-mg lozenge was tested in one multicentre and placebo-controlled trial for smoking cessation over 52 weeks with lozenge use up to 12 and (ad libitum) 24 weeks [11]. The two lozenge strengths were distributed according to the grade of dependency (FTND). The 28 day abstinence at 6 weeks dose-dependent (29 vs. 46.0 and 48.7% abstinence; OR = 2.10, CI: 1.59–2.79 and 3.69, CI: 2.74–4.96; $p <$ 0.001; placebo vs. 2- and 4-mg lozenge) [11].

11.1.8
Treatment and Dosage

Treatment with nicotine products may be given over a period of 2–3 months. *Nicotine patches* provide mean transdermal delivery over 16 or 24 h of 0.9 mg nicotine/h. Lower strength patches (0.6 or 0.3 mg/h) may also be used optionally at a later stage in the treatment course. Up to 16 pieces of *nicotine chewing gum* (4 mg strength) may be used over a 24-h period. If it is to be used successfully and without producing unpleasant symptoms, nicotine gum should be chewed slowly over a period of 30 min; the patient chews the gum once or twice using the molars on one side, waits for 30 s and then repeats the process using the molars on the other side. If the gum is chewed too rapidly, sufficient nicotine may be released within a few minutes to cause nausea, salivation, retching and indigestion. In future, instead of chewing gum, *sublingual tablets* may also be used, and this formulation may be especially advantageous for people who wear dentures. *Nicotine nasal spray* releases 0.5 mg per spray. One spray is recommended into each nostril (corresponding to 1 mg nicotine in total). Two (or a maximum of three) doses are recommended per hour. For details of the *inhaler*, see Sect. 11.1.5. The medical management of the ex-smoker involves estimating the extent to which the cravings diminish with time after smoking cessation in order to ensure that NRT is not halted too early and that the nicotine dose is not reduced too rapidly. As is evident from the data summarised in Fig. 11.3, no nicotine product generates the plasma nicotine concentrations achieved by cigarette smoking because the release of nicotine from these products (while most rapid from the nasal spray) is slower than from a cigarette [6]. It is therefore understandable that the daily nicotine doses administered must be tailored to the individual patient's level of dependence and the number of cigarettes

Table 11.3 Stepwise schedule for smoking cessation with nicotine products (patch with transdermal release of 0.9 mg/h, 4 mg chewing gum, nasal spray containing 0.5 mg/spray and sublingual tablets containing 2 mg)

Level	Diagnostic criteria	Therapeutic schedule (daily doses)
1 Mild	FTND 1–2, 5–10 cigarettes/ day, CO: 10–15 ppm	Medical consultation to educate the smoker about the harmful effects of smoking on health and about his/her personal situation based on individual findings,[a] one piece of chewing gum, as required, when the urge to smoke a cigarette is strong
2 Moderate	FTND ≥3; <15 cigarettes/ day; CO: 10–20 ppm	Initially, up to 12 pieces of nicotine chewing gum or one nicotine patch, plus a few pieces of nicotine gum only in the initial days of treatment; depending how the ex-smoker feels, continue the treatment for 2–3 weeks, then reduce the dose as appropriate
3 Severe	FTND ≥5; 15–25 ciga-rettes/ day; CO: 15–35 ppm	One nicotine patch plus 6–12 pieces of nicotine gum, depending on urge to smoke, or nicotine nasal spray (one spray into each nostril every time there is an urge to smoke; not more than two applications/h); continue the treatment for 3–6 weeks, then reduce the dose as appropriate; supply the ex-smoker with a product (nicotine chewing gum or nasal spray) as relief for craving or strong urge to smoke during the ensuing months
4 Very severe	FTND[b] ≥7; >25–40 cigarettes/day; CO[c]: >30–45 ppm	One nicotine patch plus 10–12 pieces of nicotine chewing gum[d] plus nicotine nasal spray (one spray into each nostril) as required, until craving or the urge to smoke is relieved; continue treatment for 2–4 weeks and then discontinue one nicotine product (chewing gum); later halve the dose administered by patch, retain the nasal spray to relieve craving for up to 6 months (this will not be required at all on various days)

FTND Fagerström Test for Nicotine Dependence; *CO* carbon monoxide concentration [1]. The level of dependence is classified in four grades

[a]These consultations are also compulsory at higher dependence levels

[b]An internal correlation between the FTND and CO values has not been confirmed. The two values are only approximately linked with each other

[c]The CO levels measured are influenced by the time when smoking took place. An interval of 30 min should be observed between the last cigarette and the measurement of CO

[d]Instead of the 4 mg chewing gum, the 2 mg sublingual tablet may also be used

smoked daily (see Table 11.3). Figure 11.1 summarises the efficacy of the various nicotine products, based on published reports from the literature, with a 6-month period of abstinence from smoking being the criterion for success.

NRT is the appropriate instrument for helping the dependent smoker to achieve smoking cessation. Its effectiveness is increased 2–3-fold if the smoker wants to stop. While patches are more convenient to use than chewing gum or nasal spray, they are less effective for the relief of cravings when compared with nasal spray, in particular. Although only a few studies have been published on the combined use of two different nicotine formulations (patch + chewing gum or nasal spray, and chewing gum + nasal spray or patch + inhaler), the suppression of cravings is the crucial issue with regard to failure in many dissonant ex-smokers once smoking cessation therapy has begun. Medical management has a pivotal role to play during smoking cessation therapy [5].

Our own experiences with the treatment of several hundred smokers are set out schematically in Table 11.3. The schedule cannot be defined rigidly because while the level of dependence can be identified – it is so shaped by the patient's personality structure, including his/her own willpower – the therapist must repeatedly expect the unexpected.

Where the goal of therapy is total smoking cessation, it is important to warn patients emphatically to stop smoking completely while taking nicotine products. If the objective is reduced smoking ("harm reduction"), the number of cigarettes smoked should not exceed 10/day. In this case, nicotine therapy should be tailored accordingly.

Gender differences may play a role in the efficacy of NRTs. This was analysed in a meta-analytical review of 90 effect sizes obtained from a sample of 21 double-blind, placebo-controlled randomized studies [55]. It was shown that although NRT was more effective for men than placebo at 3-, 6- and 12-month follow-ups, the benefits of NRT for women were clearly evident only at the 3- and 6-month follow-ups. Also, giving NRT in conjunction with high-intensity nonpharmacological support was more important for women than men. It was concluded that long-term maintenance of NRT treatment gains decrease more rapidly for women than men [55].

11.1.9
Adverse Events Associated with NRT

The symptoms of nicotine toxicity range from nausea, abdominal pain and vomiting, dizziness and headache to dyspnoea, convulsions and respiratory failure. Regular cigarette smokers develop tolerance to many of the effects of nicotine, and stopping smoking is associated with various nicotine withdrawal symptoms including dysphoria, irritability, anxiety, difficulty concentrating, restlessness, insomnia, decreased heart rate and increased appetite. Withdrawal symptoms are often mistaken for adverse events (AEs) associated with NRT products.

11.1.9.1
Nicotine Chewing Gum

The most frequently reported systemic AEs with nicotine 2- and 4-mg gum are headache, dizziness, gastrointestinal discomfort, nausea and vomiting, while local AEs include sore mouth or throat. Less frequent adverse reactions include palpitations, erythema and urticaria. Atrial fibrillation and allergic reactions have been reported, but these are rare (Table 11.4). A slight throat irritation and increase in salivation may occur on commencing

Table 11.4 Adverse effects reported during treatment with nicotine replacement therapy (NRT) (cf. Sect. 11.1.9)

Formulation	Adverse effects	Frequency (%)
Patch	CNS: headache, dizziness, sleep disturbance[a]	>1
	Gastrointestinal: nausea, vomiting	
	Local: erythema, itching	
	Circulation: palpitations	0.1–1.0
	Skin: urticaria	
	Cardiovascular: atrial fibrillation	<0.1
Chewing gum	CNS: headache, dizziness	>1
	Gastrointestinal: hiccups, eructation, nausea, vomiting	
	Local: sore mouth or throat, aching jaw muscles	
	Circulation: palpitations	0.1–1.0
	Skin: erythema, urticaria	
	Cardiovascular: atrial fibrillation	<0.1
	Hypersensitivity: such as angiooedema	
Nasal spray	CNS: headache, dizziness	>1
	Gastrointestinal: nausea, vomiting	
	Local: nasal and throat irritation, cough, nose bleed, rhinitis, sneezing, watering eyes	
	Circulation: palpitations	0.1–1.0
	Cardiovascular: atrial fibrillation	<0.1
Inhaler	CNS: Headache, dizziness	>1
	Gastrointestinal: hiccups, dyspepsia, nausea, vomiting	
	Local: mouth or throat irritation, cough, pharyngitis, rhinitis	
	Circulation: palpitations	0.1–1.0
	Cardiovascular: atrial fibrillation	<0.1
Sublingual tablet	CNS: headache, dizziness	>1
	Gastrointestinal: hiccups, nausea	
	Local: sore mouth or throat, dry mouth, cough, burning sensation in mouth	
	Circulation: palpitations	0.1–1.0
	Cardiovascular: atrial fibrillation	<0.1
Lozenge	Cf. Sect. 11.1.7	[b]

[a]With the 24-h patch, worn day and night
[b]Data not yet available

treatment, and excessive swallowing of dissolved nicotine may cause hiccups. The unusual taste of nicotine gum may initially be considered unpleasant. Some local effects are related to chewing technique, and their incidence can be reduced with proper instruction.

11.1.9.2
Nicotine Patch

The most common adverse effects associated with the use of the nicotine transdermal patch applied for 16 or 24 h are local skin reactions at the site of application, such as itching, erythema, edema and contact dermatitis [23, 56–58]. A meta-analysis of 35 trials reported the overall incidence of localised skin reactions to be 25% in subjects in the active treatment group and 13% in the placebo group [59]. Skin reactions are usually transient. The incidence of systemic AEs, including nausea, vomiting, dizziness, headache, insomnia and gastrointestinal discomfort, is low and rarely causes discontinuation from treatment. Several of these symptoms (dizziness, headache, sleep disturbances) may be attributable to withdrawal symptoms. Sleep disturbance may also be attributable to therapy with the 24-h nicotine patch, as it is more common than during placebo therapy (20 vs. 7%) [60]. However, use of nicotine patch during waking hours only does not appear to cause this problem [60, 61].

Some concerns were initially raised about the safety of NRT for smokers with heart disease when, following the introduction of the nicotine patch in 1992, a small number of users experienced acute myocardial infarction. However, the US Food and Drug Administration evaluated the issue using post-marketing surveillance data and concluded that the nicotine patch did not contribute to an increase in the risk of myocardial infarction [62]. Subsequent clinical studies have confirmed that patients with coronary heart disease tolerate nicotine patches well, and no increase in either angina attacks or other cardiac events has been noted in this population [59, 63, 64].

11.1.9.3
Nicotine Nasal Spray

The most common AEs with nicotine nasal spray are local irritant effects (nasal irritation, runny nose, sneezing, throat irritation, watering eyes, cough) which occur most frequently during the first few days of treatment. Nasal irritation and runny nose have been reported by approximately 90% of users [9, 45, 47] but local irritant effects were also common in the placebo groups (the placebo spray contained black pepper to maintain blinding). The frequency of local AEs decreases within the first week of use [65] and despite the high initial incidence of local irritant effects few subjects discontinue treatment because of such effects. The most common systemic events in clinical trials were headaches or dizziness, which initially occurred among 15–20% of subjects after commencing treatment [9, 45, 47] but decreased with time (to <10% after 3 weeks). Nausea, palpitations, sweating and cold hands and feet occur infrequently. No serious cardiovascular effects have been reported with nicotine nasal spray.

11.1.9.4
Nicotine Inhaler

Local AEs are common during the first few days of treatment, but these are generally mild and diminish during repeated use. The most frequent are cough and irritation in the mouth and throat [9, 48, 52]. In clinical trials, the most common systemic AEs were headache (nicotine inhaler 26%, placebo 20%), gastrointestinal discomfort (14 vs. 8%) and nausea (10 vs. 7%).

11.1.9.5
Nicotine Sublingual Tablet

The nicotine sublingual tablet may cause irritation or soreness in the mouth or throat, hiccups, nausea, gastrointestinal discomfort, dry mouth or cough [66, 67]. Most AEs are generally mild and occur soon after commencing treatment, and the incidence diminishes as treatment continues. Use of nicotine sublingual tablets for 6 months has no adverse effect on the oral mucosa or the floor of the mouth [67].

11.1.9.6
Nicotine Lozenge

The nicotine lozenge was tested in one study with 1,818 smokers [11]. 61.8% of participants reported one or more adverse effects during 6 months. Severe adverse effects were experienced by 17% of the participants (headache, diarrhoea, flatulence, heartburn, hiccup, nausea, coughing). However, detailed information about the frequency of adverse effects will be available, if larger treatment numbers are reached.

11.1.10
Withdrawal Symptoms

Withdrawal symptoms vary in severity from person to person and may last for several weeks to months. Like alcoholics, many ex-smokers are severely at risk because the least cause (going to a restaurant and having an alcoholic drink, meeting up with smokers, stress situations) may trigger a return to smoking. Many smokers, however, "merely" miss the manual cues associated with the activity of smoking. Withdrawal symptoms are commonly misinterpreted as AEs of nicotine products (Table 11.4), especially where the symptoms are of a psychological nature.

Very rarely a drug-induced dependence reaction may also develop during the course of smoking cessation therapy with nicotine preparations. In these circumstances, ex-smokers become dependent on the nicotine preparations themselves (nasal spray > chewing gum) and then frequently continue to use these products over a period of months.

11.1.11
Drug Interactions During Smoking Cessation

No systematic studies have been conducted on *interactions* between nicotine and other concurrently administered medication. The metabolic processes in the liver are stimulated principally by the combustion products of tobacco and not by nicotine. Tobacco smoke induces the cytochrome P450 enzymes CYP1A1, CYP1A2 and possibly CYP2E1 [68]. Smokers therefore metabolise various drugs more rapidly, and the converse of this situation is that during smoking cessation the activity of the drugs in question may be increased because they are now metabolised more slowly [69]. "Overdoses" resulting from this phenomenon have been described for theophylline, imipramine, haloperidol, tacrine, caffeine, phenacetin, phenylbutazone, oestradiol and pentazocine [68]. The absorption of insulin given by subcutaneous injection is also reduced by smoking, with the result that higher doses are required in smokers. After smoking cessation, this process is reversed (reduction of the insulin dose). Similarly, because smoking is known to increase catecholamine secretion, the higher doses of β-receptor blockers required in smokers may need to be reduced after smoking cessation. Clozapine, a neuroleptic drug used in psychiatric medicine, slows the metabolism of nicotine, as has been demonstrated on the basis of raised plasma cotinine concentrations [70].

11.1.12
Contraindications for the Use of Nicotine Products

Sometimes, on the basis of misconceptions concerning the effects of nicotine on the cardiovascular system, the prescribing information for nicotine products lists numerous contraindications and warnings that require revision. The vasoconstrictor effects in the nicotine-dependent smoker are attributable more to the inhaled combustion products, including CO, than to nicotine itself [71]. The same thinking also possibly applies for the administration of nicotine products during pregnancy [72]. The contraindications listed include: recent myocardial infarction, cardiac arrhythmias, recent stroke and unstable angina. The following are currently regarded as relative contraindications: stable angina, severe hypertension, cerebrovascular disease, vasospasms, severe heart failure, hyperthyroidism, insulin-dependent diabetes mellitus, acute gastrointestinal ulceration and severe renal and hepatic impairment. Additional relative contraindications listed for nicotine chewing gum include inflammation of the mouth/throat/oesophagus. For the nicotine patch, the list includes chronic generalised dermatological disorders (psoriasis, chronic dermatitis and urticaria) and for the nicotine nasal spray nose bleed and chronic diseases of the nose.

Nicotine products are not currently recommended for use during pregnancy and lactation, unless the woman is unable to stop without nicotine products, and only after consulting a physician (however, see [73]). It was stated in many expert reviews that NRT is the agent of choice for smoking cessation in pregnancy as the safety of other therapies in pregnancy have not yet been proved [74]. However, it also needs to be mentioned that while NRT avoids exposure to the myriad compounds present in tobacco smoke, nicotine itself causes damage to the developing nervous system [75].

11.1.13
Nicotine Formulations as OTC Products

Various nicotine formulations are sold as OTC products in several European countries (e.g. patch and gum in Germany). The rationale is that smokers absorb nicotine from cigarettes in higher doses, developing higher blood levels than following administration of NRT products (see Sects. 11.1.2–11.1.6; Figs. 11.2 and 11.3). The current regulatory framework restricts access to NRT without adequately considering that the likely consequence will be the continued dependence on the use of nicotine-containing tobacco, which is extremely harmful and universally available. With the aim of achieving harm reduction in smoking children, pregnant women and patients with cardiovascular diseases or diseases of the respiratory tract (e.g. COPD), all these categories of people should be permitted to use NRT not only for smoking cessation, but also for reducing the daily cigarette consumption to an optimum of <10 cigarettes/day. A critique of the current situation in the UK was published in 2001 by McNeill et al. [76].

In one large meta-analysis, the effects of prescription and OTC settings were compared in terms of their efficacy in achieving smoking cessation. The studies compared the use of patch and gum formulations of nicotine. OTC success rates were consistently higher than prescription rates at 6 weeks for both patch (OR = 1.45; CI: 1.05–1.98) and gum (OR = 2.92; CI: 1.58–5.40), and remained significant at 6 months for the patch (OR = 3.63; CI: 1.74–7.61) but not for gum (OR = 1.37; CI: 0.73–2.58) [73]. Among OTC and prescription gum users, 16.1 vs. 7.7% were abstinent at 6 weeks and 8.4 vs. 7.7% at 6 months, respectively. Among OTC and prescription patch users, abstinence rates were 19.0 vs. 16.0% after 6 weeks and 9.2 vs. 3.0% after 6 months [77]. The authors claim that NRT use within clinical studies does not follow "real-world" prescription practices. Indeed, many physicians prescribe NRT products to their smoking patients with only a few comments concerning their administration and use. In this way, lower success rates will be achieved than if physicians provide comprehensive advice to their smoking patients over several consultations (cf. Chap. 15). In contrast, the meta-analysis is correct in concluding that there is no difference in efficacy between OTC and "real-world" prescribing. If the OTC method of supplying NRT were to be spread across larger population segments, this would dramatically increase the number of abstaining smokers, and this in turn would have a substantial public health impact. In the United States, a 20% increase in quit rates was achieved [78]. The OTC method resulted in fewer smoking-attributable deaths and in increased life expectancy [79, 80]. Worldwide, NRT must become more accessible to smokers by removing regulatory barriers (e.g. France, Australia, Brazil), and early results suggest a favourable public health impact [81]. Differences between European countries concerning the sale of nicotine formulations are listed in Table 11.5. While most nicotine formulations are OTC products, bupropion is available only on prescription.

An interesting question is whether the change in NRT sales from prescription to OTC status affected smoking cessation. To assess this issue, the 1993–1999 Massachusetts Tobacco Surveys were used to compare data from adult current smokers and recent quitters before and after the OTC switch [83]. Interestingly, no significant change over time occurred in the proportion of smokers who used NRT at a quit attempt in the past year (20.1% pre-OTC vs. 21.4% post-OTC), made a quit attempt in the past year (48.1 vs. 45.2%), or quit smoking in the past year (8.1 vs. 11.1%). Fewer non-Whites used NRT after the switch (20.7% pre-OTC vs. 3.2% post-OTC, $p = 0.002$), but the proportion of Whites using NRT did not change significantly (20.6 vs. 24.0%). It was therefore concluded that there may be no increase in smokers' rates of using NRT, making a quit attempt, or stopping smoking after NRT became available for OTC sale. There appear to be other barriers to the use of NRT besides visiting a physician, especially among minority smokers [83].

Table 11.5 Interventions to support smoking cessation in several European countries [82]

Country	Training of health professionals and medical students	Cessation clinics	Helplines	Price incentive or reduced cost for treatment	Pharmacotherapies available for cessation	Pharmacotherapies available	
						On prescription only	In pharmacies, without prescription
Austria	+	+	+	–	+	B + NNS op	+
Belgium	d.n.a.	d.n.a.	d.n.a.	d.n.a.	+	NP + B op	–
Denmark	+	+	+	+	+	B op	+
Finland	d.n.a.	+	d.n.a.	d.n.a.	+	B + NNS op	+
France	+	+	+	+	+	–	+
Germany	+	d.n.a.	+	d.n.a.	+	B + NNS op	+
Greece	+	+	–	–	+	+	+
Iceland	+	+	+	+	+	–	+
Ireland	+	+	+		+	B, NNS, NI op	+
Italy	+	d.n.a.	+	d.n.a.	+	B op	+
Luxembourg	d.n.a.	d.n.a.	d.n.a.	d.n.a.	d.n.a.	d.n.a.	d.n.a.
Monaco	d.n.a.	d.n.a.	d.n.a.	d.n.a.	d.n.a.	d.n.a.	d.n.a.
Netherlands	+	+	+	+	+	B op	+
Portugal	–	+	–	–	+	B op	+
Spain	+	+	d.n.a.	d.n.a.	+	B op	+
Sweden	+	+	+	–	+	B + NNS op	+
U.K.	+	+	+	+	+	B op	+

+ yes; – no; *d.n.a.* data not available; *B* bupropion; *op* on prescription; *NNS* nicotine nasal spray; *NI* nicotine inhaler; *NP* nicotine patch

Hughes et al. determined whether OTC NRT is pharmacologically efficacious, whether it produces abstinence rates similar to those in prescription settings, and to estimate the long term (that is, greater than 6 month) abstinence rate with OTC NRT [84]. Using a meta-analysis approach, studies were analysed that compared OTC NRT vs.OTC placebo or studies comparing OTC NRT vs.prescription NRT that reported abstinence rates and for which a full study report was available. Four studies were randomised trials of nicotine vs.placebo patch with ORs of 2.1–3.2. These outcomes were homogenous and when combined resulted in an OR favouring NRT of 2.5 (95% CI 1.8–3.6). Among the two randomised and two non-randomised trials of OTC NRT vs.prescription NRT, one small study had an OR of 0.3, two others had ORs of 1.0 and 1.4, and a fourth study had an OR of 3.6. These results were not homogenous; however, when combined via a random effects model the estimated OR was not less than 1.0 – that is, OR 1.4 (95% CI 0.6–3.3). The long-term (that is, greater than 6 months) quit rates for OTC NRT was 1 and 6% in two studies and 8–11% in five other studies. These results were not homogenous; however, when combined the estimated OR was 7% (95% CI 4–11%). It was concluded that OTC NRT is pharmacologically efficacious and produces modest quit rates similar to that seen in real-world prescription practice [84].

11.2
Bupropion

Bupropion or amfebutamone, a drug belonging to the aminoketone class, is chemically unrelated to other known antidepressants [85]. Bupropion is used in a sustained-release form for smoking cessation.

11.2.1
Pharmacodynamics

The mechanisms by which bupropion acts as an aid in smoking cessation are not known. Bupropion has been shown to block the antinociceptive, motor, hypothermic and convulsive effects of nicotine in *in vitro* tests and animal experiments [86]. It non-competitively blocks [87] the activation of $\alpha_3\beta_2$-, $\alpha_4\beta_2$- and α_7-neuronal nicotinic acetylcholine receptors (nAChRs) with some degree of selectivity [86] and it functionally inhibits nAChR sub-types of human muscle type and ganglionic receptor subtypes (see Fig. 4.1 in Chap. 4) [87]. Bupropion is thought to produce its therapeutic antidepressant effects by inhibiting the neuronal uptake of dopamine and noradrenaline and, to a small degree, of serotonin [88]. The metabolites of bupropion (hydroxybupropion and threohydrobupropion) are active in vitro and in animal models of depression, and they may contribute to the therapeutic effects of the parent compound. Hydroxybupropion probably plays a critical role in the antidepressant activity of bupropion, which appears to be associated predominantly with long-term noradrenergic effects [89]. Bupropion neither inhibits MAO in the brain nor increases the release of biogenic amines from nerve endings. In contrast to amphetamine or dexamphetamine, bupropion has low abuse potential [90, 91]. A few cases of drug dependence and withdrawal symptoms associated with immediate release bupropion have been reported. Bupropion produces feelings of euphoria and drug desirability, and a mild amphetamine-like effect has been observed (400 mg bupropion) [92].

Bupropion is devoid of cardiovascular effects (such as impaired intracardiac conduction, reduced myocardial contractility, decreased peripheral resistance, orthostatic hypotension) in both human and animal studies. However, a significant increased risk of treatment-emergent hypertension has been reported in a small number of patients. The drug is non-sedating and antagonises the effects of alcohol and diazepam. It does not produce weight gain. Activating effects may occur in susceptible patients [93].

11.2.2
Pharmacokinetic Properties

Maximum plasma concentrations (C_{max}) of sustained-release bupropion of about 140 µg/l were reached approximately 3 h after administration (150 mg) [94]. The drug is extensively degraded to three metabolites (hydroxybupropion, threohydrobupropion and erythrohydrobupropion) [94, 95]. Bupropion is converted in human liver slices in vitro to hydroxybupropion by the cytochrome P450 isoenzymes CYP1A2, CYP2A6, CYP2C9, CYP2E1 and CYP3A4; CYP2B6 is the major isoenzyme involved [92, 96]. In alcoholic liver disease, the $t_{0.5}\beta$ values are increased approximately 1.5-fold with large interindividual differences (21.1 vs.32.2 h) [97]. According to data from a recently published study in 519 outpatients, sustained-release bupropion exhibits a statistically significant dose/plasma level–response relationship for smoking cessation [98]. The efficacy of sustained-release bupropion in facilitating smoking cessation was found to be related to dose and to the mean metabolite concentration. The probability of smoking cessation increased with the administered dose. Furthermore, the occurrence of AEs such as insomnia and dry mouth was positively associated with the mean plasma concentration of erythro-amino alcohol. The highest predicted probability of quitting was observed at the highest mean plasma concentration of erythro-amino alcohol in combination with the lowest number of smoked cigarettes at baseline [98].

Genetic polymorphisms in cytochrome P450 2B6 (CYP2B6) may cause variability in bupropion pharmacokinetics since hydroxylation is known to be mediated by CYP2B6. Therefore, bupropion pharmacokinetics were studied after a single oral dose of 150 mg in 121 healthy male volunteers [99]. The amino acid polymorphisms R22C, Q172H, S259R, K262R and R487C were analysed and compared to the results of a pharmacokinetic analysis. A unimodal distribution of bupropion and hydroxybupropion kinetic parameters was detected with a mean (range) AUC of 3.64 (0.89–8.14) µmol h/l for bupropion and 25.5 (6.72–75.3) µmol h/l for hydroxybupropion. Population kinetic analysis revealed that bupropion total clearance via CYP2B6 alleles *1, *2, *5 and *6 did not differ, but clearance via allele *4 was 1.66-fold higher compared to wild-type allele *1 ($p = 0.001$). Corresponding to the high clearance of bupropion, carriers of the CYP2B6 genotype *1/*4 had significantly higher Cmax of hydroxybupropion compared to all other genotypes ($p = 0.03$). Only a minor fraction of the variability in bupropion and hydroxybupropion kinetics could be explained by the known CYP2B6 amino acid variants, in particular by the CYP2B6*4 allele. The role of this allele should also be studied in other CYP2B6 substrates, including cyclophosphamide, halothane, mianserin, promethazine and propofol [99].

11.2.3
Therapeutic Efficacy

The efficacy of sustained-release bupropion has been investigated in several double-blind randomised trials involving administration of the drug over 7 or 9 weeks in daily doses of 150 or 300 mg [12, 13, 100–104]. One study investigated the dose range of sustained-release bupropion [12], while another used the combination of sustained-release bupropion + nicotine patch [13]. In one study, sustained-release bupropion was administered over 45 weeks, after which the rate of relapse was estimated [105]. Smokers with an additional history of major depression or alcohol addiction were also included in a dose-ranging study [102]. In addition, preliminary results are available from a 12-month randomised, placebo-controlled study for the prevention of smoking relapse (cf. [98]) [104, 105].

Most of the statistical analyses were performed on an intention-to-treat basis and patients who were lost in the follow-up or who discontinued early were classified as smokers. The patients' self-reports of abstinence were confirmed by CO concentrations ≤ 10 ppm in expired air [105], a level that is sensitive for validating self-reported smoking abstinence [12–14, 106] during the previous 24 h [107]. Efficacy after 6 and 12 months has been reported as 44.2 and −29.5% (placebo 19.0 and 14.4%) [12], 30 and 29% (placebo 20 and 17%) [100, 108] or 40.6 and 31.7% (placebo 12.9 and 11.8%) [100], respectively. The observed point prevalence rates differed considerably, and in two studies [100, 103] no differences between placebo and active treatment were observed after 52 weeks (OR = 1.16; CI: 0.76–1.77) [109] or 104 weeks [104]. Furthermore, sustained-release bupropion treatment (300 mg/day) over 52 weeks improved the abstinence rate at week 78 (47.7 vs. 37.7%; bupropion vs. placebo), but not at week 104 of follow-up (41.6 vs. 40.0%; bupropion vs. placebo) [104].

A further study by Simon et al. analysed a total of 244 current smokers who were enrolled in an outpatient randomized blinded smoking cessation trial conducted at the San Francisco Veterans Affairs Medical Center, San Francisco [110]. Of the 244 participants, 121 received a 7-week course of bupropion and 123 received placebo. All participants received 2 months of transdermal NRT and 3 months of cognitive-behavioural counselling. It was shown that during treatment with bupropion vs. placebo there was a trend toward increased quit rates among participants randomized to bupropion; the self-reported end-of-medication treatment quit rates were 64% for the bupropion group vs. 57% for the placebo group ($p = 0.23$). The trend favouring bupropion persisted at 3 months of follow-up ($p = 0.12$) but was not apparent at 6 months and 1 year of follow-up (both $p > 0.78$). The 12-month quit rates, validated by either saliva cotinine or spousal proxy, were 22% in the bupropion group and 28% in the placebo group ($p = 0.31$). On the basis of biochemical validation, 19% of the bupropion group vs. 24% of the placebo group had quit smoking by 1 year ($p = 0.36$). The authors conclude that in this randomized blinded trial of mostly veteran participants, the addition of a brief 7-week bupropion trial to treatment with NRT and counselling did not significantly increase smoking cessation rates [110].

A summary of several studies [12, 13, 111, 112] with regard to smoking cessation over 12 months revealed that treatment with bupropion was successful (OR = 2.54; CI: 1.90–3.41) [16]. In one study, after 6 months of follow-up observation the success rates in the four were 21.3% (nicotine patch), 34.8% (300 mg bupropion) and 38.8% (combination bupropion + nicotine patch) compared with 18.8% (placebo) [13]. In comparison with nicotine, a more powerful effect was reported for bupropion (OR = 2.07; CI: 1.22–3.53) [13], although the study included smokers who had already had adverse experiences with nicotine products [96]. The efficacy of repeated administration of NRT products for smoking cessation has been demonstrated in medical practice in several studies, and consequently the Jorenby study [13] should not be regarded as evidence of the lack of efficacy of the nicotine patch. The combination of bupropion + nicotine patch was superior to the nicotine patch (OR = 2.65; CI: 1.58–4.40), but was not more effective than bupropion alone [16] (see Table 11.1). While it is possible to treat alcohol-dependent and/or depressive smokers with bupropion, these smokers very quickly relapse as depression increases.

Among smokers, women may be at greater risk than men for developing smoking-related diseases. Collins et al. assessed wether bupropion would reduce this gender disparity among 314 women and 241 men enrolled in a placebo-controlled, randomized trial using behavioural counselling plus 10 weeks of bupropion (300 mg) [113]. Prolonged abstinence and biochemically verified point prevalence outcomes were measured at end the of treatment (8 weeks after the quit date) and at 6-month follow-up. A logistic regression model of 6-month prolonged abstinence and a Cox regression (survival analysis) model revealed a significant gender by smoking rate by drug interaction and a main effect for marital status. This three-way interaction suggests that bupropion particularly benefited men who smoked more than one pack of cigarettes per day at baseline and, conversely, women who smoked a pack or less. The point prevalence logistic regression model showed no evidence that either gender or smoking rate modified the effect of treatment. These results suggest that bupropion treatment may reduce the gender disparity in prolonged abstinence rates among lighter smokers [113].

In conclusion, a Cochrane analysis showed that when used as the sole pharmacotherapy, bupropion (31 trials, OR 1.94, 95% CI 1.72–2.19) doubled the odds of cessation [114]. However, there is insufficient evidence that adding bupropion to NRTprovides an additional long-term benefit. Three trials of extended therapy with bupropion to prevent relapse after initial cessation also did not find evidence of a significant long-term benefit. From the available data in this Cochrane analysis, bupropion appeared to be equally effective and of similar efficacy to NRT. By contrast, pooling three trials comparing bupropion to varenicline showed a lower odds of quitting with bupropion (OR 0.60, 95% CI 0.46–0.78). There is a risk of about 1 in 1,000 of seizures associated with bupropion use. Concerns that bupropion may increase suicide risk are currently unproven [114].

11.2.4
Dosage

Unlike smoking cessation programmes with nicotine products, where it is agreed that smoking cessation should coincide directly with the start of nicotine administration for safety reasons, smokers treated with bupropion may continue to smoke initially while taking a daily dose of 150 mg and then appoint a day for themselves to stop smoking during the second week of treatment. Steady-state plasma concentrations are only achieved after 5–7 days' ingestion [92]. At this point, the daily dose is then increased to 300 mg. The course of treatment lasts for 7–9 weeks. In the USA, treatment may be extended to 6 months if the product is well tolerated [2, 92]. Total smoking cessation is naturally the objective of treatment.

11.2.5
Adverse Effects

Approximately 12% of patients complain of insomnia and approximately 8% of dry mouth [12, 115]. In the second placebo-controlled multicentre study with 12-month follow-up, the effects of bupropion were compared with those of a nicotine patch and a combination of the two in 893 subjects over a 9-week treatment period [96]. Insomnia occurred as an AE disproportionately more often in the two bupropion groups [12, 13] (42.4 and 47.5 vs. 19.5%). In both studies, however, five cases of severe depression occurred during treatment with bupropion (Table 11.6). The experiences to date with bupropion have been collected exclusively outside Germany; further research is required if its equivalent efficacy is to be demonstrated [116]. Information on other AEs is presented in Table 11.6. The 450 AEs recorded in Canada over an 11-month period following the introduction of bupropion

Table 11.6 Adverse effects of bupropion [116, 117]

Organ system	Adverse effects	Frequency [%]
Central nervous system and peripheral nervous system	Insomnia, tremor, disturbed concentration, headache, dizziness, depression, restlessness, anxiety	>1
	Confusion	>0.1–1
	Convulsive seizures [23], stroke	>0.01–0.1
Skin	Rash, pruritus, sweating, urticaria	>1
Allergic reactions	Severe hypersensitivity reactions, including angio-edema, dyspnoea/bronchospasm and anaphylactic shock Arthralgia, myalgia and fever in conjunction with skin rashes (possibly serum sickness)	
	Erythema multiforme, Stevens-Johnson syndrome	>0.01–0.1
Cardiovascular system	Tachycardia, raised blood pressure (sometimes severe), facial reddening, stroke (<0.01%)	>0.1–1
	Vasodilatation, orthostatic hypotension, syncope	>0.01–0.1
Gastrointestinal tract	Dry mouth, nausea, vomiting, abdominal pain, constipation	>1
Metabolic disorders	Loss of appetite	>0.1–1
General reactions	Fever	>1
	Chest pain, asthenia	>0.1–1
Sensory organs	Disturbed sense of taste	>1
	Tinnitus, visual disturbances	>0.1–1

come from spontaneous reports and require careful analysis in terms of establishing causality [116]. For further details, see [118]. Concerns that bupropion may increase suicide risk are currently unproven [114].

11.2.6
Contraindications and Drug Interactions

Bupropion should not be used in patients with convulsive disorders or bulimia or in those with diabetes treated with insulin or antidiabetic medication. It is also not suitable for use in alcoholics, patients with alcohol or benzodiazepine withdrawal symptoms, or in those who are dependent on opioids, cocaine or stimulants [92]. Bupropion overdosage ($\geq$450 mg/day) is associated with an increased incidence of convulsive seizures (0.4% of patients at doses up to 450 mg/day) [119, 120].

Concurrent medication with MAO inhibitors is not permitted. Caution is also required in patients simultaneously treated with antipsychotic drugs, antidepressants, theophylline and systemic glucocorticoids. Potential interactions may arise in particular because of the inhibition of CYP2D6 by bupropion and hydrobupropion. This affects agents such as desipramine. However, slowing of metabolism may also be encountered with other antidepressants (imipramine, paroxetine), antipsychotic agents (risperidone, thioridazine), β-receptor blockers (metoprolol) and class 1C anti-arrhythmic agents (propafenone, flecainide) [117]. Caution is also required when combining bupropion with antimalarials, tramadol, quinolones and antihistamines with sedative activity [92]. Where appropriate, these drugs should be administered in a reduced dose or discontinued. Alternatively, consideration should be given to halting bupropion therapy [117].

During *pregnancy*, bupropion should be used only where absolutely indicated. Since bupropion and its metabolites pass into *breast milk*, with the resultant risk of triggering seizures in the infant, discontinuation of bupropion or cessation of breastfeeding should be considered [116].

11.2.7
Summary

The effectiveness of bupropion insignificantly exceeds that of nicotine products (OR = 2.1; CI: 1.5–3.0 vs. 1.9; CI: 1.7–2.2; bupropion vs. nicotine patch) [16]. Placebo-controlled long-term studies have revealed no convincing differences after 1 [109] or 2 years [105]. Relapses could not be prevented after treatment over 1 year [105], and the mean changes in body weight differed from the placebo group by 1.3 kg after 2 years [105]. In terms of a risk-benefit calculation, people who have smoked for 2 or 3 decades may feel "healthy" and have to be convinced to stop smoking, or they may feel "ill" and are unable to stop smoking because they are addicted. Where present, the risk of adverse effects and deaths [113] with bupropion is more substantial and more serious than with NRT (cf. Tables 11.4 and 11.6). Because of the severe AEs encountered, bupropion should therefore be considered as second-line rather than first-line medication for promoting smoking cessation.

11.3
Other Pharmacotherapies

11.3.1
Varenicline

Nicotine receptor partial agonists such as varenicline may help to stop smoking by reducing smoking satisfaction (acting as an antagonist) and also maintaining moderate levels of dopamine to counteract withdrawal symptoms (acting as an agonist). In this respect, varenicline was developed as a nicotine receptor partial agonist from cytosine. It is a drug that is widely used in Central and Eastern Europe for smoking cessation. The first trial reports of varenicline were released in 2006, and further trials have now been published or are currently are underway. A Cochrane analysis published in 2008 assessed the efficacy and tolerability of nicotine receptor partial agonists, including varenicline and cytisine for smoking cessation [121]. Together with other databases the Cochrane Tobacco Addiction Group's specialised register for trials was searched and randomized controlled trials which compared the treatment drug with placebo were analysed. Comparisons with bupropion and NRT were also performed. Seven trials of varenicline compared with placebo for smoking cessation were found; three of these also included a bupropion experimental arm. Also one relapse prevention trial, comparing varenicline with placebo, and one open-label trial comparing varenicline with NRT were identified [121]. In total, the nine trials covered 7,267 participants, 4,744 of whom used varenicline. As a result, the pooled risk ratio (RR) for continuous abstinence at 6 months or longer for varenicline vs.placebo was 2.33 (95% CI 1.95–2.80). The pooled RR for varenicline vs.bupropion at 1 year was 1.52 (95% CI 1.22–1.88). The RR for varenicline vs.NRT at 1 year was 1.31 (95% CI 1.01–1.71). The two trials which tested the use of varenicline beyond the 12-week standard regimen found the drug to be well-tolerated during long-term use. The main adverse effect of varenicline was nausea, which was mostly at mild to moderate levels and usually subsided over time [121]. Post-marketing safety data suggest that varenicline may be associated with depressed mood, agitation, and suicidal behaviour or ideation. The labelling of varenicline has been amended, and the FDA is conducting a safety review.The one cytisine trial included in this Cochrane review found that more participants taking cytisine stopped smoking compared with placebo at 2 years follow up, with an RR of 1.61 (95% CI 1.24–2.08).

It can be concluded from this Cochrane analysis that varenicline increases the chances of successful long-term smoking cessation between two- and threefold compared with pharmacologically unassisted quit attempts. Also, more participants quit successfully with varenicline than with bupropion. The one analysed open-label trial of varenicline vs. NRT demonstrated a modest benefit of varenicline. The main adverse effect of varenicline is nausea, but mostly at mild to moderate levels and tending to subside over time. Possible links with serious AEs, including depressed mood, agitation and suicidal thoughts, are currently under review. It can be stated that there is a need for larger, independent community-based trials of varenicline to test the efficacy of treatment extended beyond 12 weeks [121].

11.3.2
Nortriptyline

In three studies [122], the antidepressant nortriptyline showed a significant increase in smoking cessation over 6 and 12 months (OR = 2.77; CI: 1.73–4.44), and this result was not altered where a previous history of depression was present. However, because of its pronounced AE profile, nortriptyline should be regarded only as second-line therapy and should be used only in situations where smoking cessation cannot be achieved by other means [16] [see also [2]]. Nortriptyline has not been approved anywhere for use in smoking cessation (Table 11.1).

In a 2008 Cochrane analysis [114], eight trials of nortriptyline were assesed [114]. When used as the sole pharmacotherapy, nortriptyline (four trials, OR 2.34, 95% CI 1.61–3.41) doubled the odds of cessation. There is insufficient evidence that adding nortriptyline to NRT provides an additional long-term benefit. From the available data, nortriptyline appeared to be equally effective and of similar efficacy to NRT. However, nortriptyline has the potential for serious side effects, but none have been seen in the few small trials for smoking cessation [114].

11.3.3
Clonidine

Clonidine, an α_2 agonist with antihypertensive activity, is well known for its ability to reduce the symptoms of opioid dependence. Cigarette smoking also increases plasma endorphin levels, a phenomenon which supports the dependence-producing effects of nicotine; however, this has also stimulated interest in the effects of clonidine to promote smoking cessation. Out of six validated studies, one achieved a significant effect [123]. Clonidine should be designated as effective (OR = 1.89; Table 11.1). The proportion of smokers who achieve cessation is between 9 and 14% [15, 124]. These differences between the studies, coupled with the fact that a study duration of less than 6 months does not permit any definitive conclusions regarding cessation therapy, mean that despite its demonstrated activity, clonidine does not appear to be a suitable agent for use in smoking cessation, a view that is endorsed by the numerous reports of AEs (sedation, dry mouth) [15]. Similarly, it has not been confirmed that clonidine is more effective in women than in men [125].

The latest Cochrane analysis by Gourlay et al. included six trials which met the inclusion criteria. There were three trials of oral, and three of transdermal clonidine [126]. Some form of behavioural counselling was offered to all participants in five of the six trials. There was a statistically significant effect of clonidine only in one of these trials. The pooled OR for success with clonidine vs.placebo was 1.89 (95% CI 1.30–2.74). There was a high incidence of dose-dependent side effects, particularly dry mouth and sedation. It can be concluded that on the basis of a small number of trials, in which there are potential sources of bias, clonidine is statistically effective in promoting smoking cessation. Prominent side effects limit the usefulness of clonidine for smoking cessation [126].

11.3.4
Mecamylamine

The nicotine antagonist mecamylamine (see Sects 4.2 and 4.3.4 in Chap. 4) blocks the effects of nicotine, and hence the reward system, by inhibiting nicotine-induced dopamine release, thus reducing the urge to smoke. The efficacy of mecamylamine in combination with nicotine patches has been investigated in two studies conducted by the same team. The results of the first study in 48 subjects over 7 weeks showed superiority of the combination in terms of smoking cessation even after 12 months (37.5 vs. 4.2%; mecamylamine + nicotine vs. nicotine). In a second study with mecamylamine (2.5–5 mg twice daily) + nicotine (21 mg/day), abstinence was achieved in 40% (mecamylamine + nicotine), 20% (mecamylamine) and 15% of subjects (nicotine or placebo). The results were not significant [106, 127]. Daily doses up to 20 mg mecamylamine were well tolerated, and symptoms of constipation occurred in 40% of patients. The combined administration of mecamylamine + nicotine proved beneficial, but a further study in a larger patient population should be conducted before this regimen is used on a more extensive clinical basis [128]. Mecamylamine has not been approved for smoking cessation anywhere.

11.3.5
Tranquillisers and β-Receptor Blockers

Anxiety is one symptom of nicotine withdrawal, as is an increased incidence of depression. Alongside meprobamate and diazepam, the β-receptor blockers metoprolol, oxprenolol and propranolol have also been investigated for their anxiolytic properties. On the basis of the criterion of 6 months of abstinence, the available studies (one study each) for the two tranquillisers meprobamate [129] and diazepam [130] did not reveal any significant effects. The two β-blockers metoprolol (100 mg/day) and oxprenolol (160 mg/day) exerted a slight effect on smoking cessation over 12 months (17 and 24 vs. 3%; metoprolol, oxprenolol vs. placebo), although the results were significant only for metoprolol [130]. For metoprolol, at least, the results were unexpected [16].

11.3.6
Buspirone

The pharmacological properties of this atypical anxiolytic are still unclear. It is thought to possess high affinity for the 5-HT_{1A} receptors in the central nervous system (CNS), and to display D_2 agonist activity as well as enhancing noradrenaline metabolism in the locus coerulus. Contradictory findings have been published concerning its use (30–60 mg daily) as an aid to smoking cessation. After 4 weeks of treatment, placebo-controlled studies in 61 subjects [131] and 54 subjects [132] revealed a significant effect (47 vs. 16%, active treatment vs. placebo) and no proven effect (62 vs. 52%, active treatment vs. placebo) respectively, and the withdrawal symptoms of nicotine were not reliably reduced [131]. In a further study in an even smaller patient population (37 subjects), cravings were reduced after 7 days of treatment, as well as anxiety symptoms, restlessness and excitability [133]. These and other studies are not conclusive, and a larger study over a more extended period is required in order for efficacy to be demonstrated unequivocally [16]. Buspirone is not approved anywhere for use in smoking cessation.

11.3.7
Rimonabant

Rimonabant hydrochloride represents the first drug in a new class of selective cannabinoid type 1 (CB1) receptor antagonists. This compound is showing promise in clinical trials for the treatment of obesity and related metabolic risk factors. Also, it may be of help in smoking cessation therapy. The drug may assist with smoking cessation by restoring the balance of the endocannabinoid system, which can be disrupted by prolonged use of nicotine. Rimonabant also seeks to address many smokers' reluctance to persist with a quit attempt because of concerns about weight gain. Cahill and Ussher performed a meta-analysis to determine whether selective CB1 receptor antagonists increase the numbers of people stopping smoking [134]. Three trials that met the inclusion criteria, covering 1,567 smokers (cessation: STRATUS-EU and STRATUS-US) and 1,661 quitters (relapse prevention: STRATUS-WW) were included in the analysis. At 1 year, the pooled OR for quitting with rimonabant 20 mg was 1.61 (95% CI 1.12–2.30). No significant benefit was demonstrated for rimonabant at 5 mg dosage. The AEs included nausea and upper respiratory tract infections. In the one relapse prevention trial, smokers who had quit on the 20 mg regimen were 1(1/2) times more likely to remain abstinent on either active regimen than on placebo; the OR for the 20 mg maintenance group was 1.49 (95% CI 1.09–2.04, and for the 5 mg maintenance group 1.51 (95% CI 1.11–2.07) 8,131). There appeared to be no significant benefit of maintenance treatment for the 5 mg quitters. Weight gain was reported to be significantly lower among the 20 mg quitters than in the 5 mg or placebo quitters. During the treatment, overweight or obese smokers tended to lose weight, while normal weight smokers did not. Cahill and Ussher concluded from the preliminary trial reports available that rimonabant 20 mg may increase the odds of quitting approximately 1(1/2)-fold. Whereas the risk of serious AEs was reported to be low, concerns were raised over rates of depression and suicidal thoughts in people taking rimonabant for weight control [134]. In summary, the present evidence for rimonabant in concerning tobacco abstinence and its adverse effects is inconclusive and further research is needed.

11.3.8
Various Antidepressants

The antidepressants imipramine, doxepin, fluoxetine, venlafaxine and moclobemide have also been investigated as aids to smoking cessation. Overall, while these compounds may support efforts to achieve smoking cessation, no definitive cessation effect has been demonstrated [16].

Doxepin has been investigated only in one small 3-week study, and the participants were additionally promised a financial bonus on stopping smoking. The initially good effect had disappeared within one further week [135]. Fluoxetine has been compared with dexfenfluramine and placebo in 97 subjects, but efficacy was poorer than with placebo [136]. Efficacy was poor with imipramine when compared with lobeline and dextroamphetamine [137] and with venlafaxine [138] when compared with placebo. Similarly, moclobemide was shown to possess a slight degree of efficacy in one study [139] (25 vs. 16%, active treatment vs. placebo), but the effect was no longer significant after 12 months.

The latest Cochrane metaanalsis screened six trials of selective serotonin reuptake inhibitors; four of fluoxetine, one of sertraline and one of paroxetine. None of these detected significant long-term effects, and there was no evidence of a significant benefit when results were pooled. There was one trial of the monoamine oxidase inhibitor moclobemide, and one of the atypical antidepressant venlafaxine. Neither of these detected a significant long-term benefit [114].

11.3.9
Opioid Antagonists

Opioid antagonists are used for the treatment of various forms of dependence (alcohol, cocaine, opioids), and initial studies have also been published concerning the efficacy of naloxone and naltrexone in smoking cessation. A reduction in the number of cigarettes smoked daily was shown in two placebo-controlled studies with naloxone [140, 141], but this was not confirmed in a further study [142]. Because of its longer half-life, naltrexone might be beneficial, but here too the results have not been convincing (OR = 1.34; CI: 0.49–3.63) [143, 144]. Combination of naltrexone with nicotine patches has yielded a slightly higher success rate [145]. On the basis of the results available at present, no definitive assessment is possible [146], and the effectiveness of both opioid antagonists needs to be verified in a larger patient sample.

David et al. performed a meta-analysis on opiod antagonists for smoking cessation and found out that four trials of naltrexone met Cochrane inclusion criteria for meta-analyses for long-term cessation [147]. All the four trials failed to detect a significant difference in quit rates between naltrexone and placebo. In a pooled analysis, there was no significant effect of naltrexone on long-term abstinence, and CIs were wide (OR 1.26, 95% CI 0.80–2.01). No trials of naloxone or buprenorphine reported long-term follow-up. It can therefore be concluded that on the basis of limited data from four trials it is not possible to confirm or refute whether naltrexone helps smokers quit. The CIs are compatible with both clinically significant benefit and possible negative effects of naltrexone in promoting abstinence. Data from larger trials of naltrexone are needed to settle the question of efficacy for smoking cessation [147].

11.3.10
Lobeline

Lobeline is an alkaloid possessing nicotine-like activity with attenuated central and peripheral effects. Lobeline used to be employed to promote smoking cessation. However, there are no controlled studies available [148]. Therefore, its use cannot be recommended according to a Cochrane analysis [14].

11.3.11
Silver Acetate

Silver acetate in the form of chewing gum or mouth spray has been compared with placebo in four aversive smoking studies [149], but no significant results were reported. In one triple-arm study, silver acetate and the 2-mg nicotine chewing gum formulation were compared with placebo (OR = 1.05; CI: 0.63–1.73) [150]. An additional 4% gain after 2 months is too small to be deemed a success [17].

11.3.12
Nicotine-Vaccination

There are three different companies presently that have completed Phase II clinical studies of their anti-nicotine vaccines. They are all rushing to obtain regulatory approval and to bring their vaccine candidates to the market [151].

In general, nicotine vaccines are composed of a linkage between the nicotine molecule and an adjuvant with a carrier protein. Preliminary results of the three Phase II clinical studies are encouraging. In this respect, subjects who have a high anti-nicotine antibody level also present high quit rates [152]. However, the data available are by far too preliminary to extrapolate for long-term quit rates. It can be expected that vaccines may appear on the market in 2011.

11.4
Therapeutic Monitoring in Smoking Cessation

Most physicians use the *self-report* (SR) confirmed by *carbon monoxide* (CO) readings as the method usually employed in clinical practice to determine whether "ex-smokers" are smoking tobacco during and following treatment. The combination of SR and CO was evaluated in some studies, and a close relationship between CO readings and SR was found in ex-smokers who had been informed beforehand that CO reading would be taken [153, 154]. A relatively low average false-negative rate of 6% was reported in an analysis of 12 additional intervention studies using CO confirmation [107]. Data such as these have been taken as evidence that CO evaluation can detect under-representation of smoking in self-reports. If the patient has been informed that CO reading will be taken, then the inconsistent smoking patient may stop smoking for several hours before CO reading. On the other hand, the *measurement of CO* in expired air may be problematic because increased values (>10 ppm) have been recorded in ex-smokers or in smokers who quit smoking several days prior to measurement.

A second possibility to control smoking cessation is the *analysis of cotinine* in plasma, urine, or saliva. In a sample of hospital outpatients self-report, CO and cotinine analyses were used to validate the efficacy of smoking cessation [155]. Up to 20% of claimed ex-smokers were classified as smokers by each test. The cotinine analyses were superior to CO readings, although CO also worked relatively well [155]. Because of cost considerations, the cotinine analysis should not be used routinely [155]. In only one 1-year study, the CO and cotinine monitorings were compared [156] in self-reported ex-smokers: While cotinine monitoring detected 17% smokers, CO monitoring detected smokers in only 9.8% of the reported non-smokers [156]. In a recently published smoking cessation study, the efficacy of the three parameters was compared at three time points (9, 26, and 52 weeks) from treatment initiation [157]. The results suggested the cotinine analyses in urine may lead to more accurate but lowered measured abstinence rates (49, 29, and 26 vs. 38, 26, and 25%, self-report plus CO vs. self-report plus cotinine, respectively) [157].

ETS and other environmental factors (traffic pollution, fog) may also be possible explanations for elevated CO. If an ex-smoker has not smoked for >7 days previously, plasma cotinine levels should not exceed 20 ng/ml; neither do cotinine determinations in plasma, saliva or urine indicate previous cigarette smoking.

11.5
Special Therapeutic Situations

11.5.1
Ischaemic Heart Disease

The two controlled studies conducted to date in patients with stable angina point to a favourable influence on progression or on the course of the disease. In smokers (>20 cigarettes/day) with coronary heart disease, blood flow in various myocardial regions is improved as a sign of "smoking reduction" where cigarette consumption is replaced in part by nicotine patches (14 and 21 mg strengths) [158]. With falling CO content of expired air, the underperfused myocardial regions were reduced in size and the patients' exercise capacity was increased despite higher nicotine levels (compared with controls) because cigarette consumption had fallen. One study indicated that nicotine had a "minimally harmful" effect on the circulation, because even years of smokeless tobacco use did not increase either the risk factors for the development of coronary heart disease or the atherogenic index [159].

When cigarette consumption in patients with stable angina using nicotine patches (14 and 21 mg) was gradually reduced from >20 to <7 cigarettes/day, only 3 out of 77 smokers in the active treatment group compared with 8 out of 79 smokers in the placebo group had to discontinue treatment because of cardiovascular events [64]. Transdermal nicotine administration does not increase either the frequency of angina attacks or the occurrence of nocturnal attacks, arrhythmias or episodes with ECG evidence of ST-segment depression [64]. Smoking cessation was achieved in 36 and 22% of patients (active treatment vs. placebo) [64]. Thus, the usefulness of NRT has been confirmed in smokers with stable angina. Recommendations have now also been published concerning the treatment of ischaemic heart disease [160], indicating that nicotine patches clearly reduce the primary endpoints (death, myocardial infarction, cardiac arrest, hospital admission, cardiac arrhythmias or heart failure) in CHD patients within 14 weeks (5.4 vs. 7.9%, active treatment vs. placebo) [160]. Nicotine treatment may thus be initiated as early as 2–3 days after an acute myocardial infarction, and NRT is indicated for smoking cessation in all patients with angina pectoris and cardiac arrhythmias. Dosage recommendations are available for nicotine patches

Table 11.7 Recommendations on the use of nicotine products in patients with cardiovascular disease [160]

Indication/Treatment	Proposal	Proven use
Indications		
Myocardial infarction	Nicotine may be used 2–3 days after infarction	Nicotine was used up to 2–3 weeks after myocardial infarction
Arrhythmias	Nicotine may be used in all patients	To date, no experience in patients with severe ventricular arrhythmias, second and third degree AV blocks or hospitalised for arrhythmias (up to 2 weeks afterwards)
Treatment	≥10 cigarettes/day	≥15 cigarettes/day
Nicotine patch	15 mg/16 h (8–12 weeks)	21 mg/24 h[a] in CHD patients (proven over 5–10 weeks)
Nicotine chewing gum	5–15 pieces (2 mg each)/day (12–24 weeks)	Not tested in CHD patients

[a]Based on our own experiences, the use of nicotine patches overnight is not recommended because of the occurrence of insomnia etc.

and chewing gum, whereas no findings have yet been published for the inhaler. Details are presented in Table 11.7.

11.5.2
Pregnancy

Women who smoke during pregnancy must expect their neonates to display signs of embryotoxic and foetotoxic damage [70]. Since the prescription of drugs is quite properly restricted during pregnancy and lactation, controversy surrounds the use of nicotine products because the harmful effects of the combustion products of cigarettes cannot be clearly separated from the effects of nicotine. The accumulation of nicotine in breast milk is well known, but heavy metals, CO and numerous carcinogens also pass into the mother's milk. In spite of this, it has been argued that it is better for smoking mothers to breast-feed their babies than solely to expose them to the effects of passive smoking [161]. Non-drug smoking cessation programmes should be offered first (see Sect. 10.11 in Chap. 10), but NRT should be instituted very promptly where non-drug interventions are found to be ineffective [73]. Analysis of the literature, including the results of experimental animal research, indicates that nicotine does not cause any teratogenic or embryotoxic effects. The carcinogens detected in the urine of neonates are derived from tobacco and are not metabolites of nicotine [162].

Since pregnant women who smoke are heavily dependent, they incorporate the combustion products of tobacco as well as larger amounts of nicotine which reach the foetal brain [163, 164], and the binding capacity for the alkaloid has been shown to increase in foetal brain structures between weeks 12 and 19 of pregnancy. Nicotine binding in the brainstem attains peak levels at mid-gestation, with a subsequent fall at the time of delivery, indicating that adverse effects of nicotine may be expected to occur during mid-to-late gestation [164]. Since the risk of malformations and obstetric complications is demonstrably higher in women who smoke than during smoking cessation therapy with NRT, the women in question should agree to NRT if non-drug interventions fail to achieve smoking cessation. Meticulous research into this question is required in the years ahead (see [71, 73]).

11.5.3
Weight Gain

For a variety of reasons, many smokers lose weight over the course of many years of smoking (reduced appetite, increased fatty acid oxidation, deteriorating insulin resistance, increased plasma insulin concentrations), although tobacco smoke does not appear to be an anorectic agent [165]. Conversely, smoking cessation in response to nicotine administration brings an improvement in insulin resistance with a simultaneous weight gain. This weight gain on smoking cessation is clearly associated not with the withdrawal of nicotine but of other unidentified components of cigarette smoke [166]. Moreover, the presence of nicotine has been shown to increase concentrations of leptin [167] which evidently acts to reduce body weight [168]. While changes in body weight following smoking cessation are a major concern for many smokers, the transient body weight fluctuations often balance out again within a few years [169].

In particular, women who eat more in stress situations (frequently the reason for smoking) [170, 171] or who are going through the perimenopause [172] are predestined to gain weight when they stop smoking. Dietary advice should be given at the start of smoking cessation and efforts should be made to encourage greater physical activity, since this has been shown to minimise weight gain in middle-aged women [173, 174].

11.5.4
Alcohol Consumption

A close association exists between alcohol dependence and nicotine dependence. The vast majority of alcoholics also smoke, whereas only 5–10% of smokers are alcohol-dependent. Combined dependence is associated with an increased incidence of head and neck tumours [175]. It is thought that daily cigarette consumption is increased during recovery from alcoholism [176]. In addition, tobacco is the more common cause of death in former patients of drug dependence centres [177]. According to several studies (including two controlled trials [175]), smoking cessation with/without NRT is reported to have no adverse consequences on the (absence of) drinking behaviour in former alcoholics [16]. In this context, there is evidence to suggest that NRT has no adverse consequences on simultaneously implemented alcohol withdrawal [177].

11.5.5
Organic Depression and Schizophrenia

A generally pro-smoker atmosphere dominates in psychiatric clinics [177]. The percentage of patients who smoke increases with longer hospitalisation, although this tendency was only in evidence in non-schizophrenics [178]. Basically, smoking cessation is easier for psychiatric patients, the more actively they cooperate and the more independent their behaviour is. Accordingly, ex-smokers with mental illnesses have lower Brief Psychiatric Rating Scale (BPRS) scores than smokers [179]. The analysis of data on 4,411 respondents aged from 15 to 54 years demonstrated that smokers with any history of mental illness had a self-reported quit rate of 37.1%, and smokers with past-month mental illness had a self-reported quit rate of 30.5% compared with smokers without mental illness (42.5%). The ORs for current and lifetime smoking in respondents with mental illness in the past month vs. respondents without mental illness, adjusted for age, sex and region of the country, were 2.7 (2.3–3.1) vs. 2.7 (2.4–3.2). Persons with a mental disorder in the past month consumed approximately 44.3% of cigarettes smoked by this nationally representative sample [180]. In treatment with nicotine patches, the smoking withdrawal results for 208 psychiatric outpatients were no worse than for non-patients [181]. Patients treated with antidepressants and neuroleptics consume more cigarettes than patients not treated with these substances. Clearly, the anticholinergic effect of these medicines is also at least attenuated by increased nicotine administration, or else increased cigarette consumption accelerates the hepatic metabolism of neuroleptics, thus reducing the unwanted effects.

A no-smoking policy in psychiatric clinics, with the attendant withdrawal symptoms, does not have a negative effect on mental illnesses [182]. Another compromise method is to put restrictions on the smokers in these clinics, although this does not encourage them to stop smoking [183]. It is certainly no easy matter to enforce a no-smoking policy in a psychiatric clinic, although no threatening consequences result for the patients. What does make sense is to couple smoking prohibition with NRT to facilitate smoking cessation [183].

11.5.5.1
Organic Depression

Co-morbidity of psychiatric illnesses, especially depression, in conjunction with the use of illicit drugs, is more common than was previously assumed [184, 185]. This also applies for nicotine dependence in the form of cigarette smoking.

Of a group of 120 chronic smokers, 62.3% were mentally ill (mood, anxiety, or substance abuse disorders). Although these smokers were more "stressed" at the time of treatment (high levels of nicotine dependence, depressive mood), they achieved the same level of cessation success as the non-patients [186], so that it was not possible to establish an association between smoking cessation and mental illness.

An existing depression diminishes the success of smoking cessation compared with persons not suffering from this condition [187]. According to a large Finnish study [188], the motivation for smoking cessation is reportedly stronger in depressive patients, suggesting a large pool of depressive smokers. Depressive symptoms that occur during withdrawal are of decisive significance in terms of relapses and should therefore be treated concurrently [189]. Concurrent depression was the indication for smoking cessation therapy in elderly women [190]. In these patients, it proved possible to control smoking abstinence relatively arbitrarily by means of monetary rewards set for various time periods [191]. Subsequently, however, the relapse rate was not determined by the duration of abstinence but rather by psychopathological criteria only.

Considering the effects of mental illnesses on the type of withdrawal symptoms, anxious and depressive patients, as well as patients with eating disorders, tend to experience withdrawal symptoms within the clinical framework of their illness, whereas patients with stronger nicotine dependence frequently show craving, sleep disturbances and cognitive-affective disturbances [192].

11.5.5.2
Schizophrenic Patients

Smoking cessation in schizophrenic patients is rendered difficult by a variety of affective, cognitive and social problems [193], but it can be achieved using specially designed smoking cessation programmes [194] involving a combination of group therapy with nicotine patches and neuroleptics (preferably olanzapine and risperidone). These two substances have proved superior to the classic neuroleptics (success rates of 56 vs. 22%) [195]. According to other studies, clozapine was more effective in promoting smoking cessation in schizophrenics than other typical as well as atypical neuroleptics [196, 197], besides which the antipsychotic effect of clozapine was more pronounced in smokers [198]. The reasons for these effects of clozapine [199] may involve inhibition of nicotine metabolism, especially in view of the fact that raised plasma nicotine levels are measured in smoking schizophrenics [199].

The spectrum of adverse effects of neuroleptics remains essentially unchanged in smokers. With increasing age, smokers require higher doses of neuroleptics, while non-smokers require lower doses to achieve a sufficient level of efficacy [200], although smoking does not alter plasma levels significantly. The incidence of neuroleptic-induced parkinsonism and tardive dyskinesias was not higher among smokers despite considerably higher average dosage levels [201, 202]. Smoking was reported to have a protective effect against incipient dementia in smokers [203]; cases of akathisia were observed frequently in women smokers. Neuroleptic-induced parkinsonism was observed less frequently in smokers than in non-smokers [203]. Another study found an association between high neuroleptic dosage and smoking in non-schizophrenics only [204]. Smoking reportedly does not alter plasma clozapine levels, in spite of which the individual plasma levels vary under constant dosage. Antipsychotic efficacy correlates with the dosage level [205]. Haloperidol treatment was initiated in ten smoking patients with acute schizophrenia. An increased desire to smoke was observed in a 2-h ad libitum smoking phase [197].

11.5.5.3
Interactions Between Cigarette Smoking and Administration of Psychopharmaceuticals

Tobacco smoking affects the metabolism of numerous neuroleptics and antidepressants via the cytochrome P450 system, complicating the therapy of smokers in psychiatric clinics and out-patient facilities (cf. Table 11.8). Smokers require higher doses of neuroleptics than non-smokers [198, 225–227]. The neuroleptic dosage increases with age in schizophrenic smokers [200], but decreases in schizophrenic non-smokers, apparently in association with an age-dependent reduction in D_2 receptors in the corpus striatum. Increased

Table 11.8 Pharmacokinetic interactions between smoking and drugs influencing the CNS

Drug	Interactive effects
Benzodiazepines (diazepam, lorazepam, midazolam, chlordiazepoxide)	No effect [206–208]
Bupropion	No effect [94]
Chlorpromazine	AUC $\Downarrow$ (−36%), serum concentration $\Downarrow$ (−24%); clinical significance? [209, 210]
Clorazepate	AUC $\Downarrow$, $t_{0.5}$ of N-desmethyldiazepam $\Downarrow$ [211]
Clozapine	Induction of CYP_{1A2}, clearance $\Uparrow$, plasma concentration $\Downarrow$ (−28%) [205, 212–215]
Fluvoxamine	Induction of CYP_{1A2}, metabolic clearance $\Uparrow$, AUC $\Downarrow$ (−44%), plasma concentration $\Downarrow$ (−47%) [216]
Haloperidol	Clearance $\Uparrow$ (+44%), serum concentration $\Downarrow$ (−70%). Clinical significance?, no observed differences in dose [191, 217, 218]
Imipramine	Serum concentration $\Downarrow$, no clinical effect [219]
Nortriptyline	Unclear, no clinical effect [220, 221]
Olanzapine	Induction of CYP_{1A2}, clearance $\Uparrow$ (+98%), great variability in plasma clearance over a fourfold range [222–224]

cigarette consumption in schizophrenic and non-schizophrenic patients because of administration of haloperidol was measured on the basis of reliable parameters (CO, nicotine) [200]. The combination of neuroleptics and smoking reduces the frequency of parkinsonism-like symptoms in these patients and can reduce the anticholinergic doses required in some cases. On the other hand, the efficacy of haloperidol in these patients is reduced because of raised elimination rates [228–230]. Unfortunately, this interaction is usually not taken into account when calculating the haloperidol dosage. Similarly, smoking also increases the elimination of antidepressants (amitriptyline, nortriptyline, imipramine and desipramine) [220] by inducing the hepatic breakdown of these substances via-CYP1A2. Plasma protein binding by nortriptyline is clearly reduced as a result [231].

Thus, smoking cessation can be expected to result in a paradoxical increase in the efficacy of neuroleptics and antidepressants: this is manifested most particularly in an increase of adverse effects (e.g. parkinsonoid effects of neuroleptics, seizures caused by clozapine) [232].

11.5.6
Pre-operative Smoking Cessation

Up to 10% of patients develop respiratory tract or cardiovascular complications during the post-operative period. Men and women who smoke are especially at risk in this respect [233]: they have a 3 to 6-fold increased risk of intra-operative pulmonary complications [234] and there is a 2 to 5-fold increased risk of perioperative complications in smokers with chronic cardiovascular or pulmonary disease. The consequences of cigarette smoking on the various organ systems are discussed in Chaps. 5–7.

Smoking disturbs post-operative wound healing [235–237] and increases the risk of anastomotic leakage in colorectal surgery [238]. To date, there exists only one evidence-based study confirming that pre-operative smoking cessation (1 or 6–8 weeks) eliminates the risks of peri- and post-operative tobacco-associated complications [217]. This study in 120 patients indicates that an effective smoking intervention programme 6–8 weeks before surgery reduces postoperative morbidity: the overall complication rate was 18% in the smoking intervention group and 52% in the control group ($p = 0.0003$). The median length of hospital stay was 11 (7–57) vs. 13 (8–69) days (intervention vs. controls) [217]. According to estimates in one series of studies, smoking cessation should be implemented 8 weeks prior to surgery [218]. The period before and after surgery is a good time to institute interventional measures with regard to smoking cessation. In particular, peri-operative complications can be reduced by pre-operative smoking cessation. Alongside behavioural therapy interventions, NRT is probably the method of choice.

11.6
Concluding Remarks

It is assumed that, despite pharmacotherapy, medical counselling of the smoker is necessary but that this achieves independent smoking cessation in a fraction of smokers only.

- Among the pharmacological options, numerous studies indicate that treatment with nicotine products appears to be a reliable method, leading to successful smoking cessation in 30–40% of cases (see Table 11.9 for list of products).
- The level of the nicotine dose administered initially is a critical problem area (simultaneous combination of two or three formulations may be required in the initial phase of treatment).
- Depending on the level of dependence, NRT should be continued for 4–12 weeks, decreasing the nicotine dose over time.
- Nicotine chewing gum (4 mg), nasal spray and inhaler are more suitable than the nicotine patch for the relief of craving.

Table 11.9 A selection of agents used as aids to promote smoking cessation, together with dosage details

Agent	Formulation	Daily dose [mg]
Nicotine	Patch (maximum release 1.5 mg/h)	Maximum 21[a]
	Chewing gum, 2 mg	Maximum 32[a]
	Chewing gum, 4 mg	Maximum 64[a]
	Sublingual tablet, 2 mg	Maximum 60[a]
	Nasal spray (10 mg/ml)	1–2 mg/h, maximum 30[a]
	Inhaler (10 mg cartridge)	20–40[a]
	Lozenge, 2 mg	Maximum 18–30[a]
	Lozenge, 4 mg	Maximum 36–60[a]
Bupropion	Sustained-release tablets	Maximum 2 × 150

[a]Irrespective of bioavailability

- Treatment with nicotine products makes an independent contribution to smoking cessation, and to a large extent is therefore effective independently of medical counselling. The two interventions have an additive effect.
- Currently available studies indicate that bupropion is not more effective than nicotine [239], but the likely incidence of serious adverse effects has not yet been established conclusively. Because of its smaller risk-benefit ratio, bupropion should be used as a second-line option where NRT has failed or where the patient insists on bupropion despite medical advice to the contrary.
- On the basis of data currently available, other agents such as nortriptyline, clonidine, lobeline, mecamylamine, opioid antagonists and antidepressants (including buspirone) are not to be recommended for the treatment of people who wish to stop smoking.
- In pregnant women, smoking cessation with NRT should be instituted if structured counselling does not achieve the desired goal.
- All smokers with cardiovascular disease should use NRT because nicotine in therapeutic doses does not cause vasospasm.
- In the case of "hopeless" smokers who are simultaneously risk patients, consideration should be given in the near future as to whether longer-term administration of NRT preparations ("harm reduction") might not help to lower daily cigarette consumption, and thus reduce the risk of tobacco-associated morbidity and mortality.
- Nicotine receptor antagonists increase the chances of successful long-term smoking cessation between two- and threefold compared with pharmacologically unassisted quit attempts. However, there is a need for larger, independent community-based trials to test the efficacy of treatment extended beyond 12 weeks and to assess potential adverse reactions.
- Nicotine vaccines are still under development. Some preliminary studies were promising. First compounds might appear on the market in 2011.

References

1. Haustein KO (2000) Pharmacotherapy of nicotine dependence. Int J Clin Pharmacol Ther 38(6):273–290
2. The Tobacco Use and Dependence Clinical Practice Guideline Panel, Staff, and Consortium Representatives (2000) A clinical practice guideline for treating tobacco use and dependence. JAMA 283:3244–3254
3. Anonym (2000) Treating tobacco use and dependence. U.S.Department of Health and Human Services, Public Health Service, Washington
4. The Cochrane Library (2002) The Cochrane Collaboration & Update Software Ltd, editor. [Update 2002, Issue 1], Oxford, UK
5. Silagy C, Lancaster T, Stead L, Mant D, Fowler G (2002) Nicotine replacement therapy for smoking cessation. Cochrane Database Syst Rev (1):CD000146
6. Blondal T (1989) Controlled trial of nicotine polacrilex gum with supportive measures. Arch Intern Med 149(8):1818–1821
7. Bolliger CT (2000) Practical experiences in smoking reduction and cessation. Addiction 95(suppl 1):19–24
8. Blondal T, Franzon M, Westin A (1997) A double-blind randomized trial of nicotine nasal spray as an aid in smoking cessation. Eur Respir J 10(7):1585–1590

9. Schneider NG, Olmstead R, Nilsson F, Mody FV, Franzon M, Doan K (1996) Efficacy of a nicotine inhaler in smoking cessation: a double-blind, placebo-controlled trial. Addiction 91(9):1293–1306

10. Wallstrom M, Nilsson F, Hirsch JM (2000) A randomized, double-blind, placebo-controlled clinical evaluation of a nicotine sublingual tablet in smoking cessation. Addiction 95(8):1161–1171

11. Shiffman S, Dresler CM, Hajek P, Gilburt SJ, Targett DA, Strahs KR (2002) Efficacy of a nicotine lozenge for smoking cessation. Arch Intern Med 162(11):1267–1276

12. Hurt RD, Sachs DP, Glover ED, Offord KP, Johnston JA, Dale LC, et al (1997) A comparison of sustained-release bupropion and placebo for smoking cessation. N Engl J Med 337(17): 1195–1202

13. Jorenby DE, Leischow SJ, Nides MA, Rennard SI, Johnston JA, Hughes AR, et al (1999) A controlled trial of sustained-release bupropion, a nicotine patch, or both for smoking cessation. N Engl J Med 340(9):685–691

14. Stead LF, Hughes JR (2002) Lobeline for smoking cessation. Cochrane Database Syst Rev (1):CD000124

15. Gourlay SG, Stead LF, Benowitz NL (2002) Clonidine for smoking cessation. Cochrane Database Syst Rev (1):CD000058

16. Hughes JR, Stead LF, Lancaster T (2002) Anxiolytics for smoking cessation. Cochrane Database Syst Rev (1):CD002849

17. Lancaster T, Stead LF (2002) Silver acetate for smoking cessation. Cochrane Database Syst Rev (1):CD000191

18. Schoberberger R, Kunze M (eds) (1999) Diagnostik und Therapie. Nikotinabhängigkeit. Springer, New York

19. Fiore MC, Smith SS, Jorenby DE, Baker TB (1994) The effectiveness of the nicotine patch for smoking cessation. A meta-analysis. JAMA 271(24):1940–1947

20. Silagy C, Mant D, Fowler G, Lodge M (1994) Meta-analysis on efficacy of nicotine replacement therapies in smoking cessation. Lancet 343(8890):139–142

21. Tang JL, Law M, Wald N (1994) How effective is nicotine replacement therapy in helping people to stop smoking? BMJ 308(6920):21–26

22. Stead LF, Perera R, Bullen C, Mant D, Lancaster T (2008) Nicotine replacement therapy for smoking cessation. Cochrane Database Syst Rev 23(1):CD000146

23. Tonnesen P, Norregaard J, Simonsen K, Sawe U (1991) A double-blind trial of a 16-hour transdermal nicotine patch in smoking cessation. N Engl J Med 325(5):311–315

24. Henningfield JE, Keenan RM (1993) Nicotine delivery kinetics and abuse liability. J Consult Clin Psychol 61:743–750

25. Ochs HR, Greenblatt DJ, Knuchel M (1985) Kinetics of diazepam, midazolam, and lorazepam in cigarette smokers. Chest 87(2):223–226

26. Herrera N, Franco R, Herrera L, Partidas A, Rolando R, Fagerstrom KO (1995) Nicotine gum, 2 and 4 mg, for nicotine dependence. A double-blind placebo-controlled trial within a behavior modification support program. Chest 108(2):447–451

27. Kornitzer M, Kittel F, Dramaix M, Bourdoux P (1987) A double blind study of 2 mg versus 4-mg nicotine-gum in an industrial setting. J Psychosom Res 31(2):171–176

28. Tonnesen P, Fryd V, Hansen M, Helsted J, Gunnersen AB, Forchammer H, et al (1988) Effect of nicotine chewing gum in combination with group counseling on the cessation of smoking. N Engl J Med 318(1):15–18

29. Tonnesen P, Fryd V, Hansen M, Helsted J, Gunnersen AB, Forchammer H, et al (1988) Two and four mg nicotine chewing gum and group counselling in smoking cessation: an open, randomized, controlled trial with a 22 month follow-up. Addict Behav 13(1):17–27

30. Blondal T, Gudmundsson LJ, Olafsdottir I, Gustavsson G, Westin A (1999) Nicotine nasal spray with nicotine patch for smoking cessation: randomised trial with six year follow up. BMJ 318(7179):285–288

31. Tonnesen P, Paoletti P, Gustavsson G, Russell MA, Saracci R, Gulsvik A, et al (1999) Higher dosage nicotine patches increase one-year smoking cessation rates: results from the European CEASE trial. Collaborative European Anti-Smoking Evaluation. European Respiratory Society. Eur Respir J 13(2):238–246

32. Daughton DM, Heatley SA, Prendergast JJ, Causey D, Knowles M, Rolf CN, et al (1991) Effect of transdermal nicotine delivery as an adjunct to low-intervention smoking cessation therapy. A randomized, placebo-controlled, double-blind study. Arch Intern Med 151(4):749–752

33. Daughton DM, Fortmann SP, Glover ED, Hatsukami DK, Heatley SA, Lichtenstein E, et al (1999) The smoking cessation efficacy of varying doses of nicotine patch delivery systems 4 to 5 years post-quit day. Prev Med 28(2):113–118

34. Russell MA, Feyerabend C, Cole PV (1976) Plasma nicotine levels after cigarette smoking and chewing nicotine gum. Br Med J 1:1043–1046

35. Henningfield JE, Radzius A, Cooper TM, Clayton RR (1990) Drinking coffee and carbonated beverages blocks absorption of nicotine from nicotine polacrilex gum. JAMA 264: 1560–1564

36. Hughes JR, Hatsukami DK, Skoog KP (1986) Physical dependence on nicotine in gum. A placebo substitution trial. JAMA 255:3277–3279

37. Puska P, Korhonen HJ, Vartiainen E, Urjanheimo EL, Gustavsson G, Westin A (1995) Combined use of nicotine patch and gum compared with gum alone in smoking cessation: a clinical trial in North Karelia. Tob Control 4:231–235

38. Kornitzer M, Boutsen M, Dramaix M, Thijs J, Gustavsson G (1995) Combined use of nicotine patch and gum in smoking cessation: a placebo-controlled clinical trial. Prev Med 24:41–47

39. Benowitz NL, Porchet H, Sheiner L, Jacob P III (1988) Nicotine absorption and cardiovascular effects with smokeless tobacco use: comparison with cigarettes and nicotine gum. Clin Pharmacol Ther 44(1):23–28

40. Neurath GB, Dunger M, Orth D, Pein FG (1987) Trans-3¢-hydroxycotinine as a main metabolite in urine of smokers. Int Arch Occup Environ Health 59(2):199–201

41. Prather RD, Tu TG, Rolf CN, Gorsline J (1993) Nicotine pharmacokinetics of Nicoderm (nicotine transdermal system) in women and obese men compared with normal-sized men. J Clin Pharmacol 33(7):644–649

42. Gupta SK, Hwang SS, Causey D, Rolf CN, Gorsline J (1995) Comparison of the nicotine pharmacokinetics of Nicoderm (nicotine transdermal system) and half-hourly cigarette smoking. J Clin Pharmacol 35(10):985–989

43. Gupta SK, Benowitz NL, Jacob P III, Rolf CN, Gorsline J (1993) Bioavailability and absorption kinetics of nicotine following application of a transdermal system. Br J Clin Pharmacol 36(3):221–227

44. Molander L, Lunell E (2001) Pharmacokinetic investigation of a nicotine sublingual tablet. Eur J Clin Pharmacol 56(11):813–819

45. Hjalmarson A, Franzon M, Westin A, Wiklund O (1994) Effect of nicotine nasal spray on smoking cessation. A randomized, placebo-controlled, double-blind study. Arch Intern Med 154:2567–2572

46. Schneider NG, Olmstead R, Mody FV, Doan K, Franzon M, Jarvik ME, et al (1995) Efficacy of a nicotine nasal spray in smoking cessation: a placebo-controlled, double-blind trial. Addiction 90:1671–1682

47. Sutherland G, Stapleton JA, Russell MA, Jarvis MJ, Hajek P, Belcher M, et al (1992) Randomised controlled trial of nasal nicotine spray in smoking cessation. Lancet 340: 324–329

48. Leischow SJ, Nilsson F, Franzon M, Hill A, Otte P, Merikle EP (1996) Efficacy of the nicotine inhaler as an adjunct to smoking cessation. Am J Health Behav 20(5):364–371

49. Lunell E, Molander L, Ekberg K, Wahren J (2000) Site of nicotine absorption from a vapour inhaler - comparison with cigarette smoking. Eur J Clin Pharmacol 55(10):737–741

50. Lunell E, Molander L, Leischow SJ, Fagerstrom KO (1995) Effect of nicotine vapour inhalation on the relief of tobacco withdrawal symptoms. Eur J Clin Pharmacol 48:235–240

51. Westman EC, Tomlin KF, Rose JE (2000) Combining the nicotine inhaler and nicotine patch for smoking cessation. Am J Health Behav 24(2):114–119

52. Hjalmarson A, Nilsson F, Sjostrom L, Wiklund O (1997) The nicotine inhaler in smoking cessation. Arch Intern Med 157:1721–1728

53. WHO Regional Office of Europe (2002) The European Report on Tobacco Control Policy. WHO European Ministerial Conference for a Tobacco-Free Europe (ed) Third Action Plan for a Tobacco-free Europe 1997–2001. WHO Regional Office for Europe, Copenhagen, pp, 1–54

54. Choi J, Dresler CM, Norton M, Strahs KR (2003) Pharmacokinetics of a nicotine polacrilex lozenge. Nicotine Tob Res 5(5):635–644

55. Cepeda-Benito A, Reynoso JT, Erath S (2004) Meta-analysis of the efficacy of nicotine replacement therapy for smoking cessation: differences between men and women. J Consult Clin Psychol 72(4):712–722

56. Imperial Cancer Research Fund Gereral Practice Research Group (1993) Effectiveness of a nicotine patch in helping people stop smoking: results of a randomised trial in general practive. BMJ 306:1304–1308

57. Sachs DPS, Säwe U, Leischow SJ (1993) Effectiveness of a 16-hour transdermal nicotine patch in a medical practice setting, without intensive group counselling. Arch Intern Med 153: 1781–1890

58. Transdermal Nicotine Study Group (1991) Transdermal nicotine for smoking cessation. Six-month results from two multicenter controlled clinical trials. JAMA 266(22):3133–3138

59. Greenland S, Satterfield MH, Lanes SF (1998) A meta-analysis to assess the incidence of adverse effectss associated with the transdermal nicotine patch. Drug Safety 18:297–308

60. Gourlay S (1994) The pros and cons of transdermal nicotine therapy. Med J Aust 160: 152–159

61. Mendelssohn C, Richmond RL (1994) The nicotine patch: guidelines for practice use. Mod Med 105–135

62. Benowitz NL (1999) Treatment of nicotine dependence in clinical cardiology. CVD Prevention (2):135–139

63. Joseph AM, Norman SM, Ferry LH (1996) The safety of transdermal nicotine as an aid to smoking cessation in patients with cardiac disease. New Engl J Med 335:1792–1798

64. Working Group for the Study of Transdermal Nicotine in Patients with Coronary artery disease (1994) Nicotine replacement therapy for patients with coronary artery disease. Arch Intern Med 154(9):989–995

65. Hurt RD, Dale LC, Croghan GA, Croghan IT, Gomez-Dahl LC, Offord KP (1998) Nicotine nasal spray for smoking cessation: pattern of use, side effects, relief of withdrawal symptoms, and cotinine levels. Mayo Clin Proc 73:118–125

66. Molander L, Lunell E, Fagerstrom KO (2000) Reduction of tobacco withdrawal symptoms with a sublingual nicotine tablet: a placebo controlled study. Nicotine Tob Res 2(2):187–191

67. Wallstrom M, Sand L, Nilsson F, Hirsch JM (1999) The long-term effect of nicotine on the oral mucosa. Addiction 94(3):417–423

68. Zevin S, Benowitz N (1999) Drug interactions with tobacco smoking. An update. Clin Pharmacokinet 36(6):425–438

69. Miller LG (1989) Recent developments in the study of the effects of cigarette smoking on clinical pharmacokinetics and clinical pharmacodynamics. Clin Pharmacokinet 17(2): 90–108

70. Skogh E, Bengtsson F, Nordin C (1999) Could discontinuing smoking be hazardous for patients administered clozapine medication? A case report. Ther Drug Monit 21(5):580–582

71. Haustein KO (1999) Smoking tobacco, microcirculatory changes and the role of nicotine. Int J Clin Pharmacol Ther 37(2):76–85

72. Haustein KO (1999) Cigarette smoking, nicotine and pregnancy. Int J Clin Pharmacol Ther 37(9):417–427

73. Oncken C (1996) Nicotine replacement therapy during pregnancy. Am J Health Behav 20: 300–303

74. Rore C, Brace V, Danielian P, Williams D (2008) Smoking cessation in pregnancy. Expert Opin Drug Saf 7(6):727–737

75. Pauly JR, Slotkin TA (2008) Maternal tobacco smoking, nicotine replacement and neurobehavioural development. Acta Paediatr 97(10):1331–1337

76. McNeill A, Foulds J, Bates C (2001) Regulation of nicotine replacement therapies (NRT): a critique of current practice. Addiction 96(12):1757–1768

77. Shiffman S, Rolf CN, Hellebusch SJ, Gorsline J, Gorodetzky CW, Chiang YK, et al (2002) Real-world efficacy of prescription and over-the-counter nicotine replacement therapy. Addiction 97(5):505–516

78. Shiffman S, Gitchell J, Pinney JM, Burton SL, Kemper KE, Lara EA (1997) Public health benefit of over-the-counter nicotine medications. Tob Control 6:306–310

79. Lawrence WF, Smith SS, Baker TB, Fiore MC (1998) Does over-the-counter nicotine replacement therapy improve smokers' life expectancy? Tob Control 7:364–368

80. Oster G, Delea TE, Huse DM, Regan MM, Colditz GA (1996) The benefits and risks of over-the-counter availability of nicotine polacrilex ("nicotine gum"). Med Care 34:389–402

81. Shiffman S, Gitchell JG (2000) Increasing quitting by increasing access to treatment medications. Tob Control 9:230

82. Ochs HR, Greenblatt DJ, Burstein ES (1987) Lack of influence of cigarette smoking on triazolam pharmacokinetics. Br J Clin Pharmacol 23(6):759–763

83. Thorndike AN, Biener L, Rigotti NA (2002) Effect on smoking cessation of switching nicotine replacement therapy to over-the-counter status. Am J Public Health 92(3):437–442

84. Hughes JR, Shiffman S, Callas P, Zhang J (2003) A meta-analysis of the efficacy of over-the-counter nicotine replacement. Tob Control 12(1):21–27

85. Laizure SC, DeVane CL, Stewart JT, Dommisse CS, Lai AA (1985) Pharmacokinetics of bupropion and its major basic metabolites in normal subjects after a single dose. Clin Pharmacol Ther 38(5):586–589

86. Slemmer JE, Martin BR, Damaj MI (2000) Bupropion is a nicotinic antagonist. J Pharmacol Exp Ther 295(1):321–327

87. Fryer JD, Lukas RJ (1999) Noncompetitive functional inhibition at diverse, human nicotinic acetylcholine receptor subtypes by bupropion, phencyclidine, and ibogaine. J Pharmacol Exp Ther 288(1):88–92

88. Tella SR, Ladenheim B, Cadet JL (1997) Differential regulation of dopamine transporter after chronic self-administration of bupropion and nomifensine. J Pharmacol Exp Ther 281(1):508–513

89. Ascher JA, Cole JO, Colin JN, Feighner JP, Ferris RM, Fibiger HC, et al (1995) Bupropion: a review of its mechanism of antidepressant activity. J Clin Psychiatry 56(9):395–401

90. Griffith JD, Carranza J, Griffith C, Miller LL (1983) Bupropion: clinical assay for amphetamine-like abuse potential. J Clin Psychiatry 44(5 Pt 2):206–208

91. Miller L, Griffith J (1983) A comparison of bupropion, dextroamphetamine, and placebo in mixed-substance abusers. Psychopharmacology (Berl) 80(3):199–205

92. Anonym (2001) Zyban, bupropion hydrochloride; 150 mg sustained-release tablets. GlaxoSmithKline, Greenville, NC, pp 1–23

93. Preskorn SH, Othmer SC (1984) Evaluation of bupropion hydrochloride: the first of a new class of atypical antidepressants. Pharmacotherapy 4(1):20–34

94. Hsyu PH, Singh A, Giargiari TD, Dunn JA, Ascher JA, Johnston JA (1997) Pharmacokinetics of bupropion and its metabolites in cigarette smokers versus nonsmokers. J Clin Pharmacol 37(8):737–743

95. Findlay JW, Van Wyck FJ, Smith PG, Butz RF, Hinton ML, Blum MR, et al (1981) Pharmacokinetics of bupropion, a novel antidepressant agent, following oral administration to healthy subjects. Eur J Clin Pharmacol 21(2):127–135

96. Hesse LM, Venkatakrishnan K, Court MH, von Moltke LL, Duan SX, Shader RI, et al (2000) CYP2B6 mediates the in vitro hydroxylation of bupropion: potential drug interactions with other antidepressants. Drug Metab Dispos 28(10):1176–1183

97. DeVane CL, Laizure SC, Stewart JT, Kolts BE, Ryerson EG, Miller RL, et al (1990) Disposition of bupropion in healthy volunteers and subjects with alcoholic liver disease. J Clin Psychopharmacol 10(5):328–332

98. Johnston JA, Fiedler-Kelly J, Glover ED, Sachs DP, Grasela TH, DeVeaugh-Geiss J (2001) Relationship between drug exposure and the efficacy and safety of bupropion sustained release for smoking cessation. Nicotine Tob Res 3(2):131–140

99. Kirchheiner J, Klein C, Meineke I, Sasse J, Zanger UM, Murdter TE, Roots I, Brockmoller J (2003) Bupropion and 4-OH-bupropion pharmacokinetics in relation to genetic polymorphisms in CYP2B6. Pharmacogenetics 13(10):619–626

100. Gonzales DH, Nides MA, Ferry LH, Kustra RP, Jamerson BD, Segall N, et al (2001) Bupropion SR as an aid to smoking cessation in smokers treated previously with bupropion: a randomized placebo-controlled study. Clin Pharmacol Ther 69(6):438–444

101. Hays JT (2000) Tobacco dependence treatment in patients with heart and lung disease: implications for intervention and review of pharmacological therapy. J Cardiopulm Rehabil 20(4):215–223

102. Hayford KE, Patten CA, Rummans TA, Schroeder DR, Offord KP, Croghan IT, et al (1999) Efficacy of bupropion for smoking cessation in smokers with a former history of major depression or alcoholism. Br J Psychiatry 174:173–178

103. Rigotti NA, Thorndike AN, Durcan MJ, White JD, Niaura R, Gonzales D, et al (2001) Attenuation of post-cessation weight gain in smokers taking bupropion: the effect of gender. Nicotine Tob Res 2(3):304–305

104. Hays JT, Hurt RD, Rigotti NA, Niaura R, Gonzales D, Durcan MJ, et al (2001) Sustained-release bupropion for pharmacologic relapse prevention after smoking cessation. A randomized, controlled trial. Ann Intern Med 135(6):423–433

105. Hays JT, Hurt RD, Wolter TD, Buist AS, Niaura R, Rigotti N, et al (2000) Bupropion-SR for relapse prevention. Nicotine Tob Res 2(3):295–296

106. Rose JE, Behm FM, Westman EC (1998) Nicotine-mecamylamine treatment for smoking cessation: the role of pre-cessation therapy. Exp Clin Psychopharmacol 6(3):331–343

107. Velicer WF, Prochaska JO, Rossi JS, Snow MG (1992) Assessing outcome in smoking cessation studies. Psychol Bull 111(1):23–41

108. Tashkin D, Kanner R, Bailey W, Buist S, Anderson P, Nides M, et al (2001) Smoking cessation in patients with chronic obstructive pulmonary disease: a double-blind, placebo-controlled, randomised trial. Lancet 357:1571–1575

109. Puska PMJ, Brath H, Astbury C, Hider AE, Jones S Bupropion SR (2001) (Zyban) is an effective and well-tolerated aid to smoking cessation in a population of healthcare professionals. Nicotine Tob Res 4:237

110. NEU Simon JA, Duncan C, Carmody TP, Hudes ES (2004) Bupropion for smoking cessation: a randomized trial. Arch Intern Med 164(16):1797–1803

111. Ferry LH, Robbins AS, Scariati PD (1992) Enhancement of smoking cessation using the antidepressant bupropion hydrochloride [Abstract 2670]. Circulation 86(Suppl 1):I-671

112. Ferry LH, Burchette RJ (1994) Efficacy of bupropion for smoking cessation in non depressed smokers [Abstract]. J Addict Dis 13:249

113. Collins BN, Wileyto EP, Patterson F, Rukstalis M, Audrain-McGovern J, Kaufmann V, Pinto A, Hawk L, Niaura R, Epstein LH, Lerman C (2004) Gender differences in smoking cessation in a placebo-controlled trial of bupropion with behavioral counseling. Nicotine Tob Res 6(1):27–37

114. Hughes JR, Stead LF, Lancaster T (2007) Antidepressants for smoking cessation. Cochrane Database Syst Rev (1):CD000031

115. Goldstein MG (1998) Bupropion sustained release and smoking cessation. J Clin Psychiatry 59(Suppl 4):66–72

116. Anonym (2000) Bupropion: update. Canad ADR Newsletter 10:3–7

117. Anonym (2000) Fachinformation zu Zyban (R): Darstellung der Eigenschaften von Bupropion. 5 S.Bundesverband der Pharmazeutischen Industrie e.V., (ed). Glaxo-Wellcome, Aulendorf

118. Haustein KO (2003) Bupropion: pharmacological and clinical profile in smoking cessation. Int J Clin Pharmacol Ther 41(2):56–66

119. Dunner DL, Zisook S, Billow AA, Batey SR, Johnston JA, Ascher JA (1998) A prospective safety surveillance study for bupropion sustained-release in the treatment of depression. J Clin Psychiatry 59(7):366–373

120. Johnston JA, Lineberry CG, Ascher JA, Davidson J, Khayrallah MA, Feighner JP, et al (1991) A 102-center prospective study of seizure in association with bupropion. J Clin Psychiatry 52:450–456

121. Cahill K, Stead LF, Lancaster T (2008) Nicotine receptor partial agonists for smoking cessation. Cochrane Database Syst Rev (3):CD006103

122. Hall SM, Reus VI, Munoz RF, Sees KL, Humfleet G, Hartz DT, et al (1998) Nortriptyline and cognitive-behavioral therapy in the treatment of cigarette smoking. Arch Gen Psychiatry 55(8):683–690

123. Glassman AH, Stetner F, Walsh BT, Raizman PS, Fleiss JL, Cooper TB, et al (1988) Heavy smokers, smoking cessation, and clonidine. Results of a double-blind, randomized trial. JAMA 259(19):2863–2866

124. Hao W, Young D, Wei H (1988) Effect of clonidine on cigarette cessation and in the alleviation of withdrawal symptoms. Br J Addict 83(10):1221–1226

125. Glassman AH, Covey LS, Dalack GW, Stetner F, Rivelli SK, Fleiss J, et al (1993) Smoking cessation, clonidine, and vulnerability to nicotine among dependent smokers. Clin Pharmacol Ther 54(6):670–679

126. Gourlay SG, Stead LF, Benowitz NL (2004) Clonidine for smoking cessation. Cochrane Database Syst Rev (3):CD000058

127. Rose JE, Behm FM, Westman EC, Levin ED, Stein RM, Ripka GV (1994) Mecamylamine combined with nicotine skin patch facilitates smoking cessation beyond nicotine patch treatment alone. Clin Pharmacol Ther 56(1):86–99

128. Lancaster T, Stead LF (2002) Mecamylamine (a nicotine antagonist) for smoking cessation. Cochrane Database Syst Rev (1):CD001009

129. Schwartz JL, Dubitzky M (1968) One-year follow-up results of a smoking cessation program. Can J Public Health 59(4):161–165

130. Dow RJ, Fee WM (1984) Use of beta-blocking agents with group therapy in a smoking withdrawal clinic. J R Soc Med 77(8):648–651

131. West R, Hajek P, McNeill A (1991) Effect of buspirone on cigarette withdrawal symptoms and short-term abstinence rates in a smokers clinic. Psychopharmacology (Berl) 104(1): 91–96

132. Robinson MD, Pettice YL, Smith WA, Cederstrom EA, Sutherland DE, Davis H (1992) Buspirone effect on tobacco withdrawal symptoms: a randomized placebo-controlled trial. J Am Board Fam Pract 5(1):1–9

133. Hilleman DE, Mohiuddin SM, Del Core MG, Sketch MH Sr (1992) Effect of buspirone on withdrawal symptoms associated with smoking cessation. Arch Intern Med 152(2):350–352

134. Cahill K, Ussher M (2007) Cannabinoid type 1 receptor antagonists (rimonabant) for smoking cessation. Cochrane Database Syst Rev (4):CD005353

135. Edwards NB, Murphy JK, Downs AD, Ackerman BJ, Rosenthal TL (1989) Doxepin as an adjunct to smoking cessation: a double-blind pilot study. Am J Psychiatry 146(3):373–376

136. Spring B, Wurtman J, Wurtman R, el Khoury A, Goldberg H, McDermott J, et al (1995) Efficacies of dexfenfluramine and fluoxetine in preventing weight gain after smoking cessation. Am J Clin Nutr 62(6):1181–1187

137. Jacobs MA, Spilken AZ, Norman MM, Wohlberg GW, Knapp PH (1971) Interaction of personality and treatment conditions associated with success in a smoking control program. Psychosom Med 33(6):545–556

138. Frederick SL, Hall SM, Sees KL (1997) The effect of vanlafaxine on smoking cessation in subjects with and without a history of depression. NIDA Res Monogr 174:208

139. Berlin I, Said S, Spreux Varoquaux O, Launay JM, Olivares R, Millet V, et al (1995) A reversible monoamine oxidase A inhibitor (moclobemide) facilitates smoking cessation and abstinence in heavy, dependent smokers. Clin Pharmacon Ther 58:444–452

140. Gorelick DA, Rose J, Jarvik ME (1988) Effect of naloxone on cigarette smoking. J Subst Abuse 1:153–159

141. Karras A, Kane JM (1980) Naloxone reduces cigarette smoking. Life Sci 27:1541–1545

142. Nemeth-Coslett R, Griffiths RR (1986) Naloxone does not affect cigarette smoking. Psychopharmacology (Berl) 89:261–264

143. Sutherland G, Stapleton JA, Russell MA, Feyerabend C (1995) Naltrexone, smoking behaviour and cigarette withdrawal. Psychopharmacology (Berl) 120:418–425

144. Wewers ME, Dhatt R, Tejwani GA (1998) Naltrexone administration affects ad libitum smoking behavior. Psychopharmacology (Berl) 140:185–190

145. Hutchison KE, Monti PM, Rohsenow DJ, Swift RM, Colby SM, Gnys M, et al (1999) Effects of naltrexone with nicotine replacement on smoking cue reactivity: preliminary results. Psychopharmacology (Berl) 142:139–143

146. David S, Lancaster T, Stead LF (2001) Opioid antagonists for smoking cessation (Cochrane Review). Cochrane Database Syst Rev (3):CD003086

147. David S, Lancaster T, Stead LF, Evins AE (2006) Opioid antagonists for smoking cessation. Cochrane Database Syst Rev (4):CD003086

148. Schwartz JL (1969) A critical review and evaluation of smoking control methods. Public Health Rep 84(6):483–506

149. Hajek P, Stead LF (1999) Aversive smoking for smoking cessation (Cochrane Review). Cochrane Database Syst Rev (2)

150. Hymowitz N, Eckholdt H (1996) Effects of a 2.5-mg silver acetate lozenge on initial and long-term smoking cessation. Prev Med 25(5):537–546

151. Cerny EH, Cerny T (2008) Anti-nicotine abuse vaccines in the pipeline: an update. Expert Opin Investig Drugs 17(5):691–696

152. Maurer P, Bachmann MF (2007) Vaccination against nicotine: an emerging therapy for tobacco dependence. Expert Opin Investig Drugs 16(11):1775–1783

153. Colletti G, Supnick JA, Abueg FR (1982) Assessment of the relationship between self-reported smoking rate and Ecolyzer measurement. Addict Behav 7:183–188

154. Glynn SM, Gruder CL, Jegerski JA (1986) Effects of biochemical validation of self-reported cigarette smoking on treatment success and on misreporting abstinence. Health Psychol 5:125–136

155. Jarvis MJ, Russell MA, Benowitz NL, Feyerabend C (1988) Elimination of cotinine from body fluids: implications for noninvasive measurement of tobacco smoke exposure. Am J Public Health 78:696–698

156. Murray RP, Connett JE, Lauger GG, Voelker HT (1993) Error in smoking measures: effects of intervention on relations of cotinine and carbon monoxide to self-reported smoking. The Lung Health Study Research Group. Am J Public Health 83:1251–1257

157. Gariti P, Alterman AI, Ehrman R, Mulvaney FD, O'Brien CP (2002) Detecting smoking following smoking cessation treatment. Drug Alcohol Depend 65(2):191–196

158. Mahmarian JJ, Moye LA, Nasser GA, Nagueh SF, Bloom MF, Benowitz NL, et al (1997) Nicotine patch therapy in smoking cessation reduces the extent of exercise-induced myocardial ischemia. J Am Coll Cardiol 30(1):125–130

159. Bolinder G, Noren A, de Faire U, Wahren J (1997) Smokeless tobacco use and atherosclerosis: an ultrasonographic investigation of carotid intima media thickness in healthy middle-aged men. Atherosclerosis 132(1):95–103

160. anonym (2000) Don't forget nicotine replacement therapy in smokers with cardiovascular disease. Drugs Therap Perspect 16:4–6

161. McConnochie KM, Roghmann KJ (1986) Breast feeding and maternal smoking as predictors of wheezing in children age 6 to 10 years. Pediatr Pulmonol 2(5):260–268

162. Lackmann GM, Salzberger U, Tollner U, Chen M, Carmella SG, Hecht SS (1999) Metabolites of a tobacco-specific carcinogen in urine from newborns. J Natl Cancer Inst 91(5):459–465

163. Cairns NJ, Wonnacott S (1988) [3H](-)nicotine binding sites in fetal human brain. Brain Res 475(1):1–7

164. Kinney HC, O'Donnell TJ, Kriger P, White WF (1993) Early developmental changes in [3H] nicotine binding in the human brainstem. Neuroscience 55(4):1127–1138

165. Perkins KA (1993) Weight gain following smoking cessation. J Consult Clin Psychol 61(5):768–777

166. Assali AR, Beigel Y, Schreibman R, Shafer Z, Fainaru M (1999) Weight gain and insulin resistance during nicotine replacement therapy. Clin Cardiol 22(5):357–360

167. Nicklas BJ, Tomoyasu N, Muir J, Goldberg AP (1999) Effects of cigarette smoking and its cessation on body weight and plasma leptin levels. Metabolism 48(6):804–808

168. Froom P, Kristal-Boneh E, Melamed S, Gofer D, Benbassat J, Ribak J (1999) Smoking cessation and body mass index of occupationally active men: the Israeli CORDIS Study. Am J Public Health 89(5):718–722

169. Mitchell SL, Perkins KA (1998) Interaction of stress, smoking, and dietary restraint in women. Physiol Behav 64(1):103–109

170. Pirie PL, McBride CM, Hellerstedt W, Jeffery RW, Hatsukami D, Allen S, et al (1992) Smoking cessation in women concerned about weight. Am J Public Health 82(9):1238–1243

171. Burnette MM, Meilahn E, Wing RR, Kuller LH (1998) Smoking cessation, weight gain, and changes in cardiovascular risk factors during menopause: the Healthy Women Study. Am J Public Health 88(1):93–96

172. Danielsson T, Rossner S, Westin A (1999) Open randomised trial of intermittent very low energy diet together with nicotine gum for stopping smoking in women who gained weight in previous attempts to quit. BMJ 319(7208):490–493

173. Kawachi I, Troisi RJ, Rotnitzky AG, Coakley EH, Colditz GA (1996) Can physical activity minimize weight gain in women after smoking cessation? Am J Public Health 86(7):999–1004

174. Miller NS, Gold MS (1998) Comorbid cigarette and alcohol addiction: epidemiology and treatment. J Addict Dis 17(1):55–66

175. Hurt RD, Offord KP, Croghan IT, Gomez-Dahl L, Kottke TE, Morse RM, et al (1996) Mortality following inpatient addictions treatment. Role of tobacco use in a community-based cohort. JAMA 275(14):1097–1103

176. Saxon AJ, McGuffin R, Walker RD (1997) An open trial of transdermal nicotine replacement therapy for smoking cessation among alcohol- and drug-dependent inpatients. J Subst Abuse Treat 14(4):333–337

177. Mester R, Toren P, Ben Moshe Y, Weizman A (1993) Survey of smoking habits and attitudes of patients and staff in psychiatric hospitals. Psychopathology 26(2):69–75

178. Calabresi M, Casu G, Dalle LR (1991) [The prevalence of smoking in psychiatric patients. The effect of "institutionalization"]. Minerva Psichiatr 32(2):89–92

179. Hall RG, Duhamel M, McClanahan R, Miles G, Nason C, Rosen S, et al (1995) Level of functioning, severity of illness, and smoking status among chronic psychiatric patients. J Nerv Ment Dis 183(7):468–471

180. Lasser K, Boyd JW, Woolhandler S, Himmelstein DU, McCormick D, Bor DH (2000) Smoking and mental illness: a population-based prevalence study. JAMA 284(20):2606–2610

181. Gariti P, Alterman AI, Mulvaney FD, Epperson L (2000) The relationship between psychopathology and smoking cessation treatment response. Drug Alcohol Depend 60(3):267–273

182. Smith CM, Pristach CA, Cartagena M (1999) Obligatory cessation of smoking by psychiatric inpatients. Psychiatr Serv 50(1):91–94

183. Downey KK, Pomerleau CS, Huth AC, Silk KR (1998) The effect of a restricted smoking policy on motivation to quit smoking in psychiatric patients. J Addict Dis 17(2):1–7

184. Breslau N, Fenn N, Peterson EL (1993) Early smoking initiation and nicotine dependence in a cohort of young adults. Drug Alcohol Depend 33(2):129–137

185. Glassman AH (1993) Cigarette smoking: implications for psychiatric illness. Am J Psychiatry 150(4):546–553
186. Keuthen NJ, Niaura RS, Borrelli B, Goldstein M, DePue J, Murphy C, et al (2000) Comorbidity, smoking behavior and treatment outcome. Psychother Psychosom 69(5):244–250
187. Anda RF, Williamson DF, Escobedo LG, Mast EE, Giovino GA, Remington PL (1990) Depression and the dynamics of smoking. A national perspective. JAMA 264(12): 1541–1545
188. Haukkala A, Uutela A, Vartiainen E, McAlister A, Knekt P (2000) Depression and smoking cessation: the role of motivation and self-efficacy. Addict Behav 25(2):311–316
189. Covey LS, Glassman AH, Stetner F (1998) Cigarette smoking and major depression. J Addict Dis 17(1):35–46
190. Salive ME, Blazer DG (1993) Depression and smoking cessation in older adults: a longitudinal study. J Am Geriatr Soc 41(12):1313–1316
191. Gilbert DG, Crauthers DM, Mooney DK, McClernon FJ, Jensen RA (1999) Effects of monetary contingencies on smoking relapse: influences of trait depression, personality, and habitual nicotine intake. Exp Clin Psychopharmacol 7(2):174–181
192. Dursun SM, Kutcher S (1999) Smoking, nicotine and psychiatric disorders: evidence for therapeutic role, controversies and implications for future research. Med Hypotheses 52(2):101–109
193. Ziedonis DM, George TP (1997) Schizophrenia and nicotine use: report of a pilot smoking cessation program and review of neurobiological and clinical issues. Schizophr Bull 23(2): 247–254
194. Addington J, el Guebaly N, Campbell W, Hodgins DC, Addington D (1998) Smoking cessation treatment for patients with schizophrenia. Am J Psychiatry 155(7):974–976
195. George TP, Ziedonis DM, Feingold A, Pepper WT, Satterburg CA, Winkel J, et al (2000) Nicotine transdermal patch and atypical antipsychotic medications for smoking cessation in schizophrenia. Am J Psychiatry 157(11):1835–1842
196. Combs DR, Advokat C (2000) Antipsychotic medication and smoking prevalence in acutely hospitalized patients with chronic schizophrenia. Schizophr Res 46(2–3):129–137
197. McEvoy JP, Freudenreich O, Wilson WH (1999) Smoking and therapeutic response to clozapine in patients with schizophrenia. Biol Psychiatry 46(1):125–129
198. George TP, Sernyak MJ, Ziedonis DM, Woods SW (1995) Effects of clozapine on smoking in chronic schizophrenic outpatients. J Clin Psychiatry 56(8):344–346
199. Salokangas RK, Saarijarvi S, Taiminen T, Lehto H, Niemi H, Ahola V, et al (1997) Effect of smoking on neuroleptics in schizophrenia. Schizophr Res 23(1):55–60
200. Ebeling H, Moilanen I, Linna SL, Tirkkonen T, Ebeling T, Piha J, et al (1999) Smoking and drinking habits in adolescence - links with psychiatric disturbance at the age of 8 years. Eur Child Adolesc Psychiatry 8(Suppl 4):68–76
201. Sandyk R (1993) Cigarette smoking: effects on cognitive functions and drug-induced parkinsonism in chronic schizophrenia. Int J Neurosci 70(3–4):193–197
202. Menza MA, Grossman N, Van Horn M, Cody R, Forman N (1991) Smoking and movement disorders in psychiatric patients. Biol Psychiatry 30(2):109–115
203. de Leon J, Dadvand M, Canuso C, White AO, Stanilla JK, Simpson GM (1995) Schizophrenia and smoking: an epidemiological survey in a state hospital. Am J Psychiatry 152(3): 453–455
204. Hasegawa M, Gutierrez-Esteinou R, Way L, Meltzer HY (1993) Relationship between clinical efficacy and clozapine concentrations in plasma in schizophrenia: effect of smoking. J Clin Psychopharmacol 13(6):383–390
205. Goff DC, Henderson DC, Amico E (1992) Cigarette smoking in schizophrenia: relationship to psychopathology and medication side effects. Am J Psychiatry 149(9):1189–1194
206. Desmond PV, Roberts RK, Wilkinson GR, Schenker S (1979) No effect of smoking on metabolism of chlordiazepoxide. N Engl J Med 300:199–200

207. Pantuck EJ, Pantuck CB, Anderson KE, Conney AH, Kappas A (1982) Cigarette smoking and-chlorpromazine disposition and actions. Clin Pharmacol Ther 31(4):533–538

208. Stimmel GL, Falloon IR (1983) Chlorpromazine plasma levels, adverse effects, and tobacco smoking: case report. J Clin Psychiatry 44(11):420–422

209. Norman TR, Burrows GD, Maguire KP, Rubinstein G, Scoggins BA, Davies B (1977) Cigarette smoking and plasma nortriptyline levels. Clin Pharmacol Ther 21(4):453–456

210. Dettling M, Sachse C, Brockmoller J, Schley J, Muller-Oerlinghausen B, Pickersgill I, et al (2000) Long-term therapeutic drug monitoring of clozapine and metabolites in psychiatric in- and outpatients. Psychopharmacology (Berl) 152(1):80–86

211. Haring C, Meise U, Humpel C, Saria A, Fleischhacker WW, Hinterhuber H (1989) Dose-related plasma levels of clozapine: influence of smoking behaviour, sex and age. Psychopharmacology (Berl) 99:S38–S40

212. Seppala NH, Leinonen EV, Lehtonen ML, Kivisto KT (1999) Clozapine serum concentrations are lower in smoking than in non-smoking schizophrenic patients. Pharmacol Toxicol 85(11):244–246

213. Taylor D (1997) Pharmacokinetic interactions involving clozapine. Br J Psychiatry 171(8):109–112

214. Spigset O, Carleborg L, Hedenmalm K, Dahlqvist R (1995) Effect of cigarette smoking on fluvoxamine pharmacokinetics in humans. Clin Pharmacol Ther 58(10):399–403

215. Pan L, Belpaire FM (1999) In vitro study on the involvement of CYP1A2, CYP2D6 and CYP3A4 in the metabolism of haloperidol and reduced haloperidol. Eur J Clin Pharmacol 55(10):599–604

216. Shimoda K, Someya T, Morita S, Hirokane G, Noguchi T, Yokono A, et al (1999) Lower plasma levels of haloperidol in smoking than in nonsmoking schizophrenic patients. Ther Drug Monit 21(6):293–296

217. Rigotti NA (2002) Clinical practice. Treatment of tobacco use and dependence. N Engl J Med 346(7):506–512

218. Fiore MC, Kenford SL, Jorenby DE, Wetter DW, Smith SS, Baker TB (1994) Two studies of the clinical effectiveness of the nicotine patch with different counseling treatments. Chest 105(2):524–533

219. Perel JM, Hurwic MJ, Kanzler MB (1975) Pharmacodynamics of imipramine in depressed patients. Psychopharmacol Bull 11(10):16–18

220. McCarthy RH (1994) Seizures following smoking cessation in a clozapine responder. Pharmacopsychiatry 27(5):210–211

221. Callaghan JT, Bergstrom RF, Ptak LR, Beasley CM (1999) Olanzapine. Pharmacokinetic and pharmacodynamic profile. Clin Pharmacokinet 1 37(3):177–193

222. Fulton B, Goa KL (1997) Olanzapine. A review of its pharmacological properties and therapeutic efficacy in the management of schizophrenia and related psychoses. Drugs 53(2):281–298

223. Ring BJ, Catlow J, Lindsay TJ, Gillespie T, Roskos LK, Cerimele BJ, et al (1996) Identification of the human cytochromes P450 responsible for the in vitro formation of the major oxidative metabolites of the antipsychotic agent olanzapine. J Pharmacol Exp Ther 276(2):658–666

224. Benowitz NL (1993) Nicotine replacement therapy. What has been accomplished - can we do better? Drugs 5(2):157–170

225. Hughes JR, Hatsukami DK, Mitchell JE, Dahlgren LA (1986) Prevalence of smoking among psychiatric outpatients. Am J Psychiatry 143(8):993–997

226. Hughes JR (1993) Possible effects of smoke-free inpatient units on psychiatric diagnosis and treatment. J Clin Psychiatry 54(3):109–114

227. Jann MW, Saklad SR, Ereshefsky L, Richards AL, Harrington CA, Davis CM (1986) Effects of smoking on haloperidol and reduced haloperidol plasma concentrations and haloperidol clearance. Psychopharmacology (Berl) 90(4):468–470

228. Miller DD, Kelly MW, Perry PJ, Coryell WH (1990) The influence of cigarette smoking on haloperidol pharmacokinetics. Biol Psychiatry 28(6):529–531

229. Linnoila M, George L, Guthrie S, Leventhal B (1981) Effect of alcohol consumption and cigarette smoking on antidepressant levels of depressed patients. Am J Psychiatry 138(6): 841–842

230. Perry PJ, Browne JL, Prince RA, Alexander B, Tsuang MT (1986) Effects of smoking on nortriptyline plasma concentrations in depressed patients. Ther Drug Monit 8(3):279–284

231. Bluman LG, Mosca L, Newman N, Simon DG (1998) Preoperative smoking habits and postoperative pulmonary complications. Chest 113:883–889

232. Schwilk B, Bothner U, Schraag S, Georgieff M (1997) Perioperative respiratory events in smokers and nonsmokers undergoing general anaesthesia. Acta Anaesthesiol Scand 41: 348–355

233. Haverstock BD, Mandracchia VJ (1998) Cigarette smoking and bone healing: implications in foot and ankle surgery. J Foot Ankle Surg 37:69–74

234. Jorgensen LN, Kallehave F, Christensen E, Siana JE, Gottrup F (1998) Less collagen production in smokers. Surgery 123:450–455

235. Silverstein P (1992) Smoking and wound healing. Am J Med 93:22S–24S

236. Sorensen LT, Jorgensen T, Kirkeby LT, Skovdal J, Vennits B, Wille-Jorgensen P (1999) Smoking and alcohol abuse are major risk factors for anastomotic leakage in colorectal surgery. Br J Surg 86:927–931

237. Moller AM, Villebro N, Pedersen T, Tonnesen H (2002) Effect of preoperative smoking intervention on postoperative complications: a randomised clinical trial. Lancet 359(9301): 114–117

238. Warner MA, Offord KP, Warner ME, Lennon RL, Conover MA, Jansson-Schumacher U (1989) Role of preoperative cessation of smoking and other factors in postoperative pulmonary complications: a blinded prospective study of coronary artery bypass patients. Mayo Clin Proc 64:609–616

Primary Prevention

12

As already outlined in previous chapters, efforts to combat cigarette smoking must be directed primarily at developing useful and effective future strategies to ensure that children around the age of 10 years never start to smoke. In 1997, the Commissioner of the US Food and Drug Administration wrote an important article on smoking, "Nicotine addiction: a pediatric disease" [1], in which he described in graphic terms both the tactics of the tobacco industry as well as the adverse consequences of smoking on health. As long ago as the 1970s, two senior executives of the R.J. Reynolds Tobacco Company stated: *"Realistically, if our Company is to survive and prosper, over the long term, we must get our share of the youth market"* and *"Evidence is now available to indicate that the 14–18-year-old group is an increasing segment of the smoking population"* [1].

Essentially, if it is to dispel doubts about smoking and frustrate plans for smoking cessation, the tobacco industry has two time windows in which to generate smokers: (1) in children around the age of 10–12 years and (2) in adolescents around the age of 15–18 years. The number one goal of primary prevention is to ensure that children and adolescents never start to smoke.

In this context, a wide variety of factors come into play:

- The adolescent's character, ability to take a stand, and position in the group
- The parental home and its possible influence on smoking education
- The function of the group to which the adolescent belongs and of which he/she wishes to be a "respected" member
- Teachers as role models
- Tobacco industry initiatives (advertising)
- Temptations such as cigarette vending machines, department stores etc.

Discussion of the different preventive programmes will be preceded by a brief review of current knowledge on the problems of smoking initiation in adolescents because prevention programmes must be tailored to age at initiation.

K.-O. Haustein, D. Groneberg, *Tobacco or Health?*
DOI: 10.1007/978-3-540-87577-2_12, © Springer Verlag Berlin Heidelberg 2010

12.1
Smoking Initiation

Smoking initiation is the term used to describe the stage when the adolescent has gone beyond the experimentation phase and has started to smoke cigarettes regularly. The tobacco industry avoids clear definitions so that the influence of advertising on the different age groups cannot be demonstrated (see Chap. 13). According to one analysis conducted in 1,462 students aged between 11 and 14 years from New York State, the influence of the parental home, friends and acquaintances was the commonest reason for starting smoking (32.2%), followed by tobacco advertising (18.6%) [2].

In England 23% of 11-year-old children have already experimented with smoking and by the age of 15 years, 59% of boys and 63% of girls have tried smoking. In 1994, among 11–15-year olds, 10% of boys and 13% of girls were smokers [3]. Within a 2-year period (1994–1996), smoking prevalence in 16–24-year-old females increased by 5% and that in males of the same age rose by 2% [4]. Those children who try smoking at a young age are predestined to become smokers subsequently [5]. Nicotine dependence therefore sets in at a very early age, making smoking cessation extremely difficult to achieve [6].

A comprehensive survey of age at smoking initiation was conducted in the USA in 1995 [7]: in calculating the initiation rate per calendar year, the numerator was the sum of the weights for adolescents who reported starting smoking in a given year, and the denominator was the sum of the weights for those at risk to start smoking in that year.

As shown by the data presented in Fig. 12.1, from about 1920 onwards the number of female smokers has risen continuously, with a dramatic surge in smoking recorded in 14–17-year-old girls since 1967 [7]. Educational level (college education: yes or no) was found to be a substantial determinant of the initiation rate in 10–17-year-old girls who smoked (Fig. 12.2) [8]. Figure 12.2 also depicts expenditure on four well-known brands of US cigarettes preferred by female smokers. The differences in smoking initiation based on

Fig. 12.1 Smoking initiation rates among 14–17-year-old adolescents over a period of more than 60 years. See text for comment on the time periods shown [7]. The initiation rates were calculated from the number of adolescents who reported starting smoking in a given year, divided by the number of those at risk to start smoking in that year

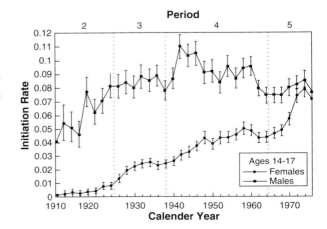

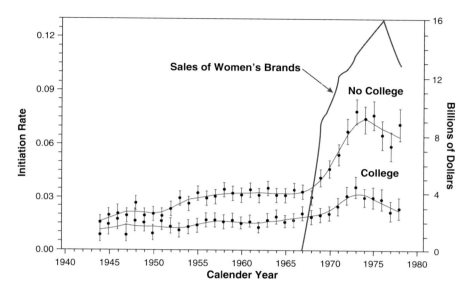

Fig. 12.2 Annual initiation rate among 10–17-year-old smoking girls as a function of educational level (college education: yes or no). Also shown, financial expenditure on "women's" cigarettes (Virginia Slims, Silva Thins and Eve) [7]

educational level are impressive. The same team has now published its findings on smoking behaviour among 14–17-year-old US adolescents for the period 1979–1989 [9].

According to the final report from the Bundeszentrale für gesundheitliche Aufklärung (BZgA; Federal Central Office for Health Education) published in 1998, 7% of 12–13-year-old children in Germany and as many as 28% of 14–15-year-olds were smokers. Among 16–17-year-old students, the figure reaches 47% [10]. Despite this trend among adolescents, the percentage proportion of never-smokers among 12–25-year-olds more than doubled from 20% in 1973 to 42% in 1997 (applies only to the former West German *Länder*) [10]. The percentage proportion of never-smokers among 12–17-year-olds has risen from 31 to 56%. In total, 20% of adolescents describe themselves as ex-smokers [11].

According to a BZgA survey among adolescents, the reasons for not smoking were related primarily to the adverse effects of smoking on health (79%), followed by responses such as "Tastes bad" (55%), "Too expensive" (47%), "Smells bad" (37%), "Makes you less fit" (36%), "Doesn't look good" (9%) and "Not allowed" (5%) [10].

Compared with the MODRUS I Study of 1998, the MODRUS II Study [12] conducted in Saxony-Anhalt in 3,087 students, 851 adults (parents) and 153 teachers revealed a further reinforcement in many respects of adolescents' tendency to be "adventurous" and "oriented towards the big wide world". The study also found a deterioration of attitudes towards sport and healthy lifestyle, while reporting that relationships with parents had become an area of increased tension. Compared with 2 years previously, greater criticism was levelled at the social environment within schools. The mean initiation age for smoking was reported to be 12.52 years, followed by 13.03 years for alcohol and 14.1 years for ecstasy. In common with numerous other studies, one particularly critical note sounded by

Table 12.1   Consumer types from the MODRUS II Study in the year 2000 [12]

Consumers of	Cigarettes	Alcohol	Cannabis	Ecstasy	Cocaine/heroin
Cigarettes	100	32	31	7	4
Alcohol	55	100	34	6	4
Cannabis	71	44	100	13	8
Ecstasy	84	41	70	100	42
Cocaine/heroin	80	46	77	74	100

All data are shown as percentages (rounded up). Example: For every 100 students who smoke, 32% drink alcohol etc.

MODRUS II was that tobacco smoking (cigarettes) is viewed as the commonest entry-level drug, potentially leading on to others ranging from alcohol to heroin (see Table 12.1) [12]. In those terms, it is essential that preventive measures be implemented to establish a smoke-free environment in schools.

12.2
Reasons for Smoking

One study in schoolchildren [13–15] indicates that smoking initiation in most European countries occurs at the age of 11 years and that by this age some 20% of boys have gained their first experiences [14]. Girls start smoking slightly later but then make up ground on boys very quickly [16], so that by the age of 15 years both sexes have the same levels of experience, with more girls than boys smoking in some countries (including Germany) [17]. It has been reported that students attempt to gain their first experience of smoking during the first 4 years in school [13, 18–20], although substantial ethnic and hence social differences have been found [21].

Initiation into tobacco consumption is initially an attempt to face up to the problems (just as much as the challenges) of daily living, to derive pleasure and to provide a coping mechanism for conflict with parents and for experiences of failure at school (being kept back a year, lack of peer recognition). Tobacco is seen as helping to eliminate symptoms of stress. Even though the (inhaled) cigarette smoke may not taste pleasant for the first 1 or 2 years, budding smokers force themselves to "enjoy" it because they need to "prove" something to friends or adults. During this initiation phase, tobacco consumption has instrumental character in psychological and sociological terms [22]. At this stage, but also over the ensuing months, tobacco consumption may be important to the adolescent for a range of reasons [11]:

- It challenges parental and social norms and values.
- It is a deliberate act against the notion of parental control.
- It demonstratively anticipates parental behaviour.
- It reflects the search for consciousness-expanding experiences.
- It gives rapid relaxation and pleasure.
- It opens up access to a circle of friends.
- It marks the smoker out as belonging to a subculture.

- It is a distraction from poor performance at school.
- It takes the smoker's mind off his/her psychological problems.
- It masks poor self-confidence and provides a boost to a vulnerable sense of self-worth.

By contrast, students who attain a higher educational level more rapidly adopt a health-conscious attitude towards cigarette smoking. People who are "smoke-free" up to the age of 20 have an overwhelming chance of remaining non-smokers for life [23]. Those who smoke in their youth are only rarely able to quit smoking during the next 2–3 decades of life. Smoking initiation in childhood is determined by external factors (instrumentalised) and is based upon the child's or adolescent's insuperable problems with self-worth [24–27].

Behavioural stabilisation increases with distance from age at initiation; people who take up smoking after the age of 20 years are relatively rare [28, 29], and conversely schoolchildren who embark on a smoking career at the age of 13–15 years are at risk of continuing to smoke for decades [23, 30–34]. The lower the age at cigarette smoking initiation, the greater the probability that the individual will become a dependent smoker before the age of 20 years [28, 29]. Early smoking initiation is the best single predictor of smoking continuity [32, 33]. This illustrates the wisdom of implementing primary tobacco-use prevention programmes as early as possible [35–37].

The perception of smoking by smokers and non-smokers is revealing. In one youth survey conducted in 1993 in 12–16-year-old students of both sexes, ten pairs of opposite attributes were each scored on a scale from 1 to 5 [38]. The results, calculated separately for female and male adolescents, revealed only quantitative differences. Some 47% of the adolescents had never smoked, while those who had tried smoking accounted for some 38%. For many of the attribute pairs, non-smokers were more critical than smokers in their perceived image of smokers ("Someone who regularly smokes cigarettes is …"): significant differences were reported for the pairs "attractive/repulsive", "in/out", "relaxed/stressed" and "interesting/boring" [38]. Compared with smoking girls, smoking boys rated regular smokers as more interesting, more relaxed and performing better [38].

12.3
Primary Prevention Programmes

The several programmes developed for primary tobacco-use prevention in schools are designed to ensure that children:

- Never start to smoke in the first place.
- At least defer the time of smoking initiation by 2–3 years or longer and thus in future do not become heavily dependent smokers like those who start at the age of 10–12 years.
- Are fully informed about the health consequences and social repercussions of smoking and also feel psychologically strengthened to resist temptations arising in the group or in other settings.

Opportunities to influence young people in this way invariably fail when scare tactics are used. Showing pictures of a bronchial carcinoma tends to make children and adolescents think that:

- This will not affect everyone in later life.
- Two, three or even four decades may pass before this happens.
- Their parents/grandparents have smoked for decades without any harm.
- Life is not much fun anyway and they do not want to live to a ripe old age etc.

Further discussions on this basis tend to remain unproductive and do not lead to the desired goal of smoking prevention.

12.3.1
Prevention Programmes for Schools

Most studies concentrate on the behaviour of children in school years 5–8 because it is during this period that children show an increasing desire to gain experience with tobacco, alcohol and illicit drugs – a finding that has also emerged from studies in other countries [12, 13, 18, 19]. As a result, prevention programmes are very much needed during the early years at school (see also [20]).

Adolescent smokers in school year 6 tend to be characterised as the self-defined type [39, 40] who can be described as "matured early, independent of authority, orientated towards peer group, risk takers" [41]. There probably needs to be fresh discussion as to whether adolescent smokers are tempted or even compelled at all to smoke as a result of group pressure. More probably, adolescents actively seek out groups whose values and norms they share. They enter into a commitment to the group that is evident in terms of externals (e.g. style of dress, shared activities etc.). If smoking is one of the shared norms of the group in this sense, it is likely that group members or adolescents, who find (generally informal) group membership attractive or wish to become members, will also smoke.

The view that children and adolescents are led astray into smoking by their peers or are driven or compelled to do so by group pressure fails to recognise that affiliation to a group is an active process of seeking out and bonding that is initiated by the attractiveness of the group based on shared norms (frequently, also based on externals such as cigarette smoking) [42]. The influence of siblings, and especially of best friends (male or female) as well as of the whole group, is relatively high and outweighs that of parents.

Adolescents should be supported in the general development of a healthy sense of self-worth [40], but it is debatable to what extent these measures contribute to smoking prevention. When imparting the requisite skills, it might be more useful as part of the programme to address pupils or class groups in a targeted manner and to communicate specific medical-psychological information designed to promote a healthy lifestyle, with particular reference to smoking [42].

According to ideas developed in the USA, effective tobacco-use prevention programmes in schools depend on the establishment of seven recommendations [43]:

1. Develop and implement a school policy on tobacco use.
2. Provide instruction about the short- and long-term negative consequences of tobacco use, social influences on tobacco use, peer norms regarding tobacco use and refusal skills.
3. Provide tobacco-use prevention education in kindergarten through 12th grade, with particularly intensive instruction in the early school grades.
4. Provide programme-specific training for teachers.
5. Involve parents and families in support of school-based programmes to prevent tobacco use.
6. Support smoking cessation efforts among students and all school staff who use tobacco.
7. Assess the tobacco-use prevention programme at regular intervals.

As well as banning tobacco advertising within schools and in school publications, efforts should be made to encourage implementation of the programme by all students and to popularise the school-based prevention scheme with parents, students and the wider community. In addition, provisions must be in place to translate the policy into action. The long-term unwanted biological, cosmetic and social consequences of tobacco use should be presented, with smoking students being criticised by non-smoking peers. The purportedly positive social image of tobacco use should be rejected. Increasing the intensity and duration of adolescents' training or instruction in terms of tobacco-use prevention enhances its effectiveness [44, 45]. Effective tobacco-use prevention should be integrated into a broader programme of prevention related to alcohol and drug abuse [46]. Over and above this, the prevention programmes should also involve the family, community organisations, anti-tobacco advertising and the adolescents' social environment. By exercising social skills [47] and using a teacher-led approach [48], the instructors of these courses can help to counteract the social pressure on adolescents to use tobacco. Seminars of this kind are time-consuming if they are to be really effective. As schools and parents work together, the subject of smoking should also be discussed at home, the ideal end result being that the adults also quit [49]. Prevention programmes for adolescents should aim at immediate smoking cessation, with attainable goals formulated and rewards also defined by agreement. Social support, coping with stress, refusal skills and avoidance of the temptation trap – all these are learnable skills [50–52]. Students should rehearse these situations in role-play sessions so that they also remain tobacco-abstinent [51, 53]. In the USA, prevention programmes already exist for kindergartens, but interventions that are too early may have an effect that is the opposite of what was intended (risk of early drug use) [54, 55].

Programmes of this type are offered in the USA by the local health departments or other health agencies (e.g. the American Cancer Society, American Heart Association or American Lung Association). Programmes with the same or similar content have also been developed in Europe (Sects. 12.4 and 12.5); for example, the "Schule 2000" programme is intended principally for school years 4 and 5 [20] and the "Be smart – don't start" programme, a project originally conceived in Finland and now used in many European countries, is intended for school years 6–8. The "Be smart – don't start" competition is sponsored by the European Commission as part of the European Union (EU) action plan "Europe Against Cancer" and is implemented in cooperation with the European Network on Young People and Tobacco (ENYPAT, Helsinki).

Prevention programmes should focus special attention on girls because their health is not merely an individual but also a social problem. Such programmes must emphasise the social role of women, their self-respect and their image in society. Younger women have a stronger tendency towards smoking cessation than older women [56]. Compared with men, it is very much more common for women to discuss social norms in regard to starting smoking. The theory of "reasoned action" forms a constructive framework for preventive strategies to-address sets of beliefs and attitudes which influence smoking by teenage girls [57].

As far as possible, primary tobacco-use prevention programmes in schools should build upon existing course work designed to promote healthy living as below:

1. In addition to the aspects of physical health, teaching should also cover psychological well-being.
2. Health education must not satisfy itself with ad hoc lessons, but must become an integral part of various curriculum subjects.
3. As well as communicating knowledge, the programme should develop a "healthy school" climate where the students can also take the facts they have been taught about health education and translate them into life skills [11].

When communicating knowledge on the subject of tobacco (and drugs, in general), it is crucial to emphasise the psychological and social consequences of use and to rehearse skills with the students (role-play, experiments, handling group pressure, awareness of personal desires and ideas about life, handling conflict, personal relaxation exercises, encouraging social responsibility). Ultimately, these instructional activities must generate a reasoned "distance from tobacco".

This mental distance from tobacco needs to attain a high threshold that will enable the individual to resist the temptation to smoke and prevent a few failures from turning into habitual use. Smokers tend to trivialise tobacco and nicotine, and while they do not consider the "product" to be non-hazardous they do "like it" very much. Distance from tobacco is built up on three levels [11]:

- Cognitively – by presenting the hazardous nature of tobacco to the extent that this aspect is perceived by the individual
- Affectively – by addressing the emotional assessment of tobacco
- Behaviourally – by communicating the idea that tobacco should not be used in the first place

Follow-up surveys in schools have in fact revealed that students with a labile, irresolute, uncertain attitude towards tobacco derived the greatest benefit from these teaching sessions, whereas hardly any influence at all was possible in students who showed less distance from tobacco [58]. Number of non-smokers in classes undergoing these instructional programmes were higher than in classes without such instruction. "Behavioural change" is therefore achieved only to a small extent.

The instructional measures only become properly effective where an entire school and not just individual classes take up and implement these programmes; it then becomes possible to create a climate in which the teaching can be "lived out". Teachers and parents also benefit from this climate, and the teachers at least should become ex-smokers themselves (see Sect. 12.8).

Two strategies have proved successful in the USA and subsequently also in Germany; the Social Influence Inoculation Strategy and the Life Skills Strategy, and these have also found expression in the projects described in later sections below [59].

12.3.1.1
Social Influence Inoculation Strategy

In the Social Influence Inoculation Strategy, adolescents are made to feel antagonistic towards social influences that encourage drug consumption; expectations and hopes linked to drug consumption are dismantled while attitudes are generated that will enable students to handle and counter group pressure. These "Say 'No' Strategies" are practised not as behaviour in isolation but as an integral part of general training in social skills in which students listen to the arguments of others but are enabled constructively to implement their own beliefs. Programmes using this social inoculation approach have been and remain successful and also produce behavioural changes [59].

12.3.1.2
Life Skills Strategy

In the Life Skills Strategy, general and specific personal and social skills are communicated, discussed and rehearsed (e.g. in role-play) so that adolescents gain a sense of social responsibility and with it develop the resources to handle the stresses of school and everyday life other than by turning to drugs. The use of drugs is viewed as a response by the student for coping with responsibilities, and the goal is to replace this attitude by other coping strategies [60, 61]. One instructional programme designed for all ages (from kindergarten through to grade 12) and used in the USA for many years now is presented in Table 12.2 [43].

The life skills programme developed in the USA is regarded as a very valuable and influential approach for health promotion in schools [60, 61]. A pivotal ingredient in this programme is the development of coping behaviours as part of the acquisition of general social skills (e.g. saying "No" when cigarettes are handed around). Although frequently used in the past, schemes to limit smoking behaviour exclusively by communicating information on smoking have not been successful [62–64].

12.4
"Be Smart: Don't Start"

The "Be smart – don't start" programme consists of three training modules for school years 1/2, 3/4 and 5/6, each comprising 20 teaching manuals: these manuals do not cross-refer to each other so that individual class years can also be instructed separately. The

Table 12.2 Instructional concepts (kindergarten through grade 12) for school health programmes to prevent tobacco use and addiction [43]

Early elementary school Knowledge: students will learn that	Later elementary school Knowledge: students will learn that
A drug is a chemical that changes how the body works	Stopping tobacco use has short- and long-term benefits*
All forms of tobacco contain a drug called nicotine	Environmental tobacco smoke is dangerous to health*
Tobacco use includes cigarettes and smokeless tobacco	Most young persons and adults do not use tobacco*
Tobacco use is harmful to health	Nicotine, contained in all forms of tobacco, is an addictive drug
Stopping tobacco use has short-term and long-term benefits	Tobacco use has short-term and long-term physiologic and cosmetic consequences
Many persons who use tobacco have trouble stopping	Personal feelings, family, peers, and the media influence decisions about tobacco use
Tobacco smoke in the air is dangerous to anyone who breathes it	Tobacco advertising is often directed toward young persons
Many fires are caused by persons who smoke	Young persons can resist pressure to use tobacco
Some advertisements try to persuade persons to use tobacco	Laws, rules, and policies regulate the sale and use of tobacco
Most young persons and adults do not use tobacco	
Persons who choose to use tobacco are not bad persons	
Attitudes: students will demonstrate	*Attitudes: students will demonstrate*
A personal commitment not to use tobacco	A personal commitment not to use tobacco*
Pride about choosing not to use tobacco	Pride about choosing not to use tobacco*
	Support for others' decisions not to use tobacco
	Responsibility for personal health
Skills: students will be able to	*Skills: students will be able to*
Communicate knowledge and personal attitudes about tobacco use	Communicate knowledge and personal attitudes about tobacco use*
Encourage other persons not to use tobacco	Encourage other persons not to use tobacco*
	Demonstrate skills to resist tobacco use
	State the benefits of a smoke-free environment
	Develop counterarguments to tobacco advertisements and other promotional materials
	Support persons who are trying to stop using tobacco
Middle school/junior high School knowledge: students will learn that	Senior high school knowledge: students will learn that
Most young persons and adults do not smoke*	Most young persons and adults do not smoke*
Laws, rules, and policies regulate the sale and use of tobacco*	
	Tobacco use has short- and long-term physiologic, cosmetic, social, and economic consequences*
Tobacco manufacturers use various strategies to direct advertisements toward young persons, such as "image" advertising*	Cigarette smoking and smokeless tobacco use have direct health consequences*

Table 12.2 (continued)

Early elementary school Knowledge: students will learn that	Later elementary school Knowledge: students will learn that
Tobacco use has short- and long term physiologic, cosmetic, social, and economic consequences*	Community organizations have information about tobacco use and can help persons stop using tobacco*
Cigarette smoking and smokeless tobacco use have direct health consequences*	Smoking cessation programs can be successful*
Maintaining a tobacco-free environment has health benefits	Tobacco use is an unhealthy way to manage stress or weight
Tobacco use is an unhealthy way to manage stress or weight*	Tobacco use during pregnancy has harmful effects an the foetus
Community organizations have information about tobacco use and can help persons stop using tobacco	Schools and community organizations can promote a smoke-free environment
Smoking cessation programs can be successful	Many persons find it hard to stop using tobacco, despite knowledge about the health hazards of tobacco use
Tobacco contains other harmful substances in addition to nicotine	
Attitudes: students will demonstrate	Attitudes: students will demonstrate
A personal commitment not to use tobacco*	A personal commitment not to use tobacco*
Pride about choosing not to use tobacco*	Pride about choosing not to use tobacco*
Responsibility for personal health*	Responsibility for personal health*
Support for others' decisions not to use tobacco*	Support for others' decisions not to use tobacco*
Confidence in personal ability to resist tobacco use	Confidence in personal ability to resist tobacco use*
	Willingness to use school and community resources for information about, and help with, resisting or quitting tobacco use
Skills: students will be able to	*Skills: students will be able to*
Encourage other persons not to use tobacco*	Encourage other persons not to use tobacco*
Support persons who are trying to stop using tobacco*	Support persons who are trying to stop using tobacco*
Communicate knowledge and personal attitudes about tobacco use*	Communicate knowledge and personal attitudes about tobacco use*
Demonstrate skills to resist tobacco use*	Demonstrate skills to resist tobacco use*
Identify and counter strategies used in tobacco advertisements and other promotional materials*	Identify and counter strategies used in tobacco advertisements and other promotional materials*
Develop methods for coping with tobacco use by parents and with other difficult personal situations, such as peer pressure to use tobacco	Develop methods for coping with tobacco use by parents and with other difficult personal situations, such as peer pressure to use tobacco*
Request a smoke-free environment	Use school and community resources for information about and help with, resisting or quitting tobacco use
	Initiate school and community action to support a smoke-free environment

*These concepts reinforce content introduced during earlier grades.

subjects "Smoking" and "Taking a stand" are not covered in years 1/2. The following life skill areas are covered in a manner commensurate with the children's age: self-image and ability to understand the situation, handling stress, communication issues, critical thinking and taking a stand, problem-solving and health-related knowledge. From school year 3 onwards, students learn about the harmful constituents of tobacco smoke and their implications for health are presented. Extensive and varied study and exercise materials are made available to the students. The programme's mascot is "Igor the Hedgehog" who says "No" to cigarettes [65].

The study was conducted in particular to establish whether students show positive changes in terms of smoking behaviour and whether they also show positive development in terms of expectations, attitudes and knowledge with regard to smoking. On the basis of a questionnaire score, the students were assessed for smoking behaviour and for its personal consequences on them. Since the teaching activities were easy to implement, the programme was very positively assessed by students and teachers [65]. A positive influence has been assumed on the psychosocial behaviour of the students: aggressive behaviour among the younger students was reduced and there was a decline in social problems among the older students in terms of delinquent and anxious, aggressive behaviour patterns [65]. However, it is important to note that only the short-term effects of the intervention were studied and that consequently no conclusions can be drawn concerning the permanence of the resulting behaviour patterns (self-worth, strength of resistance), particularly since the frequency of tobacco consumption will increase [34].

12.5
Class 2000 Health Promotion Programme

This programme also aims at the primary prevention of addiction during the early school years. Its objectives are to promote a positive attitude to health at an early stage and, by strengthening life skills, to exert an addiction-preventing influence on the children's behaviour [66], with teaching in school focusing primarily on feelings of self-worth, communication of positive body awareness, and a critical appraisal of legal drugs and substances that are harmful to health. The ability to say "No" in tempting situations is the key point. In order for this ability to be in place, knowledge has to be imparted before the first contact with the addictive substance, and the children and adolescents also have to be mentored over a longer period. Teachers take 5–10 h and specialist health educators 2–3 h in each of the first four academic years; the students are given study files, and the teachers and specialist health educators are issued with prepared lesson outlines [66]. The year groups are mentored continuously by a member of the teaching staff and parents are encouraged to become involved in the work of the school; this results in greater health awareness and this is of benefit to the children. The programme is financed through sponsorship. These "Say No" effects are reinforced during information sessions designed to prevent addiction ("advertising and happiness"), and advertising agencies have not succeeded in breaking down this attitude on the part of the students [67].

12.6
Trier University Health Programme

For the past 3 years, a programme designed to prevent cigarette smoking has been implemented in year 6 students (aged 11–12 years) from various secondary schools in the Trier region. In eight teaching sessions, the prime objective is to motivate the students not to start smoking at all. At the same time, social and personal determinants of early smoking initiation are identified so that consequences can be drawn for the programme content, which is constantly refined in the light of new data. The programme has already been described in various publications [39, 40, 68, 69] and is based on the most up-to-date social skills approaches designed primarily to modify specific social behavioural patterns of children and adolescents with regard to smoking. The programme has been integrated into the school curriculum and it comprises complementary scientific research as well as parental collaboration and public relations work. The teaching sessions have revealed that students with smoking experience are more prepared to take risks than non-smokers of the same age. They also have a considerably more positive image of smokers.

Alongside encouraging results, however, this study also revealed a fall in the number of non-smokers, although no educational or scare programme was used for which such an effect has been demonstrated. It may be that this reflects a development effect in as much as the developmental tasks facing adolescents (e.g. leaving the parental home, peer orientation) coincide with trial consumption (exploratory behaviour) [70, 71]. Clues to this may be early smoking initiation, and the connections between smoking behaviour and a tendency towards risky (forbidden) activities [42].

12.7
Long-Term Studies

Within the past 8 years, three large-scale studies have been performed to investigate the prevention of smoking initiation among adolescents: a drug abuse prevention trial in a middle-class population [60], a follow-up of smoking prevention effects in the North Karelia project [72] and the Hutchinson Smoking Prevention Project [73]. The first of these studies was a randomised trial involving 56 public schools (3,597 predominantly white, 12th grade students who represented 60.4% of the initial 7th grade sample). The schools received the prevention programme with annual provider training workshops and ongoing consultation, the prevention programme with videotaped training and no consultation, or "treatment as usual" (i.e. controls). The intervention consisted of 15 classes in 7th grade, 10 booster sessions in 8th grade, and 5 booster sessions in 9th grade. The programme taught general "life skills" and skills for resisting social influences to use drugs. The follow-up data were collected 6 years after baseline using school, telephone and mailed surveys. Six tobacco, alcohol and marijuana use self-report scales were recorded. Reductions in drug and polydrug use were found, and the strongest effects were produced for individuals who received a reasonably complete version of the intervention, resulting in 44% fewer drug users and 66% fewer polydrug (tobacco, alcohol, marijuana) users [60]. It is concluded from this study that reductions in tobacco and drug use can be achieved by teaching social resistance and general life skills, including at least 2 years of booster sessions.

The second major study described the results of a 15-year follow-up of a school- and community-based smoking prevention project in North Karelia, Finland [72]. Four intervention schools from this district and two control schools from another province were chosen for the evaluation, beginning in 1978 with 7th grade students and running through 1980, with a 15-year follow-up. In North Karelia, a community-based smoking cessation programme for adults was organised in addition. In the intervention schools, health educators and trained peer leaders led 10 sessions (3 in the 7th grade, 5 in the 8th grade, and 2 in the 9th grade). In 1993, the subjects completed a questionnaire at home and a trained nurse carried out a cardiovascular risk factor survey in a local health centre. Cohort participation was still 71% after 15 years. The prevalence of all smokers in the four intervention schools was between 28 and 32%, while that in the control schools was 36 and 41%. After 15 years, cumulative exposure to tobacco in the intervention group was 22% lower than in the

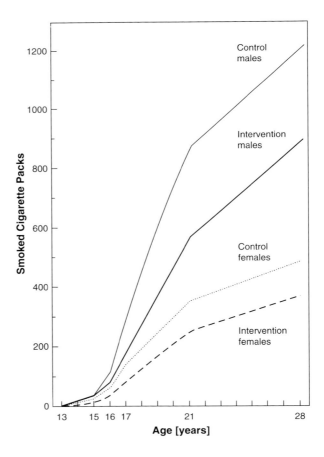

Fig. 12.3 Cumulative lifetime cigarette smoking, in packs, among male and female students in the intervention and control schools in the North Karelia Youth Project [72]. A total of 640 subjects (71% of the original cohort) participated in the final survey. Analyses of variance: school group, $p = 0.027$; sex, $p = 0.000$; school and sex interaction, $p = 0.28$

Table 12.3   Results of the Hutchinson smoker prevention programme

	Girls	Boys
Control classes ($n = 20$)	24.7% (0–41.9%)	26.7% (14.2–46.3%)
"Treated" classes ($n = 20$)	24.4% (15.5–34.2%)	26.3% (10.3–41.7%)
Difference	0.25% ($p = 0.91$)	0.33% ($p = 0.89$)

Smoking prevalence among adolescents at the end of the study [73]

control group ($p = 0.017$) when missing data points were ignored. The preventive effect measured in terms of lifetime tobacco consumption was slightly more pronounced among men than women (cf. Fig. 12.3). Men tended to smoke more heavily than women [72]. Between the ages of 13 and 28 years, the smokers in the intervention group smoked 5,500 fewer cigarettes than those in the control group. According to this study, long-term smoking prevention effects can be achieved by a prolonged but expensive social influence model in combination with community and mass media interventions [72].

The third recently published long-term study [73] reveals less optimistic results for school programmes of this type. The Hutchinson Smoking Prevention Project included 8,388 students from school years 3–12 who were mentored through a training programme with a total duration of 2,805 min, corresponding to 225–435 min per academic year. In total, 640 teachers from 72 schools were available. The social influences programme included discussions, media activities (TV, videos), social resistance skills, avoiding the temptation trap, as well as the accurate interpretation of social norms and the development of self-confidence. The smoker status of the students was verified by cotinine determinations in saliva or urine. As shown by the results at the end of the study, summarised in Table 12.3, the effect on the adolescents over several years in terms of smoking cessation was not successful when the results were compared with those in a parallel control group. Smoking prevalence at the study end was the same in all groups regardless of gender. This result gives pause for thought because exogenous factors evidently determine smoking behaviour more strongly than short-, medium- or long-term educational or training programmes [73].

12.8
Role of Teachers in Primary Prevention

Compared with other EU countries, smoking laws in Germany are very liberal [74]. The rules for students and teachers concerning smoking on school grounds are widely discrepant [75]. Smoking outside the classroom is hardly monitored at all. Infringement of the rules by students does not trigger disciplinary measures in all cases. In this respect, verbal instruction to students is provided in the minority of schools, but this has become a focal point of interest in individual schools, thanks to campaigns such as "Be smart – don't start". One major barrier to implementing school rules about tobacco use is the inclusion of tobacco consumption by the teaching staff [76]. Regulations on smoking in schools vary widely for teachers and students, as well as for students in different year groups. Teachers are permitted to smoke in almost every school and also believe that this does not influence their students' behaviour. Inconsistency such as this in any single institution can only have a negative effect on the credibility of tobacco-use prevention in the school and may even condemn such programmes to failure [74, 77]. Ultimately, teachers should act as role models for their students, and therefore tobacco consumption by teachers inevitably becomes a key determinant of student behaviour [78]. Many students report that their teachers smoke and this provides them with an alibi for their own smoking behaviour.

12.9
Prevention by Restricting Sales of Tobacco Products to Minors

In addition to health education for students, another possibility of delaying smoking initiation among minors is the statutory regulation of cigarette sales to young people below the age of 16 years by the enforcement of youth-protection legislation. Campaigns using posters (such as those depicted in Figs. 12.4 and 12.5) can also be effective in a school setting. At the same time, the numerous cigarette vending machines sited close to schools should be removed and, in conjunction with new legislation, retailers should be "educated" to recognise that the sale of cigarettes to children and adolescents (<16 years of age) is both illegal and immoral. Such action could ultimately bring about changes in adolescent smoking behaviour. Studies examining this issue have been reviewed in the USA [79]. In connection with the sale of tobacco products, the US studies showed that three questions were important: (1) whether, in response to appropriate interventions, retailers comply with the request no longer to sell cigarettes to adolescents; (2) whether adolescents quit cigarette smoking or at least cut down to some extent; and (3) whether such interventions produce a decline in smoking prevalence among adolescents.

Overall, attempts to influence retailers by verbally advising them of the legal situation have been minimally effective [80, 81]. Availability from other sources may be a decisive factor, as demonstrated by a study in 700 communities in Massachusetts [81]. More favourable results were only achieved when the interventions included personal visits to the retailers and mobilisation of assistance from the community [82]. Only a permanent warning to retailers was found to be effective, and efficacy was reduced when 4–6 checks/year were made [83]. Penalties have an important part to play where violations are found but these must be set at the right level because excessive leniency merely serves to harden retailers to the issue. The threatened withdrawal of tobacco sales licences would carry more weight if retailer compliance were to be monitored continually [84]. Where legal circumstances permit, a graduated system of warnings and fines through to licence withdrawal would be effective. Similarly, a warning system with graduated fines targeted at smoking adolescents in Woodridge was highly effective but did not meet with very wide acceptance [85]. The sanctions directed at offending tobacco retailers only hit home where a uniform policy existed in the states surrounding Woodridge [86]. Likewise, adolescent lockout devices on cigarette vending machines, such as are currently also being tested in Germany, have been less effective than removal of the vending machines altogether [87].

Fig. 12.4 Anti-smoking poster: "That's real strength" (DHM 1995-668)

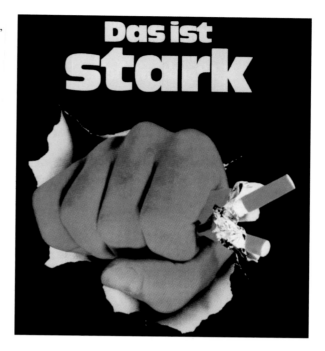

One major methodological problem is that retailers' attitudes to selling cigarettes to minors cannot be revealed even by undercover checks. Retailers recognise undercover purchasers because they behave unusually and tend to be are slightly older. In cases of doubt, they claim to sell cigarettes only to children who are known to them; alternatively, they argue that children ask grown-ups to buy the cigarettes for them [88]. The campaigns conducted to date reduce smoking behaviour among children by restricting youth access to cigarettes.

A fall in the sales of tobacco products to minors must necessarily also be reflected in a fall in sales figures. Trends such as these have been demonstrated in some communities. The study conducted in Woodridge confirms this trend when the policy is applied consistently. Also, according to data from Massachusetts, it is clear that a high inhibitory threshold has to be established in order to achieve a measurable reduction in tobacco consumption among children. The density of the retail network is also an important factor in these considerations. In the USA, despite the enactment of the Synar Amendment by Congress in 1992, not all individual states (90% so far) have yet passed appropriate legislation prohibiting the sale of tobacco products to minors [89]. Similar problems exist in the developing countries because, over and beyond the differently structured social situations, it is essential to protect children from the sale of tobacco products.

If the youth initiation rate could be reduced or completely eliminated, smoker numbers would be clearly reduced after 20–40 years [90]. According to one simulation model, if initiation among 18-year-olds had been reduced by 50% starting in 1993, the smoking rate would have fallen from 19% (48.1 million smokers) to 16.4% (44.1 million smokers) 10 years later in 2003 (Fig. 12.6), and this would have been only 3.7 million smokers fewer

Fig. 12.5 Anti-smoking poster: "Cancer is not a disease of old age" and "Cancer can strike anyone" (Chiron-Behring 8A.6.99)

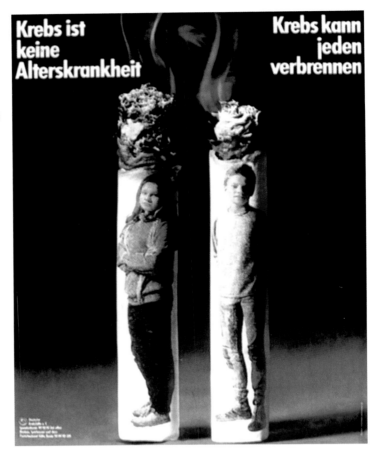

than without any policy to reduce initiation. Effective reductions in smoking prevalence would only have become apparent 20–30 years later [90]. In order to halve the number of smokers in the general population within 30 years, initiation would have to be eliminated completely, causing the smoking rate to fall from 19% (48.1 million smokers in 1993) to about 9% (25.9 million smokers in 2023) (Fig. 12.6) [90].

12.10
Role of the Mass Media in Sales of Tobacco Products to Adolescents

The mass media (TV, newspapers, radio, posters) have been recruited increasingly to deliver preventive health warnings (Fig. 12.7), particularly since they can be used to reach a high proportion of the population [91]. Children and adolescents in the USA spend twice as much time on watching TV as on their school education [92], with the result that by the age of 18 an adolescent has spent more time exposed to the media (TV) than on any other

Fig. 12.6 Effect of initiation policies on the number of smokers in the United States within 50 years. (**a**) Status quo; (**b**) 50% reduction; (**c**) 100% reduction; (**d**) 100% reduction plus 25% delayed initiation [90]

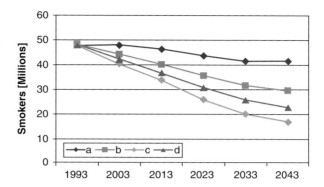

activity apart from sleeping [93]. The TV is therefore be a useful means of influencing children and adolescents with regard to acceptable social behaviour, cultural norms, issues of daily living and health-related matters [94]. In fact, several mass media campaigns have been run in the past in attempts to influence smoking behaviour among young people [95]. Specific programmes have been used for some schools [34, 79, 96, 97]. Information programmes prepared specifically for the mass media have been very much less common [98, 99], although such campaigns can actually lead to a (transient) reduction in smoking prevalence (see also Fig. 12.7) [98].

An analysis recently published by the Cochrane Group [100] warns that the results of different campaigns cannot be evaluated from a single viewpoint because the baseline situation in one study is not necessarily comparable with that in another study or campaign. Generalisation of the information obtained is complicated by a wide range of individual factors arising out of the characteristics of a community and the location of the particular school [101]. Similarly, according to a meta-analysis of other school-based prevention programmes only 16% (21 out of 131 studies) analysed their data on a statistically sound basis [102], the common failing being that changes in the control group were not consistently included in the analysis. Furthermore, the level of impartiality of the media agencies or periodicals was not always clearly defined.

According to one analysis from the USA of the impact of magazine articles on health education topics over the period from 1950 to 1983, it is clear that print media may in fact influence the initiation rate in the general population [25]. The number of educational articles on the harmful effects of smoking correlated with smoking cessation in adults but not with smoking initiation in adolescents because this latter group was not the target readership for these magazines, and greater emphasis on this aspect needs to be made in future [25]. Without doubt, broad-based PR campaigns of this type are appropriate instruments for educational purposes in those countries with a high smoking prevalence, e.g. Southern and Southeastern Europe.

According to the analysis published by the Cochrane Group [100] on the influence of mass media interventions on smoking behaviour among young people, six mass media campaigns were suitable for preventing smoking initiation in this target population, and two of these six media interventions also caused a reduction in smoking prevalence among adolescents [103–105]. Overall, efficacy has been assessed as only moderately positive to date.

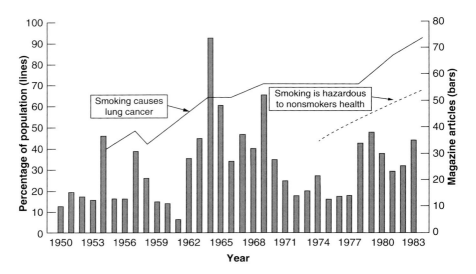

Fig. 12.7 Population beliefs on the harmfulness of smoking (left axis), and annual number of articles on smoking and health indexed in *The Reader's Guide to periodica l Literature* (right axis) [25]. In the early 1950s, there were less than 20 magazine articles on smoking and health each year. The highest peak in magazine coverage was 75 articles, which occurred surrounding the release of the 1964 Surgeon General's report. The percentage of the population believing that smoking is hazardous to non-smoker's health was below 50% in 1974, but had approached 70% by the early 1980s

In summary, media campaigns to encourage smoking cessation and discourage smoking initiation can be useful and effective provided that they are not influenced by the tobacco industry. However, the campaigns must utilise previously validated material and the programmes themselves must be designed specifically to include children as the target audience. Wherever possible, programmes should be screened on children's TV channels at the right time of day and they should be of an appropriate duration to ensure acceptance by children.

12.11
Role of Government and Community in Primary Prevention

Central government is hardly involved in the regulation of cigarette sales in the various countries within and outside Europe, not even when the issue at stake is the protection of young people from the hazards of smoking. One exception is the UK government with its "Smoking kills" campaign that has been running now for 10 years [106]: £100 million has been allocated to achieve three main goals within the next 3 years. One of these goals is to reduce smoking among adolescents (<16-years old) from 13 to 9% or less by the year 2010, with a fall to 11% by the year 2005. This is linked to a bundle of measures, such as minimal tobacco advertising in shops, tough enforcement on under-age sales, proof-of-age cards, and strong rules on the siting of cigarette vending machines. "We want children to be able go into shops without being faced with tobacco adverts or promotional materials" [106]. To ensure the achievement of these goals, the White Paper describes detailed measures that are to be implemented by central and local governments.

Since tobacco consumption is a socially determined phenomenon, changes in the social environment and social norms could become important [107]. It is entirely conceivable that a change in norms, values and behavioural patterns would increasingly discredit tobacco consumption, and that this would then be further mirrored in the social environment. This objective can be assisted by charitable organisations in many countries dedicated to the struggle for a smoke-free environment – a goal that would also include schools. School curriculum-based smoking prevention programmes might well prove highly effective [108] and local communities should help to create a positive non-smoker image [109]. A combined school- and community-based tobacco-use prevention programme clearly has the potential to reduce smoking initiation rates, as demonstrated by studies in 28-year-old non-smokers [72]. Analysis of the data by the Cochrane Group also indicates a positive result [110].

A restriction on the sale of tobacco products to minors is an important aspect of prevention. Sales to minors must be reduced in accordance with the following stipulated recommendations of the WHO: (a) minimum age 18 years, (b) licence system for tobacco retailers, (c) threat of penalties for illegal sale of tobacco goods, through to revocation of licence, (d) statutory prohibition on sales to minors, (e) no sales in health service buildings, schools or sports facilities and (f) no sales from cigarette vending machines or self-service stores [34, 111].

12.12
Concluding Remarks

- The issues surrounding primary tobacco-use prevention programmes designed to deter students from smoking in their youth need to be revisited. Children try tobacco just as they try alcohol or illicit drugs. Even though it may sound surprising, these facts cannot be altered overnight because adolescents typically want to discover what the world has to offer. Consequently, this experimentation phase can only be suppressed.
- Attempts to limit tobacco consumption by using school-based programmes, mass media campaigns or restrictions on tobacco sales to minors have been effective principally in the context of research studies. However, some of the studies conducted to date are highly complex and would be impractical in a real-life setting. The ease with which minors can obtain illicit drugs demonstrates the futility of seeking to prevent the supply of these substances. The only possible guarantee of success might be through the worldwide coordination of such efforts [97].
- Advertising encourages smoking initiation and sustains smoking (see Chap. 13), whereas advertising bans reduce the number of smokers, although the factors involved in smoking behaviour are very difficult to identify individually. The burden of proof for the effectiveness of advertising bans, however, lies with public health authorities.

- Moreover, in view of the hazardous nature of tobacco, society should accept no advertising or promotion by the tobacco industry until the absolute safety of tobacco has been confirmed beyond doubt – something that is inherently impossible. Since comprehensive advertising bans cannot currently be implemented, price increases and media campaigns should be launched to further publicise the harmful effects of smoking. In particular, heavy price rises for cigarettes in conjunction with other financial disincentives could be a key to prevention.
- The tobacco-use prevention programmes presented in this chapter are useful and effective in small groups or settings but, because they are costly in terms of time and personnel, they would be difficult to implement in a large country such as Germany, for example. Moreover, cigarette smuggling should be mentioned in this context because the cigarette companies can also earn revenue by this route. Harsh penalties should be imposed on the tobacco industry when these illegal transactions are detected. The revenue thus earned could also be funnelled back into prevention programmes, as has happened in the UK [112]. Overall, effective primary prevention will only result: (1) if a general ban is placed on advertising for tobacco products; (2) if tobacco products can only be obtained in specialist tobacco retail outlets; and (3) if sales are only made to persons over the age of 18 years, backed up by tough legislation to protect young people.
- With any tobacco-use prevention programme, it should always be remembered that it will take decades before success becomes effective and apparent in terms of a dramatic reduction in the number of smokers (Fig. 12.6).

References

1. Kessler DA, Natanblut SL, Wilkenfeld JP, Lorraine CC, Mayl SL, Bernstein IB, et al (1997) Nicotine addiction: a pediatric disease. J Pediatr 130(4):518–524
2. Delener N (1995) Assessing cigarette smoking motives of young adolescents in the US: research and health perspectives. J Smoking Relat Disord 6:81–88
3. Walters R, Whent H, Sayers M, Morgan A, Sinkler P (1996) Health update. Smoking. Health Education Authority, London
4. Health Education Authority (1997) Tobacco control in England: communication strategies of the Health Education Authority. The Health Education Authority, London
5. Oei TP, Fae A, Silva P (1990) Smoking behavior in nine year old children: a replication and extension study. Adv Alcohol Subst Abuse 8(3–4):85–96
6. Reed DO (1993) Preventing adolescent nicotine addiction: what can one do? J Amer Acad Phys Assist 6:703–710
7. Pierce JP, Gilpin EA (1995) A historical analysis of tobacco marketing and the uptake of smoking by youth in the United States: 1890–1977. Health Psychol 14(6):500–508
8. Pierce JP, Lee L, Gilpin EA (1994) Smoking initiation by adolescent girls, 1944 through 1988. An association with targeted advertising. JAMA 271(8):608–611
9. Gilpin EA, Pierce JP (1997) Trends in adolescent smoking initiation in the United States: is tobacco marketing an influence? Tob Control 6(2):122–127

10. Bundeszentrale für gesundheitliche Aufklärung. Die Drogenaffinität Jugendlicher in-der Bundesrepublik Deutschland (1998) Eine Wiederholungsbefragung der BzgA Köln. Endbericht, Köln

11. Hurrelmann K (1998) Tabakprävention und Tabakentwöhnung bei Kindern. Sucht 44:4–14

12. Chrapa M (2001) Moderne Drogen- und Suchtprävention (MODRUS II): Soziologisch-empirische Studie der Forschungsgemeinschaft für Konflikt- und Sozialstudien e.V. (FOKUS). Ministerium für Arbeit FGuSdLS-A (ed). Magdeburg, pp 1–96

13. O'Loughlin J, Paradis G, Renaud L, Sanchez GL (1998) One-year predictors of smoking initiation and of continued smoking among elementary schoolchildren in multiethnic, low-income, inner-city neighbourhoods. Tob Control 7(3):268–275

14. King A, Wold B, Tudor-Smith C, Harel Y (1996) The health of youth: a cross-national survey. WHO Reg Publ Eur Ser 69:1–222

15. Tudor-Smith C, Roberts C, Kingdon A (1999) Die Prävalenz von Alkohol- und Tabakkonsum im Jugendalter: Internationale Perspektiven. In: Kolip P (ed) Programme gegen Sucht: Internationale Ansätze zur Suchtprävention im Jugendalter. Juventa, Weinheim

16. Galanti MR, Rosendahl I, Post A, Gilljam H (2001) Early gender differences in adolescent tobacco use – the experience of a Swedish cohort. Scand J Public Health 29(4):314–317

17. Botvin GJ, Griffin KW, Diaz T, Miller N, Ifill-Williams M (1999) Smoking initiation and escalation in early adolescent girls: one-year follow-up of a school-based prevention intervention for minority youth. J Am Med Womens Assoc 54:139–143

18. Peters J, Hedley AJ, Lam TH, Betson CL, Wong CM (1997) A comprehensive study of smoking in primary school children in Hong Kong: implications for prevention. J Epidemiol Community Health 51(3):239–245

19. Zhu BP, Liu M, Shelton D, Liu S, Giovino GA (1996) Cigarette smoking and its risk factors among elementary school students in Beijing. Am J Public Health 86:368–375

20. Bölcskei PL, Hörmann A, Hollederer A, Jordan S, Fenzel H (1997) Suchtprävention an Schulen – Besondere Aspekte des Nikotinabusus. Prävention-Rehabilitation 9:82–88

21. Alexander CS, Allen P, Crawford MA, McCormick LK (1999) Taking a first puff: cigarette smoking experiences among ethnically diverse adolescents. Ethn Health 4:245–257

22. Hurrelmann K, Bründel H (1997) Drogengebrauch und Drogenmißbrauch. Darmstadt: Wissenschaftliche Buchgesellschaft

23. Khuder SA, Dayal HH, Mutgi AB (1999) Age at smoking onset and its effect on smoking cessation. Addict Behav 24:673–677

24. McCool JP, Cameron LD, Petrie KJ (2001) Adolescent perceptions of smoking imagery in film. Soc Sci Med 52(10):1577–1587

25. Pierce JP, Gilpin EA (2001) News media coverage of smoking and health is associated with changes in population rates of smoking cessation but not initiation. Tob Control 10(2): 145–153

26. Sargent JD, Beach ML, Dalton MA, Mott LA, Tickle JJ, Ahrens MB, et al (2001) Effect of seeing tobacco use in films on trying smoking among adolescents: cross sectional study. BMJ 323(7326):1394–1397

27. Hurrelmann K, Hesse S (1991) Wie ist Suchtprävention möglich? Psychomed 4:251–258

28. Conrad KM, Flay BR, Hill D (1992) Why children start smoking cigarettes: predictors of onset. Br J Addict 87(12):1711–1724.

29. Paavola M, Vartiainen E, Puska P (1996) Predicting adult smoking: the influence of smoking during adolescence and smoking among friends and family. Health Educat Res 11:309–315

30. Ellickson PL, McGuigan KA, Klein DJ (2001) Predictors of late-onset smoking and cessation over 10 years. J Adolesc Health 29(2):101–108

31. Patton GC, Carlin JB, Coffey C, Wolfe R, Hibbert M, Bowes G (1998) The course of early smoking: a population-based cohort study over three years. Addiction 93:1251–1260

32. Chassin L, Presson CC, Rose JS, Sherman SJ (1996) The natural history of cigarette smoking from adolescence to adulthood: demographic predictors of continuity and change. Health Psychol 15(6):478–484

33. Stanton WR, McClelland M, Elwood C, Ferry D, Silva PA (1996) Prevalence, reliability and bias of adolescents' reports of smoking and quitting. Addiction 91:1705–1714

34. US Department of Health and Human Services (1994) Preventing tobacco use among young people: A report of the Surgeon General. Georgia, Atlanta

35. Gulotta TP (1994) The what, who, why, where, when, and how of primary prevention. J Prim Prevent 15:5–14

36. Durlak JA (1995) School-based prevention programs for children and adolescents. Developmental clinical psychology and psychiatry. Sage, Tousands Oaks, CA

37. Durlak JA (1997) Successful prevention programs for schildren and adolescents. Plenum, New York

38. Kolip P (1995) Prävalenz des Zigarettenkonsums und Image des Rauchens im Jugendalter: Alters- und geschlechtsspezifische Aspekte. Sucht 41:323–333

39. Forster I, Schwenkmezger P, Krönig B (1997) Zigarettenkonsum bei Kindern und Jugendlichen: Entstehungsbedingungen und schulische Präventionsansätze. Prävent Rehabilitat 9:62–70

40. Schwenkmezger P, Krönig B, Forster I, Jähren B, Gläßer E (1998) Personenspezifische und soziale Determinanten eines frühen Rauchbeginns bei Schülerinnen und Schülern der 6. Jahrgangsstufe. Zschr Gesundheitspsychol 6:61–70

41. Bowen DJ, Dahl K, Mann SL, Peterson AV (1991) Descriptions of early triers. Addict Behav 16(3–4):95–101

42. Schwenkmezger P, Krönig B, Gläßer E (1999) Prävention des Zigarettenrauchens: Erfahrungen und ausgewählte Ergebnisse zu personenspezifischen und sozialen Determinanten bei Schülerinnen und Schülern des 6. Schuljahres an Gymnasien, S. 80–87. In: Rauchen und Nikotin – Eine Kontroverse? Vorträge der 2. Nikotinkonferenz Dt, Haustein KO (eds) Perfusion GmbH, Nürnberg

43. Guidelines for School Health Programs to Prevent Tobacco Use and Addiction (1994) Morb Mort Wkly Rep 43(RR-2):1–19

44. Botvin GJ, Renick NL, Baker E (1983) The effects of scheduling format and booster sessions on a broad-spectrum psychosocial approach to smoking prevention. J Behav Med 6:359–379

45. Botvin GJ, Baker E, Dusenbury L, Tortu S, Botvin EM (1990) Preventing adolescent drug abuse through a multimodal cognitive-behavioral approach: results of a 3-year study. J Consult Clin Psychol 58:437–446

46. Hansen WB, Graham JW (1991) Preventing alcohol, marijuana, and cigarette use among adolescents: peer pressure resistance training versus establishing conservative norms. Prev Med 20:414–430

47. Perry CL, Telch MJ, Killen J, Burke A, Maccoby N (1983) High school smoking prevention: the relative efficacy of varied treatments and instructors. Adolescence 18:561–566

48. Clarke JH, MacPherson B, Holmes DR, Jones R (1986) Reducing adolescent smoking: a comparison of peer-led, teacher-led, and expert interventions. J Sch Health 56:102–106

49. Perry CL, Pirie P, Holder W, Halper A, Dudovitz B (1990) Parent involvement in cigarette smoking prevention: two pilot evaluations of the "Unpuffables Program". J Sch Health 60:443–447

50. Biglan A, Glasgow R, Ary D, Thompson R, Severson H, Lichtenstein E, et al (1987) How generalizable are the effects of smoking prevention programs? Refusal skills training and parent messages in a teacher-administered program. J Behav Med 10:613–628

51. Brink SG, Simons-Morton DG, Harvey CM, Parcel GS, Tiernan KM (1988) Developing comprehensive smoking control programs in schools. J Sch Health 58:177–180

52. St Pierre RW, Shute RE, Jaycox S (1983) Youth helping youth: a behavioral approach to the self-control of smoking. Health Educ 14:28–31

53. Perry C, Killen J, Telch M, Slinkard LA, Danaher BG (1980) Modifying smoking behavior of teenagers: a school-based intervention. Am J Public Health 70:722–725

54. Masse LC, Tremblay RE (1997) Behavior of boys in kindergarten and the onset of substance use during adolescence. Arch Gen Psychiatry 54(1):62–68

55. Milberger S, Biederman J, Faraone SV, Chen L, Jones J (1997) ADHD is associated with early initiation of cigarette smoking in children and adolescents. J Am Acad Child Adolesc Psychiatry 36(1):37–44

56. Morabia A, Costanza MC, Bernstein MS, Rielle JC (2002) Ages at initiation of cigarette smoking and quit attempts among women: a generation effect. Am J Public Health 92(1):71–74

57. Faucher MA, Carter S (2001) Why girls smoke: a proposed community-based prevention program. J Obstet Gynecol Neonatal Nurs 30(5):463–471

58. Petermann H, Müller H, Kersch B, Röhr M (1997) Erwachsen werden ohne Drogen: Ergebnisse schulischer Drogenprävention. Juventa. Weinheim

59. Evans RI, Rozelle RM, Maxwell SE, Raines BE, Dill CA, Guthrie TJ, et al (1981) Social modelling film to deter smoking in adolescents: Results of a three-year field investigation. J Appl Psychol 66:399–414

60. Botvin GJ, Baker E, Dusenbury L, Botvin EM, Diaz T (1995) Long-term follow-up results of a randomized drug abuse prevention trial in a white middle-class population. JAMA 273(14): 1106–1112

61. Botvin GJ, Tortu S (1988) Preventing adolescent substance abuse trough life skills training. In: Proce RH, Cowen EL, Lorion RP, McKay JR (eds) 14 ounces of prevention. A casebook for practitioners. American Physiological Association, Washington, pp 98–110

62. Bruvold WH (1993) A meta-analysis of adolescent smoking prevention programs. Am J Public Health 83(6):872–880

63. Hansen WB (1992) School-based substance abuse prevention: a review of the state of the art in curriculum, 1980–1990. Health Educ Res 7(3):403–430

64. Tobler NC (1986) Meta-analysis of 143 adolescent drug prevention programs: quantitative outcome results of program participants compared to a control comparsion group. J Drug Issues 16:537–567

65. Asshauer M, Hahnewinkel R (1999) Lebenskompetenzförderung und Suchtprophylaxe in der Grundschule: Entwicklung, Implementierung und Evaluation primär-präventiver Unterrichtseinheiten. Zschr Gesundheitspsychol 7:158–171

66. Dupree T, Bölcskei PL (1998) Gesund ins Erwachsenenalter am Beispiel des schulischen Gesundheitsförderungsprogramms Klasse 2000. S. 69–73. Rauchen und Nikotin – Aktuelle Beiträge zur Raucherentwöhnung. In: Haustein KO (ed) Perfusion GmbH, Nürnberg

67. Philip and Morris (1997, Aug 23) Frankf Allg Ztg

68. Krönig B, Schwenkmezger P, Forster I (1997) Rauchen: Gesundheitsrisiko Nr. 1: Notwendige Prävention im Schulalter. Prävention und Rehablitation 9:48–56

69. Schwenkmezger P, Krönig B, Forster I, Jähren B, Gläßer E (1998) Erfahrungen mit einem Programm zur Prävention des Zigarettenrauchens bei Schülerinnen und Schülern der 6. Jahrgangsstufe in Gymnasien. Zschr Gesundheitspsychol 6:85–89

70. Fuchs R, Schwarzer R (1997) Tabakkonsum: Erklärungsmodelle und Interventionsansätze. In: Schwarzer R (ed) Gesundheitspsychologie. Göttingen, Hofgrefe pp 209–244

71. Silbereisen RK, Noak P, Eyferth K (1986) Places for development: adolescents, leisure settings, and developmental tasks. In: Silbereisen et al (ed) Development as action in context. Springer, Berlin

72. Vartiainen E, Paavola M, McAlister A, Puska P (1998) Fifteen-year follow-up of smoking prevention effects in the North Karelia youth project. Am J Public Health 88:81–85

73. Peterson AV Jr, Kealey KA, Mann SL, Marek PM, Sarason IG (2000) Hutchinson Smoking Prevention Project: long-term randomized trial in school-based tobacco use prevention – results on smoking. J Natl Cancer Inst 92(24):1979–1991

74. Bowen DJ, Kinne S, Orlandi M (1995) School policy in COMMIT: a promising strategy to reduce smoking by youth. J Sch Health 65:140–144

75. Denman S (1999) Health promoting schools in England – a way forward in development. J-Public Health Med 21:215–220
76. Hartland J, Tudor-Smith C, Bowker S (1998) Smoke-free policies in schools: a qualitative investigation of the benefits and barriers. Health Educ J 57:51–59
77. Smith C, Nutbeam D, Moore L, Roberts C, Catford J (1994) Current changes in smoking attitudes and behaviours among adolescents in Wales, 1986–1992. J Public Health Med 16:165–171
78. Wold B, Holstein B, Griesbach D, Currie C (2000) Control of adolescent smoking. National policies on restriction of smoking at school in eight European countries. EC BIOMED II (ed) Child & Adolescent Health Research Unit, University of Edinburgh, Edinburgh
79. Stead LF, Lancaster T (2000) Interventions for preventing tobacco sales to minors. Cochrane Database Syst Rev 2:CD001497
80. DiFranza JR, Savageau JA, Aisquith BF (1996) Youth access to tobacco: the effects of age, gender, vending machine locks, and it's the law programs. Am J Public Health 86(2):221–224
81. Siegel M, Biener L, Rigotti NA (1999) The effect of local tobacco sales laws on adolescent smoking initiation. Prev Med 29:334–342
82. Altman DG, Wheelis AY, McFarlane M, Lee H, Fortmann SP (1999) The relationship between tobacco access and use among adolescents: a four community study. Soc Sci Med 48(6): 759–775
83. Jason LA, Billows WD, Schnopp-Wyatt DL, King C (1996) Long-term findings from Woodridge in reducing illegal cigarette sales to older minors. Eval Health Prof 19(1):3–13
84. Chapman S, King M, Andrews B, McKay E, Markham P, Woodward S (1994) Effects of publicity and a warning letter on illegal cigarette sales to minors. Aust J Public Health 18(1):39–42
85. Mosher JF (1995) The merchants, not the customers: resisting the alcohol and tobacco industries' strategy to blame young people for illegal alcohol and tobacco sales. J Public Health Policy 16(4):412–432
86. Landrine H, Klonoff EA, Fritz JM (1994) Preventing cigarette sales to minors: the need for contextual, sociocultural analysis. Prev Med 23(3):322–327
87. Forster JL, Hourigan M, McGovern P (1992) Availability of cigarettes to underage youth in three communities. Prev Med 21(3):320–328
88. Rigotti NA, DiFranza JR, Chang Y, Tisdale T, Kemp B, Singer DE (1997) The effect of enforcing tobacco-sales laws on adolescents' access to tobacco and smoking behavior. N Engl J Med 337(15):1044–1051
89. DiFranza JR (1999) Are the federal and state governments complying with the Synar Amendment? Arch Pediatr Adolesc Med 153(10):1089–1097
90. Levy DT, Cummings KM, Hyland A (2000) A simulation of the effects of youth initiation policies on overall cigarette use. Am J Public Health 90(8):1311–1314
91. Redman S, Spencer EA, Sanson-Fisher RW (1990) The role of mass media in changing health-related behaviour: a critical appraisal of two models. Health Promot Int 5:85–101
92. Worden JK, Flynn BS, Solomon LJ, Secker-Walker RH, Badger GJ, Carpenter JH (1996) Using mass media to prevent cigarette smoking among adolescent girls. Health Educ Q 23:453–468
93. Davies J (1993) The impact of the mass media upon the health of early adolescents. J Health Educ 24:28–35
94. Strasburger VC (1995) Adolescents and the Media. Medical and Psychological Impact. Sage, London
95. Reid D (1996) Tobacco control: overview. Br Med Bull 52(1):108–120
96. Michell L (1994) Smoking prevention programmes for adolescents: a literatur review. Anglia and Oxford Regional Health authority (ed) Oxford
97. Reid DJ, McNeil AD, Glynn TJ (1995) Reducing the prevalence of smoking in youth in western countries: an international review. Tob Control 4:266–277

98. Flay BR (1987) Mass media and smoking cessation: a critical review. Am J Public Health 77(2):153–160

99. Flay BR (1987) Selling the smokeless society. Fifty-six evaluated mass media programmes and campaigns worldwide. American Public Health Association, Washington

100. Sowden AJ, Arblaster L (2000) Mass media interventions for preventing smoking in young people. Cochrane Database Syst Rev 2:CD001006

101. Bland JM, Kerry SM (1997) Statistics notes. Trials randomised in clusters. BMJ 315:600

102. Rooney BL, Murray DM (1996) A meta-analysis of smoking prevention programs after adjustment for errors in the unit of analysis. Health Educ Q 23(1):48–64

103. Flynn BS, Worden JK, Secker-Walker RH, Badger GJ, Geller BM (1995) Cigarette smoking prevention effects of mass media and school interventions targeted to gender and age groups. J Health Educat 26:45–51

104. Hafstad A (1997) Provocative anti-smoking appeals in mass media campaigns. An intervention study on adolescent smoking. Institute of General Practice and Community Medicine, Oslo

105. Hafstad A, Aaro LE (1997) Activating interpersonal influence through provocative appeals: evaluation of a mass media based antismoking campain targeting adolescents. Health Commun 9:253–272

106. Anonym (1999) Smoking kills. A white paper on tobacco. The Stationary Office

107. Schofield MJ, Redman S, Sanson-Fisher RW (1991) A community approach to smoking prevention: a review. Behav Change 8:17–25

108. Farquhar JW, Fortmann SP, Flora JA, Taylor CB, Haskell WL, Williams PT et al (1990) Effects of communitywide education on cardiovascular disease risk factors. The Stanford Five-City Project. JAMA 264:359–365

109. Flay BR (2000) Approaches to substance use prevention utilizing school curriculum plus social environment change. Addict Behav 25(6):861–885

110. Sowden A, Arblaster L (2000) Community interventions for preventing smoking in young people. Cochrane Database Syst Rev 2:CD001291

111. Illegal sales of cigarettes to minors (1999) Morb Mort Wkly Rep 48(19):394–398

112. Foulds J, Godfrey C (1995) Counting the costs of children's smoking. BMJ 311(7013):1152–1154

Tobacco Industry, Advertising and Advertising Bans

13

By 2020 the burden of disease due to tobacco is expected to outweigh that caused by any single disease. From its 1990 level of being responsible for 2.6% of all disease burden worldwide, tobacco is expected to increase its share to close to 10%.

G. Brundtland, World Economics Forum 1999

Over the past century, the tobacco industry has consistently been successful in advertising its products – a fact testified to ultimately by annual turnover figures of US $400 billion and annual profits of thousands of millions [1]. A slight dip in the normally stable share prices was recorded on 22 August 1997 when Geoffrey Bible, the CEO of Philip Morris, stated in a case for damages before a US court that he would halt cigarette production if a link could be proved between smoking and cancer [2]. The link is incontrovertible and yet cigarettes continue to be produced and aggressively advertised, even with apparently warning slogans [3]. It might be thought that the tobacco industry enjoys special favour with politicians in numerous countries [4].

The phenomenon of economic globalisation is a *fait accompli* in the tobacco industry and its globalised marketing and promotion of tobacco represents a threat to public health in all countries: in 1986, a total of 61% of the world's tobacco consumption was in developing countries, and by the year 2000, this figure had risen to 71% [1, 5]. By 2020, 70% of the expected 8.4 million deaths caused by tobacco will be in developing countries [6]. At present, since 70% of tobacco is grown in developing countries [5], tobacco control programmes need to be the highest priority.

If the world were a village of 1,000 people, it would include 584 Asians, 150 Europeans (of whom 55 would be from the former Soviet Republics), 124 Africans, 84-Latin Americans, 52 North Americans and 6 Australians and New Zealanders. In this 1,000-person village, 173 men and 56 women are smokers. Further, 115 of the smokers are Asian, 28 are European and 28 are African [1]. Of the 124 children in this model, 40% are exposed to environmental tobacco smoke (ETS) [7]. Of the 10 million tobacco-related deaths forecast to occur annually by 2,030, 70% will be in developing countries [7]!

In Germany, a total of DM 38.900 million was spent on smoking in 1998, representing an increase of DM 1.531 million (4.1%) over the previous year. Consumption of cigars/cigarillos and pipe tobacco plays a minor role [8]. Tobacco products are sold least commonly through specialist retail tobacconists. Instead, cigarette sales are generated predominantly in grocery stores (Fig. 13.1) [8]. In 1999, the German government received EUR 11.500 million in revenue from taxes on tobacco and this figure has increased steadily

K.-O. Haustein, D. Groneberg, *Tobacco or Health?*
DOI: 10.1007/978-3-540-87577-2_13, © Springer Verlag Berlin Heidelberg 2010

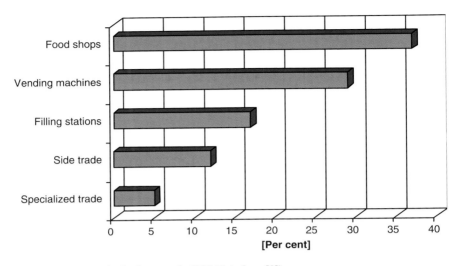

Fig. 13.1 Cigarette sales in Germany in 1998 (data from [8])

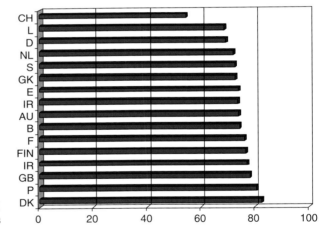

Fig. 13.2 Tax as a percentage of the retail price of cigarettes in different European countries [8]. Countries designated by international vehicle identification codes

year on year. The percentage tax share of the retail price is 69.4% in Germany and >80% in countries such as Portugal and Denmark [8]. Compared with Germany, most European Union (EU) countries impose higher taxes on tobacco (Fig. 13.2) [8].

13.1
Tobacco Advertising Strategies

The tobacco industry derives considerable advantage from its advertising campaigns for cigarettes (cinema and sporting events, sponsorship, poster campaigns, etc.; see Fig. 13.3), which help to recruit 10,000 new smokers across Europe every day. In June 1998, the EU

Fig. 13.3 Percentage breakdown of promotional expenditure by the tobacco industry in 1997: total expenditure DM 682 million. (*) Because of the advertising ban in these media, only diversification products (e.g. Camel footwear) were taken into account [8]

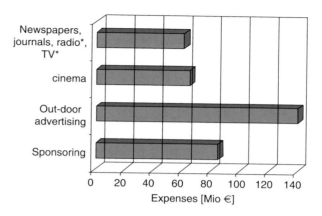

Council of Ministers issued a directive on the phased restriction of tobacco advertising and tobacco controls to prohibit promotional activities from mid-2001 onwards [9]. The directive foresees that, from 2006 onwards, tobacco advertising will only be permitted in tobacconist and kiosk outlets. It is incomprehensible that Germany, along with Austria, has done everything possible to evade this ban, alleging that it "violates the advertising industry's-freedom of speech and right to exercise its profession, and contravenes the ownership rights of the brand manufacturers." The largest sums of money are spent on outdoor advertising and sponsorship (Fig. 13.3) [8], whereas advertising spend in magazines and newspapers has seen a continuous decline over several years. In practical terms, tobacco advertising no longer plays a major role on the radio or in specialist periodicals, but continues to do so in popular magazines [8].

Increasingly, there are demands for the tobacco industry also to adopt manufacturer and product liability. There are initial signs that product liability experts are also being trained to monitor the tobacco industry and the prevailing climate of market manipulation [10].

The tobacco industry pursues several objectives in its cigarette advertising as follows:

- To encourage children and adolescents wherever possible to start smoking (and subsequently to become habitual smokers)
- To undermine smokers' motivation to quit smoking
- To encourage ex-smokers to take up the habit again
- To counteract declining sales [11, 12]

In addition, the tobacco industry wants to portray a positive image of smoking and enhance its social acceptability [11, 13].

The tobacco industry claims unjustifiably that all its advertising activities are targeted at adults and that its campaigns focus exclusively on "distribution battles" between different cigarette brands.

As illustrated in Fig. 13.4, which summarises the findings of a US group based on smoking initiation rates (calculated from the number of adolescents who started smoking regularly during a given year divided by the number of those at risk to start smoking in that year), the rise in cigarette consumption among adolescents is determined by major advertising

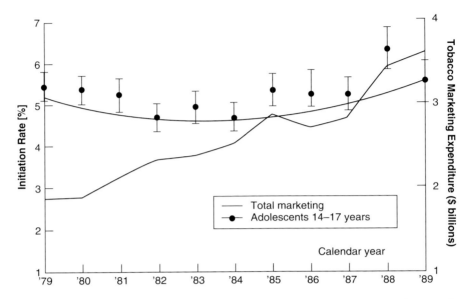

Fig. 13.4 Initiation rates (%) for adolescent smokers for the period 1979–1989, based on a study from the USA, in comparison with promotional expenditure by the tobacco industry, corrected for inflationary increases [14]

events. Overall, the initiation rate among adolescent girls correlates with the tobacco industry's advertising spend (Fig. 13.4) [14].

Direct promotion takes the form of advertisements, posters, promotional films, camouflaged advertising and Internet campaigns (such as the Philip Morris Wavenet campaign in Australia [15], which has tie-ins with dance events and nightly fashion shows for the relatively large number of registered Wave members), sales promotions and distribution of sample packs and sample cigarettes, for example, at political party meetings, many of which may be at least partly financed.

Indirect promotion (brand stretching) is evident in the appearance of cigarette brand names on other products, for instance, in the financial support provided for sports and music events and in the distribution of promotional items. In currency terms, Formula One motor racing alone swallows up 9-figure sums each year: a single grand prix event is expected to attract some 73,000 adolescents, of whom more than 9,000 will become cigarette smokers [16, 17]. The combined use of posters, cinema adverts (depicting scenes of outstanding natural beauty) and printed ads in a wide variety of magazines achieves long-term effects in future users. Furthermore, tobacco products in shops tend to be displayed in prominent positions [18]. All these activities serve to create a pro-tobacco industry attitude in politicians and the general public (see Chap. 14).

In the USA, expenditure on ads has fallen markedly since 1970s, whereas expenditure on added-value promotion (smokers purchasing a pack of cigarettes receive a second pack free or a credit voucher) has actually increased [19]. The following list summarises the principal changes in marketing forms used by the tobacco industry:

- Incentive payments to tobacco retailers [18]
- Promotional allowances in outlets in prime locations, where appropriate, using special display cabinets or stands at the point of sale [18, 20]
- Adverts in journals or daily newspapers and in cinema commercials or films with or without actors [21, 22]
- Adverts on free-standing hoardings (sometimes oversized; outdoor advertising)
- As transit system signs, financial support for sports events (Formula One motor racing; currently symbolised by Marlboro Man Michael Schumacher; sponsorship) [23]
- Using attractive model girls to distribute free sample packs either on the street at specially erected stands or, in Germany, for example, at political party meetings [10, 24–26]

In contrast with the energy and drive that characterise its advertising efforts, the tobacco industry does virtually nothing to educate people about the health hazards of continued smoking [9, 27, 28]. The industry has identified women as a prime target for its advertising: a study of 316 magazine-years has reported that women's magazines carrying cigarette advertisements have only a 5% probability of publishing an article educating their readers about the hazards of smoking [29]. The probability of smoking hazard coverage was still only 11.7% in magazines that did not carry cigarette advertisements [29].

Cigarette advertising with its large-format posters is targeted primarily at young, future smokers because older dependent smokers do not need advertising. According to comments from the R.J. Reynolds Tobacco Company: *"Kids don't pay attention to cigarette ads ... (our advertising) purpose is to get smokers of competitive products to switch ... (which is) virtually the only way a cigarette brand can meaningfully increase its business"* [30]. Even previously non-smoking groups have become preferred targets, for example, in Asia where women are starting to smoke after intensive promotion of exclusively female brands [31]. The industry does not engage in major price struggles that lead to redistribution among the various brands.

The cigarette industry does not appear to be encountering a saturated market because there is no evidence to indicate falling sales or reduced promotional expenditure [30, 32]. Advertising campaigns for cigarettes have never been directed against a fellow competitor or against a specific brand, signs that would be indicative of attempts to capture a market segment [33]. In this context, it should be recalled that the cigarette market is dominated by a small number of companies across the world, who appear to have reached agreement among themselves [33].

The compulsive need to advertise is the result of several processes as follows:

- Smokers quit the habit daily, either because they simply decide to stop or out of necessity on health grounds
- Smokers die (1,096 people/day in the USA and 309 people/day in Germany)
- New smokers have to be recruited [34] and these are to be found only among (under-age) adolescents (in Germany, about 1 million annually) [33]

In Germany, approximately 75 million EUR was spent on cigarette advertising in 1996 [35]. In the USA, the tobacco industry has spent US $6,000 million on advertising and promotion. Sums such as these are not spent if no new smokers are to be recruited. According to estimates from 1987, the aggregate profitability of brand switching was approximately US $382 million, i.e. 16% of the total promotional spend [36]. Smokers remain loyal to the same cigarette brand for years or merely switch from a stronger to a milder type of the same brand [36], so there is no reason to assume changes in the market. Fewer than 10% of smokers in the USA switch cigarette brands; moreover, since these tend to be older smokers and are beginning to report health problems, they hold little attraction in market terms. By contrast, the tobacco industry's priority is to recruit adolescents, who are just embarking on their smoking career, to make them dependent smokers who will show loyalty to the brand [30, 37]. According to internal memos from the cigarette industry: *"Young smokers represent the major opportunity group for the cigarette industry"* and *"If the last 10 years have taught us anything, it is that the industry is dominated by the companies who respond most effectively to needs of younger smokers"* [38].

The tobacco industry is extremely interested in getting its message through to adolescent consumers by siting billboards near their schools (and, if possible, by combining these with cigarette vending machines) [32, 38–40]; this is equally true in the USA, Germany and the developing countries. Radio and TV commercials in the USA are scheduled to run at times that are particularly popular with adolescents [41]; fortunately, this is not permitted in Germany [42]. Over the past 2 or 3 decades, the developing countries have become the target for the tobacco industry's promotional endeavours [43].

The cigarette industry also manufactures "youth-oriented" cigarette brands (starter brands), e.g. by including a high cocoa content (see Table 3.7) or by producing strawberry-flavoured cigarettes [44] that are certain to encourage smoking initiation [25]. In this context, mention may also be made of the popularity with young people of the Old Joe Camel ads, based on RJR Nabisco's new, specially created cartoon character [13, 45]. A smoker who is already conditioned to the habit no longer needs such advertising.

13.2
Advertising Messages

It has been found consistently that advertising messages are particularly effective when they have a visual impact within a few seconds and are consistent with the addressee's own thinking. This avoids any internal conflict with the message that might perhaps give rise to doubts. Advertising messages such as these may be directed at individuals as well as groups (peers) [11, 46, 47].

Adolescents are addressed by the following themes in advertising messages [13]:

- Independence, self-confidence, social acceptance, freedom from pressure: all these are typified by the Marlboro Man [33] and this applies equally for adolescents of either sex.
- Ritual: Smoking is depicted by the cigarette industry itself as a mark of adulthood; as such, it is associated with pleasure and with the opportunity to imitate adults [33, 38, 48] and the youthful-looking Marlboro Cowboy is often used to portray this.
- Normal behaviour: In its advertising messages, the tobacco industry links smoking with everyday living, generating the impression of something entirely normal when people smoke in familiar surroundings, e.g. drinking coffee after a work shift (a kind of self-reward).

As an ingrained activity, the combination of coffee and cigarette, in particular, is often the hardest to check in smokers who want to quit.

- Social interaction: When two or more people smoke at the same time, this makes it easier for them to socialise because the cigarette helps to create a shared identity (this situation can be compared with dog-walkers in the park who fall into conversation much more easily by means of this "vehicle" than people who are simply out walking). Adolescents find this situation pleasant because they then belong and are accepted.
- Health: While the tobacco industry cannot begin to claim that smoking is healthy in any way, it manages to create the illusion of positive associations in that cigarette ads employ actors who are young, dynamic, glowing with health and shown smoking in wonderful, visually stunning locations. The intention is to depict smoking as relatively harmless. In addition, the cigarettes are glamorised using epithets such as "mild", "light", "pure", "natural" and "fresh" (possibly with added menthol).

Many psychologists have developed theoretical models on the effectiveness of advertising in encouraging smoking initiation: problems of communication theory naturally arise in this area and these can be used to develop a deeper understanding of the reception and intellectual processing of advertising messages. The key stages are stimulus reception, stimulus processing and production of a resultant action [49].

Conversely, anti-smoking TV campaigns can achieve a marked decline in the number of smokers if they continue to be broadcast over a prolonged period (e.g. for 18 months). A series of interviews was conducted in 2,997 smokers and 2,471 ex-smokers before the intervention: after the campaign started, interviews were conducted again in 3,610 and 2,381 subjects after 6 and 18 months, respectively [50]. At study end, 9.8% of smokers had stopped smoking and only 4.3% of ex-smokers had relapsed. Applying these results to a typical control population suggests that the 12-month campaign would lead to a 1.2%-reduction in smoking prevalence [50]. Consideration is, therefore, being given in the UK to organising anti-smoking TV campaigns of this kind more frequently.

13.3
Effect of Tobacco Industry Advertising Messages

In Germany, people are exposed on all sides to tobacco industry advertising messages. Given the ubiquitous presence of these ads, many people believe that cigarette should be regarded as an essential part of common culture and that the possible harmful effects on health are exaggerated [33]. Children, in particular, are unprotected in their exposure to cigarette advertising, with the result that children and adolescents in our society experiment with cigarettes, the intensity of advertising allegedly correlating with the frequency of experimentation [51]. Figures 2.6, 2.7, 6.3 and 12.6 demonstrate the long-term effects of 20–40 years of smoking, after which the harmful effects on health can also be demonstrated epidemiologically. Nevertheless, in the future, it will still be difficult to establish reliable correlations between advertising and smoking. In particular, children and adolescents are very much more familiar with advertising messages than adults [52] who simply let many advertising messages "wash over them" as they grow older. Adolescents absorb these messages very much more avidly because, while *en route* to developing their adult identities, they monitor very much more sensitively everything that occurs in the adult world [13, 53].

A sample of 229 children aged 3 to 6 years was tested with ads featuring "Old Joe Camel": 30% of the 3-year olds and 91.3% of the 6-year olds correctly matched the "Old Joe" logo to the Camel cigarette brand [54]. It is concluded that intensive promotion of this cigarette brand resulted in this high recognition rate [54]. In a similarly designed study, recognition of the "Old Joe" logo was compared in adolescents and adults: the children were better able than adults (97 vs. 58%) to match the logo to the cigarette brand [45]. However, of much greater interest is the promotional effect of the 3-year advertising campaign: Camel's share of the children's cigarette market was initially 0.5%, rising to 32.8% 3 years later [45].

Similarly, interviews conducted in 5,040 adolescents and 24,296 adults from California revealed that perception of cigarette advertising was higher among adolescents than adults [55]. Whereas only 47% of adults named Marlboro and Camel as the most advertised brands, the figure was 70% among adolescents. The 12–13-year olds recognised Camel most often, whereas the 16–17-year olds recognised Marlboro most often [55]. Adolescent non-smokers from the same setting were interviewed about tobacco industry advertising messages. Even though they had no involvement in smoking, 84% of the sample was also able to remember one or more advertising messages [56]. The Camel advert depicted in Fig. 13.5 is directed at adolescents and adults who are already attuned and receptive to sexual innuendo. Nevertheless, this advertising message operates at a thought provoking level.

One recent study sought for an association between the number of cigarette promotional items (CPIs) owned and smoking behaviour. The two variables were studied in 10–19-year-old students, using multivariate regression analysis. Smokers were defined as students who had previously smoked 100 cigarettes or more in their lifetime, while other students were classed as never-smokers or experimental smokers [57]. Out of the 1,265 students, 406 owned CPIs: 211 owned one, 82 owned two, 57 owned three, 24 owned four, 23 owned five and 7-owned six CPIs. The study also investigated associations with educational level and family smoking behaviour. Smoking prevalence was 11.2% for students not owning a CPI, 41.5% for those owning two CPIs (OR = 3.4; 95% CI: 1.9–5.9) and 58.5% (OR = 8.4; 95% CI: 5.0–14.2) for those owning four CPIs [57]. From this, it is evident that promotional

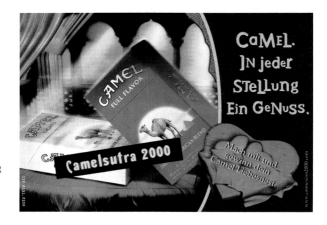

Fig. 13.5 "Camel – a pleasure whatever the position": blending smoking with sexual innuendo? Camel advert, issued in Germany in 2000

items supplied by the tobacco industry encourage smoking behaviour [57]. Conversely, consistently implemented tobacco control programmes clearly reduce the smoking behaviour of children, as has emerged from analyses in various US states [58].

Furthermore, susceptible adolescents tend to overestimate the social benefits of smoking and underestimate its risks [59], a phenomenon that may also be termed the "invulnerability syndrome" [60] and is not unknown in adults. The sheer weight of advertising is virtually bound to pre-programme misconceptions into adolescents' thinking so that they start to smoke and then are unable to free themselves from the habit [32]. Adolescents are not as capable as adults at effectively resisting these attempts of persuasion (see Chap. 12, life skills techniques) and consequently are more vulnerable than many adults to advertising strategies and sales tactics [33]. Adolescents are always looking for something novel and are also willing to try new experiences [61]. Adolescents' own insecurity and their tendency to look to a group or a leader figure provokes an opportunistic response because their recognition within, or sense of belonging to, the group may depend on this [11, 62].

A great many films from the USA and Germany portray actors smoking. One US study scrutinised every scene from 25 cinema box-office hits per year between 1988 and 1997. Those actors who smoke on screen encourage the current tobacco epidemic among young people. Cigarette and cigar smoking in the movies contribute to the characterisation of certain types: actresses who smoke often portray disreputable women embroiled in sexual affairs, involved in illegal activities and/or driving automobiles recklessly; male actors who smoke tend to portray tough guys who are frequently violent and relish dangerous situations [63]. One surprising finding was that these numerous smoker scenes account for only 2–3% of the footage [63].

According to another analysis of US films, 42% of actresses in starring roles smoked, whereas only 24% of 18–44-year-old US women are smokers. Movie smoking prevalence was just as high in films for young people as in films intended for adult viewing. The actresses generally use cigarettes in stressful situations that they wish to keep under control [64]. This movie exposure encourages young girls to accept and imitate these actresses as role models. Even Disney studio cartoon films intended solely for children's viewing depict tobacco and alcohol scenes just as frequently as ever, to judge from a comparison with a report from 1964. In 1996 and 1997, all cartoon films featured scenes of tobacco use. No film offered any verbal message highlighting the harmful effects of smoking [63].

In October 1999, British Telecom (BT) apologised for its error of judgement in supplying pagers for a Marlboro cigarette promotion aimed at young people. BT has subsequently condemned such campaigns designed to promote sales of tobacco products [65]. The background to BT's decision was that the Marlboro Company, in its promotional campaign "*Found on the Streets*" targeted at young people, was offering them leisure goods if they purchased 80-packs of cigarettes within a specified period [65]. In return for their names and addresses, young people (age > 18 years) at nightclubs were offered a free pack of Marlboro cigarettes, and later were sent glossy brochures on cigarette lighters, Lorus wristwatches, White Stuff leisure wear, Sanyo CD players and Nikon cameras [65]. Marlboro invited participants to "look around town" and "find themselves something useful." The young people were also encouraged to get their friends to telephone the Marlboro customer service department. The callers had to confirm their age in writing and attach proof of purchase to the order form. In some cases, the companies supplying the products on offer only discovered via the press that the campaign had been linked with Marlboro [65]. In terms of reprehensible advertising campaigns aimed at young people, it is my personal opinion that this represents the tip of the iceberg: after smoking 1,600 cigarettes there is a high degree of certainty that many participants in the scheme would have become dependent smokers.

13.4
Tobacco Advertising and Adolescent Smoking Initiation

It is evident from the preceding remarks that the critical time window determining whether a person will become a smoker or remain a non-smoker is the *period between 10 and 12 years of age*. Cigarette advertising has to impact this age group if it wishes to generate future customers. According to a survey conducted in 571 7th-grade students (13-years old), the likelihood of experimenting with smoking was 2.2 times greater among those who owned CPIs and 2.8 times greater among those who received mail from a cigarette company [66].

Adolescents also start smoking in response to social events and the media have a pivotal role to play here [21, 22]. Adolescents in the USA spend 2–3 h daily watching TV

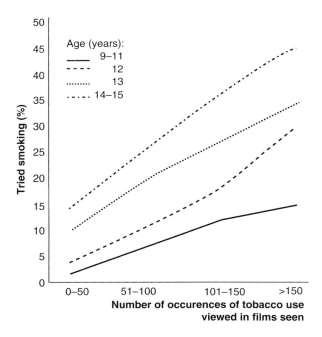

Fig. 13.6 Association between exposure to use of tobacco in films and prevalence of trying smoking by age [22]. Included were middle schools in New Hampshire and Vermont. The average participation by school was 92.5%. The final sample consisted of 4,919 schoolchildren (9–15 years of age). The authors counted occurrences of smoking in each of 601 popular contemporary films, and they asked respondents whether they had seen 50 films randomly selected from the larger pool. On the basis of the films that adolescents reported seeing, the number of occurrences of smoking seen by each survey respondent was calculated

programmes and films (Fig. 13.6). Watching just 3 films/week gives an annual total of 150 films [22]. These films include a large number of smoker scenes featuring film stars of both sexes, and adolescents are also enticed into cigarette smoking by these role models (Fig. 13.6) [22], with socio-demographic factors and social influences determining future behaviour.

Susceptibility to tobacco advertising was determined in a telephone campaign in 3,536 adolescent never-smokers. The survey was designed to discover the adolescents' attitudes towards possessing tobacco-related promotional items and their recognition of advertising messages and preferred brands. The survey also examined the extent to which the adolescents were exposed to a smoking environment [56]. The key finding was that adolescents are twice as likely to start smoking if they grow up in a smoking environment (own family members or peers) as in a smoke-free environment. The extent of their own receptivity, e.g. to advertising, was a reinforcing factor (see Fig. 13.7) [56].

One Scandinavian study has impressively demonstrated the role of the social environment (parents, siblings, friends) for the future smoking behaviour of 15-year olds: 90% of the adolescents smoked where those around them smoked, compared with only 3% where those around them did not smoke [67]. According to another study, the risk of becoming a smoker was dependent on factors such as ownership of promotional items (catalogues, coupons), and increased 22-fold if adolescents were given free sample packs [68]. An assessment of non-susceptible and susceptible non-smokers has also clearly shown that tobacco advertisements are similarly liked by smokers and by susceptible non-smokers, suggesting that the tobacco industry's advertisements should seek to convert uncommitted non-smokers into smokers [69].

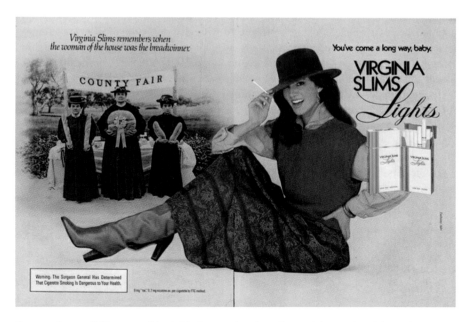

Fig. 13.7 Susceptibility to smoking initiation as a function of receptivity to advertising and exposure to smokers [56]

The available studies indicate that it is primarily adolescents who are enticed to become smokers because of advertising campaigns. The intensity of advertising increases cigarette consumption.

In each year between 1988 and 1998, advertising and promotional activities by the US tobacco companies generated 193,000 additional adult smokers who began smoking as adolescents. That decade of tobacco advertising and promotions also resulted in 46,400 smoking-attributable deaths per year and 698,400 years of potential life lost, which translates into approximately US $21.7–US $33.3 billion in total medical, productivity and mortality-related costs [70]. If all tobacco industry advertising and promotional activities were banned for the next 25 years, 60,000 smoking-attributable deaths per year could be avoided, saving 900,000 life-years, US $2.6 billion in excess medical expenses and between US $28 billion and US $43 billion in mortality costs [70].

13.5
Advertising with "Light" Cigarettes

Following the advent of light and ultralight cigarettes, many smokers who were ready to quit smoking switched to these brands because they believed that this represented a (albeit poor) compromise between health-consciousness and cigarette dependence. On the other hand, young men and women are enticed to start smoking with these "much milder" cigarettes. However, the fact remains that these cigarettes are implicated in many additional deaths [71].

Tobacco manufacturers encourage women to smoke, based on promises of glamour and attractiveness and the assurance that such behaviour is desirable [72]. In its attempts to reach women, the tobacco industry uses women's magazines as channels for its unbelievable messages in which smoking is associated with glamour, cultivated lifestyle, enjoyment, romance, sexual attractiveness, sport, sociability, relaxation, youth, emancipation, femininity, readiness to take risks and a slim figure [73]. In the EU, promotional campaigns for light cigarettes are overwhelmingly successful with middle-aged women.

Light cigarettes are sold mainly to health-conscious smokers because they are looking for less harmful cigarettes [74]. These cigarettes are most popular with women (Table 13.1). The tobacco industry (Marlboro) also believes that women associate these cigarettes with "independence" and "zest for life." In Germany, the market share for Marlboro-Light is 10.5%, though these cigarettes are less widely smoked by younger women.

In the report, *"The Changing Cigarette,"* smoking cigarettes with low condensate values was classified as reducing the risk of lung cancer, but only on the assumption that

Table 13.1 Percentage proportions of smokers of light cigarettes in the EU, classified by age (1995) [76]

Age group	Men	Women
15–24	29	36
25–44	29	48
45–64	33	60
65–	46	57
Total	31	48

the number of cigarettes smoked did not increase [75]. According to one survey in the USA, only 1 smoker in 10 knows that light cigarettes contain just as many toxic substances as "regular" cigarettes [74]. Despite this, these cigarettes can be marketed more easily to "health-conscious" smokers and are more readily accepted by women [74]. Nevertheless, surveys have revealed that where smokers are aware of the true information regarding light and ultralight cigarettes, the decision to quit smoking is taken more rapidly [74].

The market share of these low-condensate and low-nicotine cigarettes will not increase markedly, and yet action must be taken to counter the misleading advertising. According to the European Commission report [76], more than 50% of female smokers in seven EU countries (Sweden, Austria, Italy, Denmark, Ireland, Finland and France) smoke light cigarettes, and in Sweden, the percentage figure is actually 75% [76].

13.6
Tobacco Smuggling

Tobacco smuggling is "worthwhile" because the taxes on tobacco products are high (Fig. 13.8), even though considerable differences exist between the various European countries (range: 57–82%). Quasi-legal trade takes the form of sales in duty-free shops where cigarettes are available tax-free. In total, 45,000 million cigarettes (corresponding to 0.8% of all cigarettes worldwide) were sold through these channels in 1997 [77]. The European region led the way with 69%, followed by the Asia-Pacific region with 18%. The World Health Organization is extremely interested in suppressing or abolishing this form of sales (Protocol of the International Convention on the Simplification and Harmonization of Customs Procedures, 1999).

Illegal forms of "tobacco trade" are bootlegging and large-scale organised smuggling. *Bootleggers* limit themselves to buying cigarettes in countries with lower tobacco taxes and driving them by car to countries with higher tobacco tax levels without declaring these cigarettes when crossing national borders [78]. Large-scale *organised smuggling* is typical

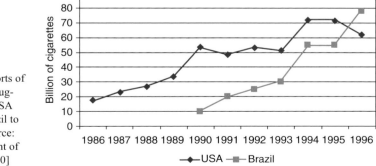

Fig. 13.8 Exports of cigarettes (smuggling) from USA and from Brazil to Belgium. Source: US Department of Agriculture [80]

of the situation in certain countries, e.g. the UK, where it accounts for 80% of total ciga-rette smuggling [79]. This smuggling benefits from transit trade because tax is not paid in the transit country on the assumption that the goods are being transported onwards. Within the EU, Belgium (port of Antwerp) is the most important receiving centre for cigarettes from the USA and Brazil where Philip Morris and BAT have built cigarette factories (Fig. 13.8) [80]. Excluding those intended for duty-free shops, these cigarettes are destined for the Third World. Here intermediate traders can buy cigarettes: the estimated total value of 100,000 million tax-free cigarettes in transit is US $14,000 million. It is these transit cigarettes that end up being sold illegally in Europe. Generally, the cigarettes are first transferred from Antwerp to Switzerland, at which point they are outside EU law. From there, they are moved to the Czech Republic, Hungary or one of the former Soviet Republics [81–83].

Over the 5-year period from 1990 to 1995, cigarette smuggling increased by 73% [84], a situation that was contributed to by the break-up of the former Soviet Union. According to reasonably reliable estimates, 303,000 million cigarettes were smuggled in this way in 1997 [85, 86]. BAT estimates that of 5.4 trillion cigarettes sold worldwide, 6% (324,000 million) are duty not paid (DNP) sales [87]. In addition, in developing countries in particu-lar, counterfeit cigarettes are being manufactured and sold, e.g. more than 50,000 million in China each year [88].

It has now been established that the multinational tobacco companies sell their ciga-rettes to dealers, and there "their responsibility ends." The dealers for their part allegedly know nothing about the country of destination of the cigarettes sold in this way. Since a gap exists between import and export, the tobacco companies and the dealers really should know something of the whereabouts of the goods. Switzerland may be thought of as a hub of the trade: Philip Morris and RJ Reynolds have their European headquarters there. And in the USA, for example, an executive of Brown and Williamson was respon-sible for trafficking in contraband cigarettes: the cigarettes were transported from a ware-house in Alabama to a private warehouse in Louisiana, were marked for off-shore vessels and thus, were tax-free and then sold to a Vietnamese organisation that smuggled them into Canada [89].

The scale of cigarette smuggling constitutes an enormous threat to general public health because (1) cigarette consumption is increased and (2) governments are deprived of thousands of millions of US$ or in tax revenue. The only possible counter-strategy depends on internationally agreed systems for regulation and tracking, and the tobacco companies should be required to operate through the prescribed trade channels. The pen-alties for tobacco smuggling should be dramatically increased by law and tobacco prod-ucts should carry a visible symbol to indicate that tax has been paid: "*An effective response to smuggling would be to keep taxes high and crack down on smuggling. Prominent tax stamps, serial numbers, special package markings, health warning labels in local lan-guages and better tracking systems are effective against smuggling*" [90]. Intermediate traders (often dealers) should have no role to play, and there should be a total ban on transit trade in tobacco products. In this regard, the World Health Organization must be even more proactive than its previous endeavours to break the resistance shown by numer-ous governments and by the tobacco companies themselves (International Framework for Tobacco Control) [91].

13.7
Effect of Advertising Bans

Although the very thought of advertising bans on its products is anathema to the tobacco industry, absolute bans should be imposed on its advertising, promotional and sponsorship activities in terms of:

- Direct and indirect advertising (the latter covers, for example, Camel footwear, Marlboro leisure clothing, Peter Stuyvesant travel, etc.).
- Advertising in all media (radio, TV, press, posters, cinema and Internet adverts, etc.).
- Financial sponsorship for national and international sporting and cultural events, etc.
- A worldwide ban on advertising which should be intensified progressively, taking account of national features in particular countries [86].

Within and outside Europe, four countries have now introduced general advertising bans on tobacco products: Norway, Finland, New Zealand and France.

These advertising bans are more extensive than the 1974 ban imposed in Germany on tobacco advertising on TV and radio. A strict ban on advertising has also existed in Poland since 1998. The advertising ban introduced in Canada has subsequently been lifted by the Supreme Court, while the existing ban on advertising in Italy cannot be assessed because of lack of data [92]. The control programmes developed in various US states [58], including restrictions on outdoor advertising [93, 94], point in the same direction with regard to a decline in smoking behaviour among children.

Community bans on advertising have also been implemented in various countries, with restrictions imposed on self-service outlets to reduce in-store advertising. Reducing consumer tobacco accessibility also has the effect of reducing shoplifting [95].

Bans on tobacco advertising in various countries have supported or encouraged several other initiatives: for example, restrictions on sales to minors, health education and health campaigns, tobacco-use prevention programmes for children and adolescents, creation of smoke-free zones, setting of legal limits for toxic substances in tobacco and pro-rata use of tobacco taxation revenue for research and health education (see Tables 13.2 and 13.3).

Table 13.2   Relationships between advertising bans in different countries and the decline in tobacco consumption, compared with Germany (D) where there is no advertising ban

Country	Introduction of advertising ban	Reference year for evaluation	Reduction in consumption by 1996	Reduction in consumption in Germany by 1996
Norway	1.7.1975	1974/1975	−26%	−13%
Finland	1.3.1978	1977	−37%	−11%
New Zealand	17.12.1990	1990; for D: 1989/1991	−21%	−14/−13%
France	1.1.1993	1992	−14%	−4%

Reduction in per-capita consumption of tobacco products in g (cigarettes, fine cut tobacco, pipe tobacco; in France, cigarettes only) [92]

Table 13.3   Reduction in percentage of adolescents who smoke daily in five countries (in Germany, the reference index shown is the percentage of adolescents who smoke regularly) [35]

Country	Introduction of advertising ban	Reference year for evaluation	Reduction in consumption among adolescents by 1996; in Germany by 1993
Norway	1.7.1975	1975	−15.8% (boys); −15.4% (girls)
Finland	1.3.1978	1978/1979	−12% (boys); −14% (girls)
New Zealand	17.12.1990	1990	−2.1%
France	1.1.1993	1992	0%
Germany	–	1993	−5.4%

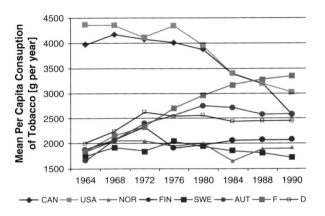

Fig. 13.9   Mean per-capita consumption of tobacco in eight different countries (Canada, USA, Norway, Finland, Sweden, Austria, France, Germany [D]) during the period 1964–1990 (adapted from [114])

Within 15 years following the general ban on tobacco advertising that has existed in *Norway* since 1975, there was a decline in the number of adolescent smokers of 5–10%, depending on age group and sex, with total smoking prevalence reductions of 10% among 16–24-year-old men and 20% among women of the same age [96, 97]. Smoking prevalence also fell among older people within 15 years, with figures of 35% for men and 32% for women being reported in 1995 [98]. Overall, per-capita tobacco consumption fell from 2,100 to 1,553 g during the period from 1975 to 1996 (Fig. 13.9) [99].

In *Finland*, the ban was implemented in two phases (in 1977 and 1994): in the second considerably more stringent phase, cigarette advertisements were also prohibited in foreign magazines, which are extremely popular in Finland. The greatest decline in smoking prevalence was recorded among men [100]. During the period 1978–1996, per-capita tobacco consumption fell from 2,134 to 1,350 g (Fig. 13.9) [99, 101].

The advertising ban introduced in *New Zealand* in 1990 resulted in a reduction in per-capita tobacco consumption from 1,957 to 1,553 g (1990 vs. 1996). Over the same period, the number of adolescent smokers fell by 1.9% [99].

In *France*, a ban on tobacco advertising has been in place since 1993. Within 4 years, per-capita tobacco consumption fell from 2,970 to 1,834 g; despite this fall, no reduction in smoking has been reported among 12–18-year olds (Table 13.3) [99].

13.8
Smoking Bans in Public Buildings and Public Spaces

The range of preventive measures should include government regulations enforcing smoking bans in public buildings, such as health centres, workplaces, schools, academic institutions, waiting rooms, restaurants, businesses and on public transport. Alongside general bans, partial bans may also be announced using appropriate signage. People wishing to smoke can be referred to special areas, a partial solution that has been employed in the USA, for example. These non-smoking policies can be supported by health education campaigns [102, 103]. Comparable regulations differ very markedly from country to country. In the USA, Australia and the countries of Northern Europe, changes have taken place as a result of legislation and general attitudes towards smoking. In other countries, the regulations are considerably more moderate [104–107].

The most effective means of achieving a smoking ban in public buildings is to issue an absolute decision on the matter, accompanied by educational programmes, dissemination of information, manager training and provision to help smokers achieve smoking cessation [102, 103]. Two studies in Baltimore hospitals have convincingly confirmed the efficacy of this approach. These models have been successfully continued in various health institutions in the USA [108], and instructions for similar campaigns are now available on the Internet [108]. In projects of this nature, it is crucial that the organisation's management takes responsibility and talks with those affected by the ban to provide education and information. It has also been found that only comprehensive measures are successful in the workplace [60, 109]. Stands displaying "No smoking" signs in public areas are minimally successful. Similarly, discussions with smokers about the harmful effects of tobacco use on health were less successful than face-to-face dialogue sessions between smokers and non-smokers. According to some studies, successful "No smoking" campaigns in the workplace have actually persuaded smokers to quit [110, 111]. In this context, it is evidently important, particularly in Germany, to issue appeals to the medical profession to ensure that there is first a reduction in the high proportion of doctors who smoke (approximately 20%). One possibility is to establish "smoke-free" hospitals, an approach that is now also being attempted in Germany (e.g. the "Berlin Heart Centre").

The implementation of "No smoking" laws is only useful if such legislation is supported by detailed regulations on enforcement [104, 106]. In France, for example, the ban on smoking in restaurants and other public buildings is largely ignored.

It remains to be established whether smoking bans in public buildings will bring about behavioural change at the individual level. Charitable organisations and anti-smoking associations must certainly strive to achieve gradual behavioural change across the whole of society, and the enforcement of existing regulations is an important challenge that must be solved.

A reduction in smoking among adolescents was reported following a concerted campaign combining restrictions on smoking at home with strict bans in public places and at school. The study, which was conducted among 17,287 students from 200 schools over 30 days, concluded that teenage smoking was reduced chiefly through restrictions on smoking at home and in public places, and to a lesser extent, in schools, and then only if the ban was strongly enforced (Table 13.4) [112].

Table 13.4 Logistic regression analysis for association of restrictions with 30-day smoking prevalence [112]

	Odds ratio (95% CI)	*p* value
Public restrictions	0.91 (0.83–0.99)	0.03
Total home ban	0.79 (0.67–0.91)	<0.001
Some home restrictions	0.85 (0.74–0.95)	<0.01
School ban	0.99 (0.85–1.13)	0.86
Enforced school ban	0.86 (0.77–0.94)	<0.001

2logL = 16 271.0, (df = 16), intracluster correlation = 0.038, cluster variance = 0.131, $p < 0.0001$. Odds ratios are adjusted for school grade, sex, race, adult smokers in home and sibling smokers; $n = 14\,746$

13.9
Concluding Remarks

- A survey of the facts and data presented by the tobacco industry and (necessarily) supplemented by government agencies (to ensure a true picture) reveals that the number of adolescent smokers can be reduced only by tough international legislation [113] to regulate a variety of issues: manufacture, trade (including cigarette smuggling), advertising and distribution of tobacco products (and promotional items), especially to young people.
- In particular, the international community and its politicians must ensure that economically weak countries do not become a target for the activities of the tobacco industry.
- Every single day, 3,000 adolescents in the USA are recruited to the ranks of smokers. If the number of smokers is not reduced in the years ahead, the lamentable fact is that 10 million people annually will die from tobacco-attributable causes worldwide by the year 2025.
- The medical profession and politicians must not stand idly and watch this trend unfold.

References

1. Yach D, Bettcher D (2000) Globalisation of tobacco industry influence and new global responses. Tob Control 9(2):206–216
2. Philip Morris (1997, Aug 23) Tabakhersteller spricht von den Gefahren des Rauchens. Frankf Allg Z [195], 1. 1997
3. Anonym (1999) Bitte kaufen Sie unser Produkt nicht! Welt
4. Haustein KO (1999) Smoking: health care and politics in flux. Rauchen: Gesundheitswesen und Politik im Wechselspiel. Z Arztl Fortbild Qualitatssich 93:355–361
5. MacKay J, Crofton J (1996) Tobacco and the developing world. In: Doll R, Crofton J (eds) Tobacco and health. Royal Society of Medicine, London, pp 206–221
6. Murray C, Lopez A (1996) The global burden of disease: a comprehensive assessment of mortality and disability from disease, injuries, and risk factors in 1990 and projected to 2020. Harvard University, Boston

7. World Bank (1999) Curbing the epidemic: governments and the economics of tobacco control. The World Bank (ed), Washington D.C. Development in Practice Series

8. Junge B (2002) Tabak – Zahlen und Fakten zum Konsum. Jahrbuch Sucht 2002. Neuland, Geesthacht, pp 32–62

9. Whelan EM, Sheridan MJ, Meister KA, Mosher BA (1981) Analysis of coverage of tobacco hazards in women's magazines. J Public Health Policy 2:28–35

10. Hanson JD, Kysar DA (1999) Taking behavioralism seriously: some evidence of market manipulation. Harv Law Rev 112:1420–1572

11. Eicke U (1992) Stellungnahme aus aus werblich-wissenschaftlicher Sicht zum Abschlußbericht der Pilotstudie "Auswirkungen der Tabakwerbung und der Zigarettenautomaten auf das Konsumverhalten, insbesondere von Kindern und Jugendlichen". Bonn

12. US-Department of Health and Human Services (1989) Reducing the health consequences of smoking: 25 years of progress. A report of the surgeon general. Washington

13. Lynch BS, Bonnie RJ (1994) Growing up tobacco free. Preventing nicotine addiction in children and youths. National Academy, Washington DC

14. Gilpin EA, Pierce JP (1997) Trends in adolescent smoking initiation in the United States: is tobacco marketing an influence? Tob Control 6:122–127

15. Harper T (2001) Marketing life after advertising bans. Tob Control 10(2):196–198

16. Charlton A, While D, Kelly S (1997) Boys' smoking and cigarette-brand-sponsored motor racing. Lancet 350:1474

17. Sadler PA (1998) Tobacco sponsorship of formula one motor racing. Lancet 351:451–452

18. Feighery EC, Ribisl KM, Achabal DD, Tyebjee T (1999) Retail trade incentives: how tobacco industry practices compare with those of other industries. Am J Public Health 89:1564–1566

19. Bartecchi CE, MacKenzie TD, Schrier RW (1995) The global tobacco epidemic. Sci Am 272:44–51

20. Feighery EC, Ribisl KM, Schleicher N, Lee RE, Halvorson S (2001) Cigarette advertising and promotional strategies in retail outlets: results of a statewide survey in California. Tob Control 10(2):184–188

21. Sargent JD, Tickle JJ, Beach ML, Dalton MA, Ahrens MB, Heatherton TF (2001) Brand appearances in contemporary cinema films and contribution to global marketing of cigarettes. Lancet 357(9249):29–32

22. Sargent JD, Beach ML, Dalton MA, Mott LA, Tickle JJ, Ahrens MB, et al (2001) Effect of seeing tobacco use in films on trying smoking among adolescents: cross sectional study. BMJ 323(7326):1394–1397

23. Siegel M (2001) Counteracting tobacco motor sports sponsorship as a promotional tool: is the tobacco settlement enough? Am J Public Health 91(7):1100–1106

24. Capman S, Cohen A, Nelson B, Woodward S (1993) A boycott of tobacco-sponsored cars? Tob Control 2:159

25. Richards JW, DiFranza JR, Fletcher C, Fischer PM (1995) RJ Reynolds "Camel Cash": another way to reach kids. Tob Control 4:258–260

26. Slade J (1993) High participation rates in cigarette brand promotions. Tob Control 2: 248–249

27. Amos A, Jacobson B, White P (1991) Cigarette advertising policy and coverage of smoking and health in British women's magazines. Lancet 337:93–96

28. Minkler M, Wallack L, Madden P (1987) Alcohol and cigarette advertising in Ms. magazine. J Public Health Policy 8:164–179

29. Warner KE, Goldenhar LM, McLaughlin CG (1992) Cigarette advertising and magazine coverage of the hazards of smoking. A statistical analysis. N Engl J Med 326:305–309

30. Pollay RW, Siddarth S, Siegel M, Haddix A, Merrit RK, Giovino GA, et al (1996) The last straw? Cigarette advertising and realized market shares among youth and adults, 1979– 1993. J Market Theory Pract 60:1–16

31. Roemer R (1993) Legislative action to combat the world tobacco epidemic, 2nd edn. WHO, Geneva
32. US-Department of Health and Human Services (1994) Preventing tobacco use among young people. A report of the surgeon general. Washington
33. Pollay RW (1997) Hacks, flacks and counter-attacks: cigarette advertising, research and controversies. J Social Issues 53:53–74
34. Kessler DA, Myers ML (2001) Beyond the tobacco settlement. N Engl J Med 345(7):535–537
35. Junge B (1997) Tabak – Zahlen und Fakten zum Konsum. Jahrbuch Sucht '98. Neuland, Geesthacht, pp 19–42
36. Siegel M, Nelson DE, Peddicord JP, Merritt RK, Giovino GA, Eriksen MP (1996) The extent of cigarette brand and company switching: results from the Adult Use-of-Tobacco Survey. Am J Prev Med 12:14–16
37. Coeytaux R, Altmann DG, Slade J (1995) Tobacco promotions in the hands of youth. Tob Control 4:253–257
38. Pollay RW, Lavack A (1993) The targeting of youth by cigarette marketers: archival evidence on trial. In: McAlister L, Rotschild ML (eds) Advances in consumer Research 20:266–271
39. Glantz SA, Slade J, Bero LA, Hanauer P, Barnes DE (1996) The cigarette papers. University of California, Berkeley
40. Pollay RW (1995) Targeting tactics in selling smoke: youthful aspects of 20th-century cigarette advertising. J Market Theory Pract 3:1–22
41. Pollay RW (1994) Exposure of US youth to cigarette television advertising in the 1960s. Tob Control 3:130–133
42. Pollay RW (1994) Self regulation of US cigarette broadcast advertising in the 1960s. Tob Control 3:134–144
43. Dagli E (1999) Are low income countries targets of the tobacco industry? Plenary lecture given during the Conference on Global Lung Health and 1997 Annual Meeting of the International Union Against Tuberculosis and Lung Disease, Palais des Congres, Paris, France, 1–4 October 1997. Int J Tuberc Lung Dis 3:113–118
44. Anonym (1999) Zigaretten mit Erdbeergeschmack. Welt
45. DiFranza JR, Richards JW, Paulman PM, Wolf-Gillespie N, Fletcher C, Jaffe RD, et al (1991) RJR Nabisco's cartoon camel promotes camel cigarettes to children. JAMA 266:3149–3153
46. Borzekowski DL, Flora JA, Feighery E, Schooler C (1999) The perceived influence of cigarette advertisements and smoking susceptibility among seventh graders. J Health Commun 4: 105–118
47. Zajonc RB (1980) Feeling and thinking: preferences need no inferences. Am Psychol 35: 151–175
48. Goebel K (1994) Lesbian and gays face tobacco targeting. Tob Control 3:65–67
49. Baacke D, Sander U, Vollbrecht R (1993) **Kinder und Werbung. Bd. 12. Kohlhammer. Schriftenreihe des Bundesministeriums für Frauen und Jugend, Stuttgart
50. McVey D, Stapleton J (2000) Can anti-smoking television advertising affect smoking behaviour? controlled trial of the Health Education Authority for England's anti-smoking TV campaign. Tob Control 9(3):273–282
51. Botvin GJ, Goldberg CJ, Botvin EM, Dusenbury L (1993) Smoking behavior of adolescents exposed to cigarette advertising. Public Health Rep 108:217–224
52. Rombouts K, Fauconnier G (1988) What is learned early is learned well? A study of the influence on tobacco advertising on adolescents. Eur J Commun 3:303–322
53. Hawkins K, Hane AC (2000) Adolescents' perceptions of print cigarette advertising: a case for counteradvertising. J Health Commun 5(1):83–96
54. Fischer PM, Schwartz MP, Richards JW Jr, Goldstein AO, Rojas TH (1991) Brand logo recognition by children aged 3 to 6 years. Mickey Mouse and Old Joe the Camel. JAMA 266: 3145–3148

55. Pierce JP, Gilpin E, Burns DM, Whalen E, Rosbrook B, Shopland D, et al (1991) Does tobacco advertising target young people to start smoking? Evidence from California. JAMA 266:3154–3158
56. Evans N, Farkas A, Gilpin E, Berry C, Pierce JP (1995) Influence of tobacco marketing and exposure to smokers on adolescent susceptibility to smoking. J Natl Cancer Inst 87: 1538–1545
57. Sargent JD, Dalton M, Beach M (2000) Exposure to cigarette promotions and smoking uptake in adolescents: evidence of a dose-response relation. Tob Control 9(2):163–168
58. Wakefield M, Chaloupka F (2000) Effectiveness of comprehensive tobacco control programmes in reducing teenage smoking in the USA. Tob Control 9(2):177–186
59. Bonnie RJ, Lynch BS (1994) Time to up the ante in the war on smoking. Issues Sci Technol 11:33–37
60. Greening L, Dollinger SJ (1991) Adolescent smoking and perceived vulnerability to smoking-related causes of death. J Pediatr Psychol 16:687–699
61. Loudon DL, Della Bitta AJ (1993) Consumer behaviour: concepts and applications. McGraw-Hill, New York
62. Stacey BG (1982) Economic socialization in the pre-adult years. Br J Social Psychol 21: 159–173
63. Escamilla G, Cradock AL, Kawachi I (2000) Women and smoking in Hollywood movies: a content analysis. Am J Public Health 90(3):412–414
64. Goldstein AO, Sobel RA, Newman GR (1999) Tobacco and alcohol use in G-rated children's animated films. JAMA 281:1131–1136
65. Die WHO lobt Telekommunikationsriesen wegen seiner Distanzierung von Zigarettenwerbung (1999)
66. Schooler C, Feighery E, Flora JA (1996) Seventh graders' self-reported exposure to cigarette marketing and its relationship to their smoking behavior. Am J Public Health 86:1216–1221
67. Aaro LE, Hauknes A, Berglund EL (1981) Smoking among Norwegian schoolchildren 1975–1980. II. The influence of the social environment. Scand J Psychol 22:297–309
68. Altmann DG, Levine DW, Coeytaux R, Slade J, Jaffe R (1986) Tobacco promotion and susceptibility to tobacco use among adolescents aged 12 through 17 years in a nationally representative sample. Am J Public Health 86:1590–1593
69. Unger JB, Johnson CA, Rohrbach LA (1995) Recognition and liking of tobacco and alcohol advertisements among adolescents: relationships with susceptibility to substance use. Prev Med 24:461–466
70. Emery S, Choi WS, Pierce JP (1999) The social costs of tobacco advertising and promotions. Nicotine Tob Res 1(Suppl 2):S83–S91
71. Warner KE, Slade J, Sweanor DT (1997) The emerging market for long-term nicotine maintenance. JAMA 278:1087–1092
72. Winstanley M, Woodward S, Walker N (1995) Tobacco in Australia. Victorian Smoking and Health Program, Carlton South
73. Amos A, Bostock C, Bostock Y (1998) Women's magazines and tobacco in Europe. Lancet 352:786–787
74. Kozlowski LT, Goldberg ME, Yost BA, White EL, Sweeney CT, Pillitteri JL (1998) Smokers' misperceptions of light and ultra-light cigarettes may keep them smoking. Am J Prev Med 15:9–16
75. US-Department of Health and Human Services (1981) The health consequences of smoking. The changing cigarette. A report of the surgeon general. Rockville
76. Europe Network for Smoking Prevention (1999) Manche mögens "Light". Frauen und Rauchen in der Europäischen Union. Europa-Bericht
77. Marketing Tracking International (1998) World tobacco file 1998. Marketing Tracking International (ed). DMG Buissiness Media, London

78. Joossens L, Naett C, Howie C (1992) Taxes on tobacco products – a health issue. European Bureau for Action on Smoking Prevention. Brussels
79. ASH. **Taxation in the 2001 Budget. 2001. Action on Smoking and Health
80. Joossens L, Raw M (1998) Cigarette smuggling in Europe: who really benefits? Tob Control 7:66–71
81. Tobacco: World Markets and trade (1997)** Circular Series, August 1997. US Department of Agriculture
82. Committee of inquiry into the Copmmunity transit system. (4 volumes) (1997) European Parliament, Brussels
83. Bonner R, Drew C (1997, Aug 25) Cigarette makers are seen as aiding rise in smuggling. New York Times
84. World tobacco file: emerging markets in Asia 1997 (1997) DMG Business Media. Market Tracking International, London
85. Joossens L, Raw M (2000) How can cigarette smuggling be reduced? BMJ 321(7266): 947–950
86. Joossens L (2000) From public health to international law: possible protocols for inclusion in the Framework Convention on Tobacco Control. Bull World Health Organ 78(7):930–937
87. ash.org.uk (2000) BATCo global five-year plan 1994–1998. www.ash.org.uk/smuggling/048.pdf
88. Yuan HA (1997) Cigarette production down: contraband and counterfeits flourish. Tobacco Reporter [April], 32
89. Former B&W executive convinced of cigarette smuggling (1997) Associated Press
90. Chaloupka F (2001) Press Release 2001/027/S. http://www.who.int/inf-pr-2000/en/pr2000-53.html
91. Persson LGW, Andersson J (1997) Cigarette-smuggling. Swedish National Police College, Stockholm
92. Hanewinkel R, Pohl J (1998) Werbung und Tabakkonsum. Wirkungsanalyse unter besonderer Berücksichtigung von Kindern und Jugendlichen. IFT-Nord. Expertise im Auftrag des BMG. Kiel
93. Bidell MP, Furlong MJ, Dunn DM, Koegler JE (2000) Case study of attempts to enact self service tobacco display ordinances: a tale of three communities. Tob Control 9(1):71–77
94. Pucci LG, Joseph HM Jr, Siegel M (1998) Outdoor tobacco advertising in six Boston neighborhoods. Evaluating youth exposure. Am J Prev Med 15:155–159
95. Lee RE, Feighery EC, Schleicher NC, Halvorson S (2001) The relation between community bans of self-service tobacco displays and store environment and between tobacco accessibility and merchant incentives. Am J Public Health 91(12):2019–2021
96. Rimpela MK, Aaro LE, Rimpela AH (1993) The effects of tobacco sales promotion on initiation of smoking - experiences from Finland and Norway. Scand J Soc Med Suppl 49:5–23
97. Bjartveit K (1990) Fifteen years of comprehensive legislation: results and conclusions. Proceedings of the 7th World Conference on Tobacco and Health, Perth. Australia, pp 71–80
98. Kraft P, Svendsen T (1997) Tobacco use among young adults in Norway, 1973–95: has the decrease levelled out? Tob Control 6:27–32
99. Joossens L (1997) The effectiveness of banning advertising for tobacco products. International Union Against Cancer; UICC/ECL Liaison Office, Brüssel, 15 pp
100. Piha T (1995) New provisions for tobacco control in Finnland. Ministry of Social Affairs and Health (ed), Helsinki
101. Pekurinen M (1991) Economic aspects of smoking. Research reports 16. Ministry of Social Affairs and Health, Helsinki, 271–273
102. Becker DM, Conner HF, Waranch HR, Stillman F, Pennington L, Lees PS, et al (1989) The impact of a total ban on smoking in the Johns Hopkins Children's Center. JAMA 262:799–802

103. Stillman FA, Becker DM, Swank RT, Hantula D, Moses H, Glantz S, et al (1990) Ending smoking at the Johns Hopkins Medical Institutions. An evaluation of smoking prevalence and indoor air pollution. JAMA 264:1565–1569

104. Bonfill X, Serra C, Lopez V (1997) Employee and public responses to simulated violations of no-smoking regulations in Spain. Am J Public Health 87:1035–1037

105. Forster JL, Hourigan ME, Kelder S (1992) Locking devices on cigarette vending machines: evaluation of a city ordinance. Am J Public Health 82:1217–1219

106. Rigotti NA, Stoto MA, Bierer MF, Rosen A, Schelling T (1993) Retail stores' compliance with a city no-smoking law. Am J Public Health 83:227–232

107. Serra C, Bonfill X, Lopez V (1997) Consumo y venta de tabaco en lugares pùblicos: evaluaciòn del cumplimento de la normativa vigente. Geceta Sanitaria 11:55–65

108. US Dept of Health and Human Services (1996) Making your workplace smokefree – a decision maker's guide. Centres of Disease Control and Prevention Office on Smoking and Health, CDC

109. Dawley HH Jr, Morrison J, Carol S (1985) The discouragement of smoking in a hospital setting. Int J Addict 20:783–793

110. Borland R, Owen N, Hill D, Chapman S (1990) Changes in acceptance of workplace smoking bans following their implementation: a prospective study. Prev Med 19:314–322

111. Eriksen MP, Gottlieb NH (1998) A review of the health impact of smoking control at the workplace. Am J Health Promot 13:83–104

112. Wakefield MA, Chaloupka FJ, Kaufman NJ, Orleans CT, Barker DC, Ruel EE (2000) Effect of restrictions on smoking at home, at school, and in public places on teenage smoking: cross sectional study. BMJ 321(7257):333–337

113. Satcher D (2001) Why we need an international agreement on tobacco control. Am J Public Health 91(2):191–193

114. Stewart MJ (1993) The effect of advertising bans on tobacco consumption in OECD countries. Int J advert 12:155–180

Society, Politics and the Tobacco Industry **14**

The question arises if the death toll from tobacco does not constitute a crime against humanity, susceptible to prosecution in the international criminal court of the United Nations.

N. Francey, *Tobacco Control* 1999

When people speak of the globalisation of industry, they usually mean worldwide networking between firms, in many cases involving the merger of complete sectors of industry. The consequences of these economic processes are not always beneficial. Some typical examples of globalisation are brand names such as Coca-Cola® or McDonald's®, and the cigarette industry can also be added to this list, being led by a small number of worldwide tobacco groups (e.g. Philip Morris, British American Tobacco (BAT), RJ Reynolds, Brown & Williamson). Especially in the case of the cigarette industry, globalisation is seen by many as a double-edged sword; for instance, causing Gro Harlem Brundtland, the Director General of the WHO, speaking in February 1999 in Davos, to describe the "operations" of the tobacco industry as a serious threat to the health of nations [1].

In the light of currently around 800,000 smoking-related deaths in the European Union, a majority of doctors in the EU frequently ask themselves what is preventing a majority of politicians from (1) imposing a ban on advertising for tobacco products in the EU, (2) gradually putting an end to the subsidies for tobacco cultivation in the EU of currently EUR 1 billion and (3) using this money to establish primary and secondary prevention programmes [2].

The Europeans, including the Germans, "tolerate" the damage to health caused by smoking because the cigarette industry in Germany alone not only provides a number of jobs (in 1996, 13,794 [3] out of a total 10.995 million people employed in manufacturing industry), but also brings the German state annual tax revenues from the sale of cigarettes totalling 11.5 billion [4]. With 192.46 billion cigarettes produced in 1996, domestic sales revenue amounted to EUR 13.32 billion [3]. In other words, each employee in the tobacco industry accounted for sales revenue of EUR 1.1 million [3], a figure which is unattainable in any other industry. With their hazardous side effects, cigarettes would have long since been taken off the market if they were classified as a pharmaceutical rather than as a foodstuff.

Even compared with the other main causes of death, alcoholism and obesity, smoking is the front runner by a long way (Table 14.1). The damage to health caused by smoking is therefore a problem of highest priority, and should be accorded the same priority by the politicians (dealing with health).

K.-O. Haustein, D. Groneberg, *Tobacco or Health?*   411
DOI: 10.1007/978-3-540-87577-2_14, © Springer Verlag Berlin Heidelberg 2010

Table 14.1 Comparison of mortality for known risk factors, and economic cost analysis [97]

Risk factor	Mortality[a]	Years of life lost[b]	Costs of illness		Loss of earnings[e]	Total costs
			Direct[c]	Indirect[d]		
Smoking	416,829	5.3	20.8	6.9	40.3	68.0
Obesity	162,191	2.1	23.0	5.6	13.4	41.0
Alcohol	105,000	1.0	6.8	27.4	27.5	66.5

[a]All premature deaths in a year because of risk factors
[b]Based on US live statistics data and years of life lost through illnesses due to the risk factors
[c]Costs caused by illnesses due to the risk factors (billion US $)
[d]Equivalent for working hours lost or time lost in the household (billion US $)
[e]Future income lost through premature death (billion US $)

Cigarette smoking causes extremely severe damage to the health of a large proportion of the population. According to a study by the Atomic Research Centre in Karlsruhe, smokers in Germany exhale 7,500 tonnes of hydrocarbons annually, equivalent to the maximum permitted emission figure for ten new waste incineration plants [5].

14.1
Tobacco Industry, Governmental and Non-governmental Organisations

In the past years, the tobacco industry has consistently avoided agreements with the state or other relevant organisations aimed at making redress for the harm caused by smoking through specific future measures or through financial compensation for the victims.

With the "Master Settlement Agreement," which was signed by the tobacco industry in 1998, 46 US states brought legal action, seeking to obtain recompense for tobacco-related health spending and to hold the tobacco industry to account for the decades of harm it had caused. The aim of the agreement was (1) to restrict the contact of young people with tobacco marketing, (2) to implement comprehensive smoking prevention programmes, and (3) to counter the marketing effects of the tobacco industry on children. Under the agreement, the tobacco industry was supposed to pay US $206 billion over a period of 25 years if the advertising restrictions were to be observed and a national institute for public health information on smoking was to be established [6]. In fact, however, the agreement was never implemented, and advertising by the tobacco industry has, if anything, even been intensified.

In a separate move from this agreement, the WHO in Geneva, together with representatives from 150 countries, put forward a proposal in October 2000 for a first international Framework Convention on Tobacco Control (FCTC), which is supposed to be in place by 2003. The goal of this is to put a brake on the increase in tobacco consumption by a range of national and international measures [7]. The tobacco industry has already announced that it will put up heavy opposition to this and seek to prevent or delay implementation of the FCTC [8]. In the year 2000, a meeting was held with people from the overwhelming majority of countries, representing 92% of the world population, to discuss this document.

Because of its huge profits, the tobacco industry is able to support a wide range of sporting and cultural activities of the state. It remains questionable whether the state or other bodies should accept such money, for which a "return" is naturally expected from politicians and state institutions. In 2002 the German government reached an agreement with the tobacco industry, under the terms of which the latter is to make a "no strings" payment of 12.6 million to the government over a period of 3 years for the implementation of prevention programmes among children to discourage them from taking up smoking at an early age. This form of collaboration is always suspect: the scientists engaged in future work of this kind are free only to a limited extent because they are "taking tobacco research Euros." An analogous situation existed when BAT announced that it would fund an International Centre for Corporate Social Responsibility at Nottingham University in the UK for the sobering sum of £3.8 million [9, 10] (see Sect. 14.3).

A few years ago, a very far-reaching law, the so-called "Tobacco Deal," was planned in the USA. This law proposed to increase tobacco duty (from $1 to $10 per pack over a period of 5 years), to impose sharp restrictions on tobacco advertising, and to set up a special fund for the treatment of smoking-related diseases ($20 billion per year). In return, the tobacco industry would be "sheltered" by the state from individual legal actions. However, in connection with elections in the year 1998, the tobacco industry gave $50 million in campaign donations to the Republicans, who at that time held a majority in Congress, and at the same time ran an advertising campaign on television, all of which had the desired effect. The law was brought down by the votes of the Republicans [11].

According to internal discussions of the German Cigarette Industry Association (VdC), the tobacco industry is pursuing several strategic goals to secure its sales markets [12]. One of its primary goals is to prevent a ban on tobacco advertising worldwide, in the EU and Germany by, for instance, obstructing the discussion and passage of bills in the European Parliament and/or preventing laws from coming into force through court action. To do this, the tobacco industry conducts talks with politicians of all parties and also seeks to exert pressure, through business and trade union representatives, on the members of the EU Parliament, with the aim of bringing 314 members of the European Parliament "onto the tobacco industry's side." The ostensible argument used against a ban on advertising was the "freedom of (advertising) information," backed by large-scale placard and advertising activities prior to the vote [13].

In a recently published comprehensive report [14], the WHO has documented in detail that the tobacco industry

- Is seeking to distract attention from tobacco abuse through sidetracking activities
- Has tried to reduce the WHO's tobacco-related budgets and mobilise other UN organisations against the WHO
- Has sought to convince developing countries that the WHO's anti-tobacco programme would be at their expense
- Has misrepresented the results of important scientific studies [14]

The tobacco industry has also laid down a strategy in a confidential document (position paper) – though this has now been published on the Internet – on ways of influencing the activities of the WHO [15].

14.2
Politicians and Their Attitude to Smoking

Smoking is seen by many people as a demonstration of strength and superiority, and cigars even as a symbol of power (as evidenced by caricatures of capitalists). Some typical examples of cigar smokers are Churchill, Clinton, Erhard and Schröder. Politicians are supposed to be independent people who decide solely according to their conscience; in fact, however, they are usually embedded in social lobby groups, who also generate the voter potential for future elections [16, 17]. Most studies on smoking, and the statements made in them on the "more or less significant risks" caused by smoking, come from the laboratories and advertising agencies of the cigarette industry, which in terms of influence on public opinion have even more importance in the USA than in Germany [18–20]. Despite an appeal by the Medical Advisory Board of the Bonn organisations to the German chancellor to abandon the government's opposition to the EU directive banning cigarette advertising, the government felt it necessary to fight the "resolutions of the EU Commission as they would put jobs at risk" and to put a brake on the "witch hunt" against advertising by the tobacco industry [21].

In 1998, the *British government* launched a nationwide "Smoking kills" campaign, with the aim of reducing smoking among juveniles from 13 to 9%, among adults from 28 to 24%, and especially among women from 23 to 15%, within a period of 10 years [22]. For the first 3 years of this campaign, the British government has made £60 million available [22].

In *Germany*, as in many other EU countries, there is still a kind of "stalemate" situation, with "powerless" politicians and journalists – a lot of whom smoke – on the one side, and the social security contributors, who ultimately have to pay for the costs of smoking-related disease, on the other side, including a potential majority of the population who would vote in favour of tough measures to protect non-smokers and for a complete ban on cigarette advertising. This scenario indicates failure on the part of many politicians [23]. Depending on whether they decide "for" or "against" a ban on advertising and the protection of non-smokers, politicians stand to lose credibility among their respective voter groups. The refusal of politicians to take a clear stand on these issues is a misrepresentation of the will of the people [24]. The politicians prefer to accept the proven damage to health caused by smoking, which can add up to billions in only a few years, rather than make a clear decision. Also, the politicians in *Germany* have so far adopted no effective measures to protect children at home. At present, there might exist some improvement concerning public protection for non-smokers, but research into this field still receives hardly any support.

Where specialist advice is called in prior to taking legislative decisions, the cigarette industry is always able to present "experts" from a range of disciplines who cast doubt on the findings of studies, generating a general atmosphere of uncertainty and in this way ultimately exercising an inhibiting effect on the intended legislative measures [25–27]. The tobacco industry is also able, by threatening to claim for damages – including court costs running into millions – to paralyse any activity, as happened in the case of CBS, the radio and TV broadcaster, in the USA [28].

14.3
Scientists and the Tobacco Industry

One perennial important issue is whether scientists should accept money from the tobacco industry for their work. Ignaz Semmelweis, director of the Gynaecology Clinic in Budapest in the mid-nineteenth century, once made the famous statement, on being asked whether he had accepted money from a condom firm, which was after all immoral: *"This is no cause for reproach: I have a machine into which I put dirty money at the top and take out clean money at the bottom."* But it is surely evident that a scientist cannot take the view that it is not where money comes from that counts, but only what it is used for.

In 1954, the US tobacco industry founded the *Council for Tobacco Research* (CTR), which provides large sums of money for research work: US $83 million for 865 research projects in 279 medical facilities at universities, hospitals and research institutes [29]. While initially the funding was given for work on the subject of "smoking and health," a research group was formed which was devoted to biomedical research without any reference to smoking. The influence of the CTR on research projects has been variously assessed, with no bias being found in many instances. In these cases, the aim of the CTR was to appear as a donor of equal standing with the American Cancer Society, the National Science Foundation, the National Institutes of Health and other leading research bodies [29], and in this way to acquire equal status with them by riding "piggy-back," as it were. It is ultimately a question of conscience whether money can be accepted from an industry which is responsible for >1,000 smoking-related deaths a day in the USA alone.

In Germany, the "Smoking and Health" research council, the *"Rauchen und Gesundheit mbH"* research company in Hamburg and the *"Verum"* (Behaviour and Environment) foundation in Munich, advised by the physiologist K. Thurau and/or the clinical medical specialist F. Adlkofer, have sought to do scientific work in this field [30, 31]. Their results have been the subject of very severe criticism [30]. The Danish physician T. Voss was paid US $3,500–6,500 a month by Philip Morris for speaking publicly against anti-smoking groups. The Swedish physician T. Malmfors of the Karolinska Institute also worked for Philip Morris, presenting the risks of passive smoking as unproven, for which they received the equivalent of DEM 60,000 [32].

Around the year 1990, INFOTAB, a think tank supported by the tobacco industry, published "A guide for dealing with anti-tobacco pressure groups" [33], in which an early warning system was established for setting up WHO bureaux and for holding regional workshops of anti-smoking groups and non-smoker organisations and coalitions. These initiatives were accompanied by activities aimed at delaying the establishment of anti-tobacco programmes. After BATCo had studied the WHO programmes, scientists were enlisted and paid by BATCo who, acting as private persons, cast doubt on the WHO programmes. These scientists included, for instance, Paul Dietrich, at that time president of the Institute for International Health and Development, and Bob Tollison from the Centre for Study of Public Choice. The former played down the tobacco issues in a publication planned for the New York Academy of Sciences, and the latter wrote similar articles for the *International Herald Tribune*. The essence of these articles was that the WHO should concern itself more with combating infectious diseases (malaria and cholera) in the Third

World, rather than with issues such as safety belts or cigarettes and alcohol [34]. If these misrepresentations of the WHO are repeated internationally often enough, they come to be accepted as facts.

The questionable sponsoring of researchers at universities for studies sympathetic to the tobacco industry should be reconsidered. Also in the USA, readers' letters on the low or non-existent risks of passive smoking have, according to the journal *Science*, been paid for with sums up to US $10,000 and evidenced on the payrolls of the tobacco industry [35]. The Munich medical journal (*Münchner Medizinische Wochenschrift*) carried, in a supplement, a study on passive smoking by the well-known statistician K. Überla, entitled "Liberty and responsibility – discussed with special reference to passive smoking," which was funded by the *Peutinger-Collegium*, a body closely affiliated to the tobacco industry [35]. This institute has, since its foundation, been run by G. B. Gori, an adviser to the tobacco industry, who also acts as its adviser in public. In the years 1992/1993, Gori received over US $20,000 for five letters to scientific journals (*J Natl Cancer Inst*) and daily newspapers (*Wall Street Journal*) [36–39].

Critical notice has also been drawn to the University of Nottingham, which opened an International Centre for Corporate Social Responsibility with financial support from BAT [40]. This decision by the university aroused considerable protest and controversial discussion in scientific quarters and raised the question as to whether an action of this kind was ethically and morally justifiable in view of the major damage to health caused by the tobacco industry's products [41, 42]. It ought to be impossible for physicians to conduct research work with the aid of subsidies from the tobacco industry (see Sect. 14.1)!

14.4
"Subsidised" Tobacco Growing

The cultivation of tobacco as a lucrative business for farmers is shown by a US list of income that can be obtained by the cultivation of various agricultural products (see Fig. 14.1) [12].

The world's best tobaccos are grown outside of Europe; in the European Union, only Greece (3% share) is able to produce tobacco of superior quality [43]. The EU subsidises the tobacco industry to the tune of >1 billion annually, including 25.6 million for the German tobacco growers [44]. In 1997, European tobacco farmers earned approximately 4,090 per hectare, a price which is below the average income for European farmers. However, as this production is subsidised, it nevertheless continues. In the Greek part of Macedonia, the farmers used to grow wheat, but because of the subsidies they switched to tobacco, especially as the annual subsidies in Greece rose, between 1986 and 1995, to >409 million [43], i.e. approximately five times the market value. The costs of smoking to the national economy (health care, social security, illness-related loss of production), on the other hand, are about three times higher than the profit earned from tobacco growing [43].

Altogether, the tobacco industry employs some 200,000 people in the EU, whereby the tobacco processing plants are also located in rural regions and support the economy there.

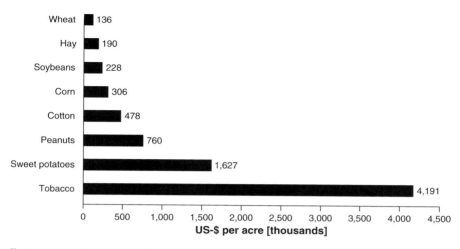

Fig. 14.1 Agricultural value of selected crop products for the year 1995 [12]. Tobacco ranked seventh in terms of frequency throughout the USA, behind the crops shown above. Tobacco earned income of US $2.3 billion in the USA [12]

On the other hand, the value of the harvested tobacco only amounts to about 20% of the subsidies paid for it [45] – a state of affairs which cannot be tolerated indefinitely.

If these jobs were "destroyed" through abolition of the subsidies, the result would be high social costs. At the same time, however, the EU tobacco is either exported as "inferior" quality or is only used to make up bulk. The EU (and especially Germany) imports 80% of the tobacco it needs for production. In other words, a product *is having* to be subsidised which cannot even be subsequently used properly. The only solution to this problem would be

- For the employees to be gradually moved to other jobs
- To pay compensation to the tobacco growers for them to give up cultivation and so reduce the amount of land under production (purchase of quotas; see also EEC Directive No. 2,079/92)
- To intensify controls on the amount of land under cultivation so as to ensure compliance with EC laws

The goal of achieving quality improvements in the tobacco grown ("non-harmful" tobacco qualities) is likely to be a long way in the future [45]. At best, tobacco plants should be used to extract the nicotine for medicinal purposes. As other branches of industry in the EU have also had to be restructured, it should be possible for the politicians to develop practicable concepts in this field. The WHO has, however, stated, that the claimed effects on employment are exaggerated and that it is prepared to initiate aid measures for tobacco growers in poor countries; in other words, there should be no obstacles to restructuring [46].

Paradoxically, world food aid programmes are supporting tobacco growing in various countries with financial donations, e.g. Ghana. The arguments used to justify this run more or less as follows: "*Tobacco is a traditional source of enjoyment and brings a little luxury and pleasure into life.*" In order to be able to grow tobacco in these countries, it is necessary to clear woodland. Moreover, because of the poor quality of the soil and the shortage of fertiliser, the land obtained in this way can only be used for a few years and then has to be replaced by new land [47]. According to UNO calculations, one tree has to be felled for every 300 cigarettes produced.

The British government has rejected a report by the Commission, which was co-initiated by the tobacco industry, to the Council on the joint marketing organisation for raw tobacco [48] and spoken out against further subsidies for tobacco growing. Its proposals were, however, not accepted [48].

An altogether indefensible attitude towards tobacco growing is that of the Swiss government: the federal government charges a kind of special tobacco duty of 2.6 *rappen* per packet of cigarettes. The SFr 20 million of revenue this generates is not put into smoking prevention, however, but is paid in subsidies towards tobacco cultivation [49]!

14.5
Governmental Control of Toxic Tobacco Constituents

In most countries in Europe (38 countries), national regulations specify maximum yields for tar and nicotine in tobacco products. In 12 countries regulations for additives exist, while the content of CO is regulated in only six countries. The limits for tar and nicotine are 12 and 1.2 mg per cigarette, respectively [50]. A 2001 EU directive will reinforce the regulation of the constituents and ingredients of tobacco products and tobacco smoke (for details, see Chap. 3.4, Tables 3.1–3.3). The data summarised in Table 14.2 indicate that there are still a few EU countries that are lagging behind because they have not yet produced any national

Table 14.2 National action plans and coordinating bodies in selected European countries [50]

Country	National tobacco control action plan	Specific targets on tobacco in action plan	National coordinating body for tobacco control
Austria	No	No	No
Belgium	No	No	No
Denmark	Yes	Yes	Yes
Finland	Yes	Yes	Yes
France	Yes	Yes	Yes
Germany	No	No	No
Greece	No	No	Yes
Ireland	Yes	Yes	Yes
Italy	Yes	Yes	No
Netherlands	Yes	Yes	Yes
Portugal	Yes	Yes	Yes
Spain	Yes	Yes	Yes
Sweden	Yes	Yes	Yes
United Kingdom	Yes	Yes	Yes

action plan for tobacco control and also have no organised national body for the coordination of such action plans [50].

By 2004 the new standards will stipulate yields for tar and nicotine of 10 and 1 mg per cigarette, respectively. By 2003 all EU member states will require manufacturers and importers to submit a list documenting all ingredients and their quantities used in the manufacture of tobacco products, by brand name and type. The list of all ingredients will be published.

The proposal, discussed within the EU since 1999, concerning the harmonisation of the legal and administrative requirements relating to the manufacture, packaging and sale of tobacco products (1999/0244 COD; KOM 1999-594) [50] envisages that, with effect from 2003, the yields of tar and nicotine per cigarette will be lowered to 10 and 1 mg respectively, and that the CO content per cigarette will be <10 mg with effect from 31 December 2003. It is also planned to include other constituents of cigarette tobacco in this control system. The warnings printed on cigarette packs are also to be regulated. The manufacturers and importers of tobacco products will be required to list for their cigarette brands the non-tobacco ingredients and constituents with quantitative details. The use of misleading labels such as "light," "mild" and "ultralight" will be prohibited. It is a recurring complaint that inadequate information and the lack of toxicology data make it impossible for the appropriate authorities in EU countries to arrive at a meaningful estimate of the health risks of tobacco products for the consumer. The lack of such information prevents the bodies responsible from ensuring a high level of health protection. It is to be hoped that this directive will also be implemented in all EU countries in the near future.

14.6
Tobacco Taxes

There have been duties and taxes on tobacco consumption in some countries for over 200 years (cf. Chap. 1). Today, the taxes on tobacco products are much higher than the actual sales value of the products themselves. Price increases are one effective instrument for reducing tobacco consumption, at least temporarily. As the data summarised in Fig. 13.2 shows, the various tobacco taxes and duties levied in the EU are equivalent to about 66% of the consumer prices [51]. In the European Union, the aim is for a minimum tax rate of about 70% of the retail end price [52]. Germany is just below this level, lying in second-last place (Fig. 13.2). While the cigarette price in Germany, allowing for inflation, rose by 4.1% from 1987 to 1993, it has risen in Great Britain by 25% since May 1997. The example of the United Kingdom illustrates that as tobacco tax rises, revenue rises too over 2–3 decades (Fig. 14.2).

There is an inverse relationship between the cigarette price and the level of consumption, with the latter falling as the former rises. On average, a 10% increase in price causes cigarette consumption among adults to drop by 3–7% [53]. Naturally, such price increases have a far bigger effect on consumption among children and juveniles, allowing a 2–3 times higher decrease in cigarette consumption to be reckoned with [54]. A doubling of the cigarette price would trigger a significant drop in cigarette consumption, provided tobacco smuggling could be effectively stopped. A price increase on this scale would also result in

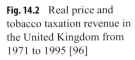

Fig. 14.2 Real price and
tobacco taxation revenue in
the United Kingdom from
1971 to 1995 [96]

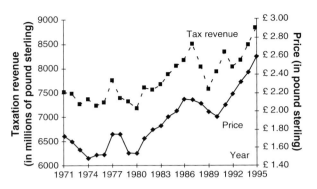

substantial health gains among the socially weaker groups [55]. Initial experience with an
approach of this kind could be gained in Canada in the years from 1982 to 1991: the sharp
rise in tobacco duty during this period resulted in a 40% decrease in tobacco consumption,
smuggling included [56]. An even bigger drop was observed in New Zealand [57].
However, such measures only take effect after several years [58]. In the case of juveniles,
such tax increases can be seen to produce a decreasing interest in cigarettes over an extended
period of time [59, 60]. Initial fears of loss of revenue by the state and an increase in smuggling prove only limited, because the tax revenue per pack increases considerably [61].
However, these increased revenues should be devoted to tobacco-related health projects.
Small rises in tobacco duty of the kind that came into force in Germany at the start of the
year 2002 have only little effect. Moreover, the German finance minister justified the tax
increase by stating that the revenue would be devoted to "improving internal security"
– a highly immoral argument as it could make smokers think that by consuming heavily,
they are performing a public duty.

14.7
Regulations on Smoking

A primary goal of tobacco regulation is to reduce smoking-related diseases and the general
harm to society arising from smoking. This includes the earlier mortality of smokers, the
damage to the health of non-smokers, and ultimately also the costs to business and the
economy as a whole. Tobacco regulation therefore has three important objectives:

- To stop people from starting smoking
- To help people to stop smoking or to at least substantially reduce their tobacco
  consumption
- To protect non-smokers from the risks of passive smoking (ETS)

The results achieved in many industrialised countries, including Germany, have so far
been unsatisfactory and inadequate [62].

In March 2000, the International Society Against Cancer and the Association of
European Leagues to Combat Cancer put forward a further proposal for an EU directive on

the control of tobacco products (COM (99) 594) which contains several crucial points on tobacco regulation:

- Restrictions on advertising and effective warning of the health risks
- Deglorification of the image of smokers
- Regulation of the substances contained in tobacco to limit damage to health
- Protection of minors by restricting their access to tobacco products
- Increase in the retail prices through higher duties and taxes
- Combating the influx of cheap smuggled cigarettes
- Eliminating the subsidies for tobacco growers
- Requiring the industry to pay compensation for damage to smokers' health
- Support for special lifestyle campaigns to dissuade young people from smoking
- Advice, assistance and treatment to help people who want to stop smoking

How this directive can be implemented is as yet unclear [63]. However, many countries have implemented a variety of restrictions.

In England, smoking was banned in indoor public places, including workplaces, bars, clubs and restaurants, on 1 July 2007. Some places, such as certain smoking hotel rooms, nursing homes, prisons, submarines, offshore oil rigs, and stages/television sets (if needed for the performance) were excluded. Palaces were also excluded. Members of the House of Commons and the House of Lords agreed to ban all smoking in the Palace of Westminster. The on-the-spot fine for smoking is varying and smoking will be allowed to continue anywhere outdoors.

With some of Europe's highest smoking rates, Germany has a patchwork of smoking bans because of its federal structure with 16 states. In general, smoking is banned on public transport, hospitals, airports and in public and federal buildings, including the parliament.

Italy was one of the first countries in the world to enact a nationwide smoking ban. Since January 10 2005 it is forbidden to smoke in all public indoor spaces, including bars, restaurants and clubs/discos. However, special smoking rooms are also allowed but only 1% of all public establishments have opted for setting up a smoking room. The ban turned out to be very popular. It is strictly enforced.

France tightened an existing ban on smoking in public places on 1 February 2007. Smoking is banned in all public places (stations, museums, airports). However, there is an exception for special smoking rooms fulfilling strict conditions. Also, special exemptions were made for cafés and restaurants, clubs, casinos, bars, etc. until 1 January 2008. Opinion polls suggested that 70% of people support the ban.

Since all the United Nations properties are not the subject of any national jurisdiction, the United Nations have their own smoking and non-smoking policies. Following the gradual introduction of partial smoking bans between 1985 and 2003, Secretary General Kofi Annan introduced in 2003 a total ban on smoking at UN Headquarters.

In the USA and Australia, the number of smokers and the number of cigarettes smoked at the workplace has been observed to decline when workplaces are declared smoking-free [64]. In the USA, the smoking policy is determined at the state or at the municipal level, but not by the federal administration. Therefore, smoking policies are clearly instituted at the state or local level. Over 50% of Americans are covered by a ban ordinance of some degree. The bans vary from total smoking bans (even outdoors), to no ban at all.

President Obama has an impressive legislative record concerning tobacco control prior to the presidential election. In this respect, as a senator Obama joined nine U.S. Senate colleagues in calling on President Bush to send to the Senate for ratification the FCTC, the world's first public health treaty. Obama was also one of the original cosponsors of pending landmark legislation providing the Food and Drug Administration with authority to regulate tobacco products and tobacco marketing.

14.8
Bans on Advertising in Various Countries

In some countries, there are increasing numbers of people who advocate a ban on smoking and on tobacco advertising and who are gaining growing public support. Some related facts have already been discussed in Chap. 13. However, there are already restrictions on tobacco advertising in all 24 OECD countries, which in the course of 20 years have resulted in a measurable reduction in tobacco consumption (Fig. 13.9). But only six countries have prohibited advertising completely: Iceland (1972), Norway (1976), Finland (1979), Portugal (1984), Italy (1984) and Canada (1989) [23].

A list has been published showing the average consumption in grams per person in most European countries for the years 1964 to 1990 [23]. Those countries with a ban on advertising can also record a decline in tobacco consumption (Fig. 13.9).

In many big cities of *China*, including Beijing, smoking has been restricted or prohibited in public buildings and on public transport since the 1980s [65] and, in view of the growing number of cancer cases, the Medical University of Zhejiang will no longer accept students who smoke [66]. In *Norway*, the "Anti-Nicotine Act," which was passed in 1995 and came into force at the beginning of 1996, seeks to reduce smoking in public, with bans on smoking in schools and other public places (restaurants, cafes, shopping centres, airports, cinemas; Fig. 14.3). The high price for cigarettes (4.75 for 20 cigarettes) is also a deterrent to purchase, while juveniles have to provide proof of age when buying cigarettes. Cigarette vending machines are prohibited, as is advertising [67]. Also in *Israel* there are now restrictions in place on tobacco advertising, and adverts may not show either people or animals. In addition, every cigarette packet must bear a health warning [68]. In *Poland*,

Fig. 14.3 Time-dependent differences in the increase of the mean price and in the tax *revenue* of one cigarette *(cent) in Germany*. The portion of the mean tax *revenue* decreased from 1984 to 2000 continuously from 66.7 to 59.5% (data from the Statistisches Bundes-amt, Wiesbaden)

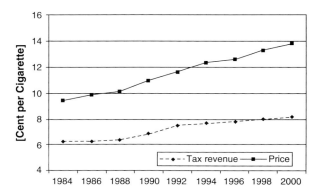

an anti-tobacco law was passed almost unanimously in August 1995; this prohibits the sale of tobacco products to young people (<18) as well as in schools, hospitals and at sporting events, makes cigarette vending machines illegal, bans smoking in public places, except in special designed areas, and at the workplace, and contains a general prohibition on advertising for tobacco products in public buildings, in the media and at health, cultural and sporting events [69]. Anyone found smoking in a hospital or a school can be fined up to 1,250 [70]. Since 1998, health warnings have been required to be placed on cigarette packets and must cover 30% of the total area on each side [71].

In *Great Britain*, a ban on tobacco advertising in the press and on hoardings came into force in December 1999. This prohibition also includes shops and newspaper kiosks. Additionally, all sponsoring by the tobacco industry is banned from July 2003 [72]. Smokers who are caught dropping a cigarette in the street in the London borough of Westminster are subject to on-the-spot fines in an amount equivalent to 40 [73]. Moreover, several British insurance companies offer a special discount for non-smoking drivers who can give a declaration that they have not smoked for at least 1 year [74]. The thinking behind this is that the eyes of drivers who smoke water more; the drivers therefore blink more often, which reduces their attention to the road [74]. They also suffer from chronic CO intoxication, with all its consequences (cf. Chap. 6). In *Italy*, a government decree came into force in January 1996 that prohibits smoking in all public buildings, meaning in this case ministries, local government offices, post offices, railway stations, etc. [75].

At its recent meeting in Seville, the *International Automobile Federation* (FIA) adopted a general ban on tobacco advertising, including a prohibition on sponsoring, with effect from the end of 2006 [76]. This decision is remarkable insofar as an FIA resolution of this kind was considered unthinkable as recently as only a year ago, but has now been taken in consultation with the WHO.

A resolution to ban tobacco advertising had been adopted at *EU* level, but the governments of Germany and Austria have launched – on the instigation of the tobacco industry – legal action against this at the European Court of Justice in Luxembourg. In the meantime, this EU directive had been declared void by the Irish Attorney General, N. Fennelly, on grounds that "*the EU has quite simply no jurisdiction to issue a ban on tobacco advertising.*" Advertising spending worth 200 million and sponsoring worth 100 million was dependent on this decision [77]. However, tobacco advertising bans spread to a large number of countries meanwhile. In this respect, these advertising bans parallel the increasing number of public smoking bans (see Sect. 14.7).

14.9
Tobacco Industry: Playing Down the Risks of Smoking and Passive Smoking

At the start of each year, many people adopt a resolution to lead a healthier life and stop smoking, and at exactly the same time, the tobacco industry intensifies its advertising [78, 79]. According to unofficial figures, worldwide spending on cigarette advertising in 1987 amounted to nearly 1 billion EURO. In Germany, tobacco advertising has for some years involved slogans such as "*I just enjoy smoking,*" "*The best thing about temptation is giving in to it*" or "*Every cigarette you don't consciously enjoy is one too many*" [80]. One message of the cigarette industry that is especially dangerous is that people should "*smoke in moderation.*" How is an alcohol addict, for instance, supposed to drink in moderation? The nicotine in cigarettes leads many people to increase their intake, with all the hazards associated with the combustion products. In this context, attention is once again drawn to the confidential position paper issued by the tobacco industry, which has been mentioned before [15].

In light of the various legal actions against the tobacco industry, Philip Morris has now adopted a new policy. The Department of Justice wishes to claim compensation for the costs incurred annually by Medicare for the treatment of smoking-related disease. "*For over 45 years, the cigarette firms have been conducting their business with no regard for the truth, the law, or the health of the American population,*" as Janet Reno, the former US Attorney General, put it [81]. For this reason, Philip Morris is now using the slogan: "*Smoking can make you ill*" [82]. The company's advertising also adopts a similar vein: "*Don't smoke our cigarettes*" is one advertising message that has even been shown on US television [83]. The director of BAT, Martin Broughton, stated in March 2002 to *The Times* newspaper: "*I think smoking does involve health risks.*" He himself does not smoke, he said, apart from an occasional after dinner cigar, because he is afraid of the risk of illness through smoking. He has also advised his two children against smoking cigarettes [84].

A highly typical example for the obfuscation of scientifically substantiated facts is the activities of the tobacco industry concerning the harmfulness of environmental tobacco smoke (ETS) [85]. In this case, the tobacco industry has got together a network of scientists who claim that ETS has not been proved to cause damage to health. The tobacco industry has set up ostensibly independent research institutes which concern themselves with the ETS problem. Examples of such institutes are the "Project Viking," the Tobacco Action Committee (TAC), the "Whitecoat," the Centre for Indoor Air Research (CIAR), the Occupational Health and Safety Association (OHSA) etc. Between 1965 and 1993 alone, these and various other bodies organised 11 symposia on ETS, of which six were overtly funded by the tobacco industry [86].

14.10
Smoking and Non-smoking: Weighing the Benefits

One claim that smokers and sympathisers of the tobacco industry have been making for decades is that smokers are the cheapest citizens because they die younger, tend to contract illnesses that quickly lead to death, and therefore cost less in the way of pension payments. This often used argument is untrue and needs refuting [87]. As long ago as 1999, the World Bank showed that while the life of a smoker is shorter, it is also more expensive than that of a non-smoker if the costs of health care and the loss of working days are also taken into account [88].

According to the calculations of a group working in Heidelberg, the costs for reproduction and loss of resources caused by smoking are significantly higher than those caused by alcohol, obesity and even road traffic (Table 14.3) [87]. On conservative estimates, the costs to the economy caused by smokers amount to 40 billion (11.75 through work

Table 14.3   Costs to the economy through damage to health in Germany, with attribution to the various causes

Cause	Reproduction costs[a]	Costs of lost resources[b]	Total
Smoking	15.7	19.6	35.2
Alcohol	0.9	4.2	5.1
Sugar, meat animal fats	7.1	4.1	11.2
Road traffic	5.6	25.2	30.8
Total	29.2	53.2	82.4

Figures in billion € per year [87]
[a]Costs of medical treatment, including administrative costs
[b]Loss of economic production because of illness, injury or death

disability, 6.75 through excess mortality and 21 through premature invalidity), while the revenues of the state from tobacco duties and taxes amount to only 11.5 billion. It should also be taken into account in this context that

- Considerable portion of the cigarettes smoked were smuggled into the country, thereby reducing the state's revenues
- The treatment of smoking-related diseases is paid for not out of tobacco tax revenues but by the health insurance funds into which everybody pays contributions [62]; the costs for such treatment from tobacco duties and taxes by 6–7 billion [89]

The state uses the money from tobacco tax for all kinds of activities, but not for the health system. According to a study by the Umwelt-Prognose-Instituts Heidelberg e.V., an environmental forecasting body, the costs for the treatment of smoking-related diseases amounted to 15.65 billion in 1997 [90]. In view of this, the demands of the health insurance funds that part of the tobacco tax revenues should be used to finance the treatment of smokers appear highly justified: the Deutsche Angestelltenkasse (German Health Insurance Fund for Salaried Employees), for instance, has demanded that 30% of the revenues from the duty on tobacco and spirits tax should be put towards the treatment of smoking-related diseases [91]. If health levies were imposed on alcoholic beverages and tobacco, they would, even at moderately rising rates, be able to generate revenues of up to 65 billion per year, which would even allow the contribution rates to the health insurance funds to be reduced from 14% of wages to 8.5% [90]. At the same time, this would mean a reduction in ancillary wage costs of 40% [90]. With 192.5 billion cigarettes produced in the year 1996 [3], a "cigarette penny" would already produce revenues of 98.42 million, which could be put towards health expenditure.

If the costs for the treatment of a patient with ischaemic heart disease or lung cancer are compared with the costs of therapy to enable people to stop smoking, the difference in is considerable. Even including several consultations with a doctor, nicotine replacement therapy could amount to at most 650 a head, while the costs for treating a patient with coronary heart disease or lung cancer, who will then probably die anyway, is estimated at 49,340 (heart attack) and 41,785 (lung cancer) [92]. If patients were themselves to pay for the nicotine instead of for the cigarettes they smoked, the costs for medical consultation in Germany would amount to 200–250 at most.

Each employee in the tobacco industry accounts for annual sales revenue of 1 billion [3]. If the purchasing power of smokers was diverted from cigarettes-to other products of our economy, many times the number of jobs would be created in other industries, because these generate much less sales revenue per employee: according to 1996 figures, the amount of purchasing power volume that would have to be diverted would be at most 15.13 billion [3].

At the end of this section, here are just a few remarks on an analysis of a kind which will certainly already have been done before by health insurance funds, insurance companies and politicians, with the aid of actuaries: namely, the study carried out in the Czech Republic by Philip Morris in the year 2000. The aim of the study, conducted by the firm of A. D. Little on behalf of Philip Morris, was to find out whether, taking the revenues from tobacco tax and duties and the expenditure on health and social costs into account, the Czech state makes a "profit" or a "loss" from smokers. For the period of the study, the year 1999, the study shows the Czech state to have made a profit of $\pm 5,815$ million Czech crowns (CZK) (confidence interval: CZK $\pm 1,347$ to $\pm 13,650$ million, equivalent to US $147.1 million). In the analysis, it is shown that the negative effects of smoking (increased health and social costs) are outweighed by the positive effects (tobacco duty and value added tax on tobacco products). This therefore means that smoking has a positive effect on the state balance sheet. *"This conclusion would hold even if the indirect positive effects of smoking were neglected."* After being submitted to the government of the Czech Republic, this study was immediately analysed and several accounting errors found [93, 94]. The central message of the Philip Morris study, namely that *"smoking has a positive effect,"* is indicative of the unethical character of the study with its unacceptable disregard for fundamental human values, and Philip Morris ought to make a public apology for it [95].

14.11
Concluding Remarks

On the basis of the problems outlined above, the following measures are necessary:

- Ban on all advertising for tobacco products.
- Effective primary and secondary prevention measures, taking into account the fact that the majority of smokers are to be found among people with lower intellectual ability or lower school qualifications, so that the programmes must therefore be designed accordingly.
- Increase in tobacco duty, which has always been an important regulative for reducing tobacco consumption among the population (see Fig. 14.4) and may be more effective than public health information programmes [87].
- Ban on the sale of cigarettes to young people under 18 years, and abolition of cigarette vending machines.
- Increase in health insurance premiums for smokers, taking the latest developments in the health system into account.

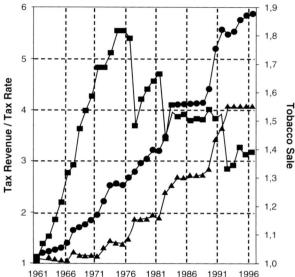

Fig. 14.4 Increase in sales turnover from tobacco (*filled box*), tax revenues (*filled circle*) and tax revenues (*s*) (from 1961 to 1996); base year: 1960 (= 1) [87]

- Financial support for the activities of the health insurance bodies towards preventing smoking among young people and helping adults to give up smoking.
- Commitment by members of the medical profession to reduce smoking among their own ranks and to update their own knowledge about smoking and the substances contained in nicotine, with their effects on the human body.
- Urgent appeal to politicians to reconsider their attitude towards the tobacco industry, to take a stand against smoking in public and to adopt measures to benefit non-smokers, who form the majority of the population.
- Implementation of directives on tobacco control and full recognition of deleterious effects.
- Recognition of nicotine as an addictive substance.

References

1. Brundtland GH (1999, Jan 30) Health for the 21st Century. Davos, Switzerland, World Economics Forum
2. Roemer R (1993) Legislative action to combat the world tobacco epidemic (2. Aufl). 24. Genf
3. Anon (1997) Zahlen aus der Tabakwirtschaft. Die Tabak-Zeitung
4. Internet Mitteilung vom (1998, Dec 28) Statistisches Bundesamt Wiesbaden
5. Odenwald M (1993) Wie der Regenwald im blauen Dunst aufgeht. Nature 6:28–34
6. Kessler DA, Myers ML (2001) Beyond the tobacco settlement. N Engl J Med 345(7): 535–537

7. Satcher D (2001) Why we need an international agreement on tobacco control. Am J Public Health 91(2):191–193
8. Giddens A (1999) Globalisation. BBC Reith Lecture series 1999
9. Chapman S, Shatenstein S (2001) The ethics of the cash register: taking tobacco research dollars. Tob Control 10(1):1–2
10. Thomson A (2000, Dec 5) Special reports: dealing with killer industries. Channel 4 News
11. Anonym (1998) Tabakdeal im US-Senat gescheitert. Süddt. Ztg. 26
12. US Department of Agriculture (1995) History of Budgetary Expentidures of the Commodity Credit Corporation. In: AMSaFMDASaCS (ed) Washington, US Government Printing Office
13. Strategiepapier der Tabakmafia: Vorlage zur VdC-Vorstandssitzung am (1998, Mar 03) Werberichtlinie; Strategie nach dem Ministerrat. Nichtraucher-Info 31:III/98
14. Zeltner T, Kessler DA, Martiny A, Randera F (2000) Tobacco Company Strategies to undermine tobacco control activities at the World Health Organization. Report of the Committee of Experts on Tobacco Industriy Documents, 247-pp
15. Position Paper (secret) (1977, Jun 10) http://www.pmdocs.com/Getallimg.asp?DOCID = 2501024522
16. Adams M (1994) Heroin an Süchtige? - Ein abschließender Schlagabtausch. Zschr Rechtspolitik 27:422–426
17. Wonka D (1998, Dec 11) Zum Grünen-Parteitag. Schnelle Truppe. LVZ/Leipziger Volksztg, Stadtausgabe, 1–2
18. Anonym (1999) Florida jury finds tobacco companies guilty of fraud. Br med J 319:143
19. Anonym (1998, Jun 19) Zur Vorgehensweise der Tabakmafia. Süddt Ztg
20. Freedman A, Jensen E, Stevens A (1995, Aug 24) Why ABC settled with the tobacco industry. Online Bericht der Agentur Dow Jones vom
21. Anonym (1999, Dec 28) Krebshilfe kämpft weiter für Verbot der Tabakwerbung. Gießener Anz
22. Smoking kills: A White Paper on Tobacco (1998) www-1.hel.se.pnu.com/nintogen/sin/book/white. html
23. Stewart MJ (1993) The effect of advertising bans on tobacco consumption in OECD countries. Int J Advertis 12:155–180
24. World Health Organization (1993) Tabakfreies Europa: Aktionsplan. Hamburg, für Gesundheitsförderung G. Conrad
25. Wöckel F (1990) Wes Brot ich eß, des Lied ich sing. Oeffentl Dienst 43:182
26. Fälschung bei Tabakstudie ausgemacht (1994, Dec 22) Frankfurter Rundschau
27. Hess H (1987) Geschichte, Geschäfte, Gefahren. Rauchen. Campus, Frankfurt – New York
28. Anonym (1995, Nov 14) Wallace will quit if CBS does 'it' again. Online Bericht der UPI Western US vom
29. Wolinsky H (1985) When researchers accept funding from the tobacco industry, do ethics go up in smoke? N Y State J Med 85:451–454
30. Remmer H (1999) Der Schutz des Rauchers.: Eine moralische Verpflichtung der DGPT. DGPT-Forum 24:19–23
31. Smoking and HEalth Research Activities in Europe (1990) http://www.pmdocs.com/getallimg.asp? DOCID = 20232233372/33831990
32. Anonym (2000, Sep 25) Enthüllungen über korrupte Mediziner. Thür Landesztg
33. A guide for dealing with anti-tobacco pressure groups (1999) Infotab document
34. Dietrich P (1999, Apr 03) Count of the cost of infectious diseases: financing the fight against illness has consequences for investors. International Herald Tribune [Money Section]
35. Anonym (1998) Forscher bekommen 10.000 Dollar für industriefreundliche Leserbriefe. Naturkost
36. Wadman M (1998) Dilemma for journals over tobacco cash. Nature 394:609
37. Kaiser J (1998) Tobacco consultants find letters lucrative. Science 281:895–897

38. Anonym (1998, Sep 18) Die lenkende Hand der Tabakindustrie ist deutlich auszumachen. Süddt Ztg, 13
39. Anonym (1998, Sep 09) Mängel der Studien über Passivrauchen. Süddt Ztg, 18
40. Cohen JE (2001) Universities and tobacco money. BMJ 323(7303):1–2
41. Ong EK, Glantz SA (2000) Tobacco industry efforts subverting International Agency for Research on Cancer's second-hand smoke study. Lancet 355(9211):1253–1259
42. Sweda EL Jr, Daynard RA (1996) Tobacco industry tactics. Br Med Bull 52:183–192
43. Harris JA (1997) Das Geschäft mit dem Gift: Europas Tabak-Subventionen. Reader's Digest 11:67–68
44. EU-Subvention für Tabakanbau (1998) Nichtraucher-Info 32-IV
45. Europäische Kommision: Die Reform des Tabaksektors (1998) http://europa.eu.int/comm/dg06/ publi/fact/tobacco/index_de.html
46. Tobacco controls not harmful to farmers, says UN health agency (1996, Mar 08)
47. Anonym (1995) Welthunger-Hilfe fördert Tabakanbau. 18/II. Nichtraucher-Info
48. Bericht über den Bericht der Kommision an den Rat über die gemeinsame Marktorganistion für Rohtabak (1997, Jul 19) KOM(96)0554-C4-0057/97
49. Hat der Bundesrat Angst? (1997) http://www.proaere.ch/d/info/1997/2/p01.html
50. The European Report on Tobacco Control Policy (2002) WHO European Ministerial Conference for a Tobacco-free Europe (eds) 3rd Action Plan for a Tobacco-free Europe 1997–2001. WHO Regional Office for Europe, Copenhagen, pp 1–54
51. Chaloupka FJ, Hu T, Warner K, Jacobs R, Yurekli A (2000) The taxation of tobacco products. In: Jha P, Chaloupka FJ (eds) Tobacco control in Developing Countries. Oxford University Press, Oxford, pp 237–268
52. Joossens L, Chaloupka FJ, Merriman D (2000) Issues in the smuggling of tobacco products. In: Jha P, Chaloupka FJ (eds) Tobacco Control in Developing Countries. Oxford University Press, Oxford, pp 393–406
53. Saffer H, Chaloupka F (2000) The effect of tobacco advertising bans on tobacco consumption. J Health Econ 19(6):1117–1137
54. Lewit EM, Hyland A, Kerrebrock N, Cummings KM (1997) Price, public policy, and smoking in young people. Tob Control 6(Suppl 2):S17–S24
55. Helmert U, Shea S, Bammann K (1999) Social correlates of cigarette smoking cessation: findings from the 1995 microcensus survey in Germany. Rev Environ Health 14:239–249
56. Joossens L, Raw M (1995) Smuggling and cross border shopping of tobacco in Europe. BMJ 310:1393–1397
57. Laugesen M, Scollo M, Sweanor D, Shiffman S, Gitchell J, Barnsley K, et al (2000) World's best practice in tobacco control. Tob Control 9(2):228–236
58. Novotny TE, Siegel MB (1996) California's tobacco control saga. Health Aff (Millwood) 15:58–72
59. Chaloupka FJ, Warner KE (2000) The economics of smoking. In: Newhouse JP, Cuyler A (eds) Handbook of Health Economics. Elsevier, New York, pp 1539–1627
60. Chaloupka FJ, Wechsler H (1997) Price, tobacco control policies and smoking among young adults. J Health Econ 16:359–373
61. Merriman D, Yurekli A, Chaloupka FJ (2000) How big is the worldwide cigarette-smuggling problem? In: Jha P, Chaloupka FJ (eds) Tobacco control in developing Countries. Oxford University Press, Oxford
62. Haustein KO (1999) Smoking: health care and politics in flux. Rauchen: Gesundheitswesen und Politik im Wechselspiel. Z Arztl Fortbild Qualitatssich 93:355–361
63. The International Tobacco-Control Network (2000, Mar 31) Vorschlag für eine EU-Richtlinie zur Regulierung von Tabakprodukten KOM(99)594. Briefing Notiz im Auftrag von Europäischen Gesundheitsnetzwerken, die in der Tabakprävention aktiv sind

64. Chapman S, Borland R, Scollo M, Brownson RC, Dominello A, Woodward S (1999) The impact of smoke-free workplaces on declining cigarette consumption in Australia and the United States. Am J Public Health 89:1018–1023

65. Anonym (1996, May 15) Rauchbeschränkungen auch in China. Süddt Ztg, 14

66. Anonym (1995) Chinesische Universität nimmt keine Raucher mehr auf (dpa). Stuttgarter Nachr

67. Anonym (1996) "Anti-Nikotin-Gesetz" in Norwegen. Frankfurter Rundsch, 34

68. Beschränkung der Tabakwerbung in Israel (1998) http://home.snafu./de/nichtraucherbund/ texte/L Israel.html

69. Anti-Tabak-Gesetz in Polen (1996, May 03) http://tt.dx.com.Tobacco Daily.html

70. Anonym (1996, May 03) Anti-Tabak-Gesetz in Polen. Berliner Morgenpost

71. Anonym (1998, Feb 01) Große Warnhinweise auf Zigarettenpackungen in Polen. Tabak-Ztg

72. Ab 10 (1999, Jun 17) Dezember Verbot für Tabakwerbung in Großbritannien. News vom 17.06.1999

73. Anonym (1998, Apr 12) London: Bußgeld für achtlose Autofahrer. Berliner Morgenpost

74. Anonym (1997) Autoversicherun: Wer raucht, zahlt mehr. Nature 2

75. Italiens Raucher setzen "Task forces" ein (1996, Jan 20) Frankfurter Allg Ztg, 9

76. FIA beschließt Tabakwerbeverbot ab 2006 (2000, Oct 05) http://de.sports.yahoo.com/001005/ 37/ 130xl.html

77. Paoli de N, Jennen B (2000) Generalanwalt hält Tabakwerbeverbot für unzulässig. Financial Times Dtl 11

78. US Federal Trade Commission (1994) Federal Trade Kommission report to Congress für 1992: pursuant to the Federal Cigarette Labeling and Advertising Act. Washington, DC

79. Online Beitrag (1995, Oct 30) Study says cigarette ads target smokers who quit. Reuters Financial Report

80. Kohout P (1998, May 22) Genuß gegen Muß. Sonderveröffentlichung der British American Tobacco. Die Woche [21 (Beilage)]

81. Anonym (1999) USA klagen gegen die Zigarettenindustrie

82. Philip Morris gibt zu: Es gibt keine "sichere"Zigarette (1999)

83. Bitte kaufen Sie unser Produkt nicht! Welt (1999, May 31)

84. Broughton M (2002, Mar 01) I don't like to smoke. The Times (No. 67387), p 1

85. Proctor CJ (1998) The hot air on passive smoking. BAT has not tried to discredit data on passive smoking. BMJ 317:349

86. Drope J, Chapman S (2001) Tobacco industry efforts at discrediting scientific knowledge of environmental tobacco smoke: a review of internal industry documents. J Epidemiol Community Health 55(8):588–594

87. Kostenumschichtung im Gesundheitswesen durch Anwendung des Verursacherprinzips (2000) Vorschläge für eine Finanzreform im Gesundheitswesen. 46/3. Auflage, 124. UPI-Bericht Nr. 46

88. Chaloupka FJ (1999) Curbing the epidemic: governments and the economics of tobacco control. Development in practice series. The World Bank, Washington DC

89. Welte R, König HH, Leidl R (2000) The costs of health damage and productivity losses attributable to cigarette smoking in Germany. Eur J Public Health 10(31):38

90. 30,6 Mrd (2001) DM jährliche Reproduktionskosten aufgrund von Rauchern. http://snafu.de/ nichtraucherbund/texte/UPI.html

91. Anonym (1995) DAK fordert 30% der Tabaksteuer für die Krankenkassen. Nichtraucher-Info 18-II

92. Schulenburg JM v d, Uber A, Laaser U (1997) Raucherentwöhnung durch höherdosierte Nicorette-Kaugummi: eine Kostenanalyse für Deutschland. Gesundh ökon Qual manag 2:74–79

93. Death and taxes: A response to the Philip Morris study of the impact of smoking on public finances in the Czech Republic (2001, Jul 21) Action on Smoking and Health. 2002

94. Kralikova E, Kozak J (2001, Aug 19) Comments to the Philip Morris Study concerning the economic impact of smoking in the Czech Republic by Czech NGOs
95. Parrish SC (2001, Aug 19) Wall Street Journal
96. Townsend J (1998) The role of taxation policy. In: Abedian I, van der Merwe R, Wilkins N, Jhi P (eds) The economics of tobacco control: towards an optimal policy mix. Applied Fiscal Research Centre, Cape Town
97. US Department of Health and Human Services (1989) Reducing of the health consequences of smoking: 25 Years of progress: A report of the surgeon general. Washington, Public Health Service, Centers for Disease Control, Center for Chronic Disease Prevention and Health Promotion, Office on Smoking and Health. pp 89–8411, DHHS Publ No (CDC)

Appendix: Experiences from a Smoker Counselling Centre

15

The following procedures were established at the Smoker Counselling Centre in Erfurt, Germany. The Smoker Centre aims to provide free counselling to smokers and, upon request, to help them achieve smoking cessation. The Counselling Centre, which may be seen as a model for centres, provides a phased service as follows:

- Individual counselling, free of charge over several consultations, to smokers who wish to quit.
- Smoking cessation discussions and therapy on a group basis, and telephone counselling of smokers.
- Smoker education in public lectures, specifically for adolescents in schools and for pregnant women.

15.1
Treatment Strategy

The strategy to promote smoking cessation is based on physician advice combined with administration of nicotine replacement therapy (NRT). Our experience indicates that nicotine is the drug that smokers have been taking anyway through cigarettes over a period of several decades. They may, therefore, also continue to receive it in a pure, but low-dose form for a further maximum period of 3 months (see Chap. 11). The success rates achieved in the Centre clearly surpass those reported from many other sources using non-drug methods as well as pharmacotherapy. The benefit–risk ratio is high because, in contrast to other medications, the adverse effects of treatment are invariably kept within manageable limits.

Treatment of the smoker should aim at *complete cessation*, and stopping smoking abruptly is indicated. Some 20–40% of smokers achieve this goal without any medical intervention, through willpower alone and without outside help. Because of their heavy dependence and/or considerable habituation, many smokers are unable to give up smoking completely, with the result that "*harm reduction*" or *partial cessation* is then a possible option. The goal here is for smokers (simultaneously patients at risk) to cut their consumption to <10 cigarettes/day with pharmacological support. After a longer period of reduced cigarette consumption, some smokers may possibly themselves recognise the sense of quitting completely.

K.-O. Haustein, D. Groneberg, *Tobacco or Health?*
DOI: 10.1007/978-3-540-87577-2_15, © Springer Verlag Berlin Heidelberg 2010

The smoker's own determination to quit is the crucial prerequisite for success in smoking cessation therapy. Discordant smokers are more suitable as patients. In principle, given the many and well-known harmful effects of smoking, any intervention to achieve smoking cessation is to be recommended (for details of indications, see Sect. 10.1 in Chap. 10).

15.2
The Counselling Process

During the initial consultation, the patient's history is taken and information is elicited concerning any concurrent illnesses that might be relevant in terms of smoking cessation. The Fagerström Test is administered to determine the degree of nicotine dependence (Table 4.5 in Chap. 4). Smokers undergo a situational analysis to determine how easily they can be provoked to smoke, and the CO content in expired air and forced expiratory volume in 1 s (FEV_1) are measured. They are informed in detail about the harmful effects of smoking, and the effects of nicotine and those of tobacco smoke and its constituents are discussed separately. The mode of action of the various nicotine products is then explained. Once smokers have consented to NRT, one or perhaps two nicotine products are prescribed, depending on the extent of smoking, the Fagerström Test score and CO levels in expired air.

Future ex-smokers are issued with an information booklet written in the Institute and are referred to the nearest pharmacist with a private prescription and precise instructions on how the nicotine products are to be used. Patients are told to start using the nicotine products that same day in the form supplied. A date is also fixed for the next appointment. The initial consultation lasts for 1-h, giving smokers the opportunity to outline their motives for smoking. Information sessions in dialogue format have been assessed positively.

The appointment schedule for individual smokers who wish to quit depends on the progress made. Weekly appointments are made initially, followed later by appointments every 2 weeks and then every 4 weeks. Interim telephone counselling is often considered helpful. In all cases, the target is for the ex-smoker to report an outcome of tobacco abstinence after 6 months. The number ($n = 6–12$) and duration of subsequent counselling sessions will depend upon the success of therapy.

Contrary to what is stated in the prescribing information, nicotine products are used in double or triple combinations, depending on the assessed severity of dependence (see Table 11.3 in Chap. 11). Additional individual counselling for smokers is essential and boosts the success rate. The duration of treatment is guided by the active and successful cooperation of the ex-smoker and may range from 4 to 12 weeks. The nicotine dose administered initially is reduced as rapidly as possible: this means that the patient's cravings should be extremely minimal or abolished altogether. Nicotine patches with a nicotine release rate of 1.5 mg/h are prescribed to be worn only for 16 h during the day. The patch dose is reduced by halving the patch – though this is only possible with Nicorette patches. Nicotine chewing gum and/or nasal spray are used in addition, with treatment supplemented by both products together in exceptional cases only (see Table 11.3 in Chap. 11).

If smokers who wish to quit do not receive NRT with nicotine doses that are similar to those obtained from cigarette smoking, they relapse at once. Naturally, these high initial doses must be reduced as rapidly as possible, but in a way that reliably prevents relapses. The risk of adverse effects through to intoxication exists only if ex-smokers additionally smoke larger quantities of cigarettes during this period.

15.3
Experiences with Outpatient Smoker Counselling

In the 2.5 years since the Centre has been in existence, a total of >1,000 smokers, primarily from Thuringia (but also from other regions of Germany), have enrolled with the intention of quitting smoking. History-taking revealed that these patients were highly dissatisfied with their smoker status, and many of them admitted that for years they had wanted to quit the habit, but had been prevented from doing so by their degree of dependence. Over the intervening period, smokers for whom smoking cessation is an urgent necessity on medical grounds have also been referred to the Centre by their doctors. After an initial consultation, patients from other German *regions* have then undergone telephone counselling and successfully achieved smoking cessation. Among the patients at the Centre, five had already withdrawn from alcohol and successfully remained tobacco-abstinent for 6 months.

On average, female smokers have smoked 20 cigarettes/day for 17 years, while male smokers have smoked 25 cigarettes/day for 20–25 years. The very heaviest smokers consume 80–100 cigarettes/day. Attempts at smoking cessation initiated by the smokers themselves have lasted for a maximum 4 weeks in women and generally for only 1 week in men.

The Fagerström Test in women has revealed scores of 4–6 for the most part, with scores of 7–10 in isolated cases only, whereas in men scores of 4–6 or 7–10 were recorded with equal frequency. At the start of treatment, the smokers had an average CO level in expired air of 21 ppm. On the completion of successful treatment, levels of 5 ppm were recorded. CO levels of 80 ppm were measured initially in four cases. For ex-smokers, the measurement of this variable was an important marker of success in cases where smoking cessation was achieved.

Further appointments with ex-smokers at weekly or fortnightly intervals are useful, particularly at the start of treatment. Approximately 25% of smokers who attend a first appointment fail to return subsequently. A further 25% give up the treatment after 4–8 weeks because they have relapsed. Also of importance is the patients' experience of leaving the first consultation – supplied with NRT products – without having the craving to smoke. This abstinence from smoking was also confirmed by virtually all ex-smokers (97%) during the following week and should be interpreted as a key experience: "The feeling that it is not necessary to smoke." In this context, it is important that smokers obtain their nicotine products immediately from a nearby pharmacy. If the continuous supply of nicotine is not guaranteed immediately after the first consultation, patients turn back to cigarettes and thus, start to smoke again.

15.4
Success in Smoking Cessation

An analysis of the 116 smokers attending our Centre during the first 6 months of 2,000 reveals that, of those seen for the first time, a total of 86 smokers returned for further consultations after the first session. These 86 individuals evidently intended to undergo smoking cessation therapy, whereas the remaining 30 patients attended simply to obtain information and were not included in the analysis because they did not even attempt smoking cessation. In a specific telephone interview, 21 male and 17 female patients reliably stated that they had been abstinent from cigarettes for at least 6 months (corroborated by CO measurements). The calculated success rate was, therefore, 44.7% for males (21 out of 47) and 43.6% for females (17 out of 39). These percentages are clearly higher than the success rates of 20–30% reported in the literature. In the meantime, we included 200 smokers into a controlled study to evaluate the efficacy of NRT under standardized conditions. The results will be evaluated in the beginning of 2003.

15.5
Concluding Remarks

- PR campaigns and notices in the press should be used repeatedly to reinforce the existence and availability of Smoker Counselling Centres.
- Smoking cessation therapy is successful particularly if the physician simultaneously shows "strong support" for the patient (in terms of counselling input) and initiates NRT with sufficiently high nicotine doses. It is also important for smokers to realise that they can leave the counselling session in the afternoon without smoking a cigarette afterwards.
- In addition, patients should be supplied promptly with nicotine replacement drugs from a nearby pharmacy to ensure that the decision to quit smoking is not frustrated right at the outset by an organisational obstacle.

Initial consultation (Day 0):

. . . .

Family name: .... **First name:** ....
Patient no.: [_|_|_]   Date of birth: [_|_].[_|_].[_|_]

Address: ....   Tel.: ..../...................

Height [cm]: [_|_|_]   Body weight [kg]: [_|_|_]

Health insurance scheme: ....

Medical history

	Yes*	No	Not known
Angina pectoris			
Myocardial infarction			
Hypertension			
Cardiac arrhythmias			
Peripheral vascular disease			
Recent gastrointestinal ulceration			
Skin disease			
Chronic infection (tuberculosis, hepatitis)			
Metabolic disease (diabetes mellitus, gout)			
Allergic reactions			
Diseases of internal organs (liver, kidneys)			
Other diseases, elective hospitalisation			
Receiving regular medication*			
Abuse of alcohol and other drugs			
Use of smokeless tobacco (snuff or chewing tobacco)			

* If yes, provide details.

Medication history (with dosage details):
. . . .
. . . .

Blood pressure (BP) and heart rate (HR) readings: yes
(Readings to be taken after the patient has sat quietly for 10 minutes)

Reading	BP$_{sys}$ [mmHg]	BP$_{dia}$ [mmHg]	HR [1/min]
1	[_I_I_]	[_I_I_]	[_I_I_]
2	[_I_I_]	[_I_I_]	[_I_I_]
3	[_I_I_]	[_I_I_]	[_I_I_]

Mean readings: [_I_I_]/[_I_] mmHg   [_I_I_]/min

ECG   **(optional)**   **yes/no**

Conduction times (mean of 3 R-R intervals)	PQ QRS QT	[__I__I__] ms [__I__I__] ms [__I__I__] ms

                                                        Yes   No

Abnormalities?
If **yes**, specify details:

Smoker history

For how many years have you smoked?   [_I_]
How old were you when you started smoking?   [_I_]
How often have tried to quit smoking?   never   [_]
                                           once   [_]
                                           several times   [_]

What method did you use? ....

Discordant smoker: .... yes: .... no: ....
Carbohydrate dependence: .... yes: .... no: ....
....
Chronic bronchitis or COPD:.. yes: .... no: ....

. . . .
. . . .
. . . .

Fagerström Test for Nicotine Dependence

	Questions	Responses		Scores
1	How soon after you wake up do you smoke your first cigarette?	Within 5 minutes 6–30 minutes 31–60 minutes After 60 minutes		3 2 1 0
2	Do you find it difficult to refrain from smoking in places where it is forbidden? (e.g., in the cinema, in meetings etc.)	Yes No		1 0
3	Which cigarette would you hate most to give up?	The first in the morning Any other		1 0
4	How many cigarettes per day do you smoke?	10 or less 11–20 21–30 31 or more		0 1 2 3
5	Do you smoke more frequently during the first hours after awakening than during the rest of the day?	Yes No		1 0
6	Do you smoke if you are so ill that you are in bed most of the day?	Yes No		1 0
		Total score:		[_|_]

Cravings

Situational analysis: I can go without smoking ... (How certain are you?)

		1	2	3	4	5
1.	When I feel anxious	○	○	○	○	○
2.	When I get annoyed	○	○	○	○	○
3.	When I'm with smokers	○	○	○	○	○
4.	When I have cigarette cravings	○	○	○	○	○
5.	When I drink wine or beer	○	○	○	○	○
6.	After eating	○	○	○	○	○
7.	When I'm nervous	○	○	○	○	○
8.	When I've done something great	○	○	○	○	○
9.	When I'm occupied with difficult problems	○	○	○	○	○
10.	When I'm "down"	○	○	○	○	○

1: Not certain at all, 2: Rarely certain, 3: Often certain, 4: Mostly certain, 5: Absolutely certain

Taste	○	○	○	○	○
Smell	○	○	○	○	○
Performance (physical)	○	○	○	○	○
Subjective mood produced by smoking	○	○	○	○	○
Cough	○	○	○	○	○
Mucus	○	○	○	○	○

Degree of impairment/presence: 1: Extreme, 2: Considerable, 3: Moderate, 4: Hardly any, 5: None (i.e., symptom-free or not present)

CO content in expired air
Reading [ppm]: [_|_]
(measured with Bedfont Micro II Smokerlyzer)

FEV_1 [l]: [_],[_][_]

Standard information provided on the hazards of smoking: yes/no

Treatment proposal discussed with patient: yes/no

Medication issued during the consultation after informing the patient about the effects of nicotine:

Patient given   [_] nicotine patches, each containing 24.9 mg,
    plus   [_] pieces of nicotine chewing gum, each containing 4 mg,
    or/plus   [_] spray doses of nasal spray totalling ..... mg.

Patient intends to stop smoking immediately:	yes/no
Patient intends to stop smoking within 2–3 days:	yes/no
Patient intends to stop smoking after 1 week	yes/no
Patient does not intend to stop smoking and is unable to decide whether to have the treatment	O

The following have been prescribed or recommended for subsequent treatment:
    [_] [_] Nicorette chewing gum 2 mg (O) or 4 mg (O)
    [_] [_] Nicorette membrane patch 16.6 mg (O) or 24.9 mg (O)
    [_] [_] Nicorette nasal spray 10 ml

Further treatment measures: ....
....
Date of next appointment: ....

Follow-up appointments   after 1, 2, 3 weeks on ....
(Use the same forms for all consultations)
Patient attended appointment   yes/no
Patient telephoned to cancel   yes/no
Smoking history: smoked: yes (○) – no (○); number of cigarettes: .... per day

Feels: very well · – well ☺ – satisfactory ♨ – unwell ☒
Cravings: yes (○) – no (○)

CO in expired air: .... ppm CO

· ·

Situational analysis: I can go without smoking … (How certain are you?):

		1	2	3	4	5
1.	When I feel anxious	○	○	○	○	○
2.	When I get annoyed	○	○	○	○	○
3.	When I'm with smokers	○	○	○	○	○
4.	When I have cigarette cravings	○	○	○	○	○
5.	When I drink wine or beer	○	○	○	○	○
6.	After eating	○	○	○	○	○
7.	When I'm nervous	○	○	○	○	○
8.	When I've done something great	○	○	○	○	○
9.	When I'm occupied with difficult problems	○	○	○	○	○
10.	When I'm "down"	○	○	○	○	○

1: Not certain at all, 2: Rarely certain, 3: Often certain, 4: Mostly certain, 5: Absolutely certain

Adverse effects during treatment with nicotine products (<u>underline</u>):
Patch: Skin redness, tingling, inflamed skin, itching, burning;
Chewing gum: Nausea, mucosal redness, bleeding in the mouth, irritation at back of throat;
Nasal spray: Sneezing, runny nose, nosebleed, watering eyes, headache.

Tobacco withdrawal symptoms:	**yes**	**no**
Depression	yes	no
Concentration disturbances	yes	no
Reduced performance	yes	no
Bad mood	yes	no
Irritable reactions	yes	no
Worried, anxious	yes	no
Insomnia	yes	no
Increased appetite	yes	no
Body weight increase	yes	no
by .... kg in .... weeks/months		

Blood pressure (BP) and heart rate (HR) readings: **yes**
(Readings to be taken after the patient has sat quietly for 10 minutes)

Reading	BP_{sys} [mmHg]	BP_{dia} [mmHg]	HR[1/min]
1	[_I_I_]	[_I_I_]	[_I_I_]
2	[_I_I_]	[_I_I_]	[_I_I_]
3	[_I_I_]	[_I_I_]	[_I_I_]

Mean readings: [_I_I_] / [_I_] mmHg   [_I_I_] / min

The following have been prescribed or recommended for subsequent treatment:
   [__] [__]
   [__] [__]
   [__] [__]

Further treatment measures: ....

. . . .

Final consultation (after 6 months): on ....

Patient attended appointment   yes/no
Patient telephoned to cancel   yes/no
Smoking history: smoked: yes/no
Patient feels: very well   well   satisfactory   unwell
Cravings: yes/no; Number of cigarettes smoked: .... per day

CO in expired air: .... ppm CO

FEV$_1$ [l]:   [_],[_][_]

Fagerström Test for Nicotine Dependence

	Questions	Responses		Scores
1	How soon after you wake up do you smoke your first cigarette?	Within 5 minutes 6–30 minutes 31–60 minutes After 60 minutes		3 2 1 0
2	Do you find it difficult to refrain from smoking in places where it is forbidden? (e.g., in the cinema, in meetings etc.)	Yes No		1 0
3	Which cigarette would you hate most to give up?	The first in the morning Any other		1 0
4	How many cigarettes per day do you smoke?	10 or less 11–20 21–30 31 or more		0 1 2 3

5	Do you smoke more frequently during the first hours after awakening than during the rest of the day?	Yes No		1 0
6	Do you smoke if you are so ill that you are in bed most of the day?	Yes No		1 0
		Total score:		[_l_]

Situational analysis: I can go without smoking … (How certain are you?)

		1	2	3	4	5
1.	When I feel anxious	○	○	○	○	○
2.	When I get annoyed	○	○	○	○	○
3.	When I'm with smokers	○	○	○	○	○
4.	When I have cigarette cravings	○	○	○	○	○
5.	When I drink wine or beer	○	○	○	○	○
6.	After eating	○	○	○	○	○
7.	When I'm nervous	○	○	○	○	○
8.	When I've done something great	○	○	○	○	○
9.	When I'm occupied with difficult problems	○	○	○	○	○
10.	When I'm "down"	○	○	○	○	○

1: Not certain at all, 2: Rarely certain, 3: Often certain, 4: Mostly certain, 5: Absolutely certain

Taste	○	○	○	○	○
Smell	○	○	○	○	○
Performance (physical)	○	○	○	○	○
Subjective mood produced by smoking	○	○	○	○	○
Cough	○	○	○	○	○
Mucus	○	○	○	○	○

Degree of impairment/presence: 1: Extreme, 2: Considerable, 3: Moderate, 4: Hardly any, 5: None (i.e., symptom-free or not present)

Occasional use of nicotine replacement drugs: yes/no

Patch:	yes/no
Chewing gum (2 mg):	yes/no
Chewing gum (4 mg):	yes/ no
Nasal spray:	yes/no
Other drugs:	yes/no

Tobacco withdrawal symptoms:	yes	no
Depression	yes	no
Concentration disturbances	yes	no
Reduced performance	yes	no
Bad mood	yes	no
Irritable reactions	yes	no
Worried, anxious	yes	no
Insomnia	yes	no
Increased appetite	yes	no
Body weight increase	yes	no

by .... kg in .... weeks/months

The following have been prescribed or recommended for emergency prophylaxis:
   [__] [__]
   [__] [__]

Further treatment measures: .....:..
. . . .

Successfully abstinent over 6 months: **yes/no**

date ....../....../ 200...

                                                            ....
                              Doctor's signature

Index

Printing: Ten Brink, Meppel, The Netherlands
Binding: Stürtz, Würzburg, Germany